IADVL

Color Atlas of Dermatopathology

Indian Association of Dermatologists, Venereologists and Leprologists

IADVL Color Atlas of Dermatopathology

Editor-in-Chief

Pradeep Mahajan MD DNB (Dermatology)

Fellowship in Dermatopathology (Ackerman Academy of Dermatopathology, New York, USA)
Consultant Dermatologist and Dermatopathologist
Dr Mahajan's Dermatology and Dermatopathology Services
Pune, Maharashtra, India
Email: *pradeepmahajan@doctor.com*

Project Director and Foreword

Venkataram Mysore

MD DNB Dip RCPath (London) FRCP (Glasgow) FISHRS
Consultant Dermatologist and Dermatopathologist
Director
Venkat Charmalaya Centre for Advanced Dermatology and
Postgraduate Training Institute
Bengaluru, Karnataka, India
Project Director and President
Indian Association of Dermatologists,
Venereologists and Leprologists (IADVL)

Under the Aegis of IADVL Academy

JAYPEE The Health Sciences Publisher

New Delhi | London | Philadelphia | Panama

Jaypee Brothers Medical Publishers (P) Ltd

Headquarters
Jaypee Brothers Medical Publishers (P) Ltd
4838/24, Ansari Road, Daryaganj
New Delhi 110 002, India
Phone: +91-11-43574357
Fax: +91-11-43574314
Email: jaypee@jaypeebrothers.com

Overseas Offices

J.P. Medical Ltd
83 Victoria Street, London
SW1H 0HW (UK)
Phone: +44 20 3170 8910
Fax: +44 (0)20 3008 6180
Email: info@jpmedpub.com

Jaypee-Highlights Medical Publishers Inc
City of Knowledge, Bld. 235, 2nd Floor
Clayton, Panama City, Panama
Phone: +1 507-301-0496
Fax: +1 507-301-0499
Email: cservice@jphmedical.com

Jaypee Medical Inc
325 Chestnut Street
Suite 412, Philadelphia, PA 19106, USA
Phone: +1 267-519-9789
Email: support@jpmedus.com

Jaypee Brothers Medical Publishers (P) Ltd
17/1-B Babar Road, Block-B, Shaymali
Mohammadpur, Dhaka-1207
Bangladesh
Mobile: +08801912003485
Email: jaypeedhaka@gmail.com

Jaypee Brothers Medical Publishers (P) Ltd
Bhotahity, Kathmandu, Nepal
Phone +977-9741283608
Email: kathmandu@jaypeebrothers.com

Website: www.jaypeebrothers.com
Website: www.jaypeedigital.com

Inquiries for bulk sales may be solicited at: jaypee@jaypeebrothers.com

IADVL Color Atlas of Dermatopathology

First Edition: **2017**

ISBN: 978-93-85891-23-6

Printed at Ajanta Offset & Packagings Ltd., Faridabad, Haryana

Dedicated to

IADVL Teacher Par Excellence
Late Dr MB Gharpuray

Editorial Board

Assistant Editor

Col Aradhana Sood
MD DNB
Associate Professor
Department of Dermatology
Armed Forces Medical College and Command Hospital
Pune, Maharashtra, India

Editorial Assistants

Priyanka Patil
MD
IADVL Fellowship in Dermatopathology

Meeta Mantri
MD
IADVL Fellowship in Dermatopathology

Prathyusha Yakkala
MD
IADVL Fellowship in Dermatopathology

Pranav Raj
Senior Resident , YCM Hospital
Pune, Maharashtra, India

Nitika Deshmukh
Senior Resident , BJ Government Medical College
Pune, Maharashtra, India

Roby Bose
Senior Resident, Ruby Hall Clinic
Pune, Maharashtra, India

Contributors

Achyut Pokharel
MBBS MD (Skin and VD) FISDP
Fellowship in Dermatopathology (USA) European and International Board Certified in Dermatopathology (Germany)
Assistant Professor
Department of Dermatology
Chitwan Medical College
Bharatpur, Nepal

Alistair Robson
FRCPath Dip RCPath
Founder
LD Path Group
London, UK

Asha Kubba
MBBS Diplomate American Board of Pathology
Diplomate American Board of Pathology in Dermatopathology
Adjunct Assistant Professor
Dermatopathology Section, Department of Dermatology
Boston University Medical Center
Boston, USA
Director
Delhi Dermpath Laboratory, Delhi Dermatology Group
New Delhi, India

Atul Dongre
MD Fellowship in Dermatopathology (Germany)
Fellowship in Diagnostic Dermatology (MUHS)
Assistant Professor
Department of Skin, STD and Leprosy
KEM Hospital and SGS Medical College
Mumbai, Maharashtra, India

Chirag Desai
MBBS DVD Fellowship in Diagnostic Dermatology
Consultant Dermatologist
Hindu Sabha Hospital, Ghatkopar
Mumbai, Maharashtra, India

Col Aradhana Sood
MD DNB
Associate Professor
Department of Dermatology
Armed Forces Medical College and Command Hospital
Pune, Maharashtra, India

Col Deep Kumar Raman
MD
Associate Professor
Department of Pathology
Armed Forces Medical College and Command Hospital
Pune, Maharashtra, India

Deepa Gharpuray Pandit
MD (Path) DCP FRCPath
Consultant Histopathologist
Lancashire Teaching Hospitals NHS
Department of Cellular Pathology
Royal Preston Hospital
Preston, UK

Dipankar De
MD
Associate Professor
Department of Dermatology
Postgraduate Institute of Medical Education and Research
Chandigarh, India

Gp Capt Sandeep Arora
Professor and Senior Advisor (Dermatology)
Base Hospital, Delhi cantt and
Army College of Medical Sciences
New Delhi, India

Jag Bhawan
MD
Professor, Department of Dermatology and Pathology
Head, Dermatopathology Section
Vice-Chairman, Department of Dermatology
Boston University School of Medicine, Boston, USA

Jerad Gardner
MD
Assistant Professor
Department of Pathology and Dermatology
Bone and Soft Tissue Pathology
Program Director
Dermatopathology Fellowship Program
University of Arkansas for Medical Sciences
Arkansas, USA

KC Nischal
MD
Associate Professor
Department of Dermatology
Adichunchanagiri Institute of Medical Sciences
Bengaluru, Karnataka, India

Mani Makhija
MBBS MD DNB (Path)
Elective Rotation in Dermatopathology at Ackerman Academy of Dermatopathology
Fellow
Skin and Cancer Foundation, Australia

Mithilesh Chandra
MD (Path) FICPath
Consultant Pathologist
Pathology Consultancy Services
Noida, Uttar Pradesh, India

Mohamad Buraik
MD ICDP-UEMS
Dermatology Consultant and Dermatopathologist
Department of Dermatology and Pathology
King Fahd Hospital
Jazan, Saudi Arabia

M Ramam
MD
Professor
Department of Dermatovenereology
All India Institute of Medical Sciences
New Delhi, India

Nandakumar Gopinath
MD (Skin and Venereal Disease) MD (Path)
Additional Professor
Department of Pathology
Government Medical College
Thiruvananthapuram, Kerala, India

Nathan Lee
MD Dermatopathology Fellow
University of Arkansas for Medical Sciences
Arkansas, USA

Pradeep Mahajan
MD DNB (Dermatology)
Fellowship in Dermatopathology
(Ackerman Academy of Dermatopathology
New York, USA)
Consultant Dermatologist and Dermatopathologist
Dr Mahajan's Dermatology and
Dermatopathology Services
Pune, Maharashtra, India

Rajiv Joshi
DVD DDV MD (Skin Diseases) DNB Fellowship in Dermatopathology (USA)
Consultant Dermatologist
Department of Dermatology
Hinduja Hospital
Consultant Dermatopathologist
SRL Ranbaxy Laboratories
Mumbai, Maharashtra, India

Rathnam Attilee
MD
Consultant
Visakha Institute of Skin and Allergy
Visakhapatnam, Andhra Pradesh, India

Sara Edward
MBBS FRCpath Dip Dermpath
Consultant, Soft Tissues and Dermatopathology
Department of Histopathology
St James's University Hospital
Leeds, UK

Smita Ghate
MD (Skin and VD) DDV Fellow in Dermatopathology (USA)
Associate Professor
Department of Dermatology
Lokmanya Tilak Municipal Medical College
Mumbai, Maharashtra, India

Steven Kossard
MBBS FACD FRCPA (Hon)
American Board of Dermatopathology
Skin and Cancer Foundation
NSW, Australia

Sudhir Arora
MBBS MD
Assistant Professor
Department of Pathology
All India Institute of Medical Sciences
New Delhi, India

Sujay Khandpur
MD DNB MNAMS
Professor
Department of Dermatology and Venereology
All India Institute of Medical Sciences
New Delhi, India

Uday Khopkar
DVD MD (Skin Diseases) DNB Fellow in Dermatopathology (USA)
Professor and Head
Department of Skin, STD and Leprosy
KEM Hospital and SGS Medical College
Mumbai, Maharashtra, India

Uma Nahar Saikia
MD (Path) MNAMS FIMSA
Professor
Department of Histopathology
Postgraduate Institute of Medical Education and Research
Chandigarh, India

Venkataram Mysore
MD DNB Dip RCPath (London) FRCP (Glasgow) FISHRS
Consultant Dermatologist and Dermatopathologist
Director
Venkat Charmalaya Centre for Advanced Dermatology and
Postgraduate Training Institute
Bengaluru, Karnataka, India
Project Director and President
Indian Association of Dermatologists, Venereologists and Leprologists (IADVL)

V Ramesh
MD
Professor and Head
Department of Dermatology and STD
Vardhman Mahavir Medical College and Safdarjung Hospital
New Delhi, India

Ying Guo
MD
Dermatopathologist
Ackerman Academy of Dermatopathology
USA

Foreword

Dermatopathology is the backbone of dermatology. Sound knowledge of dermatopathology enhances the prowess of a clinician. Dermatology being a visual specialty, makes it easier for a clinician to learn dermatopathology. It is, therefore, not surprising that so many dermatopathologists are also clinical dermatologists.

The idea of an atlas in dermatopathology was conceived five years back when I was the convenor of special interest group of dermatopathology. I am happy it is being published now; this has been completed in one year, which speaks about the commitment of our authors and the hard work put in by the editor Dr Pradeep Mahajan.

The atlas seeks to fill a void; there are hardly any atlases of this type by Indian authors, and hence, I am sure it will be welcomed by all. The atlas is all encompassing with around 1,500 images. The format makes it easy to learn and will be useful to both residents and practitioners in both dermatology and dermatopathology.

In the days when basic sciences are facing existential challenges and being pushed to the background by the onslaught of cosmetic procedures, it is important that associations and teachers nurture and develop this subspecialty to ensure proper development of the subject and also training of residents for the future. This project, therefore, has been particularly satisfying to initiate and oversee.

I congratulate the editor-in-chief, all the editors and the contributors for the excellent work and hope that the book will prove useful to all.

Venkataram Mysore
MD DNB Dip RCPath (London) FRCP (Glasgow) FISHRS
Consultant Dermatologist and Dermatopathologist
Director
Venkat Charmalaya Centre for Advanced Dermatology and
Postgraduate Training Institute
Bengaluru, Karnataka, India
Project Director and President
Indian Association of Dermatologists Venereologists and
Leprologists (IADVL)

Message from IADVL Academy

It is with a sense of fulfillment that we pen this message for the *IADVL Color Atlas of Dermatopathology*. This book, edited by Dr Pradeep Mahajan, is a unique project of the IADVL Academy and the brainchild of Dr Venkataram Mysore, the outgoing IADVL President. The desire to create it was ignited by the renewed interest in this specialty, especially among our young members, and the continued realization of its importance in the diagnosis of dermatoses when the clinician is in a dilemma.

The creation of this atlas has necessitated obtaining good and typical photomicrographs of common and rare conditions from the collections of dermatopathologists from India and abroad. That it has been prepared in less than a year under exceptionally tight deadlines is a tribute to the editors. We fervently hope that this atlas encourages young dermatologists to take up this enchanting specialty as their chosen path. Its unique format will ensure that dermatologists and pathologists will be able to scan through the images to correlate them with the histopathology of lesions pertaining to their patient.

It is hoped that this book, along with the other two prepared under the aegis of the IADVL Academy this past year, would find a place in every Indian dermatologist's library. Its acceptance by our members would be the true culmination of the efforts taken towards its completion.

Col Manas Chatterjee
Chairman
IADVL Academy

Ameet Valia
Convenor and Chairperson Designate
IADVL Academy

Preface

Dermatopathology is a rapidly developing specialty in India, and this book, an IADVL Presidential Project conceived by Dr Venkataram Mysore, is a major attempt to strengthen it.

I hope this atlas reflects the science, practice and art of dermatopathology in India. While not an exhaustive display of all dermatology conditions, it showcases the histology of common skin disorders in a systematic manner.

The contents are entirely the result of the relentless efforts of eminent dermatopathologists from India and all over the globe, who sent images of a very high standard.

I am not just thankful, but indebted, to the IADVL office bearers (Dr Venkataram Mysore, IADVL President; Dr Rashmi Sarkar, IADVL Honorary Secretary General; Dr Manas Chatterjee, Chairman, IADVL Academy, and Dr Ameet Valia, Convenor, IADVL Academy), the editorial board, the assistant editor, the contributors, and my fellows and postgraduate students, who helped complete the work.

I thank Dr Bhushan Madke, who introduced us to dermatopathologists from US who contributed images of a few uncommon disorders.

I thank all my seniors, friends and students, who sent amazing clinical material whose photomicrographs are included in the atlas.

I am also thankful to Shri Jitendar P Vij (Group Chairman), Mr Ankit Vij (Group President) and Mr Tarun Duneja (Director–Publishing), especially Mr Sabarish Menon, Mr Rajesh Sharma and the team of M/s Jaypee Brothers Medical Publishers (P) Ltd, New Delhi, India, who have supported me throughout the process.

I conclude with a quote:

"I was clever yesterday,
And I wanted to improve the world
Today I am wise,
And I want to change myself!"

Pradeep Mahajan

Contents

Chapter 1. **Approach to Dermatopathology** 1
Uday Khopkar, Chirag Desai

Chapter 2. **Clues and Pitfalls in Diagnostic Dermatopathology** 15
Venkataram Mysore, Pradeep Mahajan

Chapter 3. **Psoriasiform Tissue Reaction** 27
Pradeep Mahajan, Achyut Pokharel

Chapter 4. **Lichenoid and Interface Dermatitis** 43
Mithilesh Chandra, Achyut Pokharel, Pradeep Mahajan, Uday Khopkar, Chirag Desai, Atul Dongre, Venkataram Mysore

Chapter 5. **Spongiotic Dermatoses** 71
Pradeep Mahajan, KC Nischal, Atul Dongre

Chapter 6. **Vesiculobullous Disorders** 87
Pradeep Mahajan, Nathan Lee, Jerad Gardner, Smita Ghate, Atul Dongre, Uday Khopkar, Mohamad Buraik, Nandakumar Gopinath

Chapter 7. **Granulomatous Tissue Reaction** 119
Uday Khopkar, V Ramesh, Sudhir Arora, Col Deep Kumar Raman, Pradeep Mahajan, KC Nischal, M Ramam, Nathan Lee, Jerad Gardner, Gp Capt Sandeep Arora, Col Aradhana Sood

Chapter 8. **Vasculitis and Other Vascular Reaction Patterns** 165
Uday Khopkar, Sujay Khandpur, Venkataram Mysore, Pradeep Mahajan, KC Nischal, Nathan Lee, Jerad Gardner

Chapter 9. **Disorders of Pigmentation** 185
Pradeep Mahajan

Chapter 10. **Panniculitis** 197
Pradeep Mahajan, Uday Khopkar, Chirag Desai, KC Nischal

Chapter 11. **Diseases of Collagen, Elastin and Mucin** 215
Asha Kubba, Atul Dongre, Uday Khopkar, Sara Edward, Nathan Lee, Jerad Gardner

Chapter 12. **Pilosebaceous Disorders and Cysts** 235
KC Nischal, Sujay Khandpur, Pradeep Mahajan, Venkataram Mysore, Nandakumar Gopinath

Chapter 13. **Cutaneous Deposits** 253
Rajiv Joshi, Venkataram Mysore

Chapter 14.	**Perforating Disorders** *Uday Khopkar, Chirag Desai, Atul Dongre, Nathan Lee, Jerad Gardner*	**265**
Chapter 15.	**Cutaneous Infections** *Uma Nahar Saikia, Dipankar De, KC Nischal, Pradeep Mahajan, Uday Khopkar*	**275**
Chapter 16.	**Epidermal Premalignant and Malignant Conditions** *Pradeep Mahajan, Nandakumar Gopinath, Nathan Lee, Jerad Gardner, Rathnam Attilee*	**299**
Chapter 17.	**Appendageal Tumors** *Deepa Gharpuray Pandit, Pradeep Mahajan, Nandakumar Gopinath, Jag Bhawan, Ying Guo, Asha Kubba*	**321**
Chapter 18.	**Melanocytic Lesions** *Sara Edward, Ying Guo, Steven Kossard, Mani Makhija, Alistair Robson*	**349**
Chapter 19.	**Vascular and Other Tumors** *Atul Dongre, Uday Khopkar, Pradeep Mahajan, Asha Kubba, Nathan Lee, Jerad Gardner, Jag Bhawan*	**363**
Chapter 20.	**Cutaneous Infiltrates—Nonlymphoid** *Pradeep Mahajan, Atul Dongre*	**393**
Chapter 21.	**Lymphoproliferative Disorders of Skin** *Nandakumar Gopinath, Uday Khopkar, Chirag Desai, Pradeep Mahajan, Nathan Lee, Jerad Gardner, Asha Kubba*	**411**
Chapter 22.	**Miscellaneous Conditions** *Nathan Lee, Jerad Gardner, Venkataram Mysore*	**427**
	Further Reading	*441*
	Index	*443*

1

Approach to Dermatopathology

Chapter Outline

1.1: Normal Histology
1.2: Topography
1.3: Inflammatory Cells
1.4: Basic Histopathological Reactions
1.5: Specialized Techniques
1.6: Improving Biopsy Outcome

Uday Khopkar, Chirag Desai

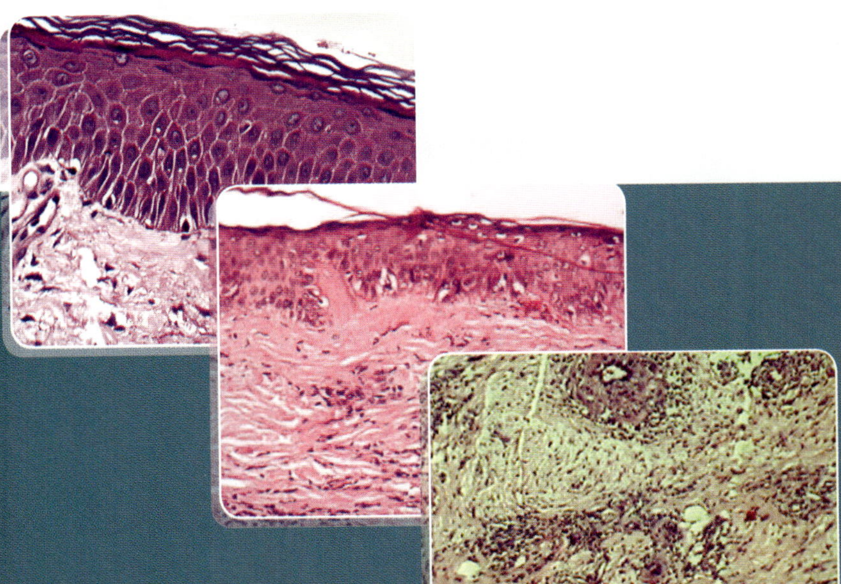

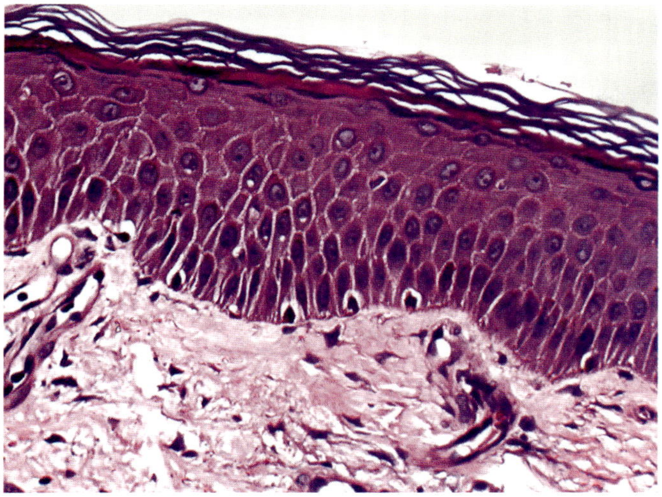

FIGURE 1.1.1.1

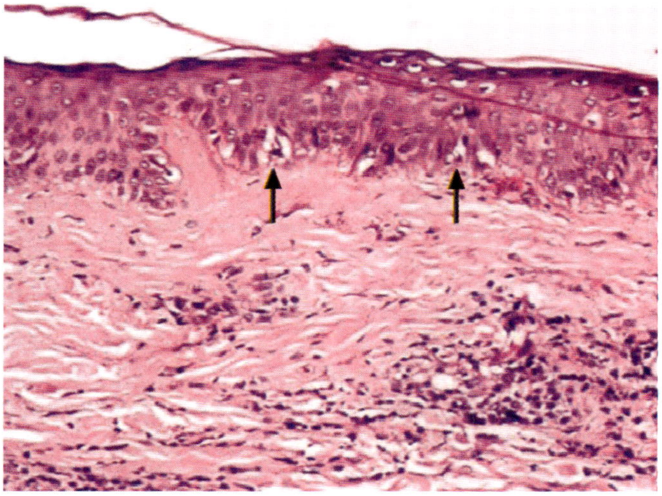

FIGURE 1.1.1.2

1.1: NORMAL HISTOLOGY

1.1.1: Epidermis

1.1.1.1: Normal epidermis with its layers (*High power view*)

1.1.1.2: Melanocytes (*Low power view*)

1.1.2: Dermis

1.1.2.1: Dermis and subcutaneous tissue (*Scanner view*)

1.1.2.2: Capillary (*High power view*)

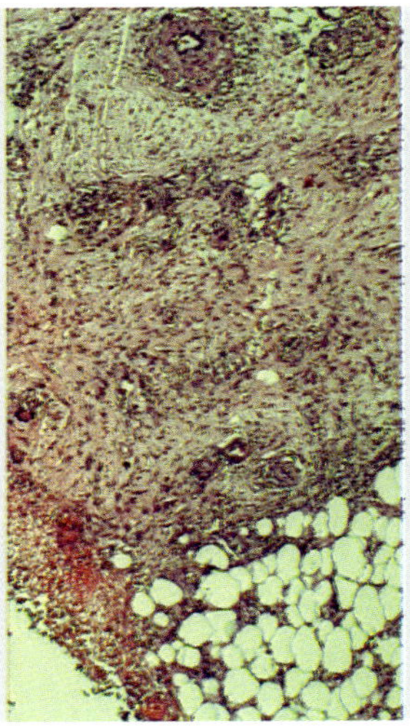

FIGURE 1.1.2.1

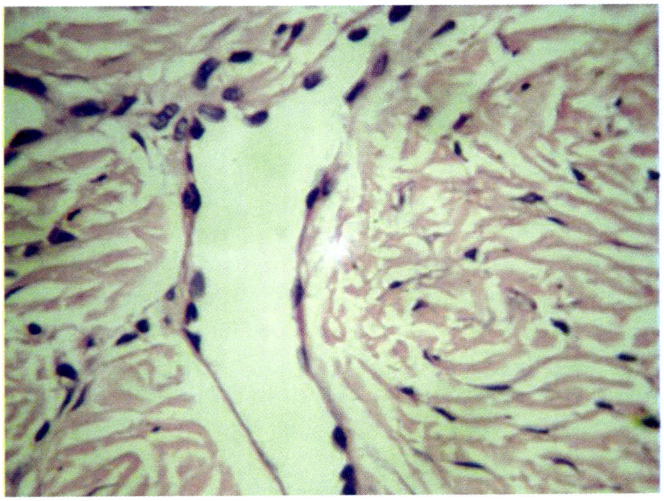

FIGURE 1.1.2.2

INTRODUCTION

Clinical dermatology without a sufficient knowledge of pathology and pathogenesis of a dermatosis would be like going on a treasure hunt without a ground map. This chapter aims to equip with images of basics of normal anatomy of skin and major tissue reaction patterns which inflammatory skin disorders follow in various dermatoses.

NORMAL HISTOLOGY

1. **Epidermis**
   The epidermis (Fig. 1.1.1.1) is stratified squamous epithelium that is terminally differentiated, renews continously and forms derivative structures like hair, sebaceous glands, sweat glands and nails. Its thickness varies between 0.4 and1.5 mm. Keratinocytes constitute more than 95% of cells, while the remainder is constituted by melanocytes (Fig. 1.1.1.2), Langerhans cells and merkel cells. Morphologically, epidermis is divided into stratum basale, stratum spinosum, stratum granulosum and stratum corneum from inside out.
2. **Dermis**
   The dermis (Fig. 1.1.2.1) is an integrated system of fibrous, filamentous and amorphous connective tissue that accommodates nerves, lymphatic and vascular networks (Figs 1.1.2.2 to 1.1.2.4) epidermally derived appendages, fibroblasts, macrophages, mast cells and other blood borne cells which enter the dermis in response to various stimuli. The dermis makes up the bulk of the skin and provides pliability, elasticity and tensile strength. Its thickness varies from 1 mm on eyelids to 30 mm on the back.
3. **Subcutaneous fat**
   The subcutaneous fat, like dermis (Figs 1.1.2.1 and 1.1.2.4), is derived from the mesenchyme, and fibroblast-like mesenchymal cells give rise to lipocytes, as well as to fibrocytes. Lipocytes manufacture so much fat in their cytoplasm that it displaces, and flattens the nucleus against the periphery of the cell. The thickness varies in different body parts, broad in the waists and nonexistent in eyelids, penis and scrotum. It mainly functions as heat insulator, shock absorber and nutritional depot which is mobilized during starvation.
4. **Hair follicles**
   The hair follicle (Fig. 1.1.3.1) and its hair are fundamentally one structure derived from undifferentiated cells of fetal epidermis. Anatomically hair can be divided into three segments: (a) infundibulum, the upper, funnel-shaped invagination that extends from the follicular orifice above to the entrance of the sebaceous duct below; (b) isthmus, the short midsection of the follicle bounded superiorly by the sebaceous duct and inferiorly by the insertion of the hair-erector muscle, and (c) inferior segment, extending from the muscle insertion to the base of the follicle. At the expanded lower part of the follicle is the hair bulb which encloses an ovoid, vascular connective-tissue papilla. The hair matrix differentiates along 6 separate lines of cells that form 3 concentric layers of inner root sheath and 3 concentric layers of hair itself. From outside inwards, these are (1) Henle's layer; (2) Huxley's layer; (3) Cuticle of inner root sheath; (4) Cuticle of hair; (5) Hair cortex, and (6) Hair medulla. Enveloping this central core is the outer root sheath comprising of glycogen filled cells. The hair cycle follow three phases: (a) anagen (growing phase); (b) catagen (involuting), and (c) telogen (resting). Describing each of them is beyond the scope of this chapter.
5. **Sebaceous glands**
   The sebaceous gland, specialized for sebum synthesis, arises embryologically as an epithelial bud from the outer root sheath at a point marking the junction of the future infundibulum and isthmus. The lobules of this gland are enveloped by a thin and vascular fibrous capsule. The peripheral germinative cells are somewhat flattened or cuboidal and have large nuclei and homogenous basophilic cytoplasm. During differentiation, lipid droplets accumulate eventually filling the cytoplasm. The more centrally located cells have a characteristic vacuolated cytoplasm and a scalloped nucleus, owing to compression by lipid globules. Function of this gland is not known.
6. **Apocrine glands**
   Histologically, the apocrine gland consists of: (1) a coiled secretory gland situated in deep dermis or in subcutaneous tissue, and (2) a straight excretory duct that empties into the infundibular part of hair follicle just above the entrance of sebaceous duct. The secretory portion is lined by cuboidal to columnar cells with convex apical borders. These cells are surrounded by myoepithelial cells. The excretory duct is composed of two layers of cuboidal cells. The type of secretion in these glands is called apocrine, due to pinching off of the apical cytoplasm into the lumen (decapitation secretion) (Fig. 1.1.4.1). These glands are present in only few areas of the body like the axilae. Function of this gland is not known.
7. **Eccrine sweat glands**
   The eccrine sweat unit comprises of (1) a coiled secretory gland (Fig. 1.1.5.1); (2) coiled dermal duct; (3) straight dermal duct, and (4) spiraled intraepidermal duct or acrosyringium. The coiled secretory gland is composed of two layers of cells, outer row of myoepithelial cells and inner row of pyramidal secretory cells cells. The secretory cells are of two types, small mucopolysaccharide containing dark cells and large gycogen containing pale cells. The eccrine dermal duct is lined by two layers of small, darkly basophilic staining cuboidal epithelial cells. Eccrine sweat is the product secreted by this gland which helps in thermoregulatory system of the body.

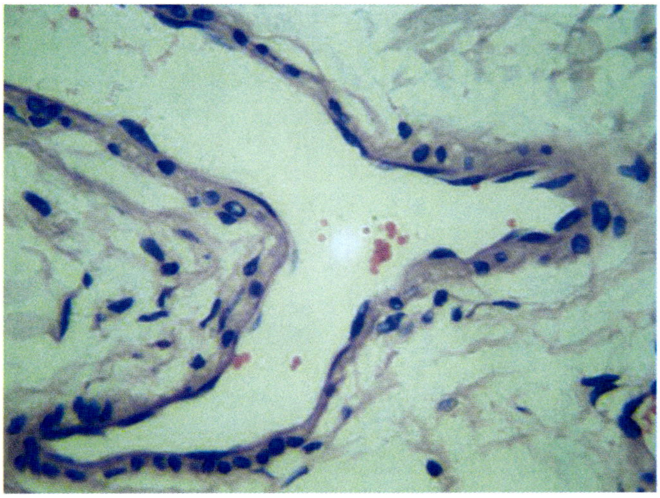

FIGURE 1.1.2.3

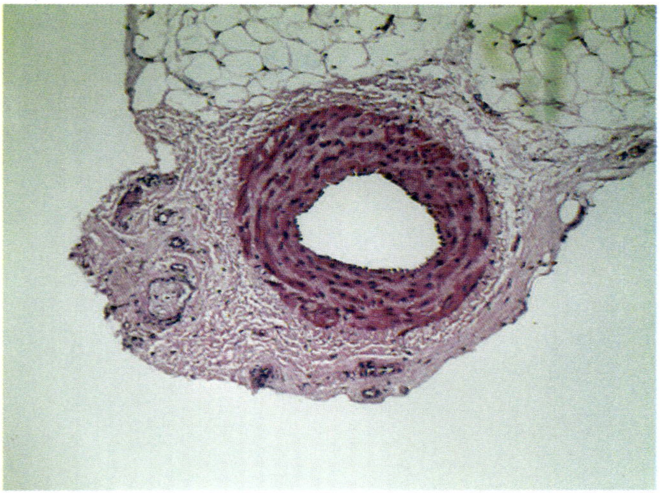

FIGURE 1.1.2.4

1.1.2.3: Venule (*High power view*)

1.1.2.4: Arteriole (*High power view*)

1.1.3: Hair Follicles

1.1.3.1: Hair follicle and sebaceous glands (*Low power view*)

1.1.4: Apocrine Glands

1.1.4.1: Apocrine gland (*High power view*)

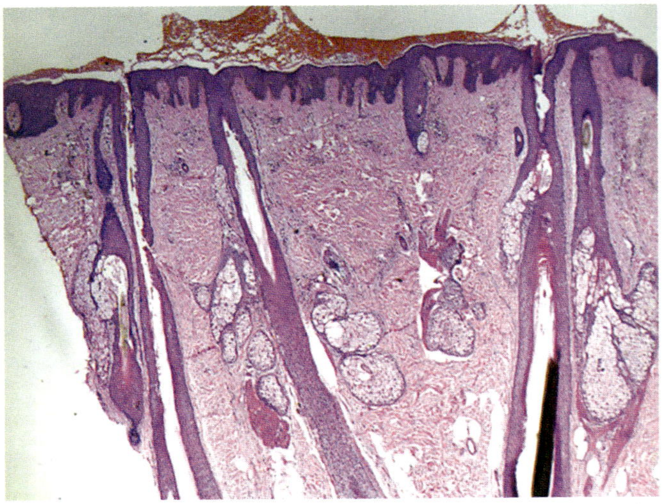

FIGURE 1.1.3.1

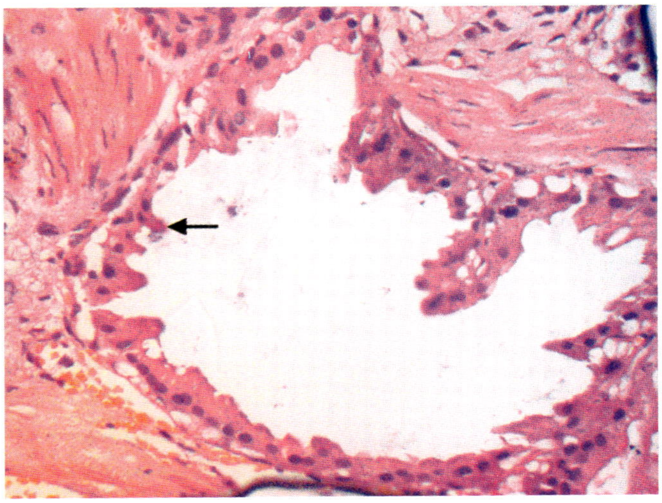

FIGURE 1.1.4.1

8. **Dermal nerves and receptors**
   The skin is a specialized neural structure (Fig. 1.1.6.1), the terminus of peripheral nervous system. Sensory receptors (Figs 1.1.6.2 and 1.1.6.3) may be free or encapsulated, myelinated or unmyelinated and are visualized with difficulty in routine H&E sections.
9. **Nail unit**
   The nail unit comprises of beginning with the superficial proximal skin and progressing around and behind and under the nail to the distal edge. Components include: (1) proximal nail fold; (2) nail matrix; (3) nail bed, and (4) hyponychium.

TOPOGRAPHY

The skin surface is intricate and varied. Regional variations in skin structure either represent adaptations to a particular function or the vestiges of pre-human life (Figs 1.2.1 to 1.2.3).

Skin surface markings develop during the third and fourth months of fetal life and becomes prominent in childhood. Swirled patterns typify palms and soles and roughly diamond-shaped outlines crisscross the rest of the body surface which is well seen in skin over the volar aspect of wrists and elbows, in the antecubital fossae, and between the knuckles.

The scalp, pubic area, axillae, beard, mustache and chest, in actuality the entire body surface, excluding acral volar skin and mucocutaneous junctions, is dotted by hairs, many of them fine and tiny.

The skin of the back is taut, mainly composed of broad collagen bundles to withstand stress of upright posture while the skin of eyelids thin and distensible, aptly designed for rapid movements necessary to protect eyes. Thus demonstrating the elasticity of skin.

At body openings, the skin is continuos with mucous membrane. However the skin here differs from the mucous membranes by possessing a cornified layer of cells without nuclei.

There are other distinguishing features of skin at different sites, describing all of them is beyond the scope of this chapter.

BASIC HISTOPATHOLOGICAL REACTIONS

Pattern analysis was first developed by Wallace Clark in 1965. Several modifications were done by A Bernard Ackerman, Martin Mihm, Murphy, John Maize, David Weedon, John Mckee, etc. till the advent of algorithmic method evolved in late 1990's.

This involves: (1) To decide the category e.g. inflammatory, neoplastic, etc.; (2) To determine tissue reaction

INFLAMMATORY CELLS (TABLE 1.1) (FIGS 1.3.1 TO 1.3.5)

Table 1.1: Inflammatory cells

Type of cell	*Dimensions/ nucleus/ cytoplasm*	*Salient features*
Neutrophil	10 to 20 microns/multilobed nucleus/ amphophilic granules in cytoplasm	• 50 to 70% of circulating WBCs • Major function is ingestion and elimination of foreign bodies and infective organisms (phagocytosis)
Eosinophil	Bilobed nucleus/eosinophilic granules in cytoplasm	• Phagocytosis • Role in immediate hypersensitivity reaction by inactivating some of mast cell's most potent products
Lymphocyte	Size varies from small (5 to 8 microns), medium (8 to 12 microns) and large (12 to 30 microns)/dark stained or slightly indented round nucleus/thin rim of cytoplasm	• T(thymus influenced) and B(bursa dependent) lymphocytes are two major types • T cells are essential for cell mediated immunity • B cells are precursors for antibody producing plasma cells
Plasma cell	Ovoid cells with eccentric round or oval nuclei/perinuclear halo/cart wheel appearance of nucleus/deeply purple cytoplasm	• Russel bodies are accumulations of glycoprotein as an eosinophilic globule in the cytoplasm • Secretion of immunoglobulins that are produced in endoplasmic reticulum
Mast cell	8 to 15 microns/central round or ovoid dark nucleus/ tiny amphophilic granules in cytoplasm	• Storage and release of chemical mediators of inflammatory reactions (histamine, ECF-A, NCF-A, SRS-A, PAF)
Histiocyte	15 to 25 microns/large and pale reniform or deeply indented nucleus/ abundant cytoplasm	• Mainly functions as a scavenger • Concentration and retention of a small amount of immunogen for subsequent presentation to the lymphocyte

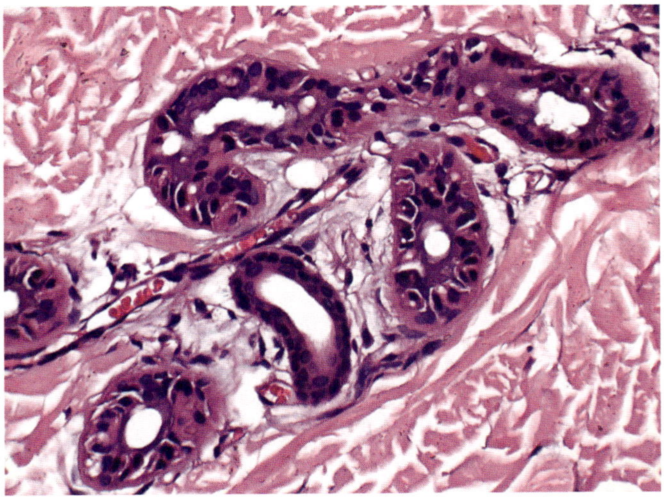

FIGURE 1.1.5.1

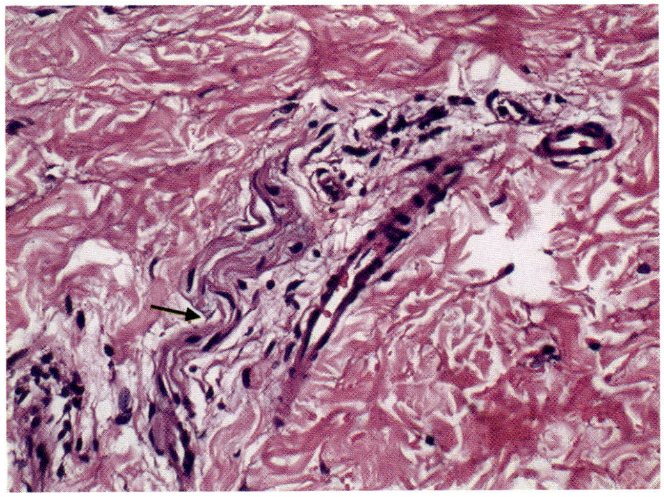

FIGURE 1.1.6.1

1.1.5: Eccrine Sweat Glands

1.1.5.1: Eccrine unit (*High power view*)

1.1.6: Dermal Nerves and Receptors

1.1.6.1: Dermal nerve (*High power view*)

1.1.6.2: Meissner's corpuscle (*High power view*)

1.1.6.3: Pacinian corpuscle (*Low power view*)

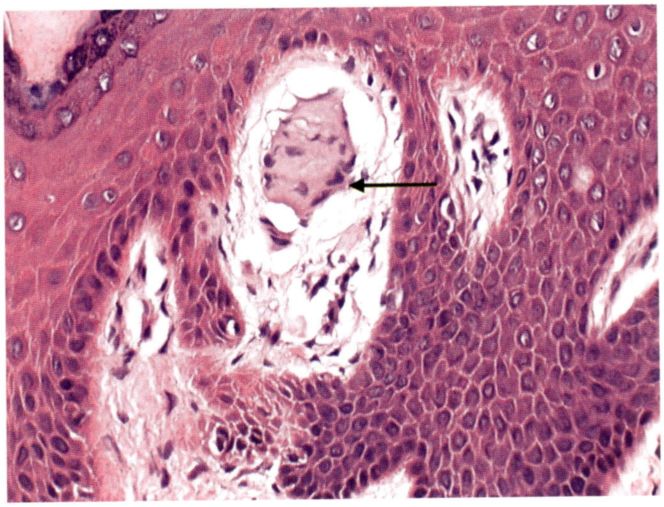

FIGURE 1.1.6.2

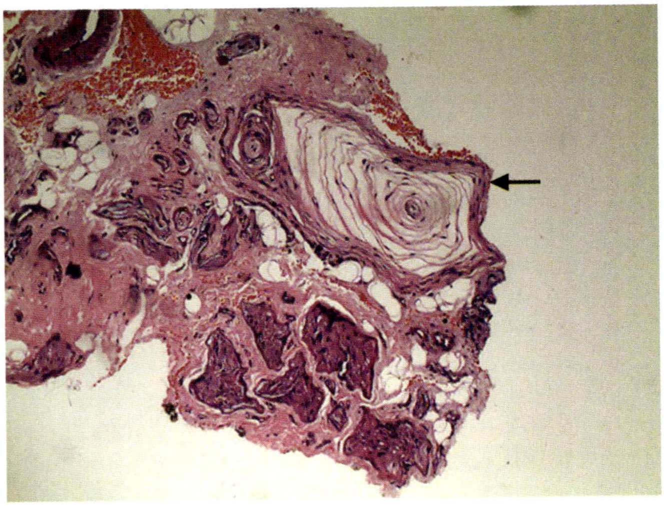

FIGURE 1.1.6.3

pattern; (3) Epidermal changes; (4) Inflammatory cell (Table 1.1), and (5) Specific changes of the disease

Tissue reaction patterns are important morphological patterns and the majority of inflammatory dermatoses can be categorized into six different patterns.

1. **Spongiform pattern**: The spongiotic reaction pattern is characterized by intraepidermal intercellular edema or spongiosis. It is recognised by the presence of widened intercellular spaces between the epidermal cells, with elongation of intercellular bridges. The spongiosis varies from microscopic foci to grossly visible vesicles. Inflammatory cells are present in the dermis and their distribution and type may help in arriving at a specific diagnosis.
   For example, allergic contact dermatitis, nummular dermatitis, etc.
2. **Psoriasiform pattern**: The psoriasiform reaction pattern is defined as epidermal hyperplasia in which there is elongation of rete ridges, usually in a regular manner. However, early lesions of certain diseases such as psoriasis may not have significant hyperplasia. Rather, dilated papillary dermal vessels and overlying suprapapillary scale are dominant features in this condition. The concept of "squirting dermal papilla" clearly explains this in early lesions.
   For example, psoriasis, Reiters syndrome, pityriasis rubra pilaris, etc.
3. **Lichenoid pattern**: The lichenoid pattern is characterized by epidermal basal cell damage, manifested by cell death and/or basal vacuolar change. The dead basal cells form shrunken eosinophilic tiny globules called the civatte bodies. Lichenoid pattern is also sometimes referred to as "Interface dermatitis".
   For example, lichen planus and its variants, lichenoid keratosis, lichenoid drug eruption, etc.
4. **Blistering pattern**: This pattern comprises of vesicles or bullae at any level within the epidermis or at the dermoepidermal junction. Specific diagnosis can be made by assessing 3 features: (a) anatomical level of split; (b) underlying mechanism; (c) nature of infiltrate. The anatomical split can be subcorneal, within stratum malpighii, suprabasal or subepidermal. The mechanism responsible would be exaggerated spongiosis, intracellular edema and ballooning or acantholysis.
   For example, pemphigus vulgaris, pemphigus vegetans, bullous pemphigoid, etc.
5. **Granulomatous pattern**: This pattern of inflammation is characterized by localized collections of epitheloid cells, admixed with giant cells, lymphocytes, plasma cells, fibroblasts, and non-epitheloid macrophages. Five types depending on constituent cells and other changes include—sarcoidal, tuberculoid, necrobiotic, suppurative and foreign body.
   For example, sarcoidosis, tuberculosis, blastomycosis, mycetoma, granuloma annulare, etc.
6. **Vasculopathic pattern**: This group includes diseases with pathological changes in blood vessels. The most important entity in this group is 'vasculitis' which is defined as the inflammatory changes in the walls of blood vessels of any size.
   For example, leukocytoclastic vasculitis, urticarial vasculitis, purpura, etc.
7. **Fibrosing dermatitis**: Fibrosing dermatitis results from alteration in formation of fibrous tissue in dermis.
   For example, hypertrophic scars, scleroderma, lichen sclerosus, etc.
8. **Folliculitis:** Inflammation of hair follicles is called as folliculitis while that of perifollicular connective tissue is called perifolliculitis.
   For example, acne vulgaris, rosacea, perforating folliculitis, etc.
9. **Panniculitis:** Inflammatory changes in subcutaneous fat comprises of panniculitis. There are two major types: (a) Lobular panniculitis: wherein the inflammatory cells are present mainly in the lobules with some septal involvement, and (b) Septal panniculitis: where the septae are mainly involved although some spilling over may occur in the lobules. Thus, these two types may overlap.
   For example, erythema nodosum, erythema induratum, lupus panniculitis, etc.
   Details of these reaction patterns follow in subsequent chapters.

SPECIALIZED TECHNIQUES

a. **Special stains:** Following are the common histochemical stains used in dermatopathology (Figs 1.4.1.1 and 1.4.1.2). Can be done using formalin-fixed, paraffin-embedded sections (Table 1.2).
b. **Direct immunofluorescence:** Valuable diagnostic tool for many autoimmune and inflammatory skin conditions (Fig. 1.4.2.1). Requires transport medium and fresh frozen section (Table 1.3).
c. **Immunohistochemistry (Table 1.4)**: Following are common antigens that can be detected in formalin-fixed, paraffin-embedded sections (Fig. 1.4.3.1).

IMPROVING BIOPSY OUTCOME

As a clinical dermatologist following are important points to remember before and while taking a skin biopsy, in order to enable the dermatopathologist to arrive at a correct diagnosis or a differential diagnosis.

- The need to take a biopsy must be established and discussed with the patient.
- If appropriate lesion is not present postpone the biopsy informing the patient about its necessity at a later date.

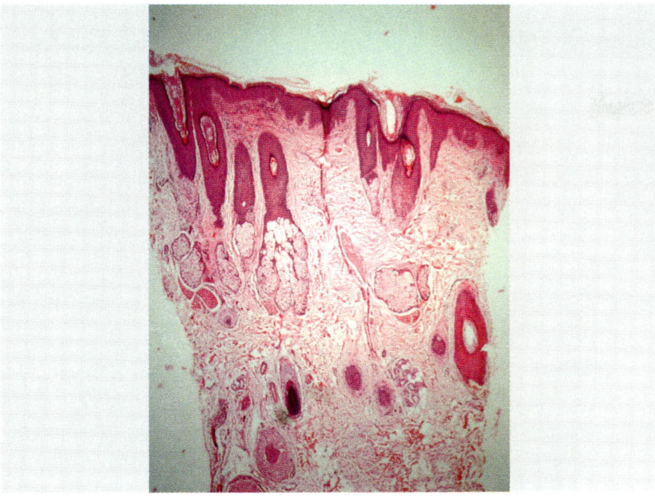

FIGURE 1.2.1

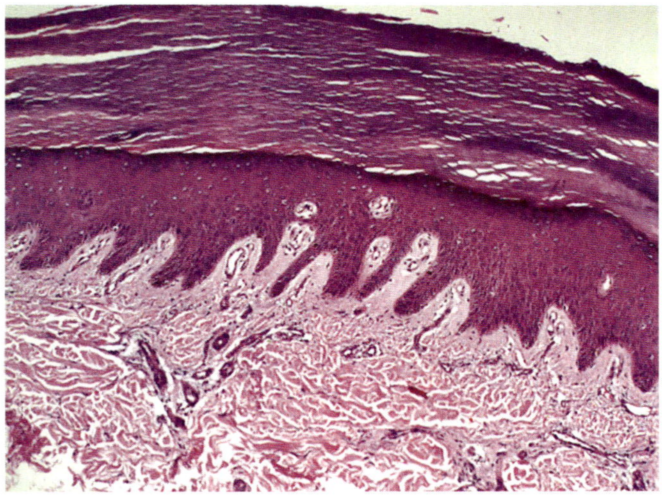

FIGURE 1.2.2

1.2: TOPOGRAPHY

1.2.1: Scalp skin (*Scanner view*)

1.2.2: Palmar skin (*Low power view*)

1.2.3: Mucosal epithelium (*High power view*)

1.3: INFLAMMATORY CELLS (TABLE 1.1)

1.3.1: Neutrophil (*High power view*)

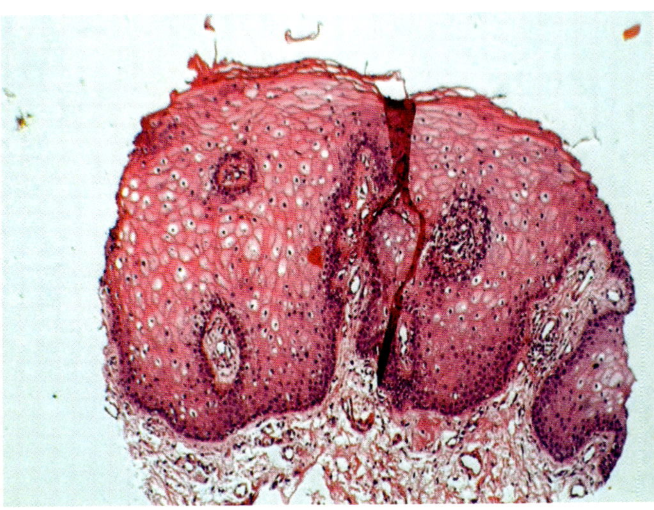

FIGURE 1.2.3

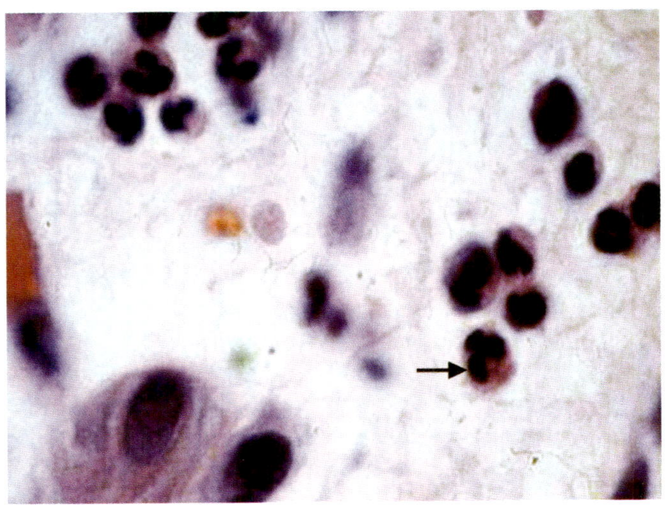

FIGURE 1.3.1

Table 1.2: Special stains

Stain	Purpose of stain	Results
Hematoxylin-eosin	Routine	Nuclei: blue; cytoplasm: pink
Periodic acid-Schiff (PAS)	Glycogen, neutral mucopolysaccharide, fungi	Glycogen: red; diastase labile. Neutral MPS, fungi: red; diastase resistant
Masson trichrome	Collagen	Collagen: blue or green. Nuclei, muscles, nerves: dark red
Verhoeff-van Gieson	Elastic fibers	Elastic fibers: black Collagen: red
Fontana-Masson	Melanin	Black
Methanamine silver	Fungi, Donovan bodies, Frisch bacilli, basement membranes	Black
Grocott	Fungi	Fungal cell walls: black
Alcian blue	Mucopolysaccharide	Blue
Toluidine blue	Mucopolysaccharide	Blue
Colloidal iron	Mucopolysaccharide	Blue
Giemsa	Mast cell granules (MCG), Mucopolysaccharide, myeloid granules, Leishmania	MCG and mucopolysaccharide: metachromically purple. Myeloid granules and Leishmania: red
Gram's stain	Bacteria	Positive—blue Negative—pink
Fite	Acid-fast bacilli	Red
Congo red	Amyloid	Pink-red; green birefringence in polarized light
Von kossa	Calcium	Black
Scarlet red	Lipids	Red
Oil red O	Lipids	Red
Warthin Starry	Spirochetes	Black

Table 1.3: Direct immunofluorescence

Condition	Pattern
Pemphigus vulgaris	IgG and C3 on epidermal ICS (chicken wire pattern). More superficial in pemphigus foliaceous than *P. vulgaris*
Bullous pemphigoid	C3 and IgG or C3 alone deposited on the basement membrane. Deposits are localized on the roof of the split in salt split biopsy
Gestational pemphigoid	Linear C3 deposits on basement membrane zone (BMZ)
Epidermolysis bullosa acquisita	Auto-antibodies to type VII collagen in BMZ. Linear deposits at the dermal, or floor aspect of induced blister on salt split biopsy
Dermatitis herpetiformis	IgA reactive granular deposits at the tips of dermal papillae
Linear IgA dermatosis	Intense linear IgA deposits along the BMZ, but none in dermal papillae
Lupus erythematosus	Coarse, granular, continuous deposits of Igs and complement along the DEJ
Lichen planus	Large, grouped and globular deposits of immunoglobulins and complement, i.e. civatte bodies

If the case is complex, it is better to take two biopsies in the beginning.

- Choice of lesion is very important as selecting a lesion that is not representative can be misleading, e.g. in a polymorphic rash.
- Evolution of the disease as well as evolution of the lesion is available to the clinician. However, for dermatopathologist, one lesion at one point of time only is available. It is a two-dimensional freeze of a four-dimensional event.
- Never include normal skin in biopsy (important to remember when edge is being biopsied).
- Avoid excoriated or ulcerated lesions unless there is no option.
- Avoid legs: Stasis change complicates interpretation.
- Avoid bony prominences or pressure bearing areas: Non-specific lymphocytic infiltrate complicates interpretation, epidermal changes complicate interpretation, more painful to patients and takes longer to heal.

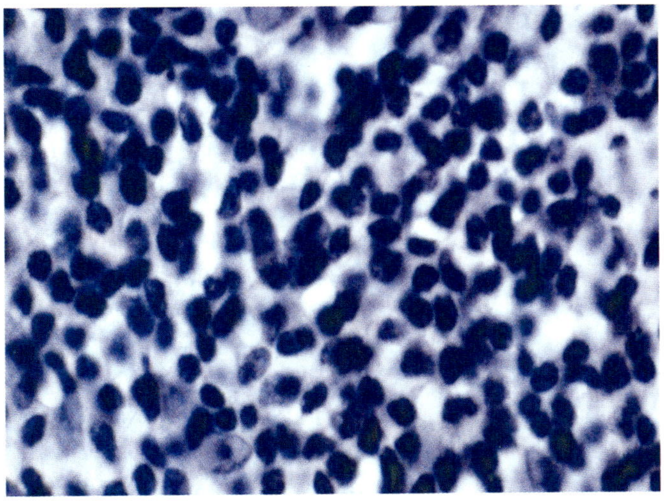

FIGURE 1.3.2

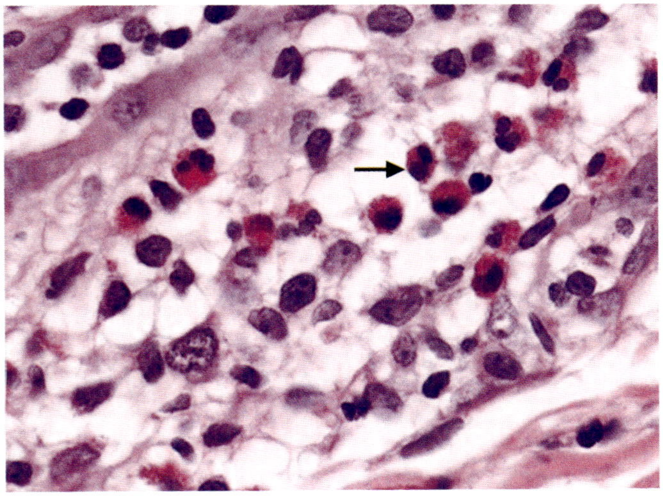

FIGURE 1.3.3

1.3.2: Lymphocyte (*High power view*)
1.3.3: Eosinophil (*High power view*)
1.3.4: Plasma cell (*High power view*)
1.3.5: Multinucleated giant cell (*High power view*)

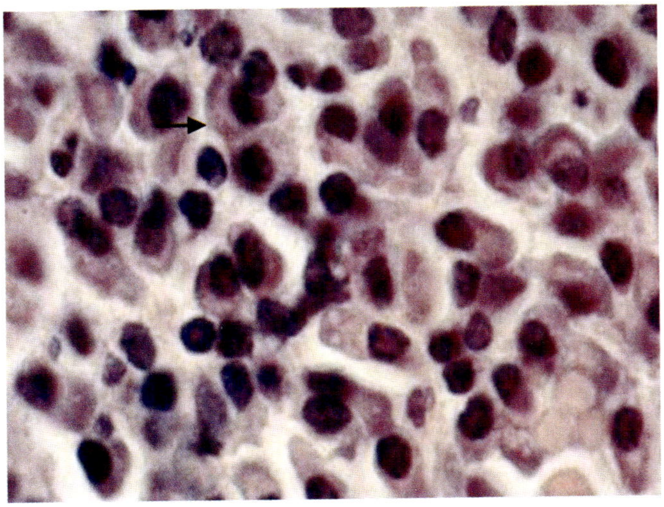

FIGURE 1.3.4

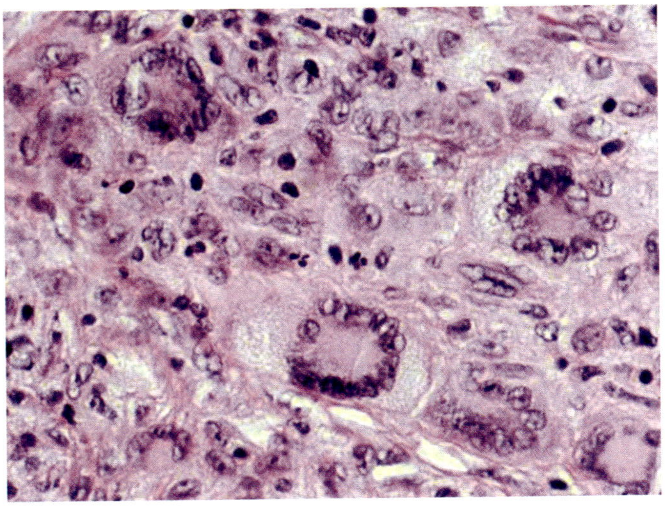

FIGURE 1.3.5

Table 1.4: Immunohistochemistry

Antigen	*Location*
Cytokeratins (AE1, AE3, CAM 5.2, CK 20)	Epidermis, appendages and epidermal tumors
Vimentin	Mesenchymal cells, melanocytes, lymphomas, sarcomas, melanomas
Desmin	Smooth and skeletal muscle, muscle tumors
Leukocyte common antigen	Benign leukocytes, lymphomas, leukemia
Epithelial membrane antigen	Sweat and sebaceous glands, carcinoma, epitheloid sarcoma
S 100	Melanocytes, Langerhans cells, eccrine and apocrine glands, and their tumors, Schwann cells, nerves, interdigitating reticulum cells, chondrocytes, melanomas, adipose tissue, liposarcomas, histiocytosis X
HMB 45	Melanoma cells and some nevus cells
CD 31	Endothelial cells
CD 34	Endothelial cells, bone marrow progenitor cells, cells of dermatofibrosarcoma protuberans
CD 4	T-helper cells, monocytes, macrophages, Langerhans cells, peripheral T cell lymphoma, mycosis fungoides, HTLV-1 associated adult T cell leukemia/ lymphoma
CD 8	T cytotoxic/suppressor cells, NK cells, T cell lymphomas
CD 20	B cells, B cell lymphomas
CD 30	Activated lymphoid cells, anaplastic large cell lymphoma, lymphomatoid papulosis
CD 68	Histiocytes, myeloid cells, mast cells and their neoplasms
CD 45 RO	T cells, histiocytes, myeloid cells, T cell lymphomas, histiocytic neoplasms, myeloid leukemias
Factor XIIIa	Dermatofibromas, certain fibrohistiocytic cells

- Choice of punch
  - 3 mm, 4 mm or 5 mm
  - Bigger the better; but not always necessary
  - In cosmetically, important area 3 mm or even 2.5 mm punch gives equally good results with a well trained dermatopathologist
  - Proper handling after biopsy
  - Inform the technician
- While taking the biopsy: Stretch the skin across relaxed skin tension lines (Langer's lines) this small maneuver makes biopsy wounds smaller and elliptical, it is easier to take a suture, faster to heal and leaves behind a better scar.

For a dermatopathologist to arrive at a correct diagnosis or a differential diagnosis here are some useful tips:

- Take serial deep cut sections or exhaust the block and try to examine every section on every slide.
- Examine sections preferably without reading clinicians differential diagnosis.
- Try to fit it into one of the patterns and come to some diagnosis.
- When the pathologist is unable to do so then try to correlate clinically.
- If not then ask for additional sections or consult directly with the clinician and discuss.
- If diagnosis is not possible then give descriptive reports and specify about the type of pattern. For example, lichenoid reaction pattern/spongiotic reaction pattern/ granulomatous reaction pattern, etc.
- If one wishes to comment further or to speculate, he can add a note in which he can discuss differential diagnosis and offer his interpretations as probabilities or possibilities.

To summarize, dermatopathology requires years of training and practice, but is exciting and challenging. There seems to be an endless number of potential diagnoses. However if this systematic approach is adopted, the great majority of skin biopsies can be diagnosed specifically.

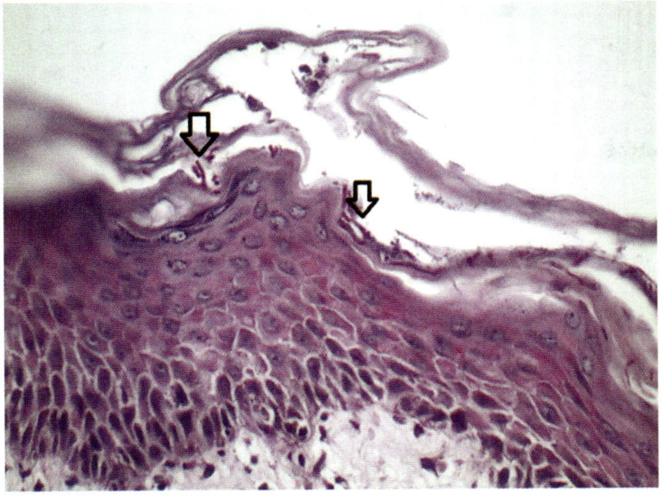

FIGURE 1.4.1.1

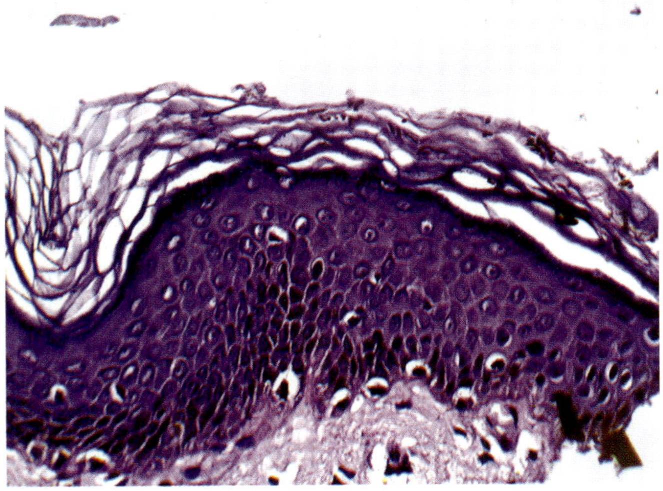

FIGURE 1.4.1.2

1.4: SPECIALIZED TECHNIQUES

1.4.1: Special Stains (Table 1.2)

1.4.1.1: PAS stain dermatophyte (*High power view*)

1.4.1.2: PAS stain pityriasis versicolor (*High power view*)

1.4.2: Direct Immunofluorescence (Table 1.3)

1.4.2.1: Direct immunofluorescence (*High power view*)

1.4.3: Immunohistochemistry (Table 1.4)

1.4.3.1: Immunohistochemistry (*High power view*)

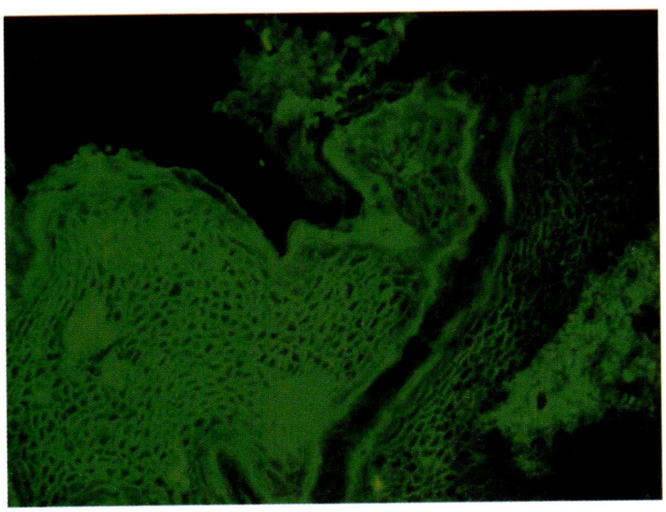

FIGURE 1.4.2.1

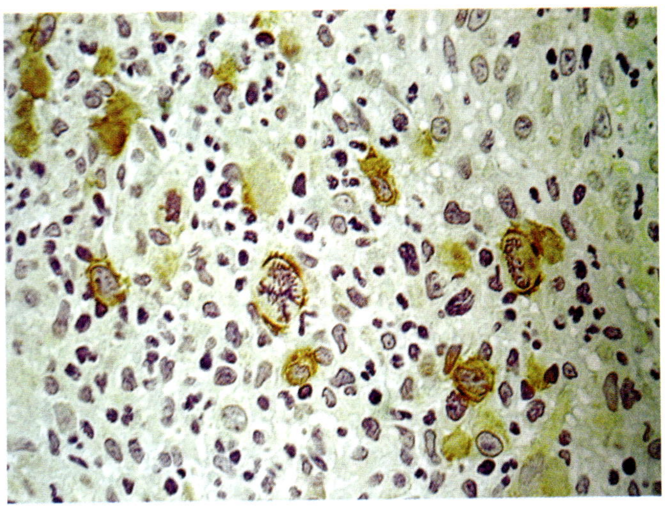

FIGURE 1.4.3.1

Clues and Pitfalls in Diagnostic Dermatopathology

2

Chapter Outline

2.1: Hyperkeratosis
2.2: Parakeratosis
2.3: Cornoid Lamellation
2.4: Papillomatosis
2.5: Church Spires
2.6: Acantholysis
2.7: Dyskeratosis
2.8: Dermal Polymorphonuclear Infiltrate
2.9: Epidermal Eosinophilic Infiltrates (Eosinophilic Spongiosis)
2.10: Dermal Eosinophilic Infiltrate
2.11: Foam Cells
2.12: Clues to Early Diagnosis of Mycosis Fungoides
2.13: Extravasated RBCs
2.14: Keratinocyte Pallor
2.15: Increased Mitotic Activity
2.16: Artifacts and Thermal Changes
2.17: Special Stains

Venkataram Mysore, Pradeep Mahajan

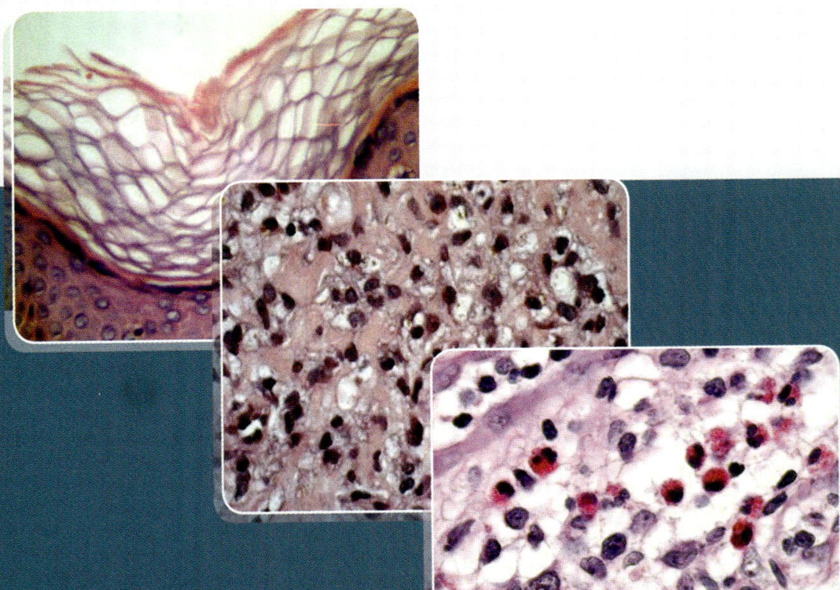

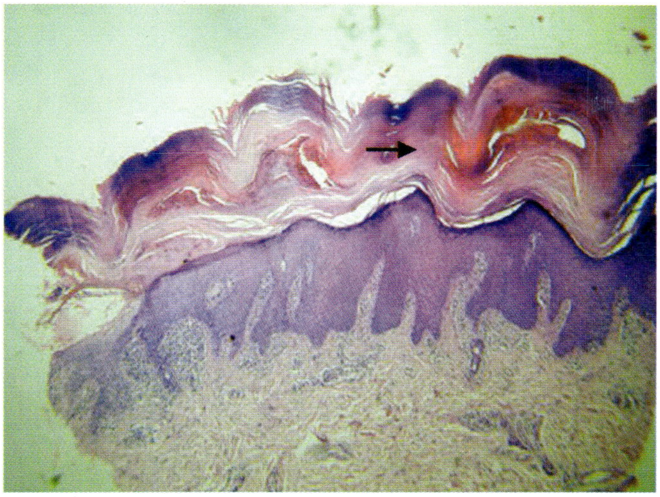

FIGURE 2.1.1

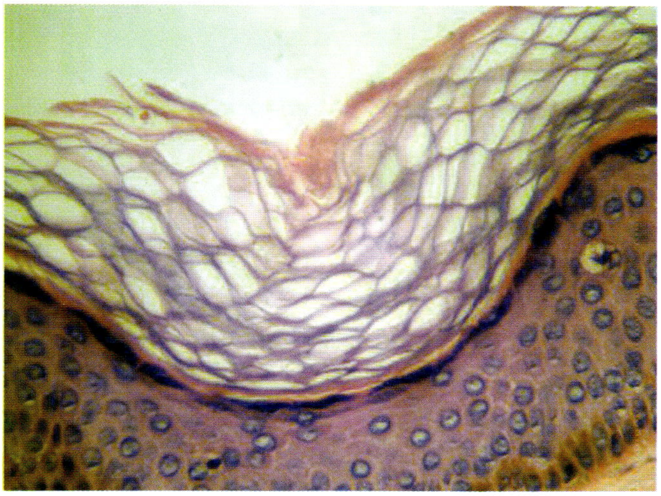

FIGURE 2.1.2

2.1: Hyperkeratosis

2.1.1: Compact hyperkeratosis (*Low power view*)

2.1.2: Basket weave hyperkeratosis (*High power view*)

2.2: Parakeratosis (*High power view*)

2.3: Cornoid lamellation (*Low power view*)

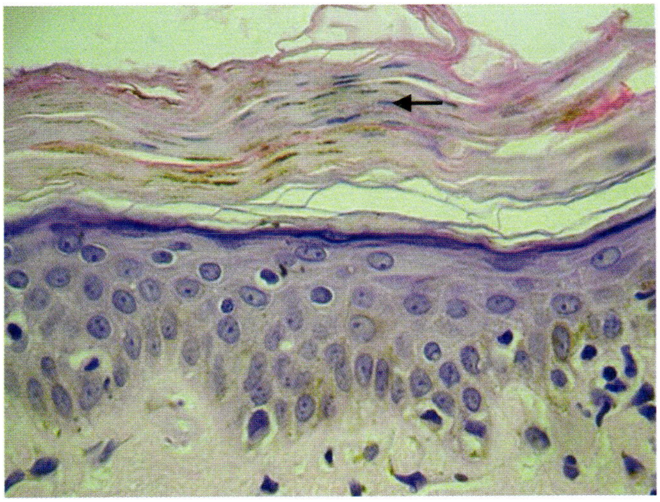

FIGURE 2.2

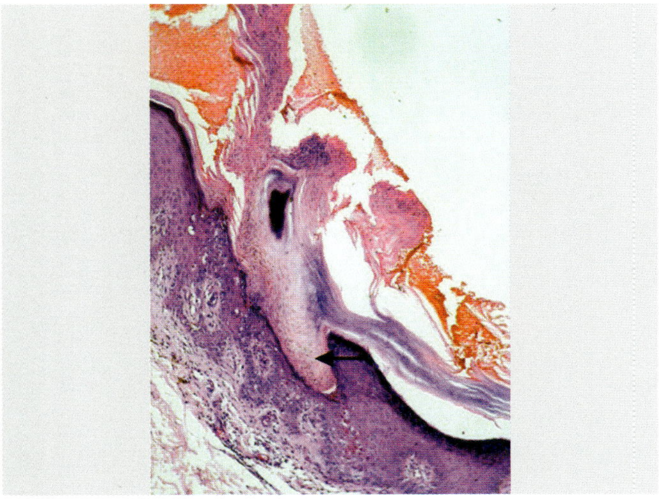

FIGURE 2.3

INTRODUCTION

- Histopathological findings under the microscope many a times differ from the classic reaction patterns and may not be diagnostically specific always.
- Some useful points may assist in reaching a correct diagnosis.
- Dr A Bernard Ackerman has contributed to many of these clues than anyone else.
- But remember that these are not the absolute criteria for diagnosis.

2.1: Hyperkeratosis (Figs 2.1.1 and 2.1.2)

Thickened stratum corneum to more than 1/3rd of the total thickness of epidermis is referred to as hyperkeratosis.

Orthokeratosis is hyperkeratosis with normal stratum corneum and stratum granulosum. It may be basket weave as in retention type of ichthyosis (ichthyosis vulgaris) or compact as in lichen simplex chronicus.

2.2: Parakeratosis (Fig. 2.2)

Retention of nuclei in stratum corneum is parakeratosis, which indicates delayed maturation process and altered keratinization.

There is diminished or absent granular layer which accompanies parakeratosis (the only condition in which parakeratosis is seen with normal granular layer is axillary granular parakeratosis).

Parakeratosis is:

1. Focal and scattered as in dermatitis.
2. Focal and cap-like as in lichen nitidus.
3. Alternating with hyperkeratosis and vertically arranged: as in viral warts, inflammatory linear verrucous epidirmal nevus (ILVEN), psoriasis.
4. Horizontally alternating as in actinic keratosis.
5. Horizontal as well as vertical alternating as in PRP.
6. Punctate as in pityriasis lichenoides chronica.
7. With polymorphonuclear cells, as in psoriasis.

2.3: Cornoid Lamellation (Fig. 2.3)

It is keratin filled invagination of the epidermis at an angle from the center of which arises a parakeratotic column.

Seen in:

- Porokeratosis
- Verruca vulgaris
- Actinic keratosis
- Porokeratotic eccrine duct nevus.

2.4: Papillomatosis (Fig. 2.4)

Gross hyperplasia of epidermis, with elongated dermal papillae pushing up the epidermis, in the form of finger like processes is papillomatosis.

It is seen in various conditions like:

Inflammatory diseases: Verrucous skin lesions, such as verrucous tuberculosis, subcutaneous fungal infections, pemphigus vegetans, pyoderma vegetans, milker's nodule, viral warts, and acrokeratosis verruciformis of Hopf.

Tumors: Seborrheic keratosis, hypertrophic form of actinic keratosis, some cases of intradermal nevi, epidermal nevi, nevus sebaceous.

2.5: Church Spires (Fig. 2.5)

Refer to hyperkeratosis and papillomatosis with elevations of epidermis resembling church spire.

Seen in:

- Acrokeratosis verruciformis of Hopf
- Seborrheic keratosis
- Verruca vulgaris.

2.6: Acantholysis (Fig. 2.6)

It is loss of cohesion (due to loss of intercellular bridges) of keratinocytes leading to seperation of cells with formation of clefts and/or bulla.

Acantholytic cells appear rounded with central condensed nucleus.

Acantholysis may be:

1. Primary:
   a. Pemphigus vulgaris—suprabasal
      Pemphigus foliaceous—subcorneal
   b. Hailey-Hailey disease
   c. Darier's disease
   d. Transient acantholytic dyskeratosis
   e. Warty dyskeratoma.
2. Secondary to cell degeneration; in subcorneal pustular dermatosis, viral blisters (herpes simplex and zoster).
3. Neoplastic acantholysis: some cases of actinic keratosis, squamous cell carcinoma.

2.7: Dyskeratosis (Fig. 2.7)

Abnormal and premature individual cell keratinization of cells, which appear as deeply pinkish cells, with small dark nucleus.

Seen in:

a. *Acantholytic dyskeratosis*: in Hailey-Hailey disease, Darier's disease (corps ronds and grain).
b. *Neoplastic dyskeratosis*: Bowen's disease, actinic keratosis, and squamous cell carcinoma.
c. Genodermatoses such as incontinentia pigmenti.

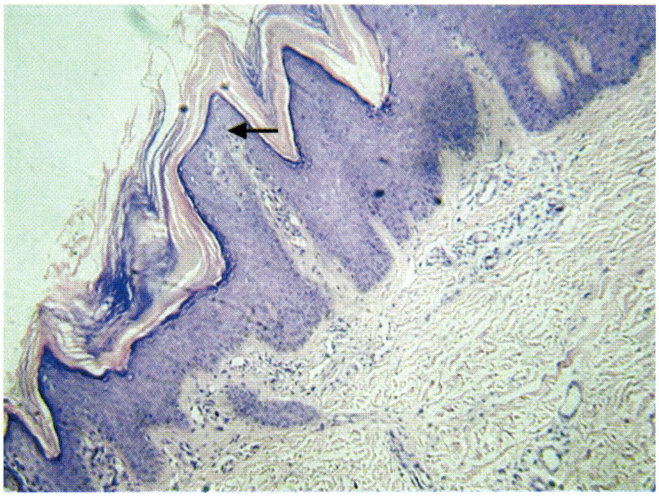

FIGURE 2.4

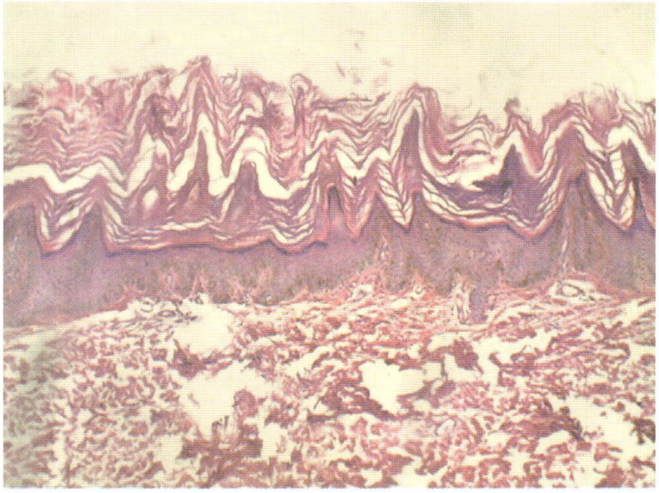

FIGURE 2.5

2.4: Papillomatosis (*Low power view*)
2.5: Church spires (*Scanner view*)
2.6: Acantholytic cells (*High power view*)
2.7: Dyskeratotic cells (*High power view*)

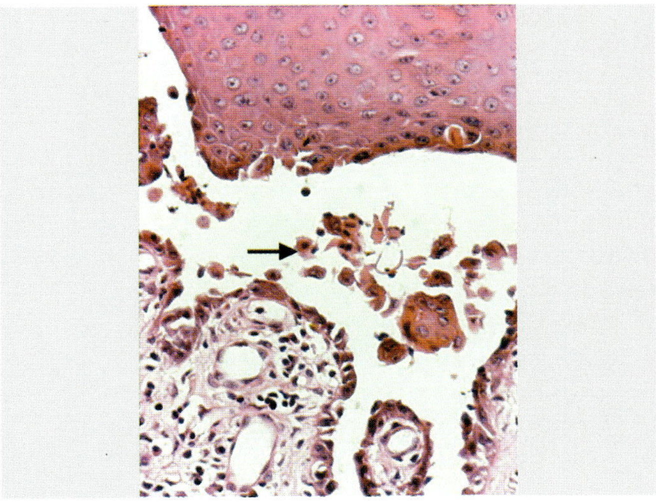

FIGURE 2.6

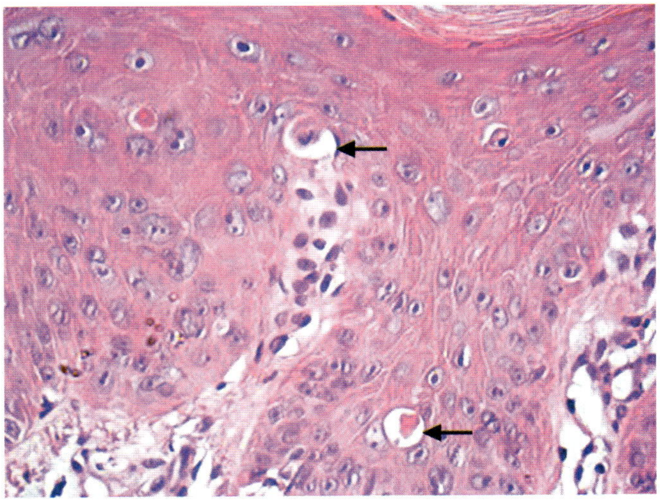

FIGURE 2.7

2.8: Dermal Polymorphonuclear Infiltrate (Fig. 2.8):

a. Leukocytoclastic vasculitis
b. Sweet's syndrome
c. Dermatitis herpetiformis
d. Erythema nodosum in early stages
e. Erythema nodosum leprosum
f. All suppurative granulomas
g. Ruptured cyst
h. Infectious processes—furuncle, cellulitis, etc.

2.9: Epidermal Eosinophilic Infiltrates (Eosinophilic Spongiosis) (Fig. 2.9)

a. Pemphigus
b. Bullous pemphigoid
c. Insect bite reactions
d. Dermatophyte infections
e. Incontinentia pigmenti
f. Eosinophillic pustular folliculitis, etc.

2.10: Dermal Eosinophilic Infiltrate (Fig. 2.10)

a. Atopic dermatitis
b. Erythroderma, particularly atopic type
c. Parasitic infestations, such as scabies, onchocerciasis, larva migrans
d. Allergic granulomatosis of Churg Strauss
e. Eosinophilic fasciitis
f. Bullous pemphigoid, herpes gestationis
g. Granuloma faciale
h. Mycosis fungoides
i. Histiocytosis X-eosinophilic granuloma
j. Urticaria, urticaria pigmentosa, etc.

2.11: Foam Cells (Fig. 2.11)

a. Lepromatous leprosy
b. Xanthomas
c. Xanthogranuloma
d. Necrobiotic xanthogranuloma
e. Panniculitis—particularly of Weber Christian type
f. Histiocytosis X
g. Atypical fibroxanthoma
h. Involuting intradermal nevi
i. Tumors—atypical fibroxanthoma, sebaceous gland tumours, etc.

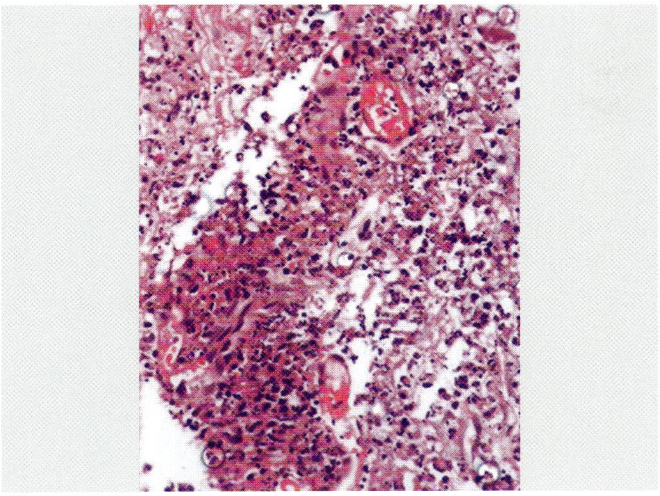

FIGURE 2.8

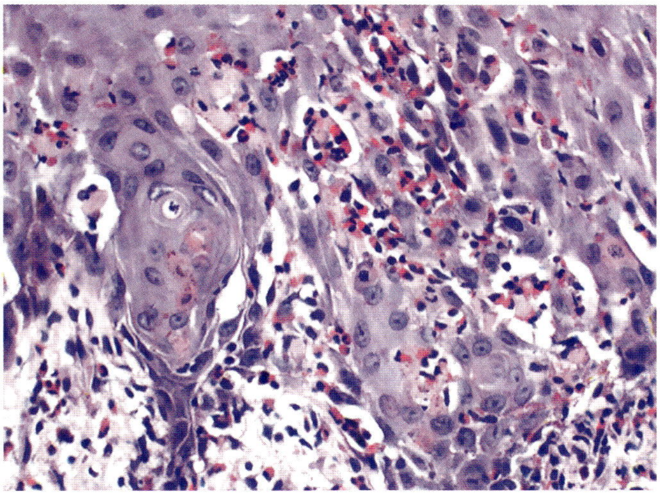

FIGURE 2.9

2.8: Dermal polymorphonuclear infiltrate (*High power view*)
2.9: Epidermal eosinophilic infiltrates (eosinophilic spongiosis) (*High power view*)
2.10: Dermal eosinophilic infiltrate (*High power view*)
2.11: Foam cells (*High power view*)

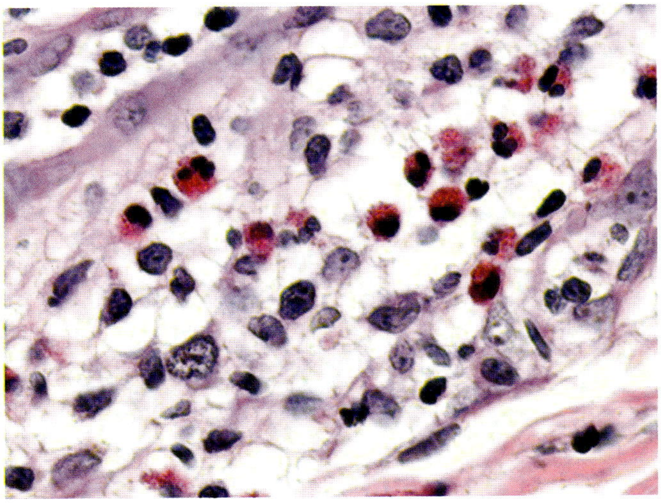

FIGURE 2.10

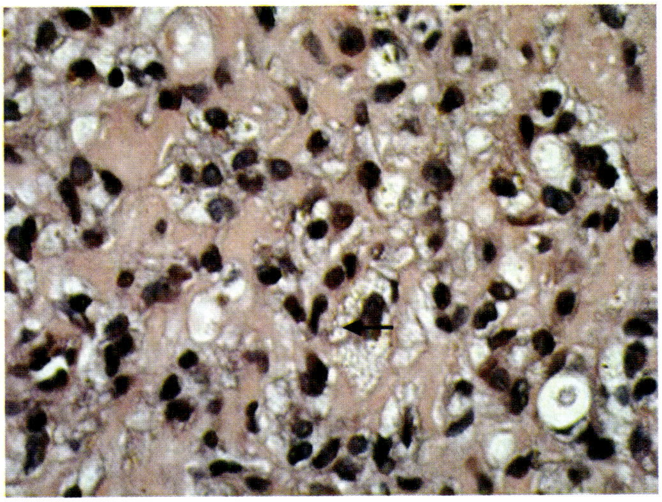

FIGURE 2.11

2.12: Clues to Early Diagnosis of Mycosis Fungoides (Fig. 2.12)

a. Elongated mounds of parakeratosis
b. Lymphocytes in the epidermis surrounded by a clear halo
c. Lymphocytes lining the basal cell layer as a single row (Toy Soldier's appearance)
d. Epidermal lymphocytes larger than dermal
e. Vertical streaks of thickened collagen in papillary dermis.

2.13: Extravasated RBCs (Fig. 2.13)

Seen in:

- Vasculitis
- PPD (Pigmented purpuric dermatoses)
- Hemorrhagic fevers
- Pityriasis rosea
- Pityriasis lichenoides
- Hemorrhage related to biopsy.

2.14: Keratinocyte Pallor (Fig. 2.14)

Along with neutrophilic infiltrate in the epidermis is seen in:

- Nutritional deficiencies like pellagra, zinc deficiency.
- Necrolytic migratory erythema (Glucagonoma syndrome)
- Keratoacanthoma.

2.15: Increased Mitotic Activity (Fig. 2.15)

Psoriasiform tissue reaction pattern is seen in many different conditions including psoriasis and dermatitis (eczemas). Important differentiating point can be demonstration of increased mitosis in psoriasis.

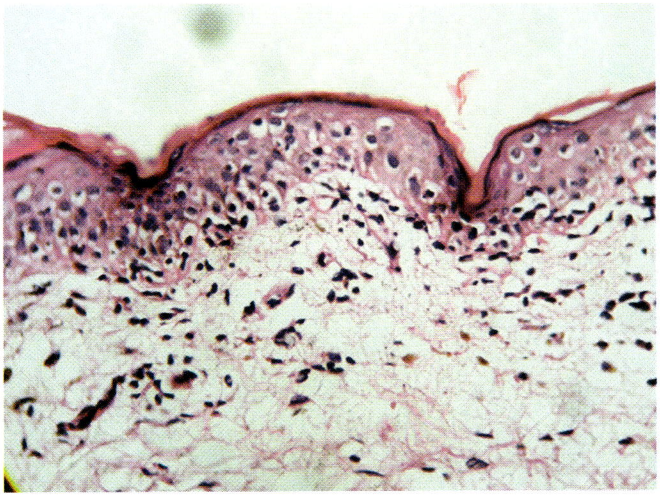

FIGURE 2.12

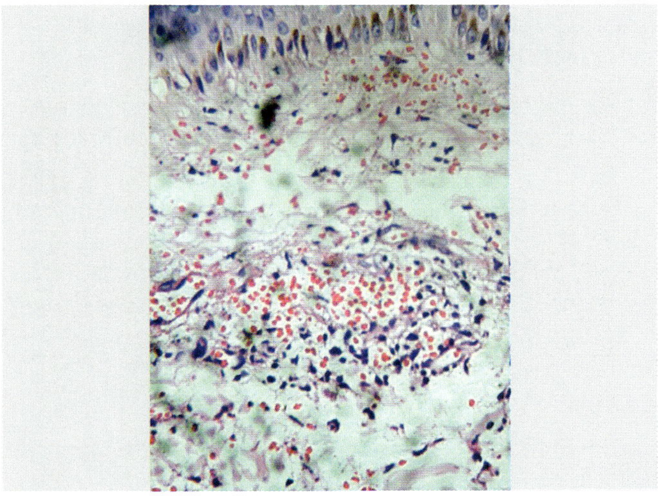

FIGURE 2.13

2.12: Clues to early diagnosis of mycosis fungoides (Toy soldier's appearence) (*Low power view*)

2.13: Extravasated RBCs (*Low power view*)

2.14: Pale keratinocytes below the stratum corneum (*Low power view*)

2.15: Increased mitotic activity (*High power view*)

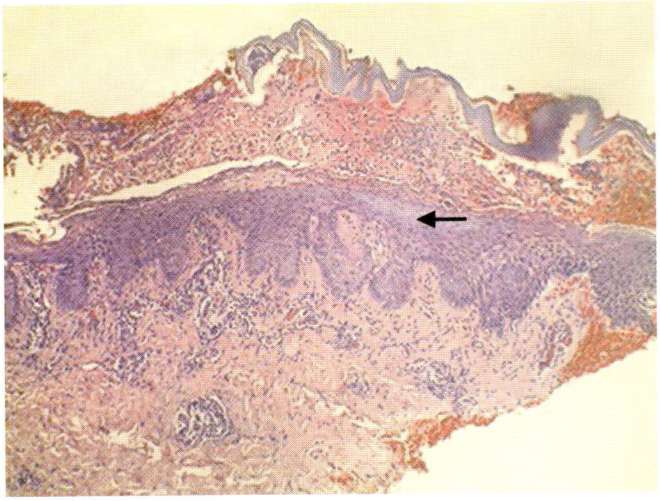

FIGURE 2.14

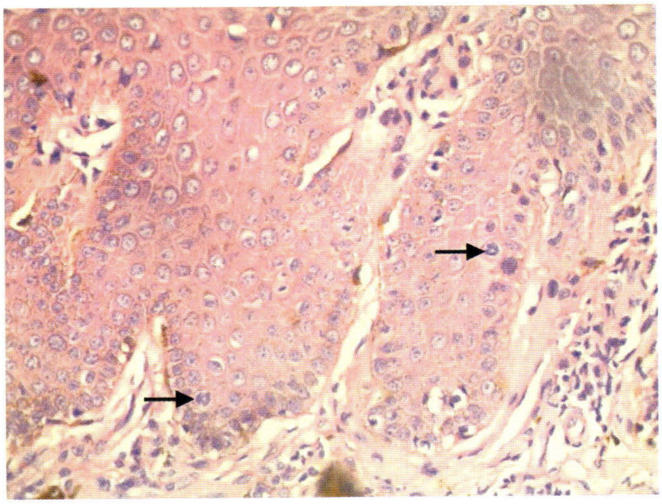

FIGURE 2.15

2.16: Artifacts and Thermal Changes (Fig. 2.16)

One should be aware of biopsy procedural or processing or staining artifacts and should not consider them pathological changes.

Similarly, biopsy done by electric cautery or radiofrequency machines (skin biopsy procedure not recommended to be done by these devises) leads to histologic changes (like elongation of nuclei of keratinocytes and necrosis of dermal collagen) which can be confusing.

2.17: Special Stains

Crystal violet stain is supposed to be better for Amyloid than Congo Red and, Colloidal Iron for mucin than Alcian Blue (but in India, these stains are done very infrequently and only at a few centers).

Summary

- Dermatopathology is interesting field when a mathematical approach through algorithm is followed.
- There are many confusing differentials.
- However, with systematic approach when a diagnosis for a clinically perplexing case is offered by dermatopathology and it helps patient get rid of his/her distress, it is a rewarding and satisfying experience.

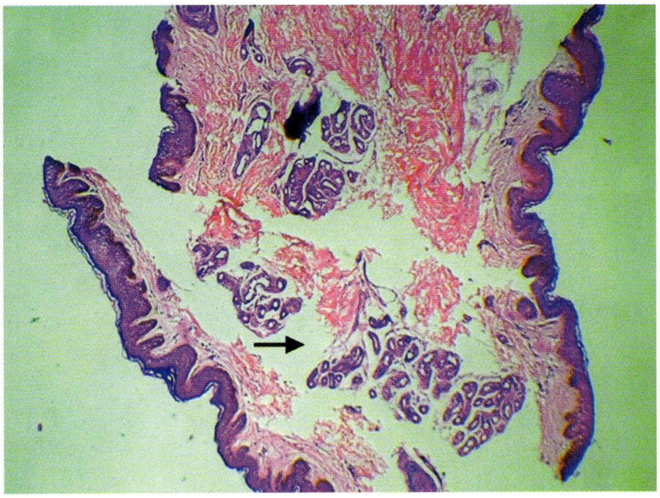

FIGURE 2.16.1

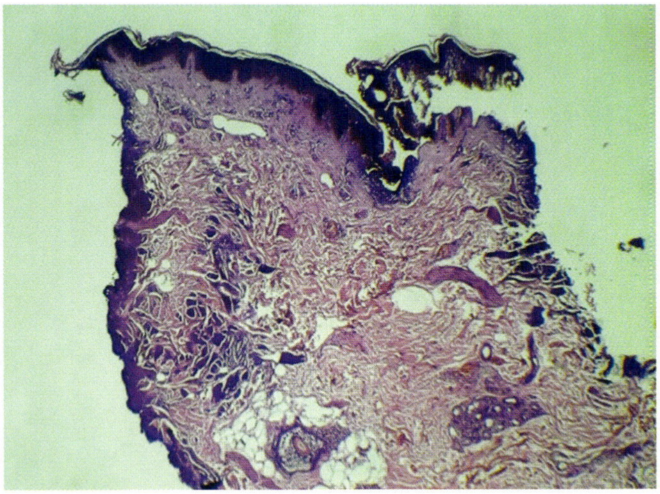

FIGURE 2.16.2

2.16: Artifacts and Thermal Changes

2.16.1: Artifacts—separation of epidermis from dermis during sectioning (*Scanner view*)

2.16.2: Artifacts—sectioning error with epidermis seen on side and top (*Scanner view*)

2.16.3: Radiofrequency changes—coagulated collagen (*Scanner view*)

2.16.4: Radiofrequency changes—elongation of keratinocytes and clefting (*High power view*)

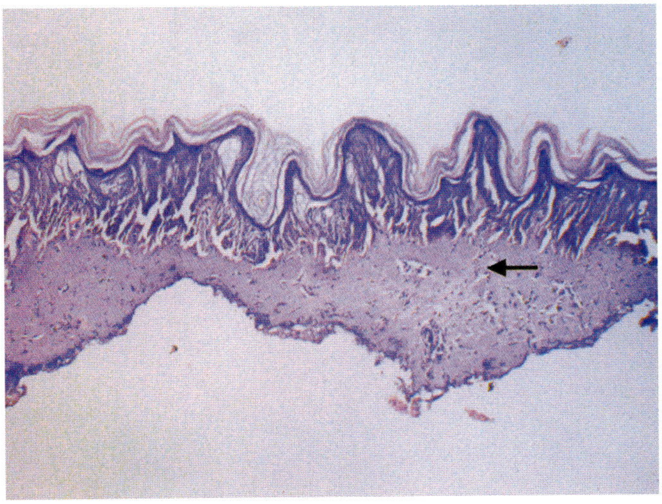

FIGURE 2.16.3

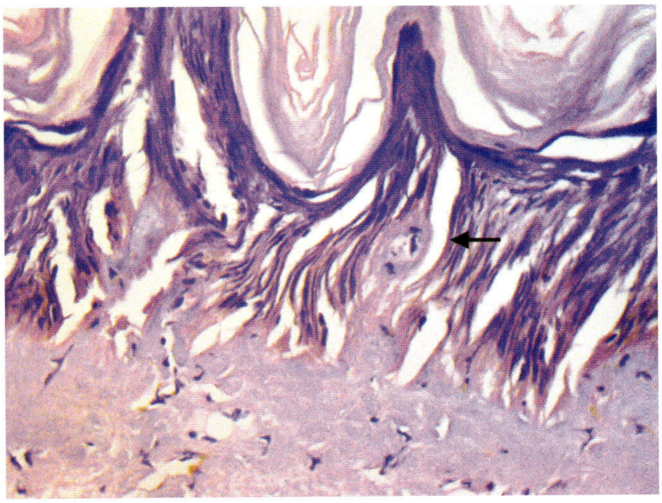

FIGURE 2.16.4

3

Psoriasiform Tissue Reaction

Chapter Outline

3.1: Psoriasis Vulgaris
3.2: Guttate Psoriasis
3.3: Pustular Psoriasis
3.4: Reiter's Disease
3.5: Pityriasis Rubra Pilaris
3.6: Lichen Simplex Chronicus/Chronic Dermatitis
3.7: Inflammatory Linear Verrucous Epidermal Nevus
3.8: Chronic Superficial Dermatitis (Small Plaque Parapsoriasis)

Pradeep Mahajan, Achyut Pokharel

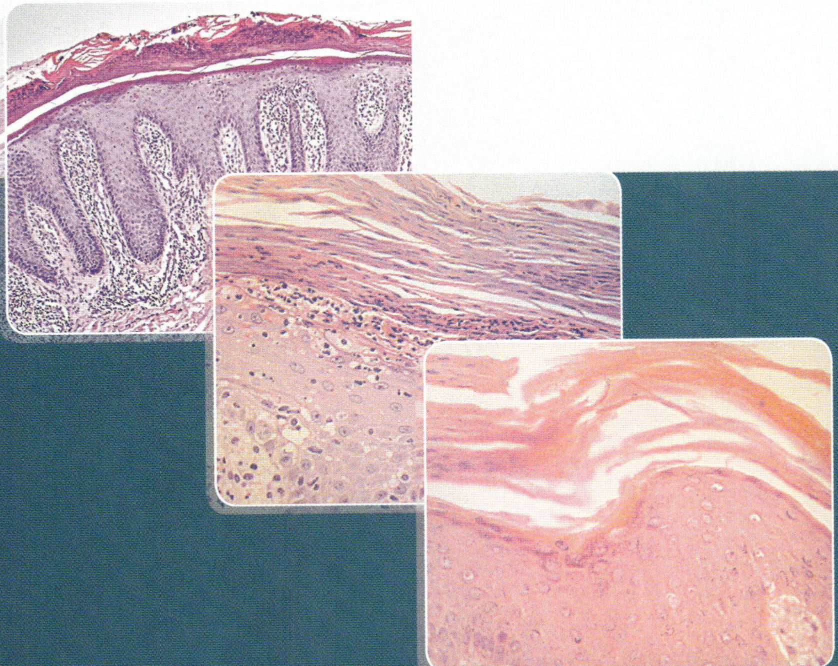

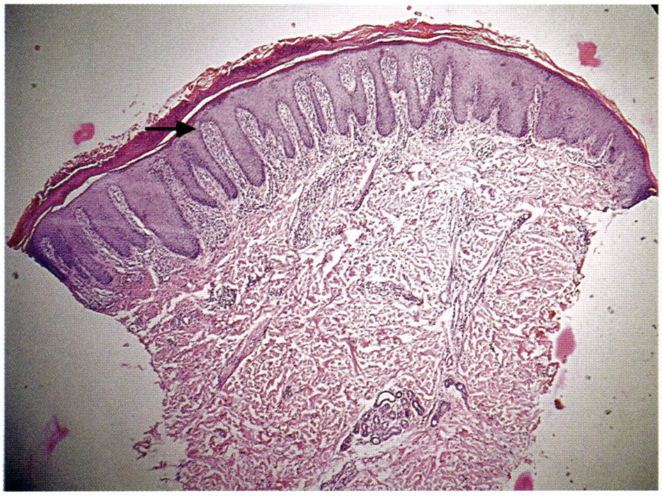

FIGURE 3.1.1

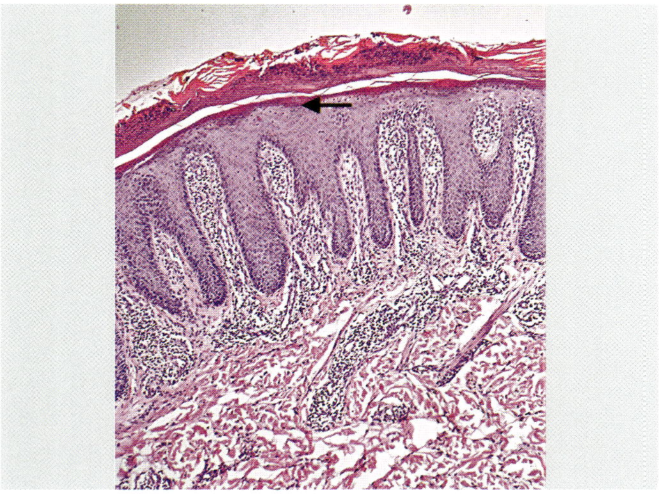

FIGURE 3.1.2

3.1: PSORIASIS VULGARIS

3.1.1: Regular elongation of rete ridges and thinning of suprapapillary plate (*Scanner view*)

3.1.2: Mounds of parakeratosis and hypogranulosis/absent granular layer (*Lower power view*)

3.1.3: Munro microabscess (neutrophilic collection in parakeratotic cornified layer (*High power view*)

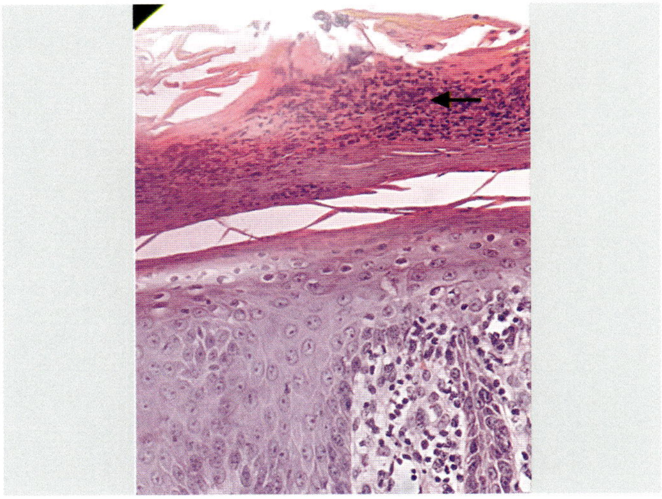

FIGURE 3.1.3

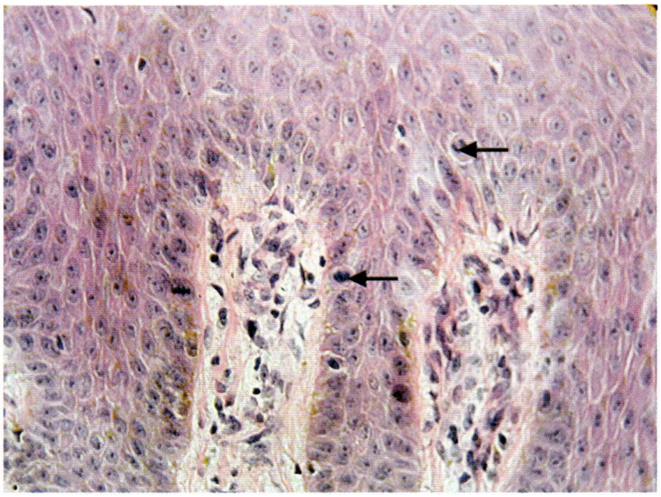

FIGURE 3.1.4

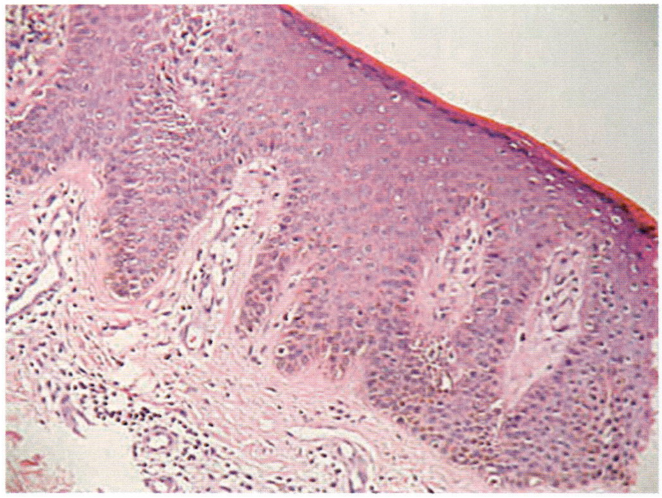

FIGURE 3.1.5

3.1.4: Increased mitotic activity *(High power view)*

3.1.5: Resolving lesion—dilated blood vessels in dermal papillae last to disappear (*Low power view*)

3.1.6: Resolving lesion—granular cell layer restored, parakeratosis disappears (*High power view*)

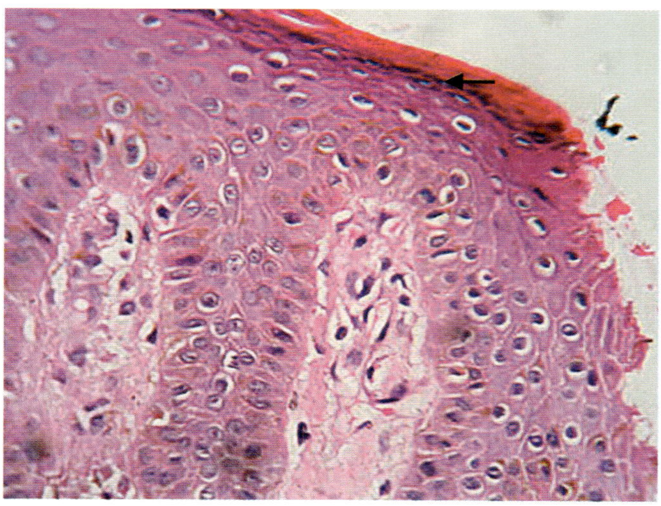

FIGURE 3.1.6

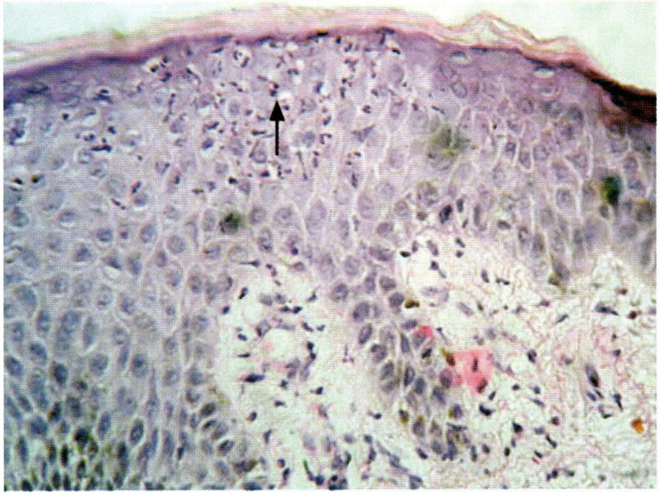

FIGURE 3.2.1

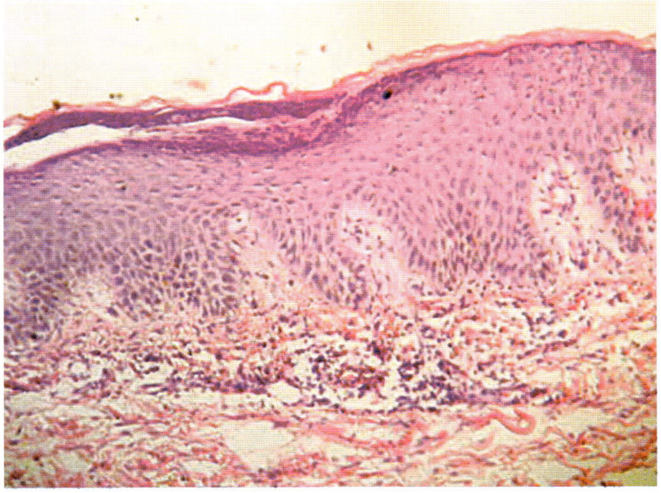

FIGURE 3.2.2

3.2: GUTTATE PSORIASIS

3.2.1: Evolving psoriatic plaque—early change—squirting dermal papilla (neutrophils from the blood vessels in the dermal papillae infiltrating the overlying epidermis) (*High power view*)

3.2.2: Epidermis shows slight acanthosis with foci of parakeratosis (*Low power view*)

3.2.3: Spongiosis is seen in early lesions with a few neutrophils (*High power view*)

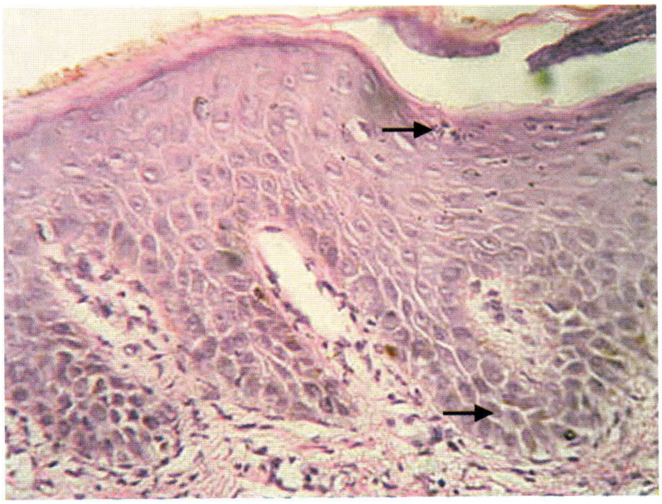

FIGURE 3.2.3

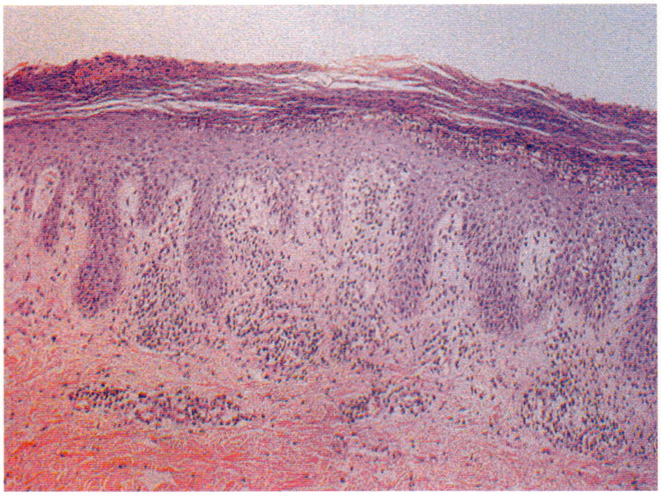

FIGURE 3.3.1

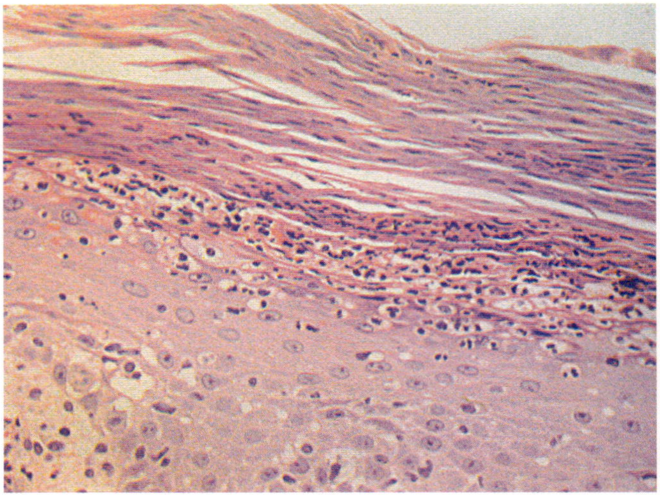

FIGURE 3.3.2

3.3: PUSTULAR PSORIASIS

3.3.1: Perivascular infiltrate of lymphocytes and a few neutrophils, psoriasiform hyperplasia and parakeratosis (*Low power view*)

3.3.2: Neutrophils and spongiosis in the upper epidermal layer (*High power view*)

3.3.3: Spongiform pustule of Kogoj—collection of neutrophils in the upper spinous layer between degenerate keratinocytes (*High power view*)

3.3.4: Munro's microabscess (*High power view*)

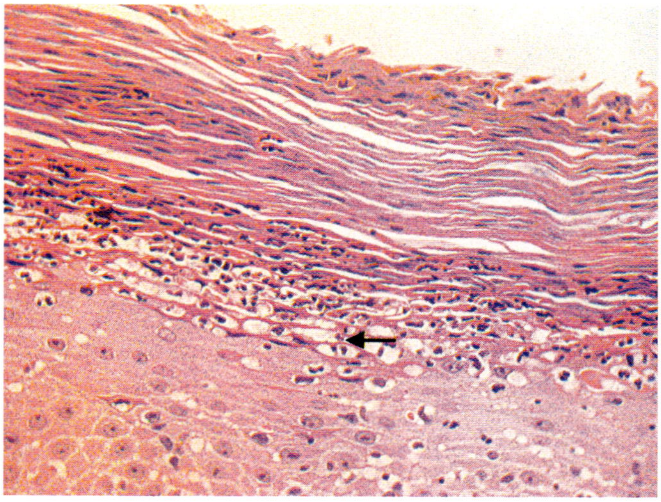

FIGURE 3.3.3

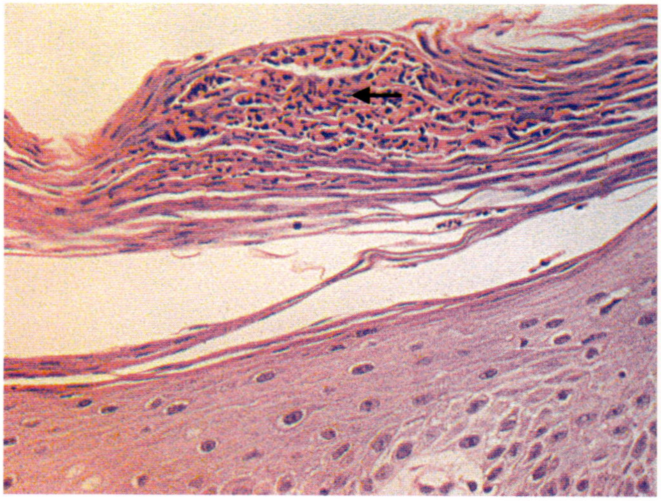

FIGURE 3.3.4

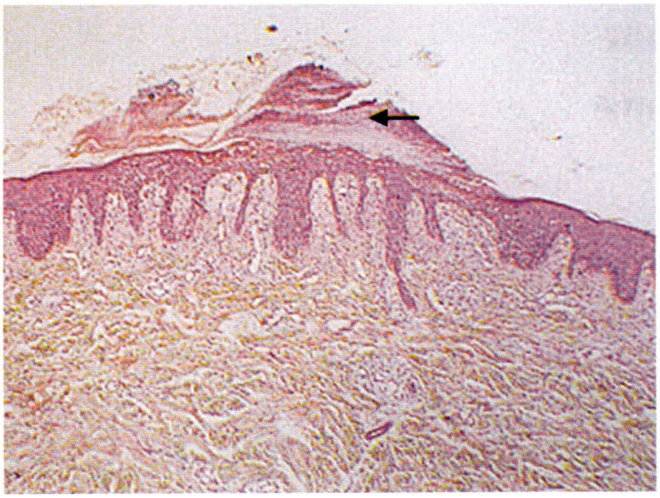

FIGURE 3.4.1

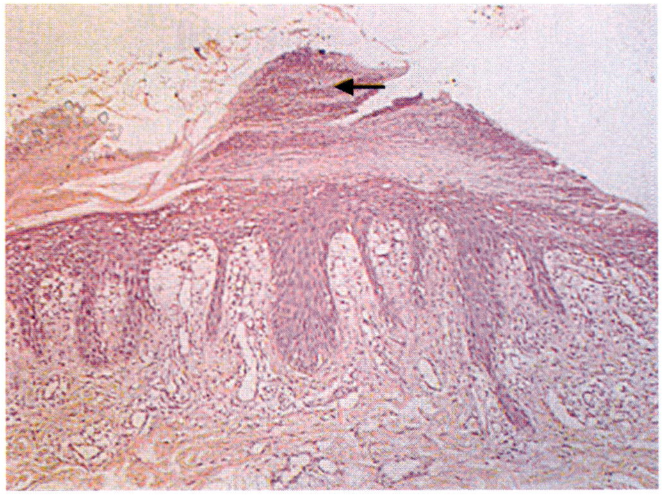

FIGURE 3.4.2

3.4: REITER'S DISEASE

3.4.1: Localized thickening of stratum corneum with psoriasiform hyperplasia (*Scanner view*)

3.4.2: Closer view showing parakeratosis and neutrophils, perivascular infiltrate of lymphocytes and a few neutrophils in the upper dermis (*Low power view*)

3.4.3: Thicker suprapapillary plate and epidermal spongiosis (*Low power view*)

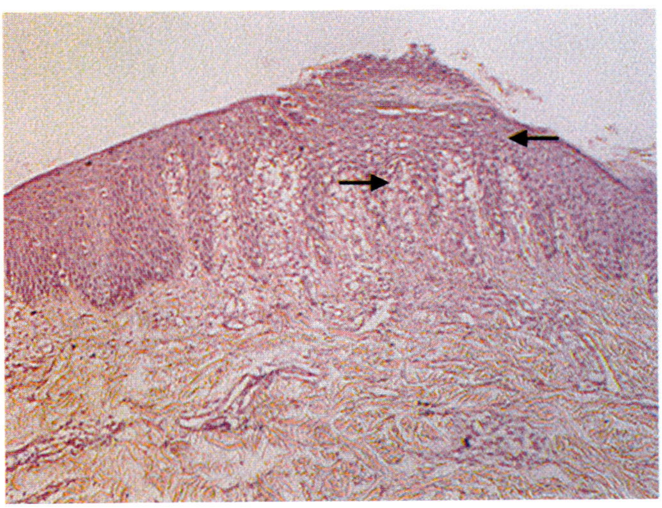

FIGURE 3.4.3

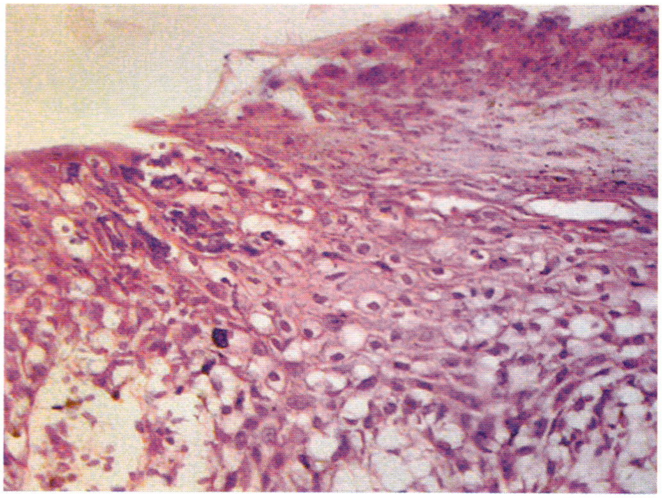

FIGURE 3.4.4

3.4.4: Spongiosis with exocytosis of neutrophils (*High power view*)

3.4.5: Spongiform pustule in upper epidermal layer (v/s pustular psoriasis—thicker horny layer, larger spongiform pustule, eczematous changes, thicker suprapapillary plate, neutrophils in the epidermis, etc.) (*High power view*)

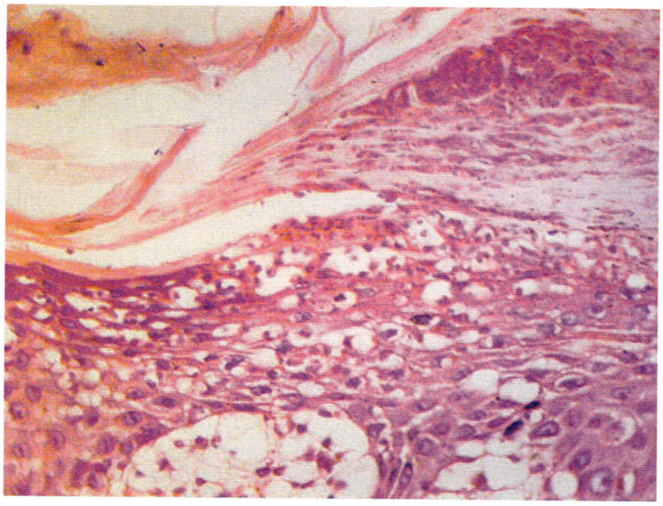

FIGURE 3.4.5

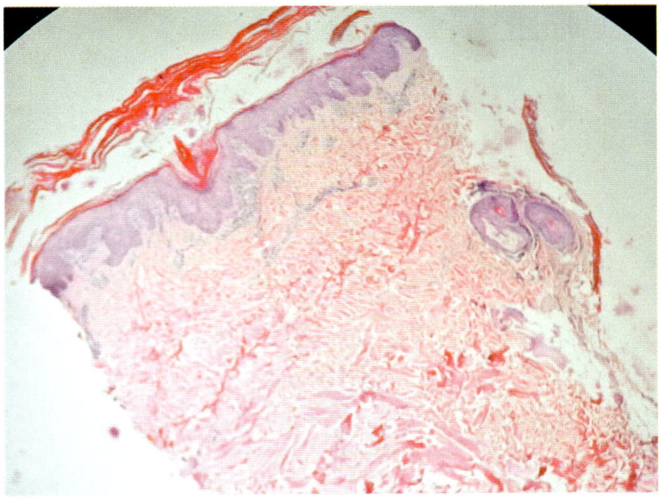

FIGURE 3.5.1

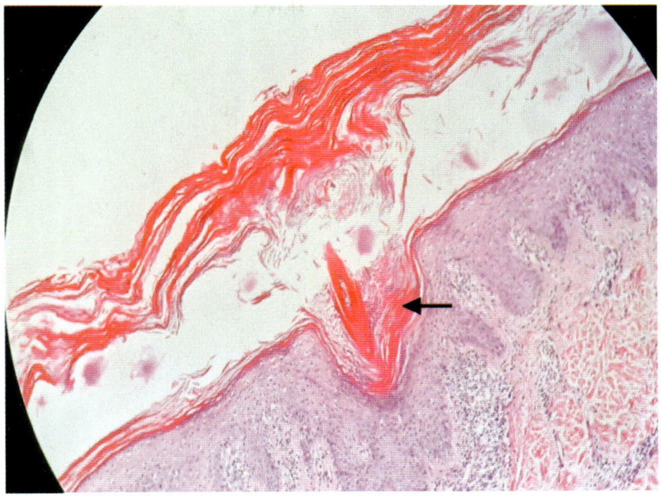

FIGURE 3.5.2

3.5: PITYRIASIS RUBRA PILARIS

3.5.1: Rete ridges broad and elongated, thick suprapapillary plates (*Scanner view*)

3.5.2: Follicular hyperkeratosis (*Low power view*)

3.5.3: Alternate horizontal and vertical bands of parakeratosis "checkerboard pattern" (*High power view*)

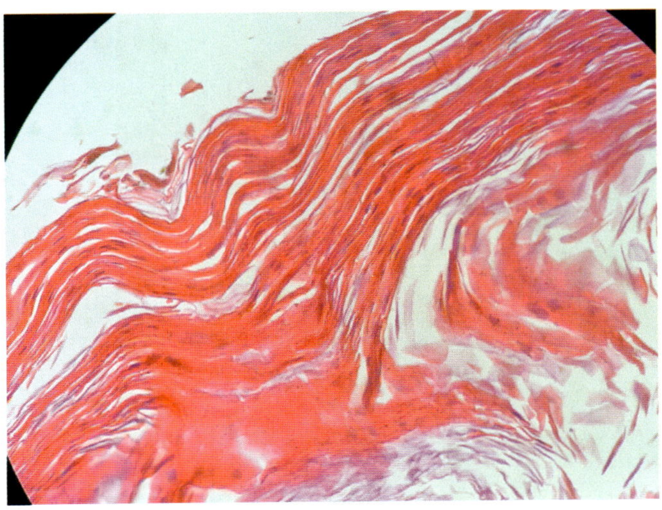

FIGURE 3.5.3

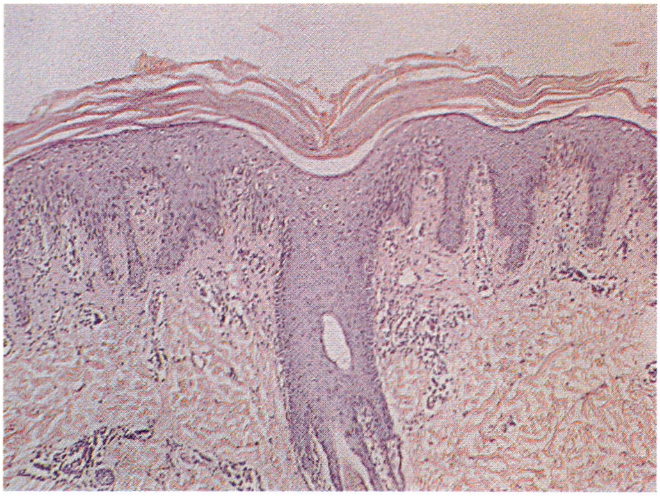

FIGURE 3.5.4

3.5.4: Another case with psoriasiform hyperplasia and follicular hyperkeratosis (*Low power view*)

3.5.5: Alternate horizontal and vertical bands of parakeratotic columns "checkerboard pattern" (*High power view*)

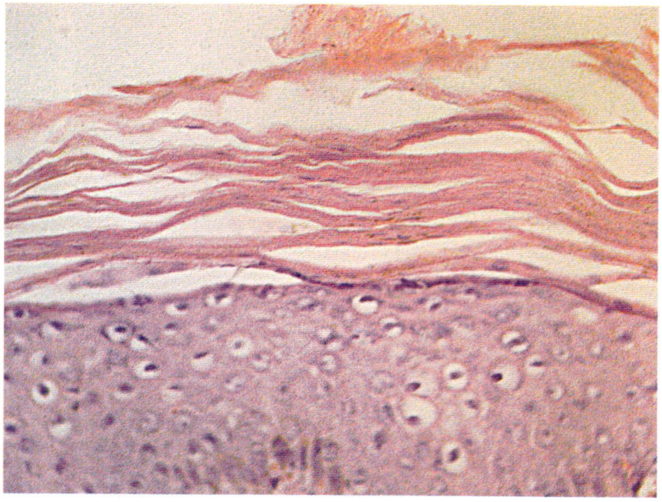

FIGURE 3.5.5

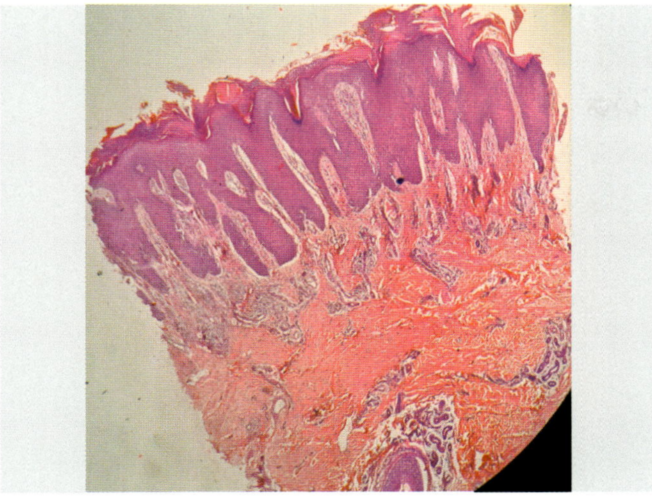

FIGURE 3.6.1

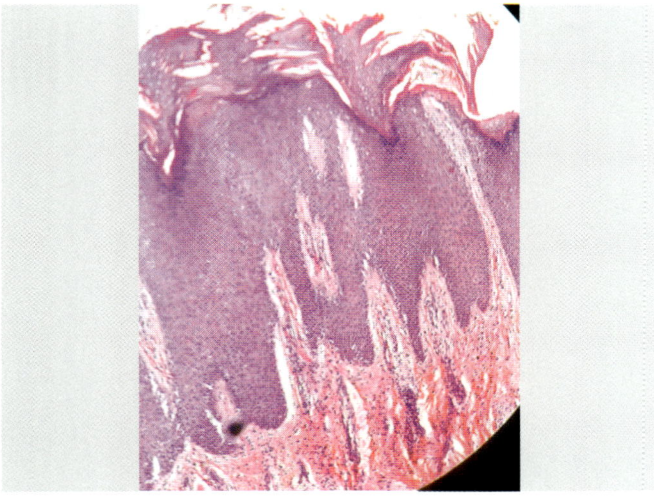

FIGURE 3.6.2

3.6: LICHEN SIMPLEX CHRONICUS/CHRONIC DERMATITIS

3.6.1: Hyperkeratosis, hypergranulosis and hyperplasia (*Scanner view*)

3.6.2: Regular elongation of Rete ridges (*Low power view*)

3.6.3: Vertical streaks of thickened collagen bundles in papillary dermis (*High power view*)

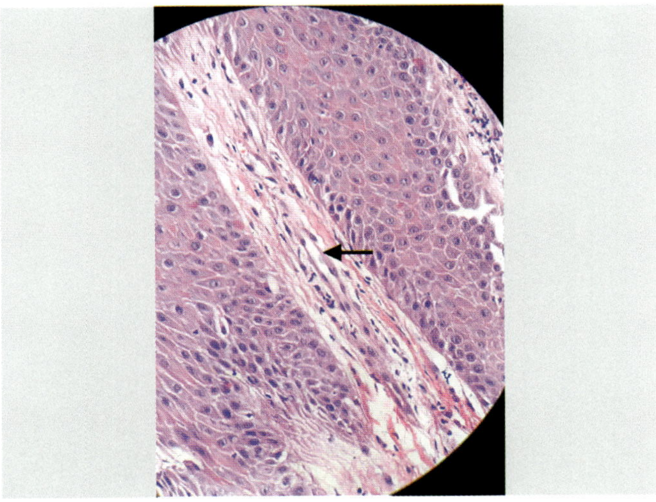

FIGURE 3.6.3

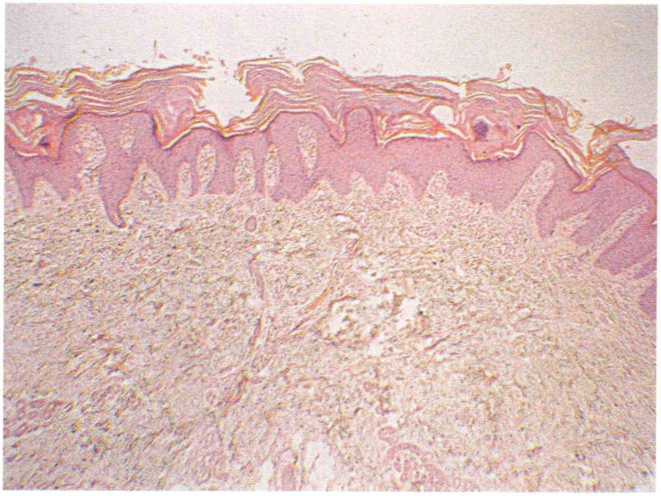

FIGURE 3.7.1

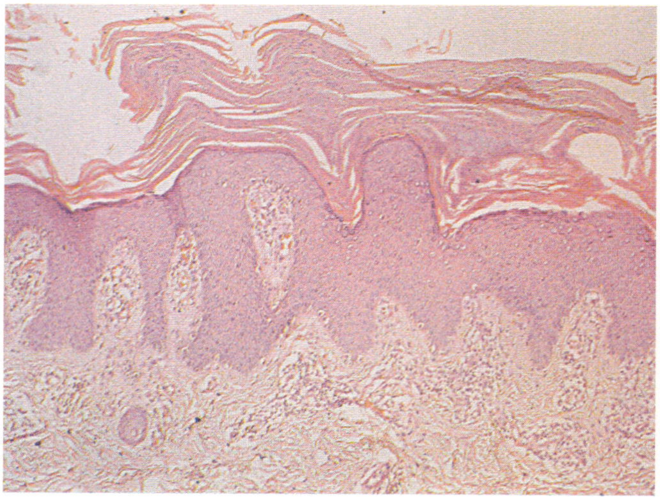

FIGURE 3.7.2

3.7: INFLAMMATORY LINEAR VERRUCOUS EPIDERMAL NEVUS

3.7.1: Epidermis shows psoriasiform hyperplasia with papillomatosis (*Scanner view*)

3.7.2: Mild perivascular lymphocytic infiltrate is seen in upper dermis (*Low power view*)

3.7.3: Alternating and parakeratotic hyperkeratosis and orthokeratotic hyperkeratosis (*High power view*)

3.7.4: Parakeratosis overlying diminished granular cell layer and hyperkeratosis overlying normal stratum granulosum (*High power view*)

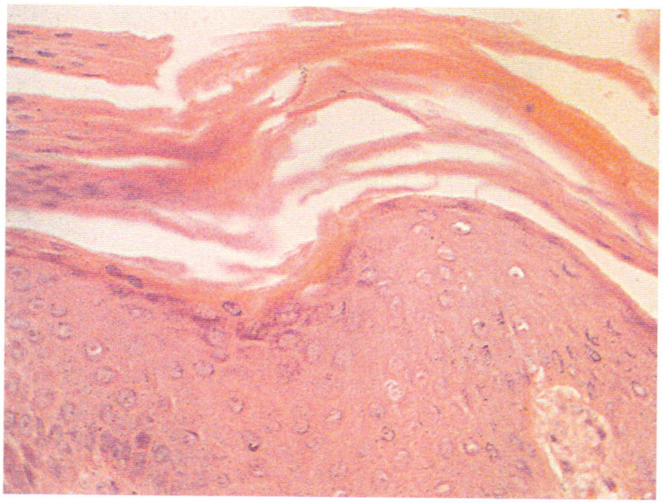

FIGURE 3.7.3

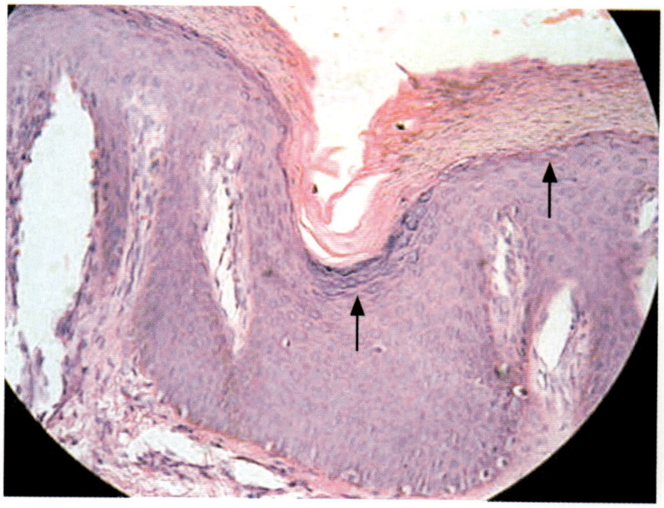

FIGURE 3.7.4

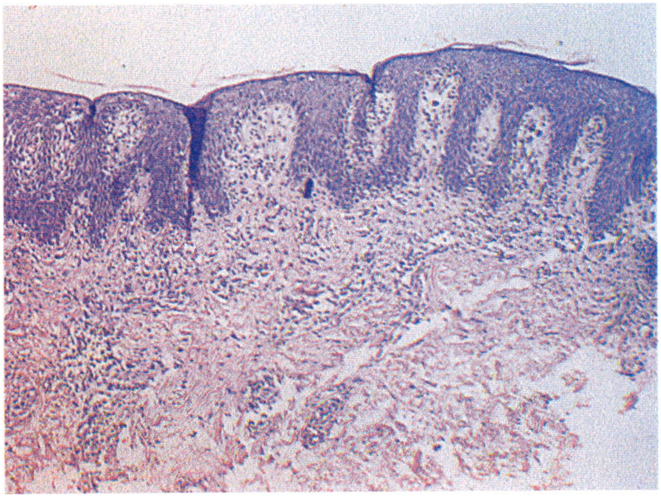

FIGURE 3.8.1

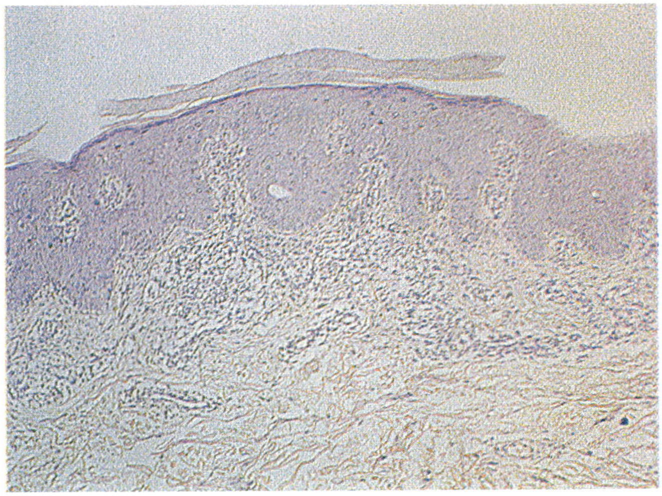

FIGURE 3.8.2

3.8: CHRONIC SUPERFICIAL DERMATITIS (SMALL PLAQUE PARAPSORIASIS)

3.8.1: Epidermal acanthosis like psoriasiform hyperplasia, infiltrate of lymphocytes around blood vessels in the superficial plexus (*Low power view*)

3.8.2: Focal parakeratosis, thick suprapapillary plates, infiltrate (*Low power view*)

3.8.3: Lymphocytes extend high in the papillary dermis, associated with exocytosis (*High power view*)

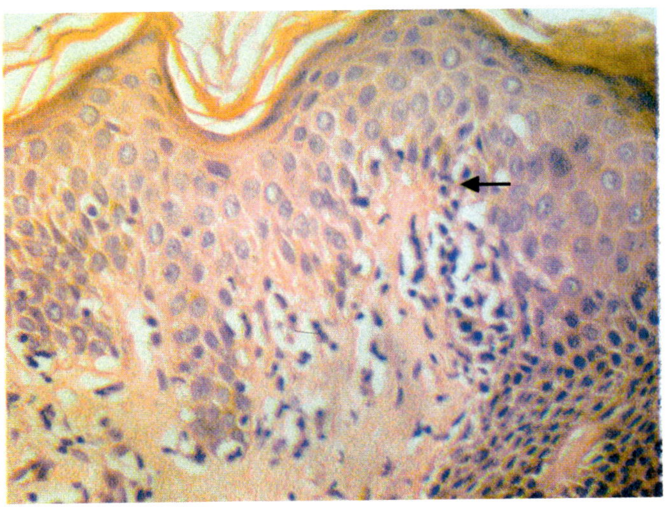

FIGURE 3.8.3

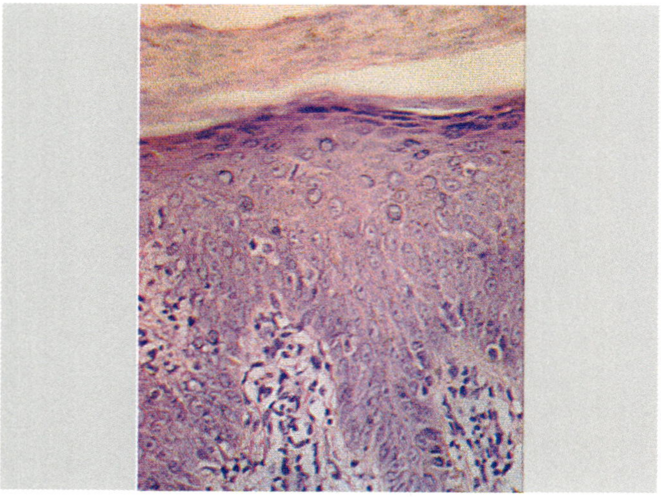

FIGURE 3.8.4

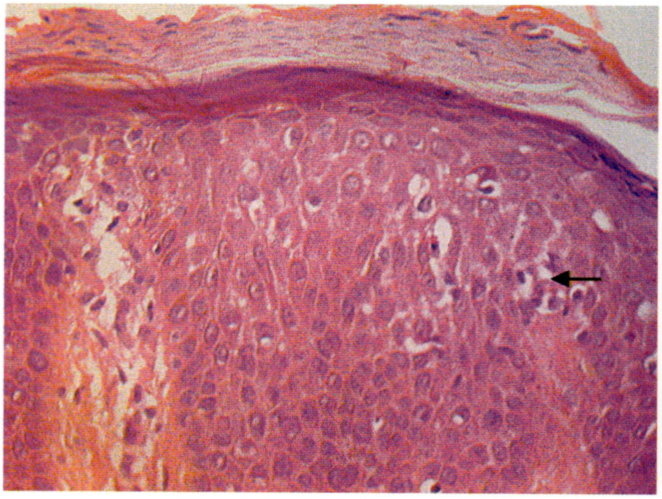

FIGURE 3.8.5

3.8.4: Parakeratosis, infiltrate high in the papillary dermis (v/s psoriasis—absence of dilated vessels in the papillary dermis and neutrophils in the epidermis) (*High power view*)

3.8.5: Exocytosis, parakeratosis and mild spongiosis (*High power view*)

3.8.6: Lymphocytes with a normal mature morphology (*High power view*)

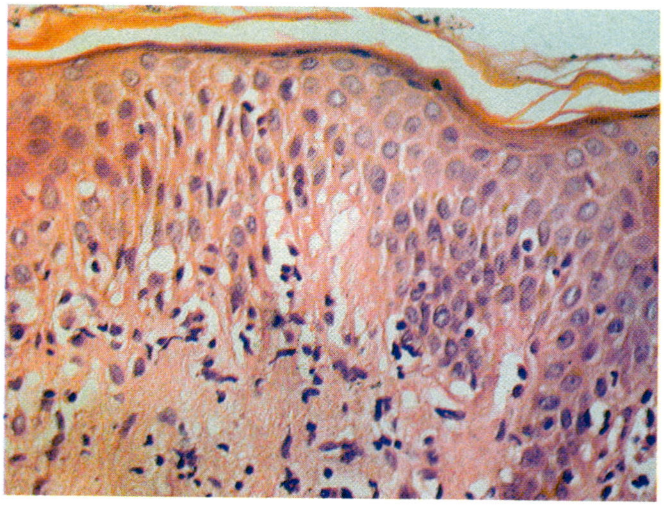

FIGURE 3.8.6

DIFFERENTIAL DIAGNOSIS

1. Bowen's disease
2. Erythroderma
3. Pellagra
4. Acrodermatitis enteropathica
5. Glucagonoma syndrome
6. Secondary syphilis
7. Lamellar ichthyosis and ichthyosis linearis circumflexa
8. Norwegian scabies
9. Clear cell acanthoma

DIAGNOSTIC PEARLS

1. In psoriasis, plasma cells and eosinophils are usually absent, but plasma cells can be present in patients with HIV infection.
2. Spongiosis can be a feature of the early lesions of psoriasis, erythrodermic psoriasis and of psoriasis occurring in regions such as the hands and feet, genital regions, nail psoriasis. But, the presence of prominent spongiosis involving the rete ridges usually rules out psoriasis.
3. In pustular psoriasis, the main diagnostic feature is the presence of intraepidermal pustules at various stages of development and a few eosinophils may be present in the infiltrate (in contrast to psoriasis vulgaris).
4. Biopsies of Reiter's syndrome are indistinguishable from pustular psoriasis but various histological features that are more suggestive of Reiter's syndrome are thicker horny layer, larger spongiform pustules, eczematous changes, thicker suprapapillary plate of epidermis, absence of clubbing of the rete ridges, presence of neutrophils in the dermis.
5. In pityriasis rubra pilaris, the changes are most marked when erythema is more, and least in biopsies of follicular papules.
6. Pellagra, acrodermatitis enteropathica and glucagonoma syndrome have characteristic upper epidermal pallor.
7. Biopsies of the ichthyosis linearis circumflexa may be misdiagnosed as congenital psoriasis.
8. In parapsoriasis, there are no interface changes as in pityriasis lichenoides chronica and no atypical lymphoid cells as in mycosis fungoides.

4

Lichenoid and Interface Dermatitis

Chapter Outline

4.1: Lichenoid Tissue Reaction
4.2: Interface Dermatitis

Mithilesh Chandra, Achyut Pokharel, Pradeep Mahajan, Uday Khopkar, Chirag Desai, Atul Dongre, Venkataram Mysore

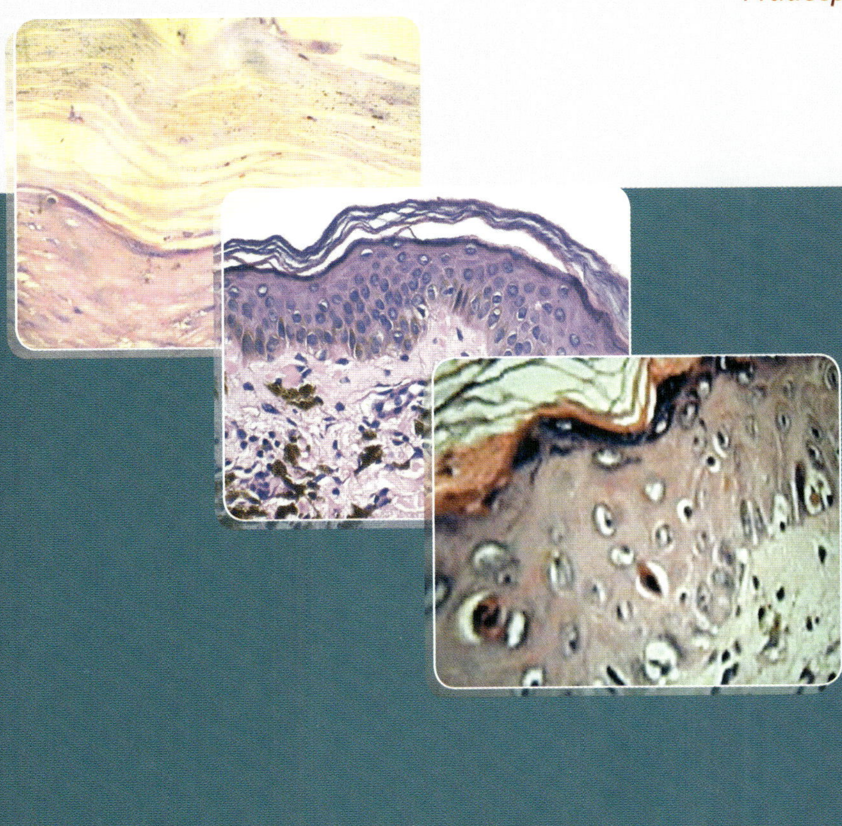

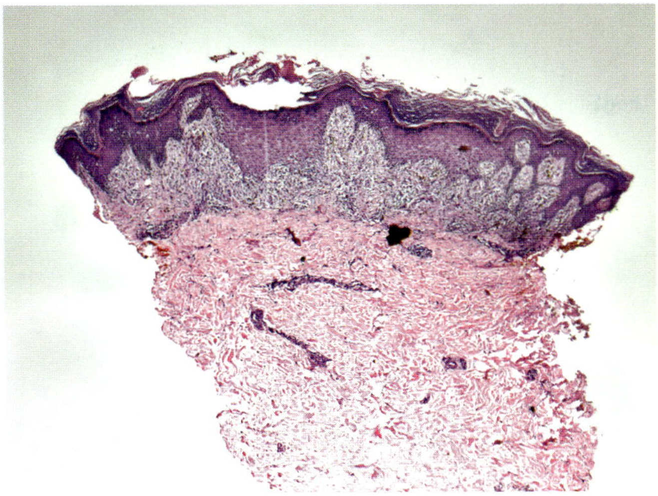

FIGURE 4.1.1.1

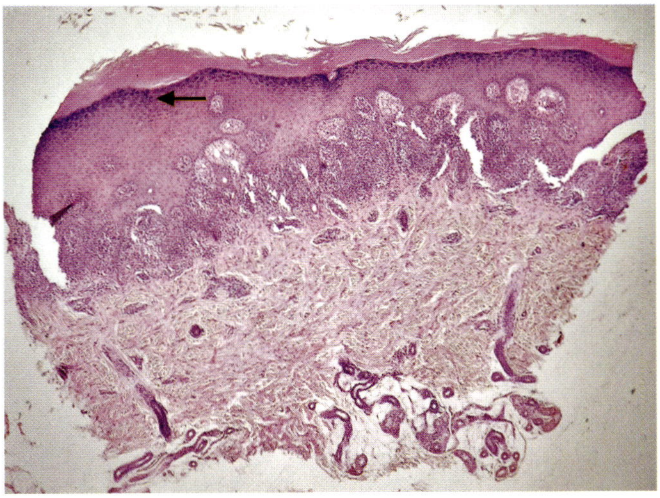

FIGURE 4.1.1.2

4.1: LICHENOID TISSUE REACTION

4.1.1: Lichen Planus and Variants

4.1.1.1: Lichen planus (LP) shows band-like infiltrate of lymphocytes in the papillary dermis that hugs the epidermis (*Scanner view*)

4.1.1.2: Another case with compact orthokeratosis and wedge-shaped hypergranulosis (*Scanner view*)

4.1.1.3: Basal cell damage, saw toothing of rete ridges, squamatization of basal cells (basal cells look like squamous cells) (*Low power view*)

4.1.1.4: Different case showing colloid or civatte bodies (oval or round homogenous eosinophilic bodies) in the epidermis as well as the dermis and pigment incontinence in the dermis (*Low power view*)

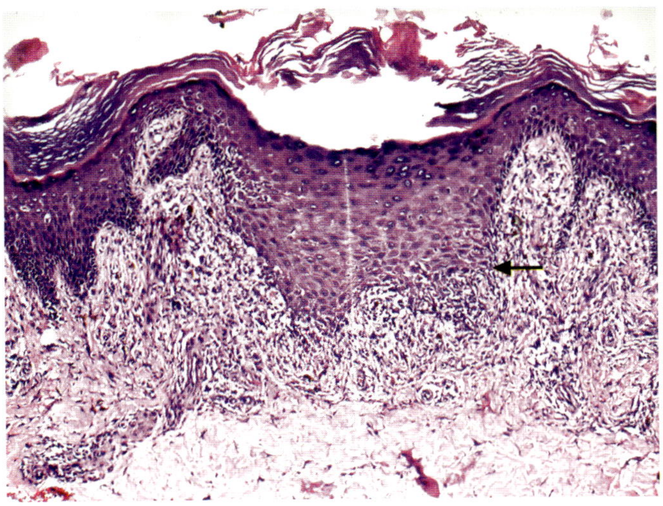

FIGURE 4.1.1.3

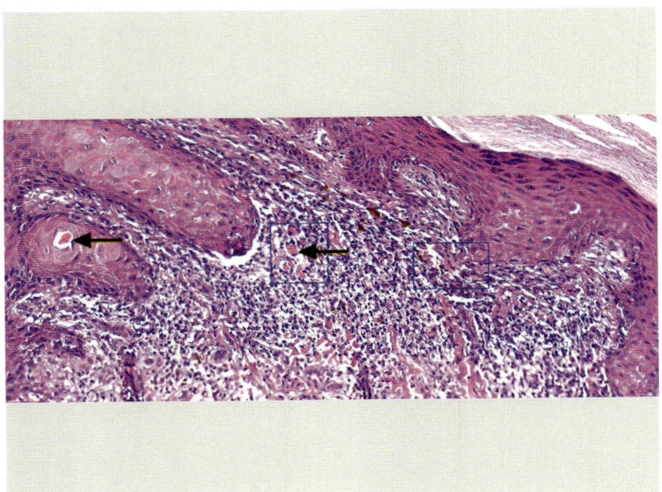

FIGURE 4.1.1.4

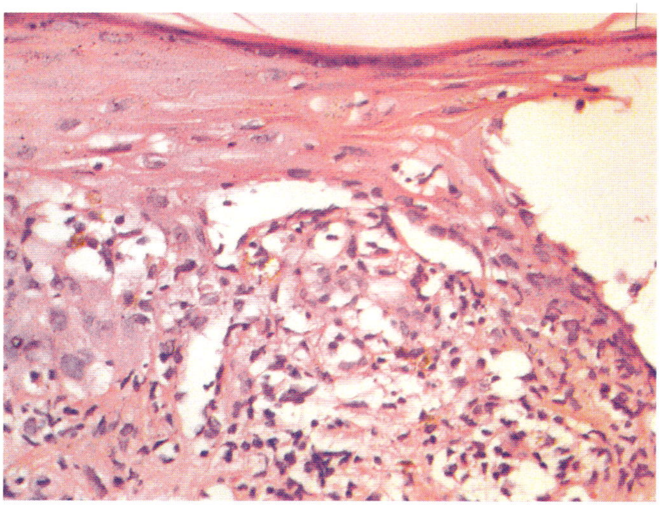

FIGURE 4.1.1.5

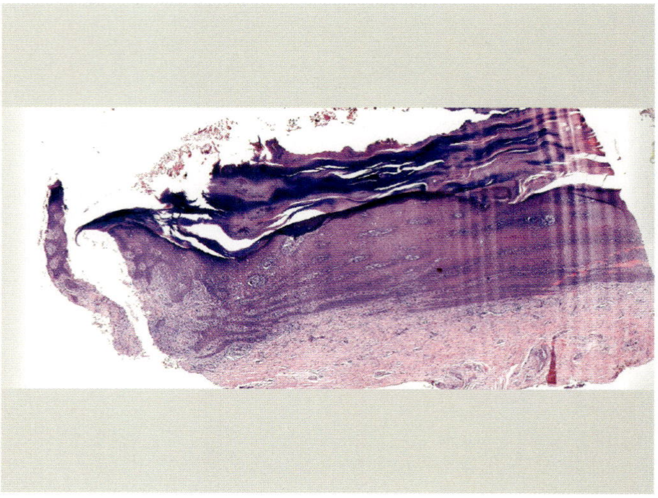

FIGURE 4.1.1.6

4.1.1.5: Max Joseph's spaces (subepidermal cleft) (*High power view*)

4.1.1.6: Nail bed lichen planus showing infiltrate at dermoepidermal junction (*Scanner view*)

4.1.1.7: Wedge-shaped hypergranulosis seen (*Low power view*)

4.1.1.8: Nail LP showing lymphocytic infiltrate and basal cell damage on the left side of the section (*High power view*)

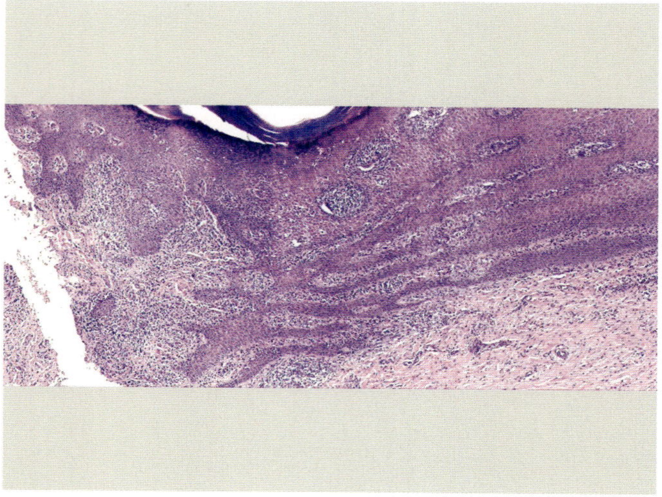

FIGURE 4.1.1.7

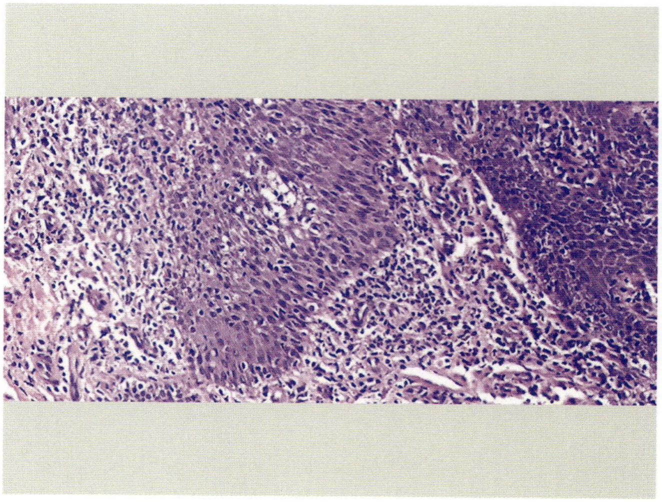

FIGURE 4.1.1.8

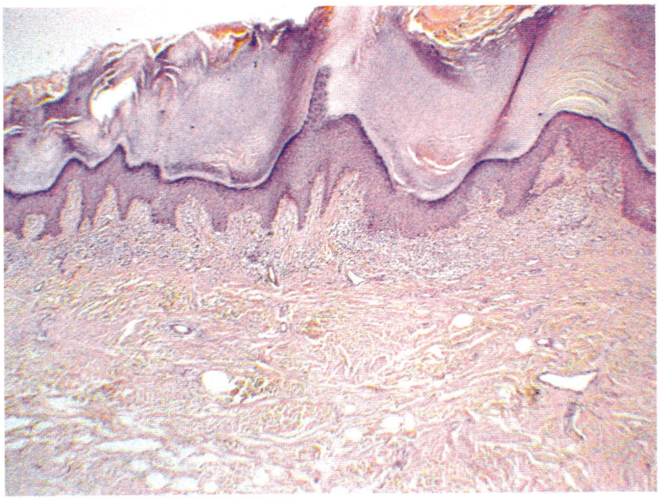

FIGURE 4.1.1.9

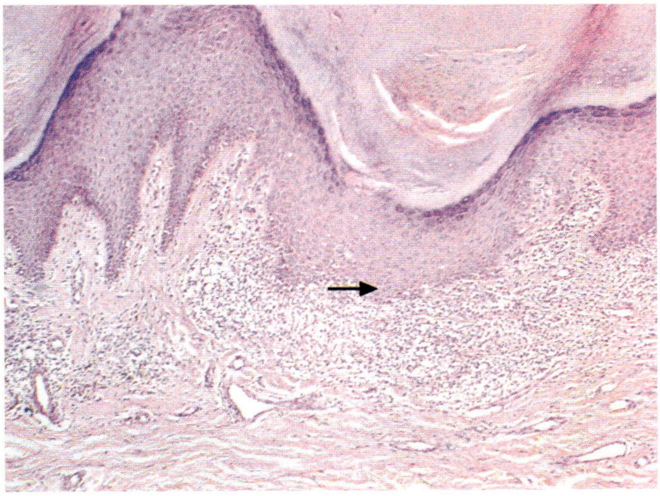

FIGURE 4.1.1.10

4.1.1.9: Lichen planus hypertrophicus—marked irregular hyperplasia and compact orthokeratosis (*Scanner view*)

4.1.1.10: Hypergranulosis and lymphocytic inflammatory infiltrate predominantly at the base (tips) of rete ridges (*Low power view*)

4.1.1.11: Epidermis above the dermal papilla pretty normal without lichenoid tissue reaction (*High power view*)

4.1.1.12: Closer view of basal cell vacuolation, lymphocytic infiltrate with pigment incontinence (*High power view*)

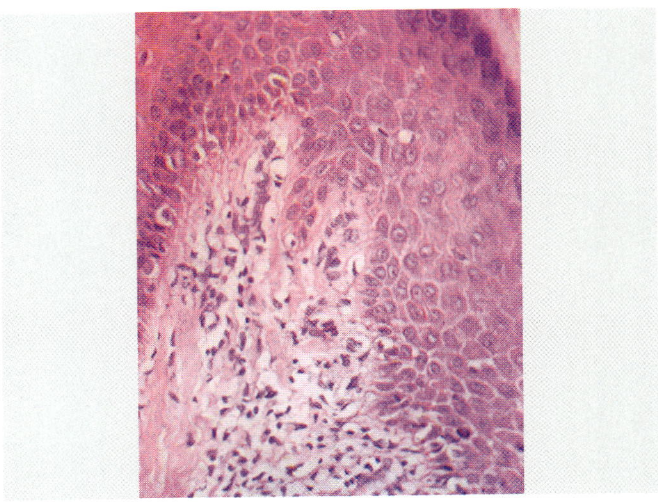

FIGURE 4.1.1.11

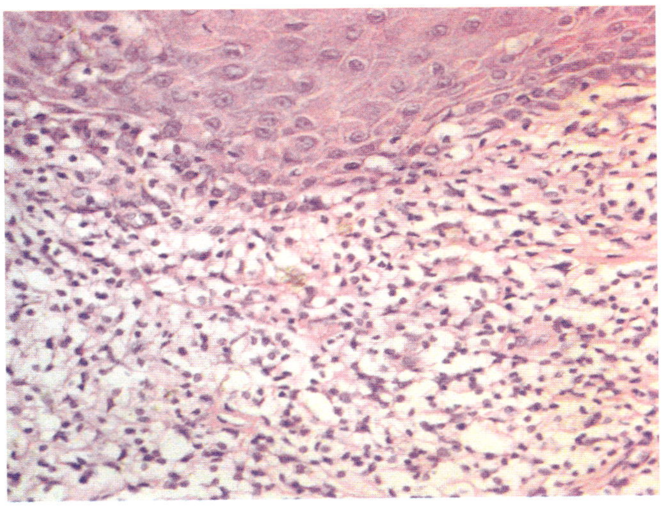

FIGURE 4.1.1.12

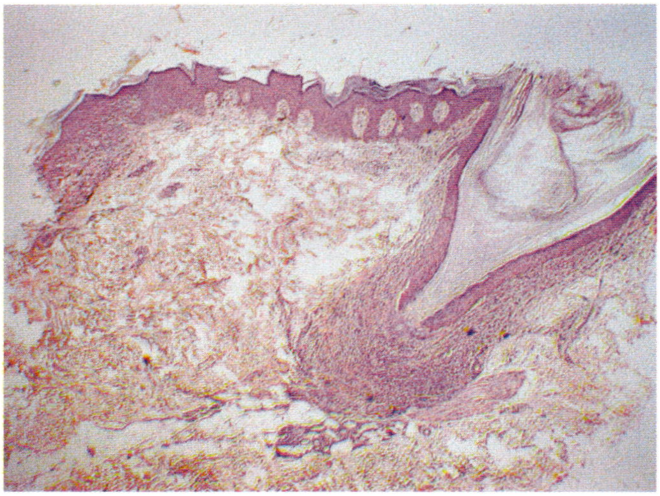

FIGURE 4.1.1.13

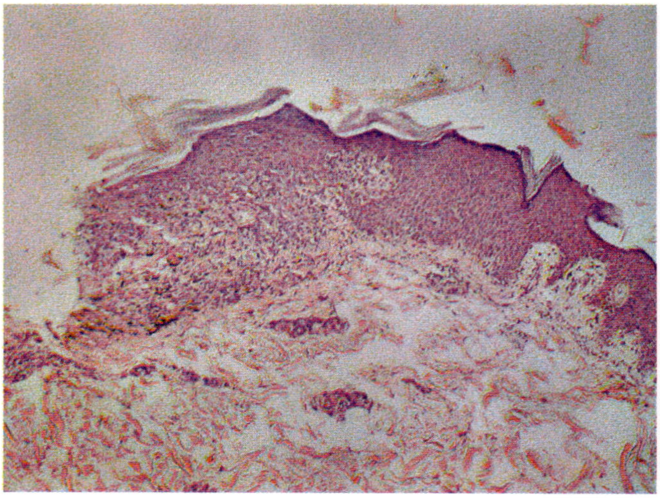

FIGURE 4.1.1.14

4.1.1.13: Follicular lichen planus—lichenoid reaction pattern involving the basal cell layer of the follicular epithelium and the adjacent epidermis (*Scanner view*)

4.1.1.14: Epidermis—lichenoid change (*Low power view*)

4.1.1.15: Band-like infiltrate at the follicular epithelium (*Low power view*)

4.1.1.16: Basal cell damage, lymphocytic infiltrate and pigment incontinence at the follicular epithelium (*High power view*)

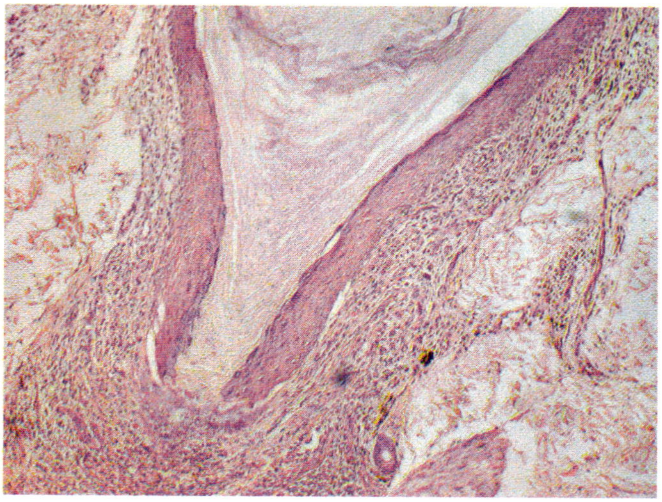

FIGURE 4.1.1.15

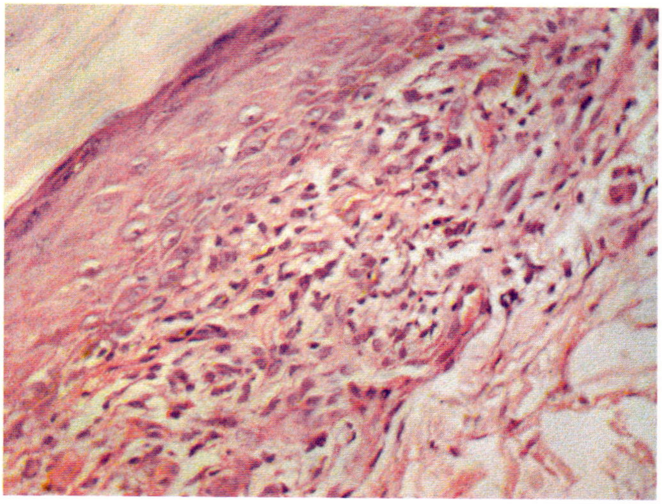

FIGURE 4.1.1.16

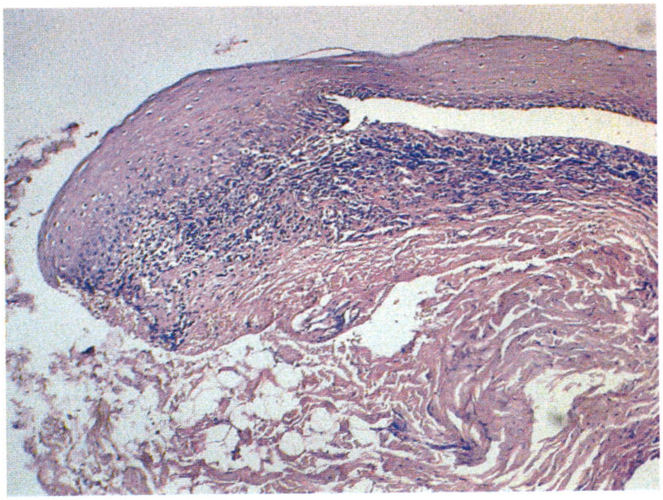

FIGURE 4.1.1.17

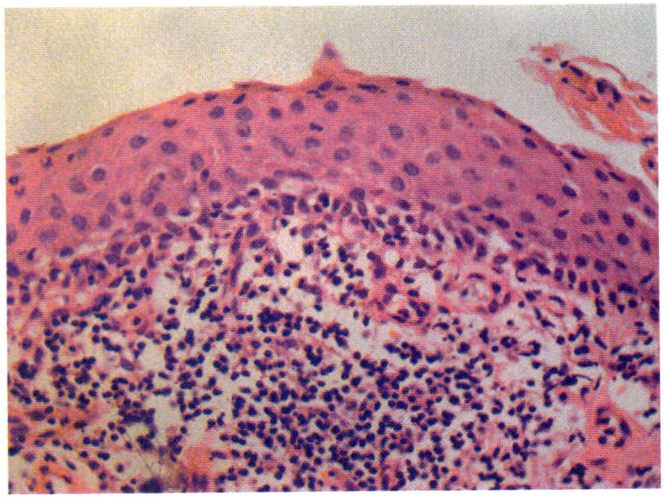

FIGURE 4.1.1.18

4.1.1.17: Oral lichen planus—band-like infiltrate with subepidermal separation (extensive in this case, usally like Max-Joseph spaces) (*Low power view*)

4.1.1.18: Closer view of mucosal epithelium, infiltrate and basal cell damage (*High power view*)

4.1.1.19: Infiltrate also contains plasma cells (*High power view*)

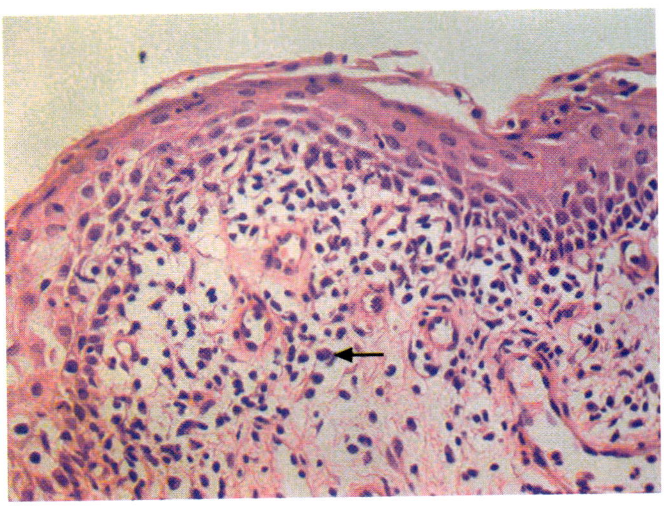

FIGURE 4.1.1.19

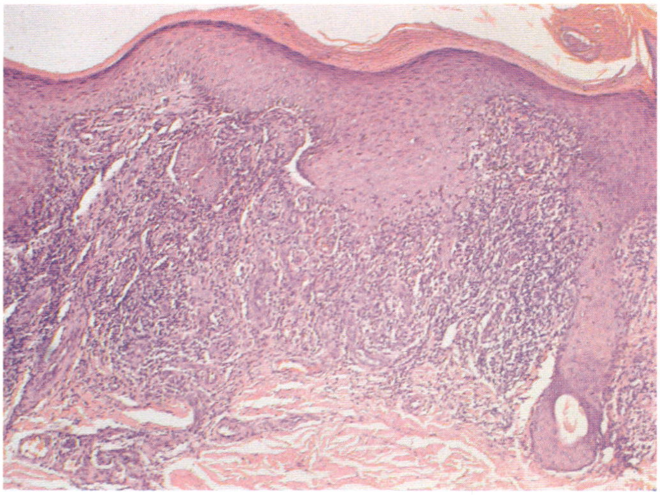

FIGURE 4.1.2.1

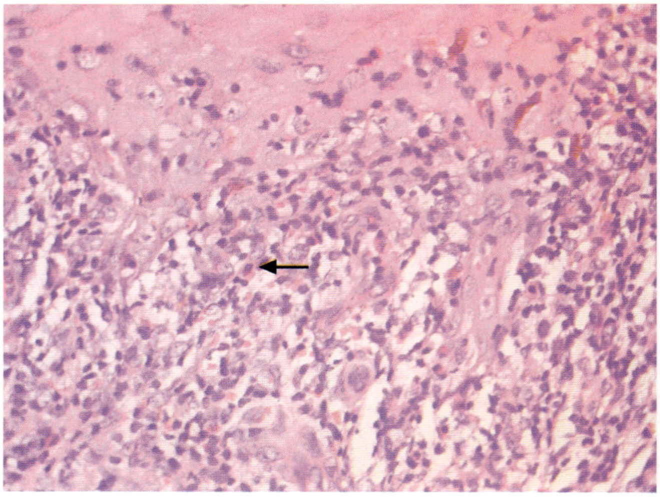

FIGURE 4.1.2.2

4.1.2: Lichenoid Drug Reaction

4.1.2.1: Lichenoid tissue reaction with basal cell damage, band-like infiltrate and overlying parakeratosis (*Low power view*)

4.1.2.2: Vacuolar change of basal cells, pigment incontinence and infiltrate composed of lymphocytes and many eosinophils (*High power view*)

4.1.2.3: Another case with parakeratosis, focal basal cell damage and variable infiltrate (*Low power view*)

4.1.2.4: Infiltrate composed of lymphocytes and many eosinophils, perivascular extension of infiltrate also (*High power view*)

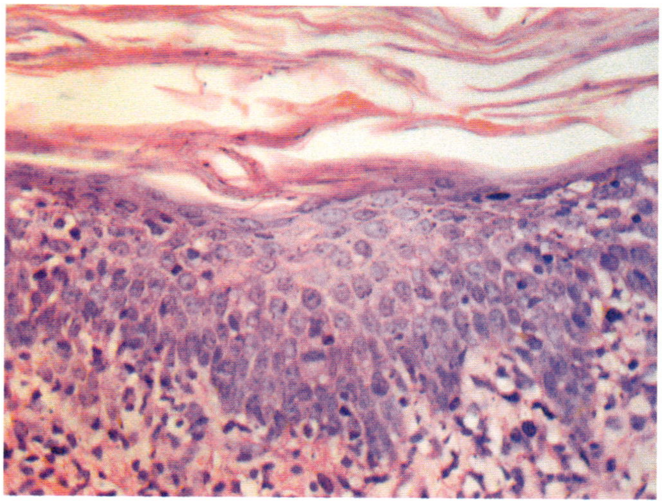

FIGURE 4.1.2.3

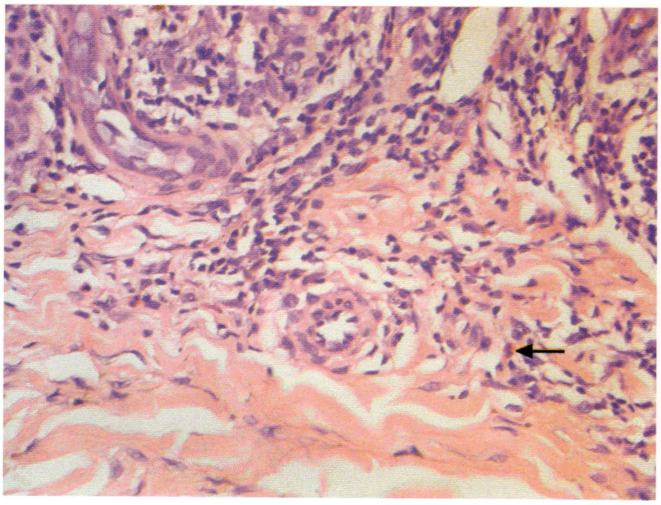

FIGURE 4.1.2.4

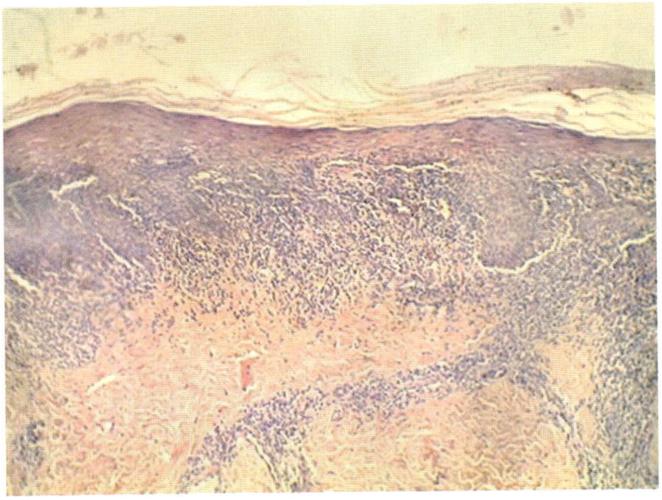

FIGURE 4.1.3.1

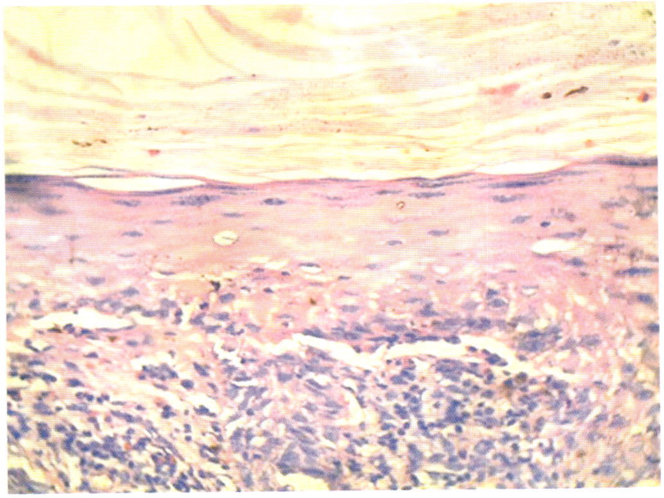

FIGURE 4.1.3.2

4.1.3: Lichen Striatus

4.1.3.1: Lichenoid tissue reaction with band-like infiltrate in upper dermis (*Scanner view*)

4.1.3.2: Closer view of basal cell damage and lymphocytic infiltrate at the dermo-epidermal junction (*High power view*)

4.1.3.3: Parakeratosis and necrotic keratinocytes (*High power view*)

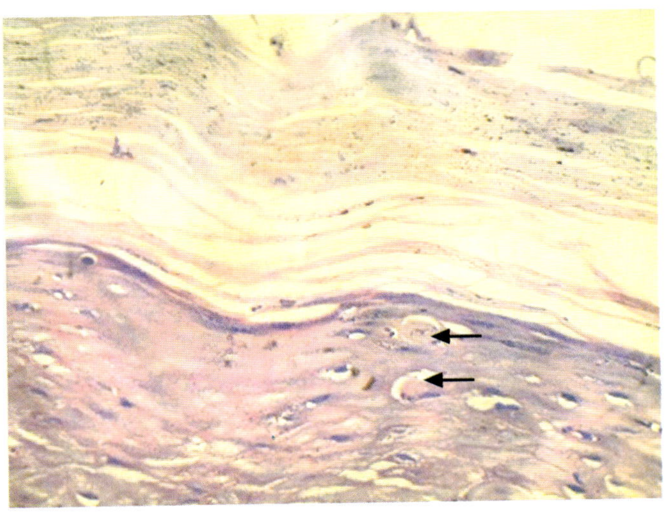

FIGURE 4.1.3.3

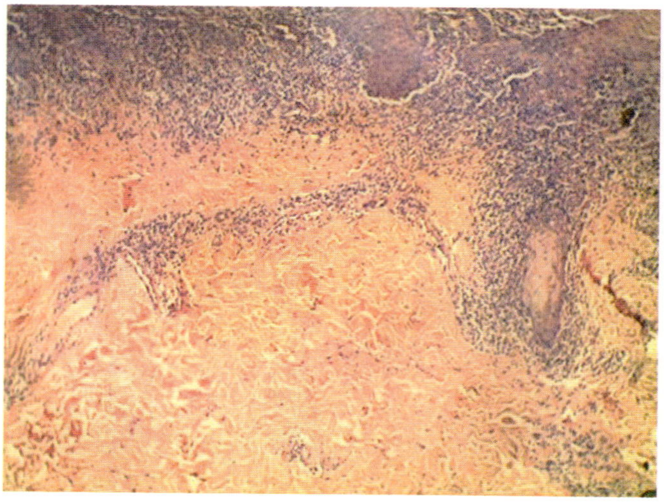

FIGURE 4.1.3.4

4.1.3.4: Extension of the infiltrate down in the dermis, shows superficial and deep perivascular and perifollicular infiltrate of lymphocytes *(Low power view)*

4.1.3.5: Closer view of infiltrate, extending around the blood vessels *(High power view)*

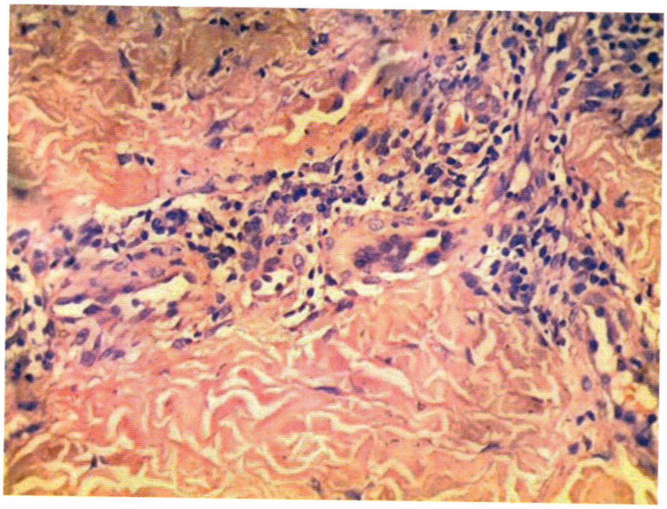

FIGURE 4.1.3.5

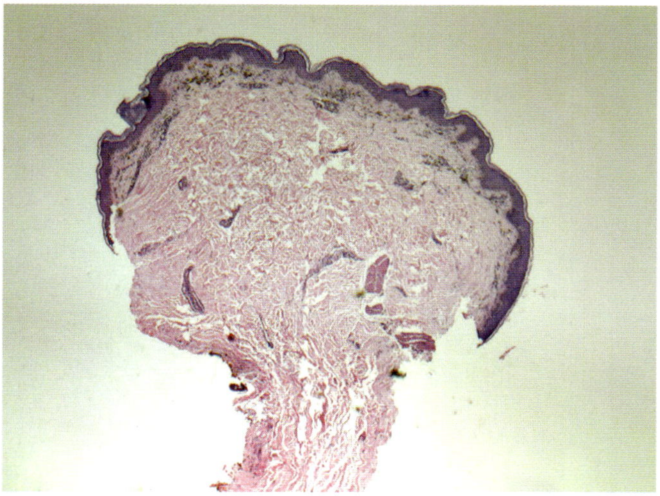

FIGURE 4.1.4.1

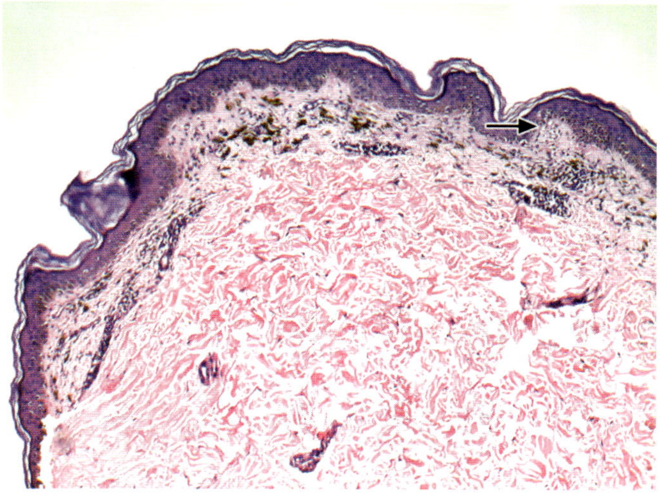

FIGURE 4.1.4.2

4.1.4: Lichen Planus Pigmentosus

4.1.4.1: Marked melanin incontinence (*Scanner view*)

4.1.4.2: Focal basal cell vacuolation (*Low power view*)

4.1.4.3: Prominent melanin incontinence, colloid bodies and perivascular lymphocytic infiltrate (*High power view*)

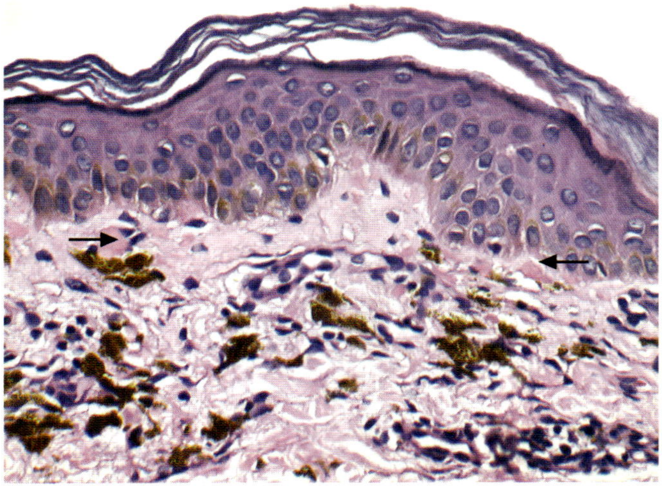

FIGURE 4.1.4.3

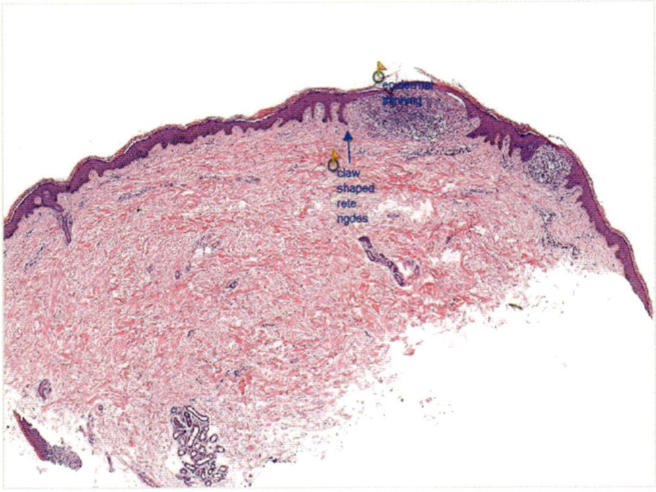

FIGURE 4.1.5.1

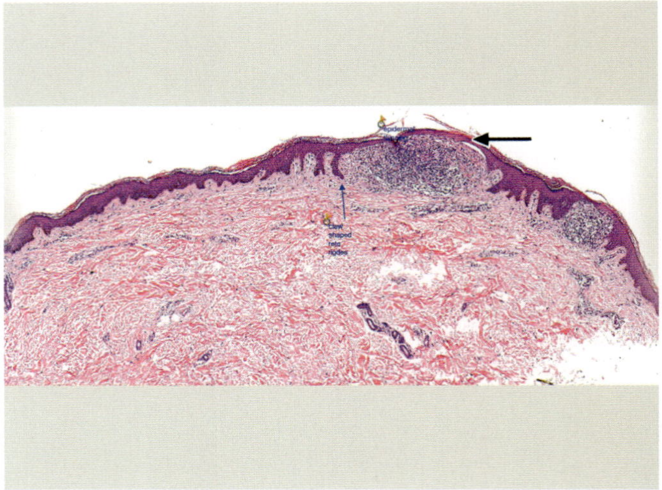

FIGURE 4.1.5.2

4.1.5: Lichen Nitidus

4.1.5.1: Circumscribed inflammatory infiltrate in the dermal papilla surrounded by claw-shaped rete ridges (*Scanner view*)

4.1.5.2: Thinning of overlying epidermis (*Low power view*)

4.1.5.3: Lichenoid tissue reaction, inflammatory infiltrate composed of lymphocytes and histiocytes, multinucleated giant cells may be seen (*High power view*)

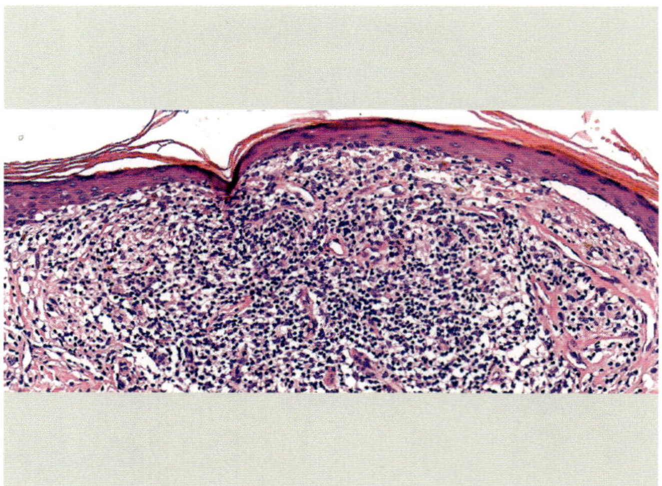

FIGURE 4.1.5.3

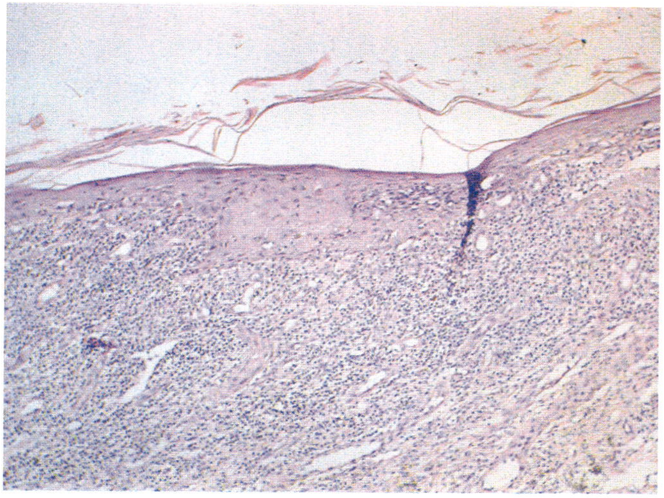

FIGURE 4.1.6.1

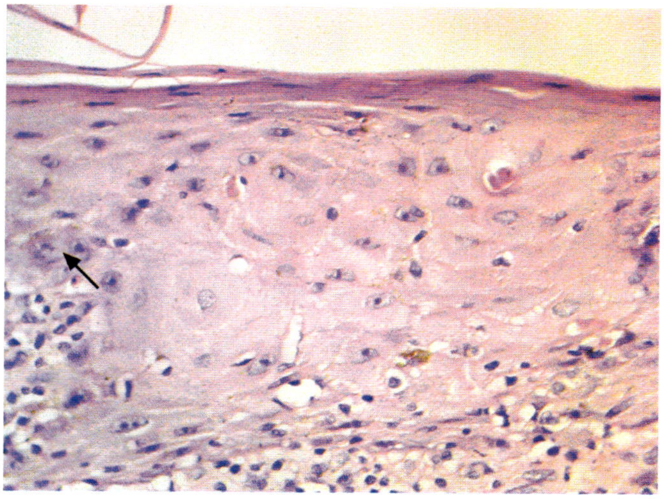

FIGURE 4.1.6.2

4.1.6: Lichen Planus-like Keratosis

4.1.6.1: Lichenoid tissue reaction with parakeratosis and diminished granular cell layer (*Low power view*)

4.1.6.2: Parakeratosis, necrotic keratinocytes with a few atypical keratinocytes (*High power view*)

4.1.6.3: Another view of lichenoid tissue reaction pattern (*Low power view*)

4.1.6.4: Parakeratosis, atrophic epidermis and apoptotic keratinocytes (*High power view*)

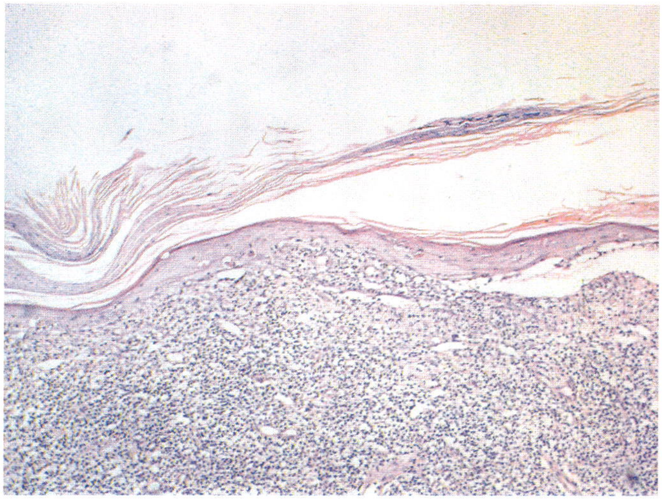

FIGURE 4.1.6.3

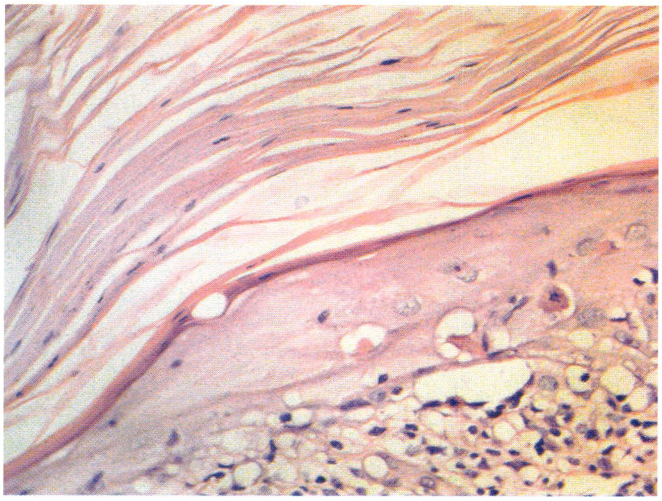

FIGURE 4.1.6.4

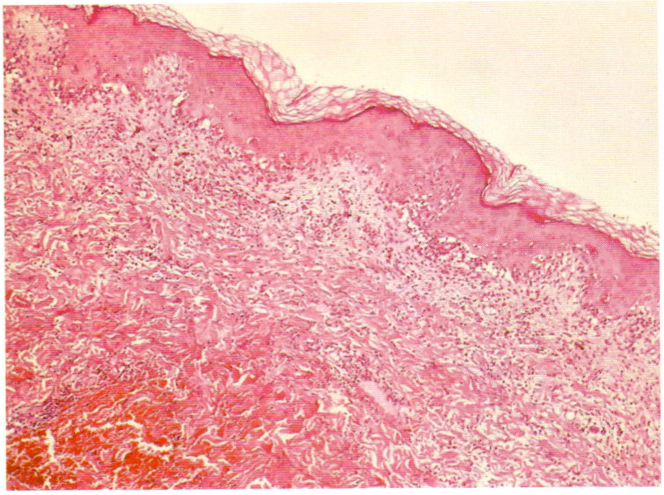

FIGURE 4.2.1.1

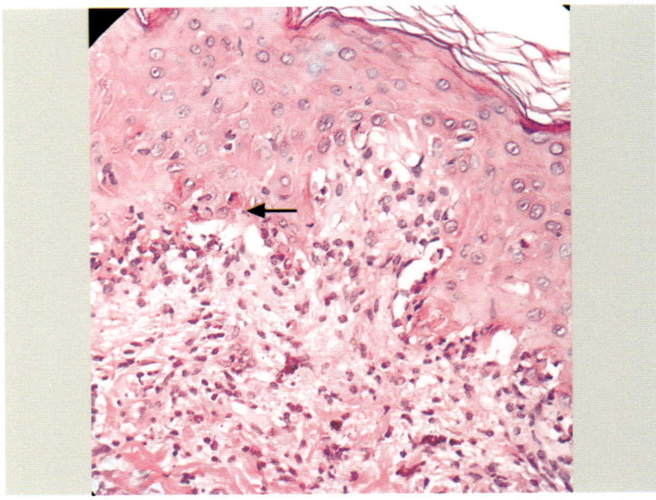

FIGURE 4.2.1.2

4.2: INTERFACE DERMATITIS

4.2.1: Erythema Multiforme

4.2.1.1: Basket weave hyperkeratosis, focal vacuolation of basal cell layer, a few lymphocytes at the dermoepidermal junction (*Low power view*)

4.2.1.2: Closer view of the same with a few necrotic keratinocytes (*High power view*)

4.2.1.3: Epidermis has necrotic keratinocytes at all levels of the epidermis (*High power view*)

4.2.1.4: Confluent necrosis of the epidermis with subepidermal separation (*Low power view*)

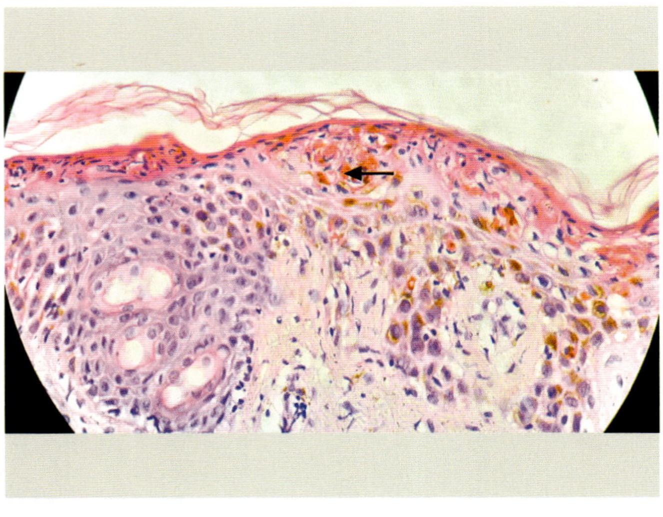

FIGURE 4.2.1.3

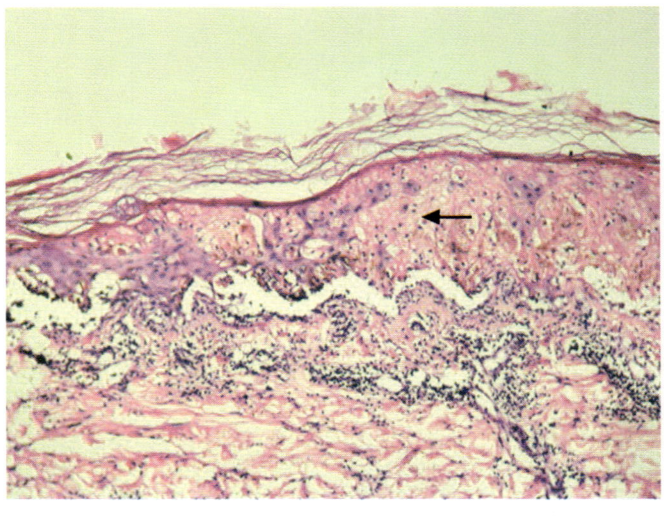

FIGURE 4.2.1.4

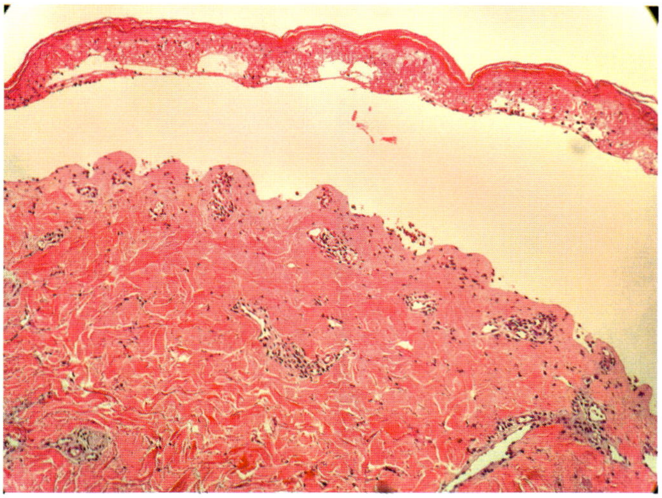

FIGURE 4.2.2.1

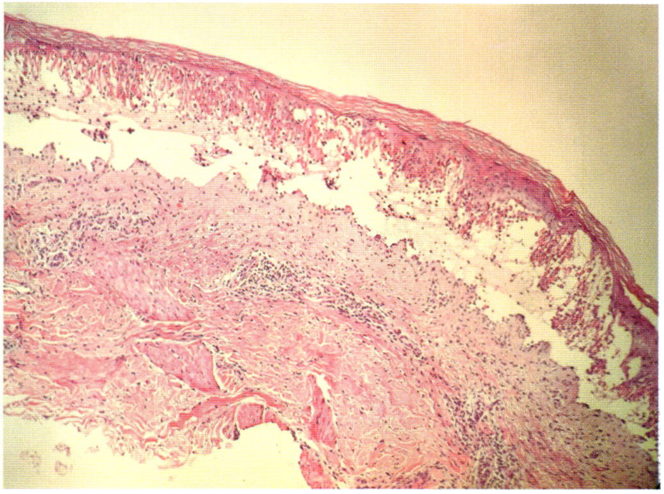

FIGURE 4.2.2.2

4.2.2: Toxic Epidermal Necrolysis and Fixed Drug Eruption

4.2.2.1: Subepidermal cell—poor blister in toxic epidermal necrolysis (*Scanner view*)

4.2.2.2: Interface dermatitis with mild perivascular lymphocytic infiltrate in superficial dermis (*Low power view*)

4.2.2.3: Individual necrotic keratinocytes (*High power view*)

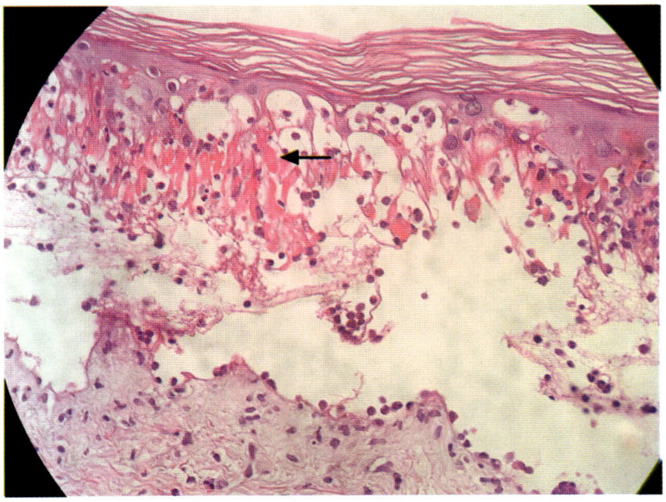

FIGURE 4.2.2.3

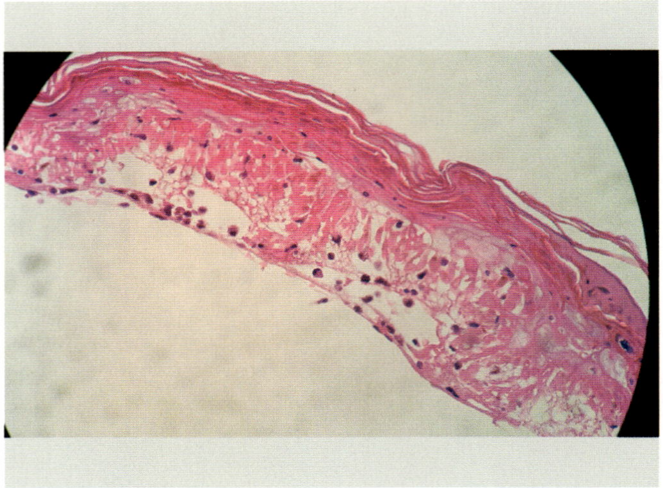

FIGURE 4.2.2.4

4.2.2.4: Confluent necrosis of epidermis (*High power view*)

4.2.2.5: Fixed drug eruption—lichenoid reaction pattern with inflammatory infiltrate, necrotic keratinocytes, pigment incontinence (*High power view*)

4.2.2.6: Another case with individual necrotic keratinocytes to confluent necrosis, subepidermal cleft, pigment, mild inflammation (*Low power view*)

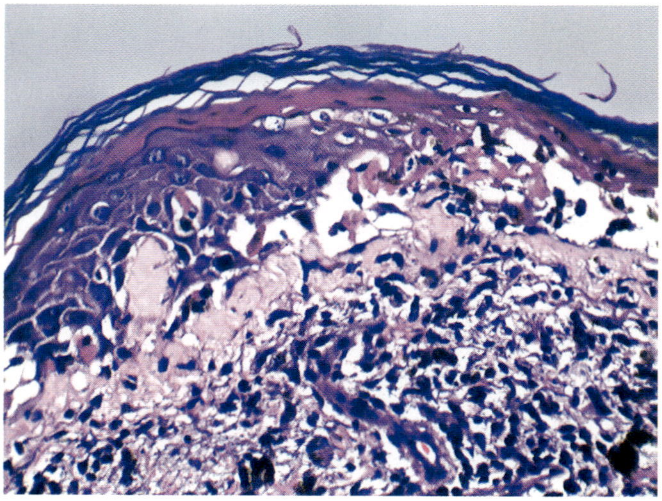

FIGURE 4.2.2.5

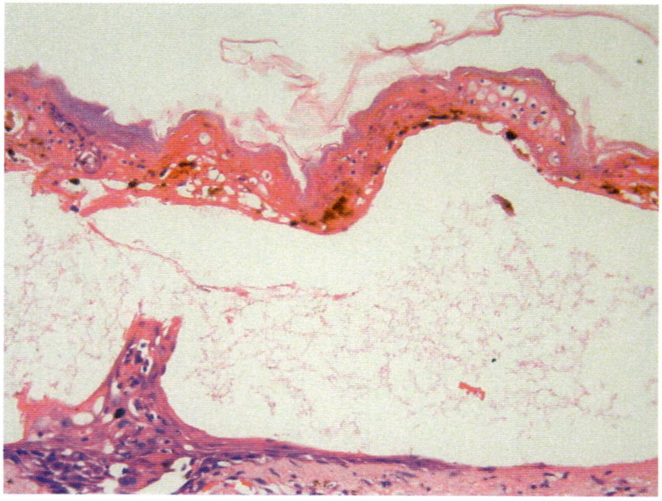

FIGURE 4.2.2.6

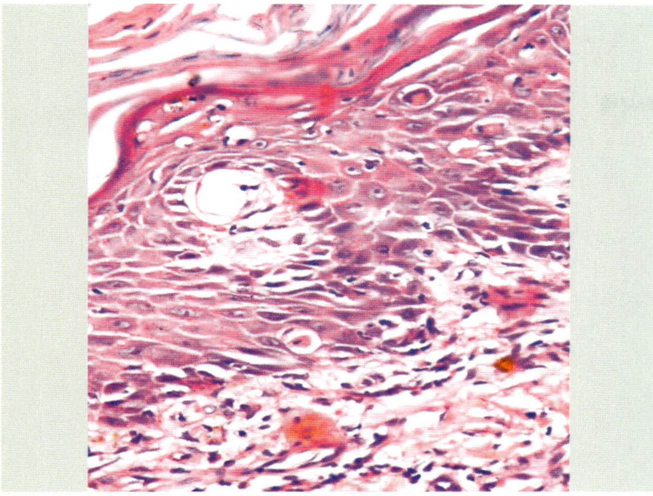

FIGURE 4.2.3.1

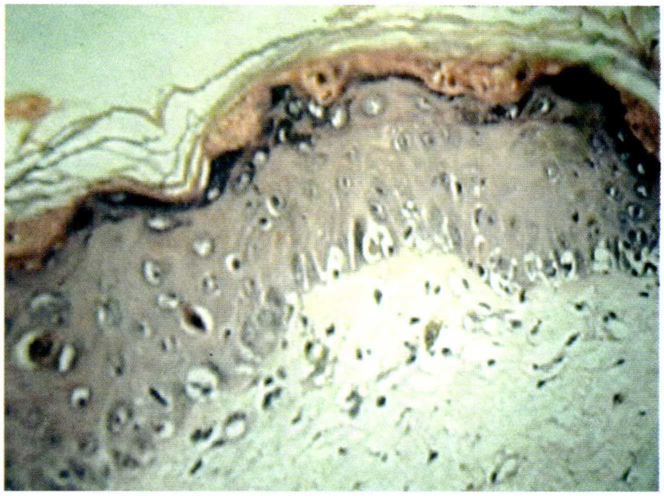

FIGURE 4.2.3.2

4.2.3: Graft-versus-Host Disease

4.2.3.1: Acute phase shows parakeratosis, focal basal cell vacuolation, subepidermal lymphocytic infiltrate (*Low power view*)

4.2.3.2: Another case with hyperkeratosis, apoptotic keratinocytes, pigment incontinence (*Low power view*)

4.2.3.3: Satellite cell necrosis—apoptotic keratinocytes surrounded by lymphocytes (*High power view*)

4.2.3.4: Chronic phase with apoptotic keratinocytes with surrounding lymphocytes, dermal sclerosis (*Low power view*)

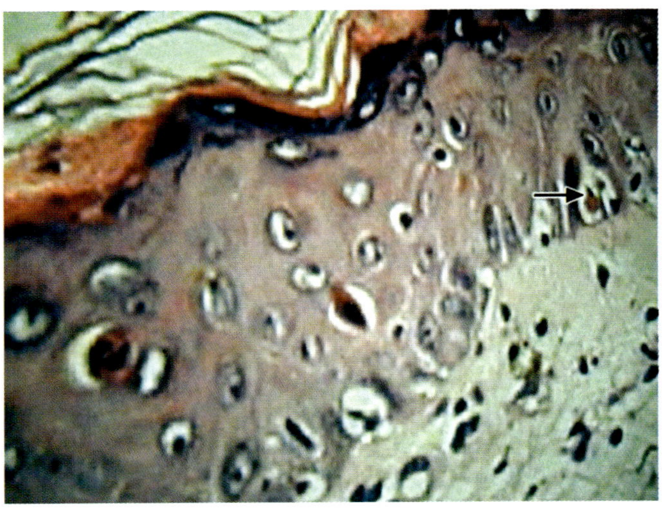

FIGURE 4.2.3.3

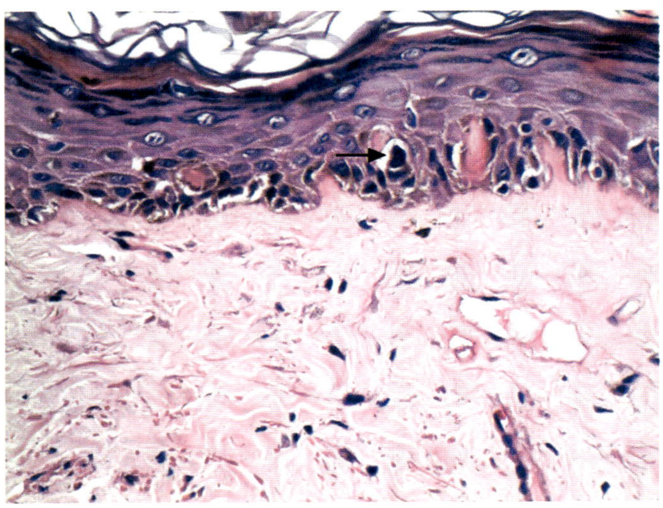

FIGURE 4.2.3.4

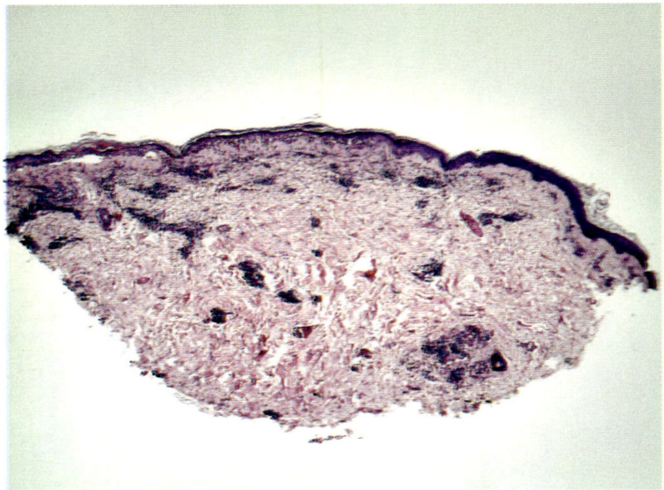

FIGURE 4.2.4.1

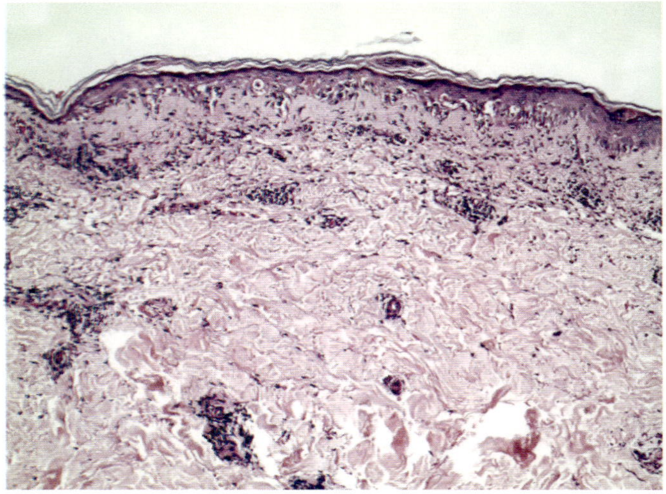

FIGURE 4.2.4.2

4.2.4: Lupus Erythematosus and Variants

4.2.4.1: Acute cutaneous lupus erythematosus—basal cell vacuolation, perivascular lymphocytic infiltrate in upper dermis (*Scanner view*)

4.2.4.2: Hyperkeratosis, focal atrophy of the epidermis, few necrotic keratinocytes (*Low power view*)

4.2.4.3: Vacuolar changes in the basal layer better appreciated along with papillary edema and mucin deposition (*High power view*)

4.2.4.4: Thickening of basement membrane H and E stain (*High power view*)

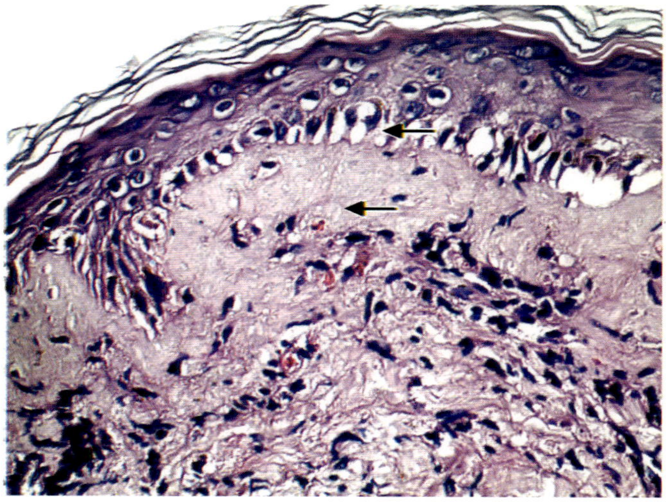

FIGURE 4.2.4.3

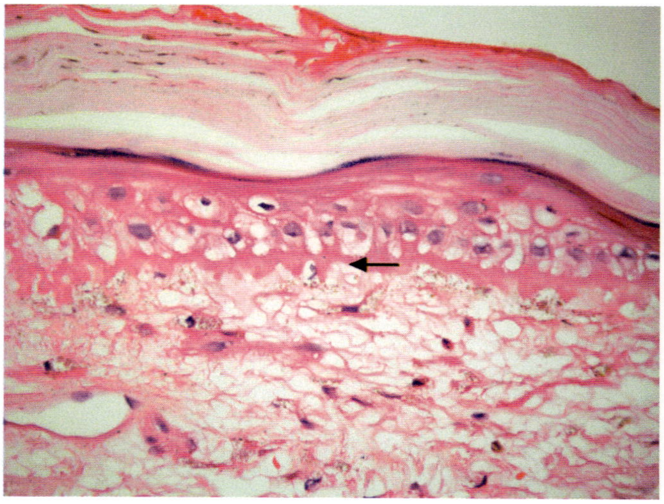

FIGURE 4.2.4.4

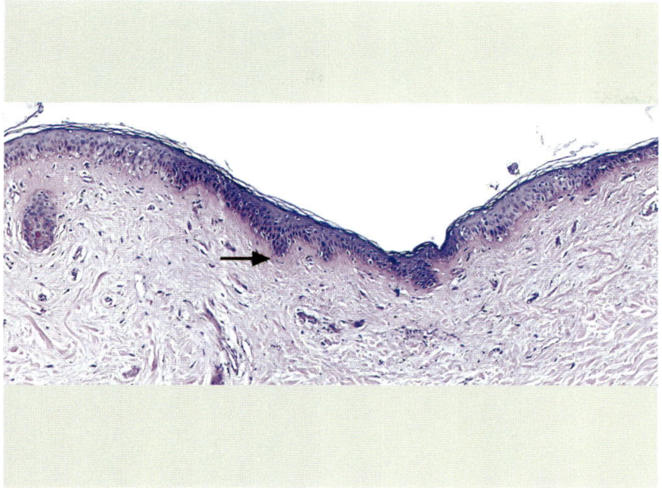

FIGURE 4.2.4.5

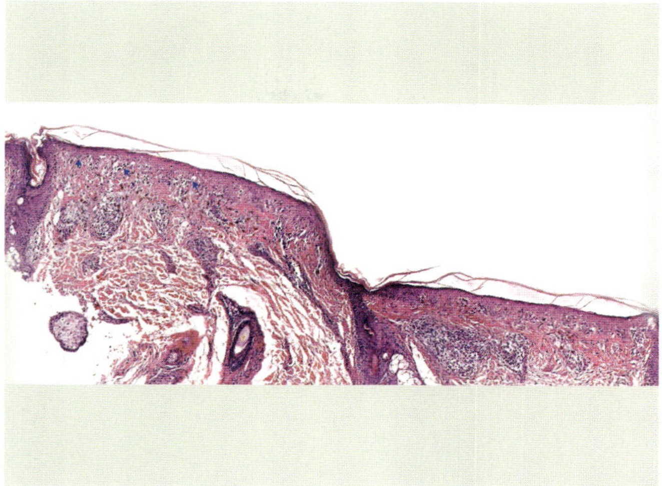

FIGURE 4.2.4.6

4.2.4.5: Periodic acid-Schiff stain highlighting basement membrane (*Low power view*)

4.2.4.6: Subacute cutaneous lupus erythematosus—epidermis is thinned out, follicular plugging, basal cell vacuolation (*Scanner view*)

4.2.4.7: Basal cell vacuolation with civatte bodies seen along with pigment incontinence and perivascular lymphocytes (*Low power view*)

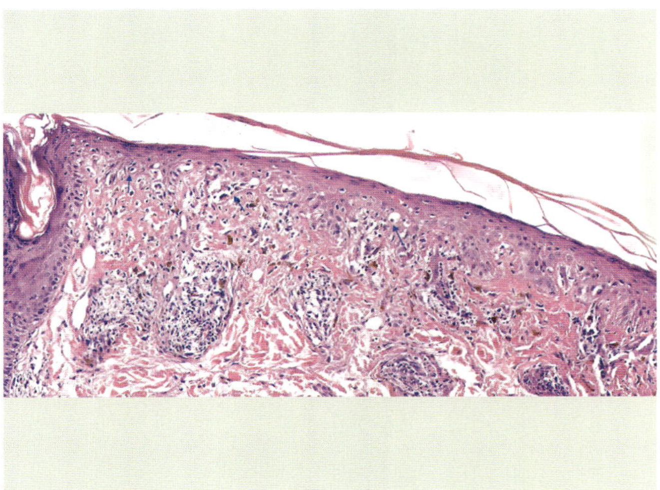

FIGURE 4.2.4.7

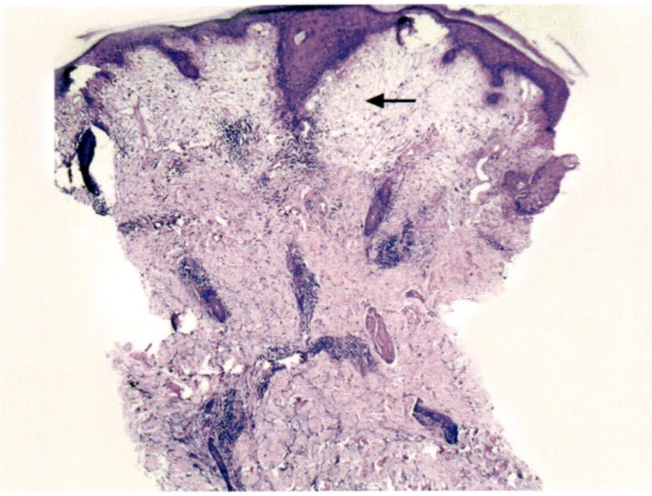

FIGURE 4.2.4.8

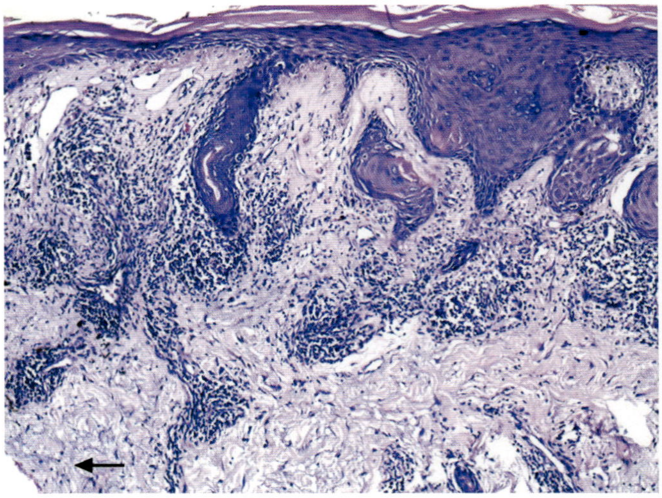

FIGURE 4.2.4.9

4.2.4.8: Discoid lupus erythematosus—epidermal hyperplasia, papillary edema and superficial and deep dermal infiltrate (*Scanner view*)

4.2.4.9: There is hyperkeratosis with focal atrophy and basal cell vacuolation, dermis shows mucin deposition and infiltrate around pilosebaceous units (*Low power view*)

4.2.4.10: Lupus profundus showing dense inflammatory infiltrate extending up to subcutaneous tissue (*Scanner view*)

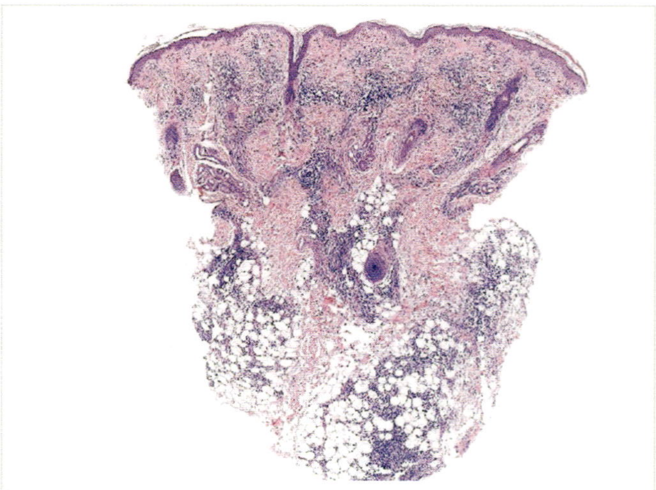

FIGURE 4.2.4.10

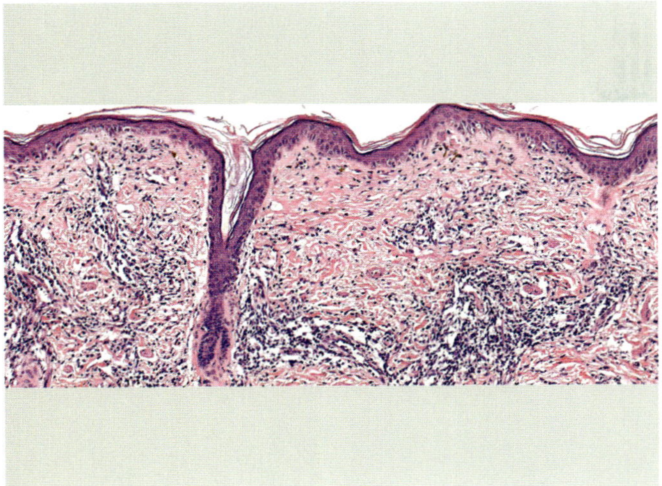

FIGURE 4.2.4.11

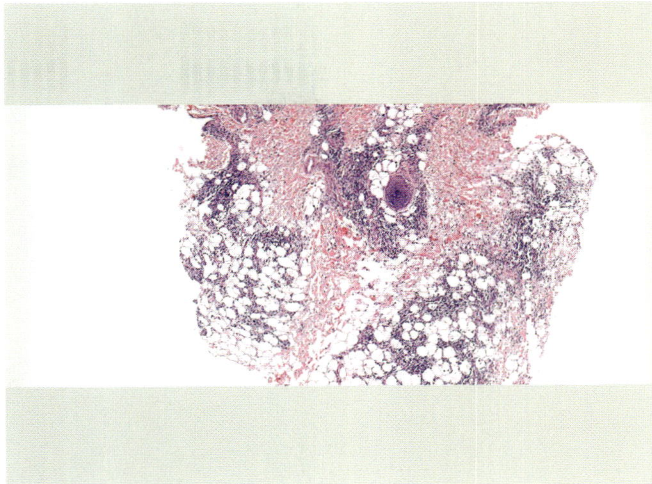

FIGURE 4.2.4.12

4.2.4.11: Epidermis shows hyperkeratosis, atrophy, follicular plugging and basal cell vacuolation. Upper dermis has mucin and infiltrate (*Low power view*)

4.2.4.12: Lobular panniculitis (*Low power view*)

4.2.4.13: Closer view of infiltrate (difficult to differentiate from other causes of lobular panniculitis like subcutaneous panniculitis-like T cell lymphoma) (*High power view*)

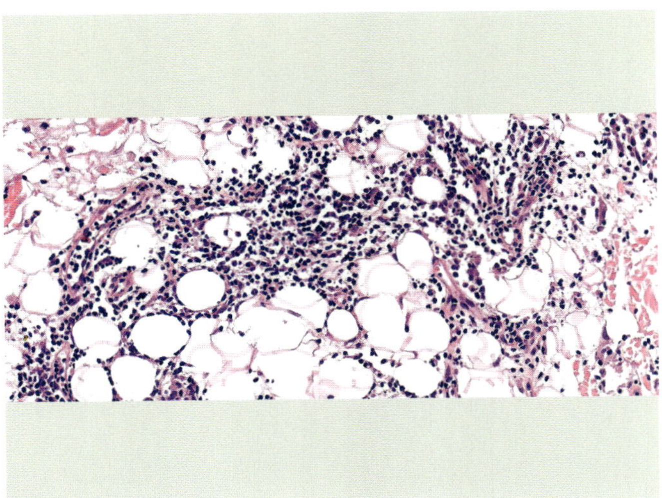

FIGURE 4.2.4.13

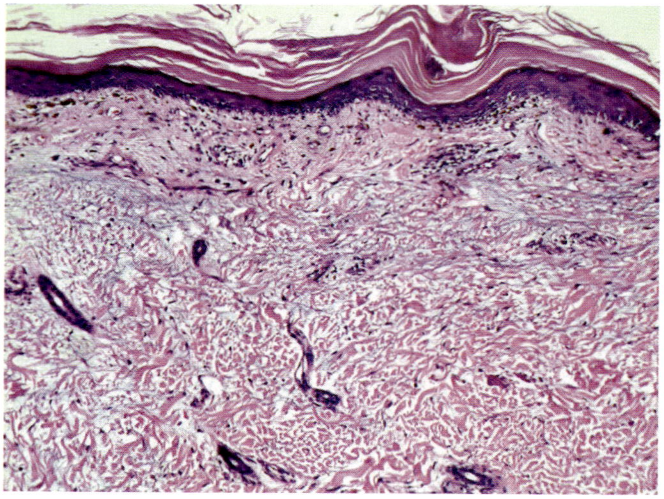

FIGURE 4.2.5.1

4.2.5: Dermatomyositis

4.2.5.1: Changes similar to lupus erythematosus but less pronounced, hyperkeratosis, atrophic epidermis, sparse superficial perivascular infiltrate (*Low power view*)

4.2.5.2: Dermal edema and mucin deposits, pigmentary incontinence (*Low power view*)

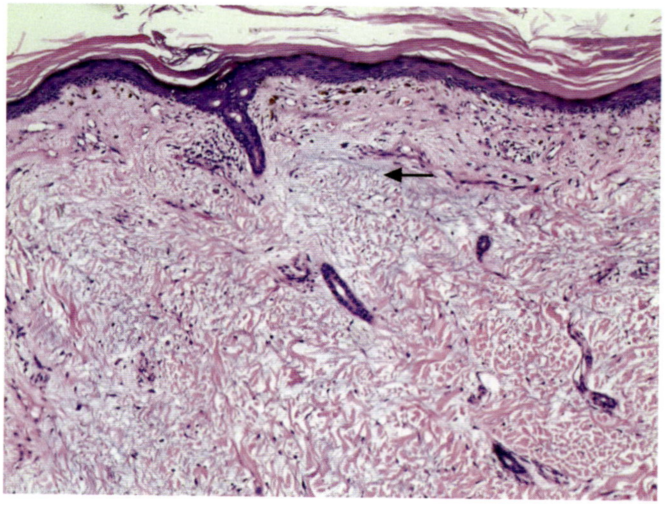

FIGURE 4.2.5.2

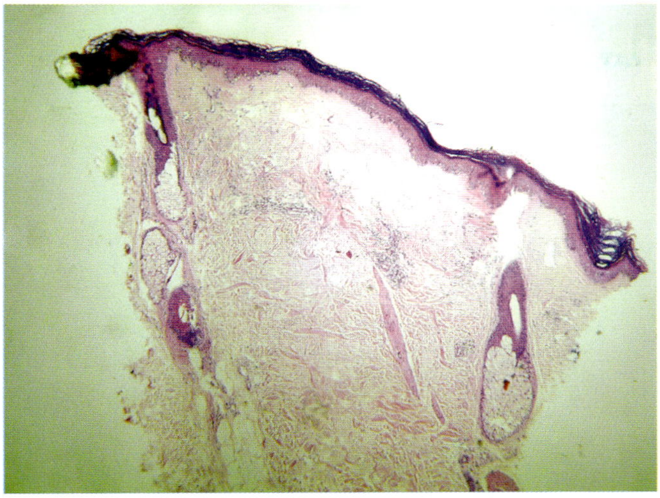

FIGURE 4.2.6.1

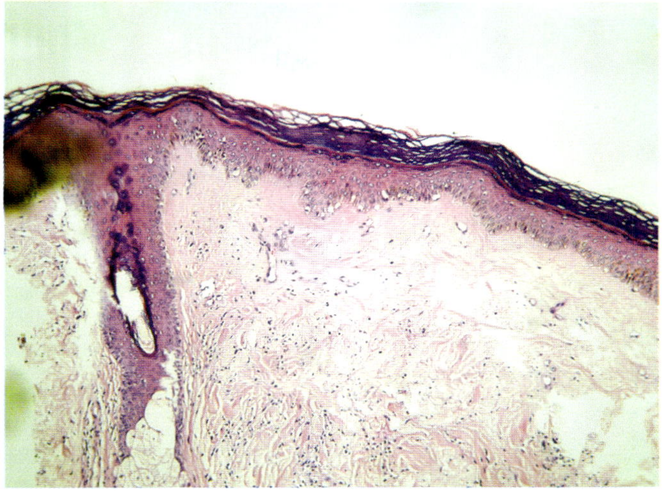

FIGURE 4.2.6.2

4.2.6: Lichen Sclerosus et Atrophicus

4.2.6.1: Atrophic epidermis, hyperkeratosis and papillary edema (*Scanner view*)

4.2.6.2: Focal basal cell vacuolation, lymphocytic infiltrate below the zone of papillary edema (*Low power view*)

4.2.6.3: Dilated capillaries and papillary edema (*Low power view*)

4.2.6.4: Lymphocytic infiltrate, dilated capillaries and follicular hyperkeratosis (*Low power view*)

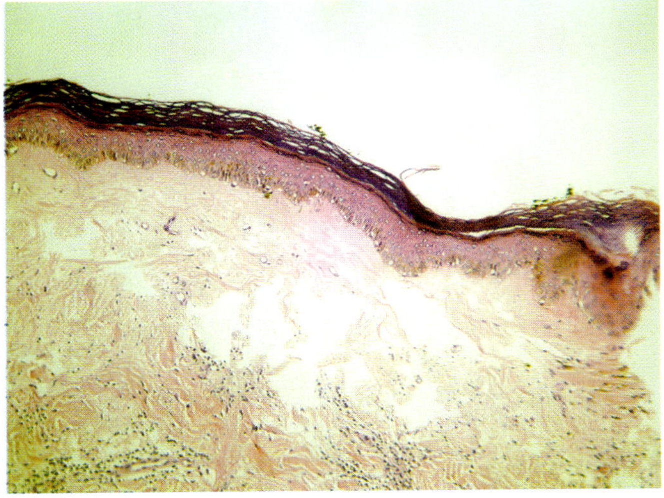

FIGURE 4.2.6.3

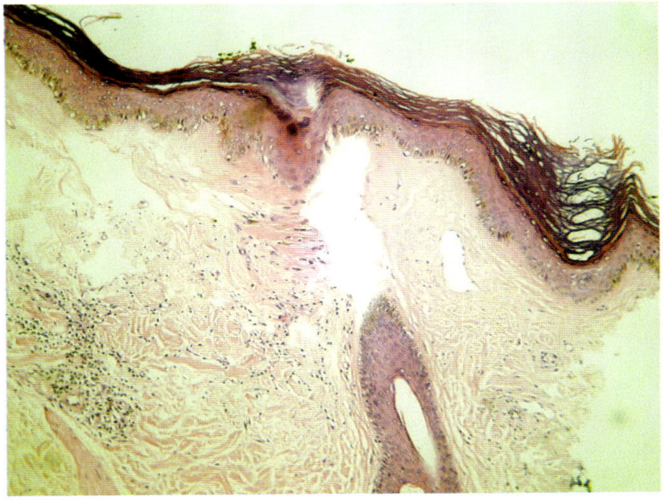

FIGURE 4.2.6.4

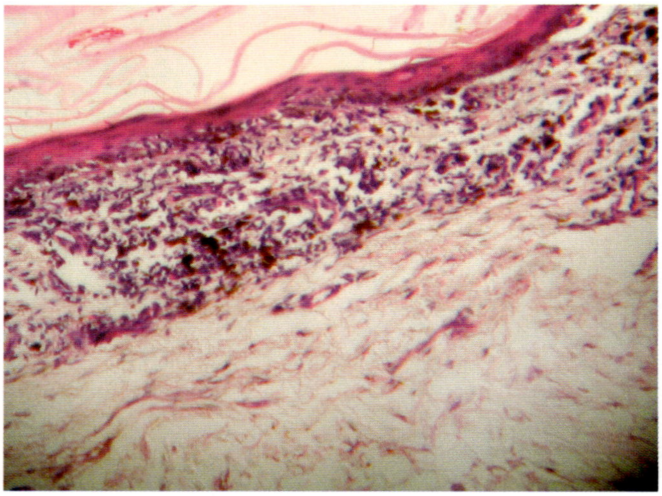

FIGURE 4.2.7.1

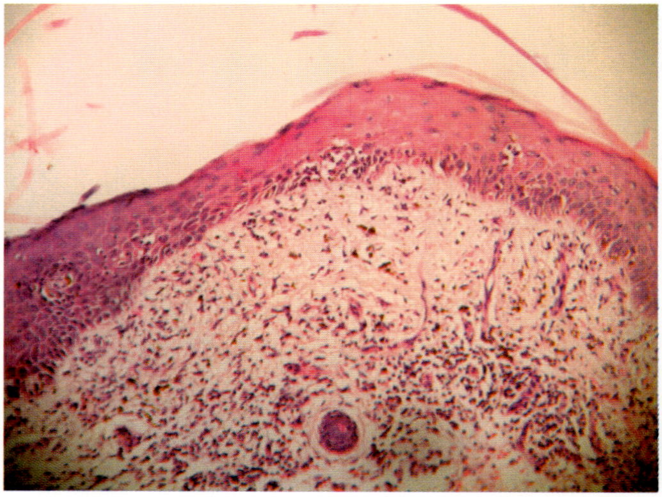

FIGURE 4.2.7.2

4.2.7: Poikiloderma

4.2.7.1: Hyperkeratosis, epidermal atrophy, lichenoid tissue reaction (*Scanner view*)

4.2.7.2: Another case with dilated capillaries and perivascular lymphocytic infiltrate (*Low power view*)

4.2.7.3: Focal basal cell vacuolation, occasional apoptotic keratinocyte, pigment incontinence (*High power view*)

4.2.7.4: Closer view of capillaries, infiltrate and pigment (*High power view*)

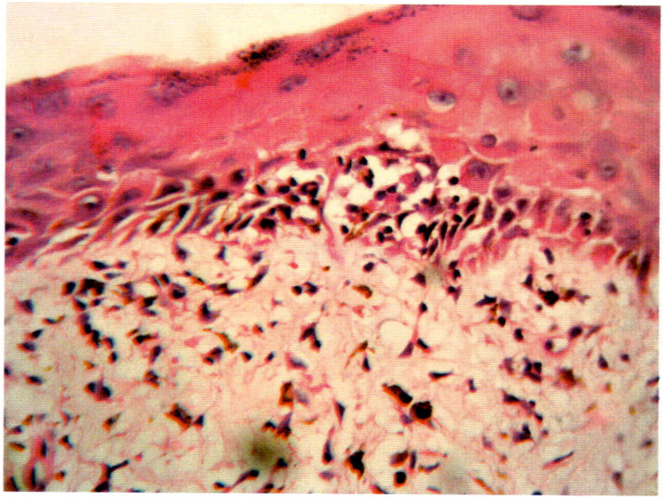

FIGURE 4.2.7.3

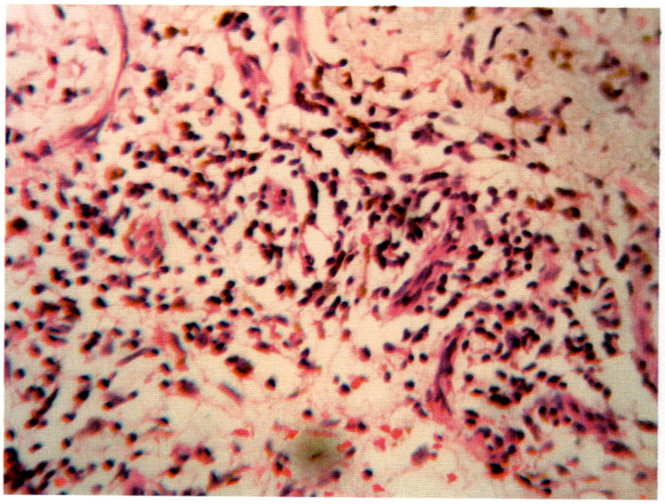

FIGURE 4.2.7.4

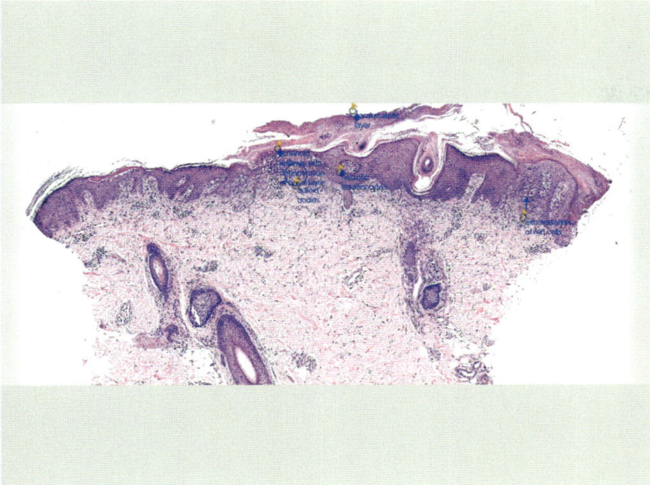

FIGURE 4.2.8.1

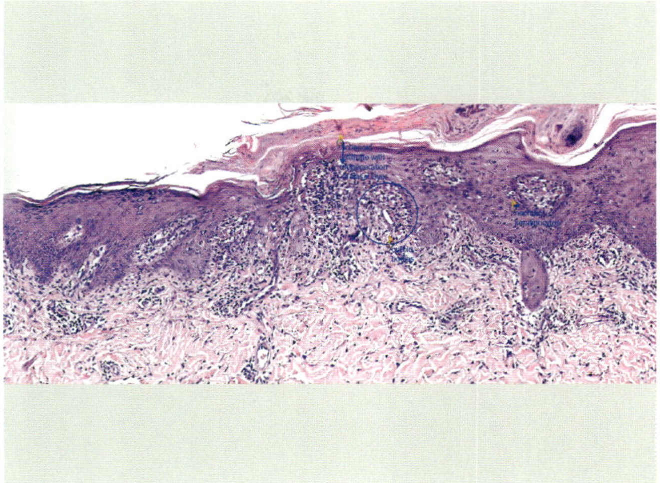

FIGURE 4.2.8.2

4.2.8: Pityriasis Lichenoides

4.2.8.1: Pityriasis lichenoides acuta shows focal parakeratosis with lichenoid infiltrate and basal cell vacuolation (*Scanner view*)

4.2.8.2: Closer view of focal change with parakeratosis and basal cell vacuolation (*Low power view*)

4.2.8.3: Migration of lymphocytes into layers of epidermis with spongiosis (*High power view*)

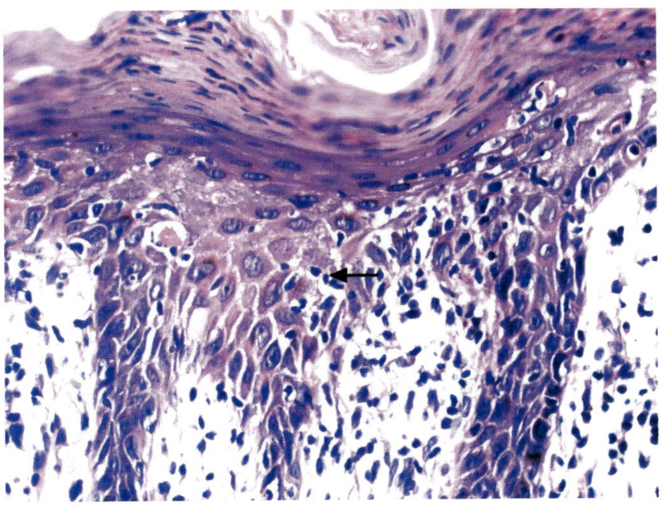

FIGURE 4.2.8.3

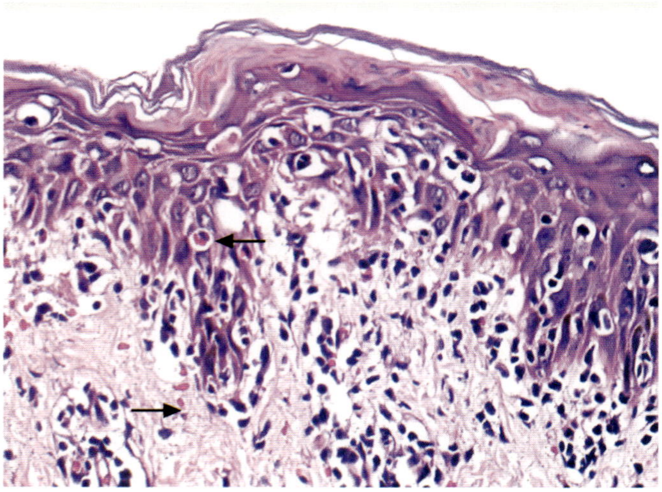

FIGURE 4.2.8.4

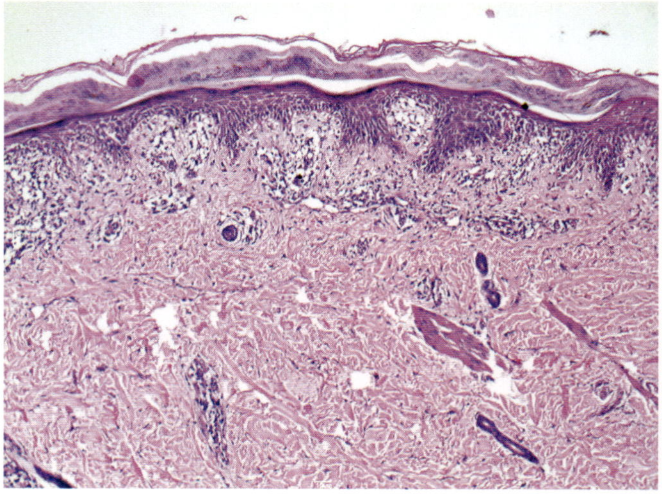

FIGURE 4.2.8.5

4.2.8.4: Extravasated red blood cells and necrotic keratinocytes (*High power view*)

4.2.8.5: Pityriasis lichenoides chronica shows similar changes but less pronounced, parakeratosis, focal basal cell damage. A superficial perivascular lymphocytic infiltrate is also seen (*Scanner view*)

4.2.8.6: Lymphocytes extending to the epidermis with mild spongiosis and an occasional necrotic keratinocyte, extravasated red blood cells (*Low power view*)

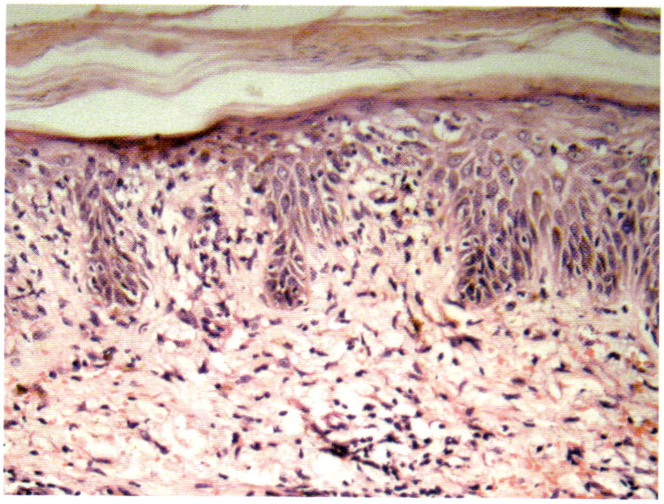

FIGURE 4.2.8.6

DIFFERENTIAL DIAGNOSIS

1. Lichenoid purpura
2. Lichenoid contact dermatitis
3. Mycosis fungoides
4. Erythroderma
5. Porokeratosis

DIAGNOSTIC PEARLS

1. Lichenoid dermatitis refers to band like infiltrate in the upper dermis obscuring dermoepidermal junction (lichen planus) and interface dermatitis refers to presence of basal cell vacuolation and apoptosis (erythema multiforme) (quoted from McKee's pathology of the skin with clinical correlations). But these terms are used interchangeably for most diseases included under this section by many dermatopathologists.
2. Older lesions of lichen planus will have minimal inflammation with many melanophages and dilated capillaries in dermis.
3. Mucous membrane lichen planus—show plasma cells which are rare in cutaneous lichen planus.
4. Early pointer to acute graft-versus-host disease (GVHD) is involvement of follicular epithelium with basal cell vacuolation.
5. The infiltrate in lichen planopilaris does not extend around blood vessels of the mid and deep plexus like lupus erythematosus (LE).
6. Lichen nitidus versus lichen scrofulosorum—the infiltrate in lichen nitidus expands the dermal papilla, the granulomas in lichen scrofulosorum do not cause widening of the papillae and are usually perifollicular.
7. Prominent basal cell vacuolation and presence of mucin are helpful in distinguishing systemic lupus erythematosus (SLE) from polymorphic light eruption.
8. In tumid lupus erythematosus, there is increased dermal mucin and epidermal involvement is uncommon.
9. Only subtle histologic changes with mucin deposition is suggestive of dermatomyositis. The histopathology may be indistinguishable from lupus erythematosus but basement membrane thickening is prominent and colloid bodies are frequent in LE than in dermatomyositis (DM).
10. Lupus band test of involved skin is positive in almost 100% of cases of SLE, while uninvolved skin from sun-exposed areas is positive in about 90% of cases.
11. Lichenoid reaction with spongiotic changes are seen in drug reactions, lichenoid contact dermatitis, lichen striatus.
12. Lichenoid change with granulomatous reaction is encounterd in lichen nitidus, lichenoid sarcoidosis, infective reactions including secondary syphilis, herpes zoster, human immunodeficiency virus (HIV) infection, tuberculosis, atypical tuberculosis and some drug reactions.
13. Lichenoid reaction with parakeratosis is a feature of pityriasis lichenoides, lichenoid drug eruptions, lichen striatus, lichen planus-like keratosis, lichen nitidus.

5

Spongiotic Dermatoses

Chapter Outline

5.1: Spongiosis with Eosinophils
5.2: Spongiosis with Neutrophils
5.3: Other Spongiotic Disorders

Pradeep Mahajan, KC Nischal, Atul Dongre

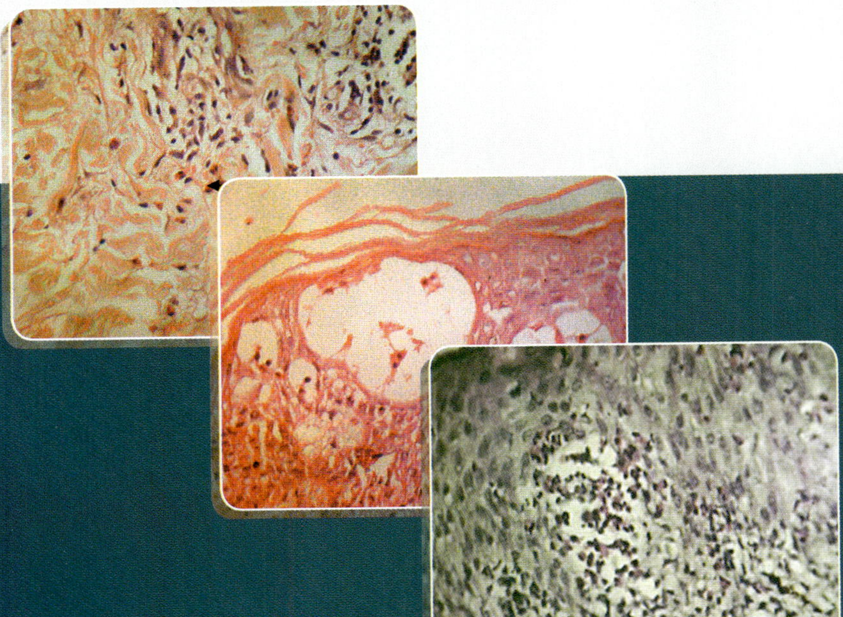

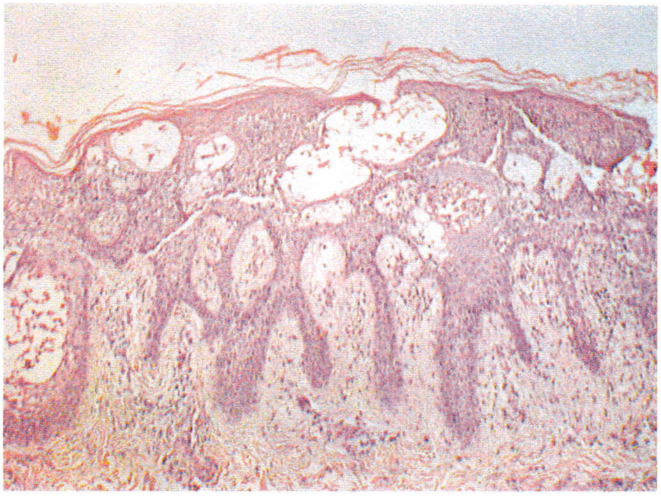

FIGURE 5.1.1.1

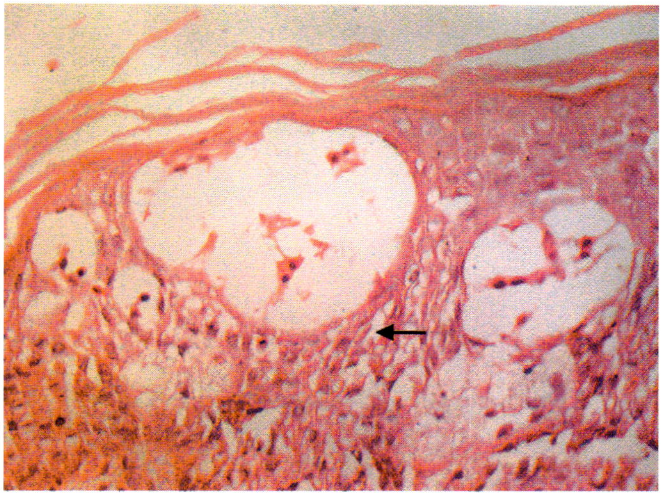

FIGURE 5.1.1.2

5.1: SPONGIOSIS WITH EOSINOPHILS

5.1.1: Allergic Contact Dermatitis

5.1.1.1: Spongiosis with multiple spongiotic microvesicles (acute dermatitis) (*Low power view*)

5.1.1.2: Closer view of spongiosis and vesicles at different levels, horizontally as well as vertically with exocytosis of lymphocytes and eosinophils (*High power view*)

5.1.1.3: Marked spongiosis with vesicles (*High power view*)

5.1.1.4: Perivascular lymphocytes and eosinophils in the dermis (*High power view*)

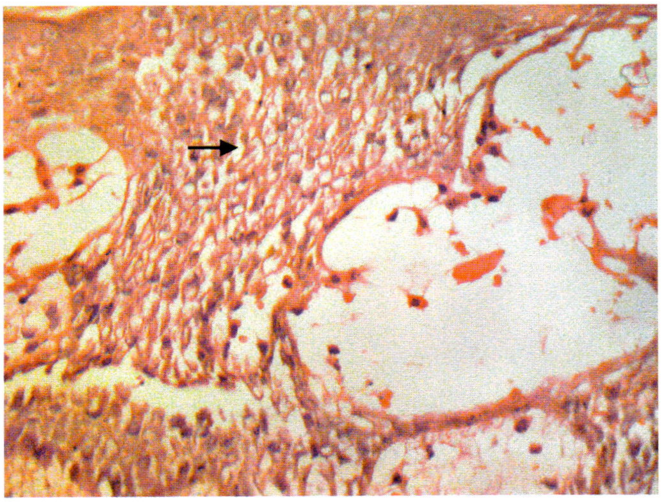

FIGURE 5.1.1.3

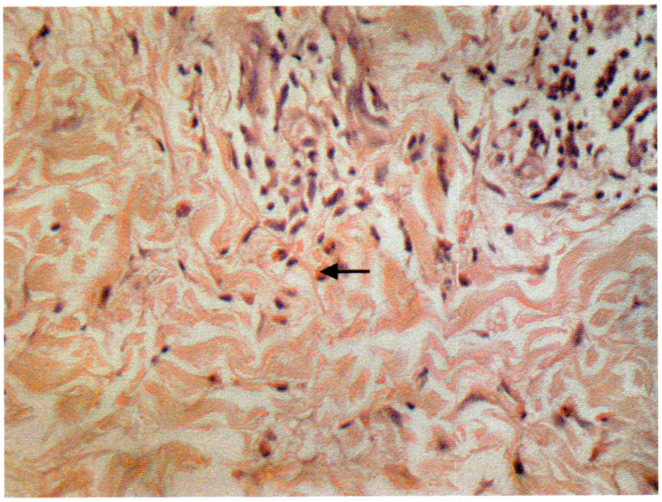

FIGURE 5.1.1.4

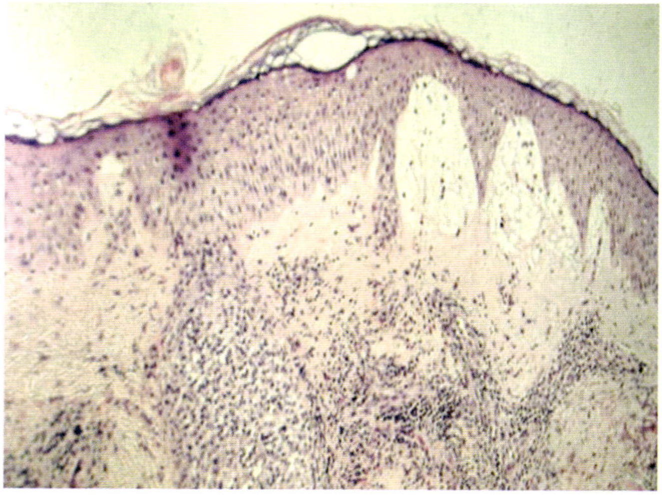

FIGURE 5.1.2.1

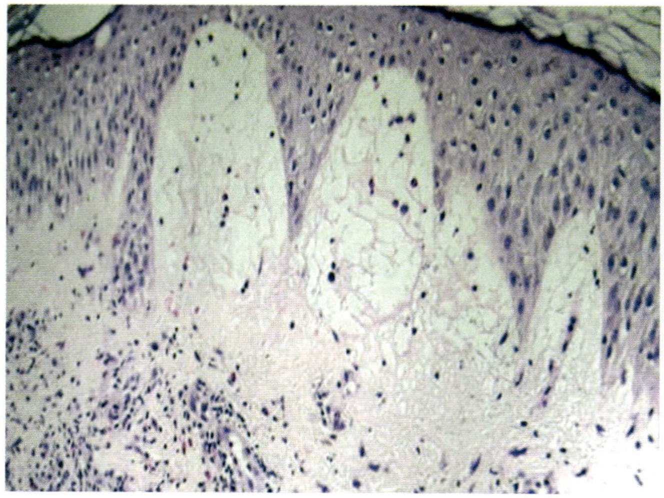

FIGURE 5.1.2.2

5.1.2: Arthropod Bite Reaction

5.1.2.1: Perivascular and interstitial inflammatory dermal infiltrate composed of lymphocytes and eosinophils with overlying focus of spongiosis (*Low power view*)

5.1.2.2: Marked papillary edema with eosinophils (*Low power view*)

5.1.2.3: Perivascular eosinophils extending to the interstitial tissue (*High power view*)

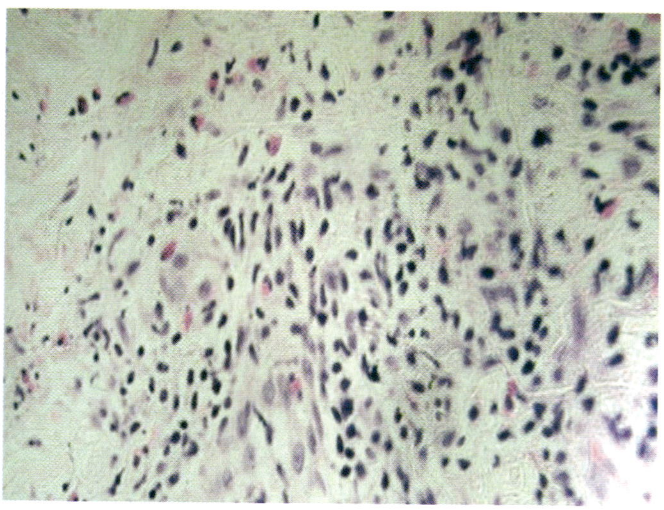

FIGURE 5.1.2.3

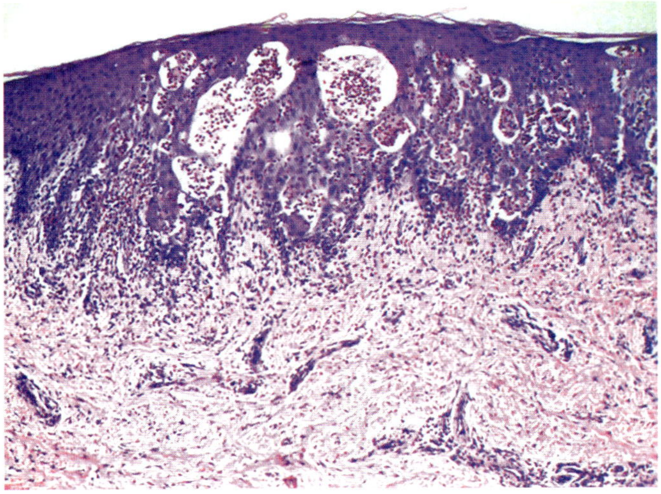

FIGURE 5.1.3.1

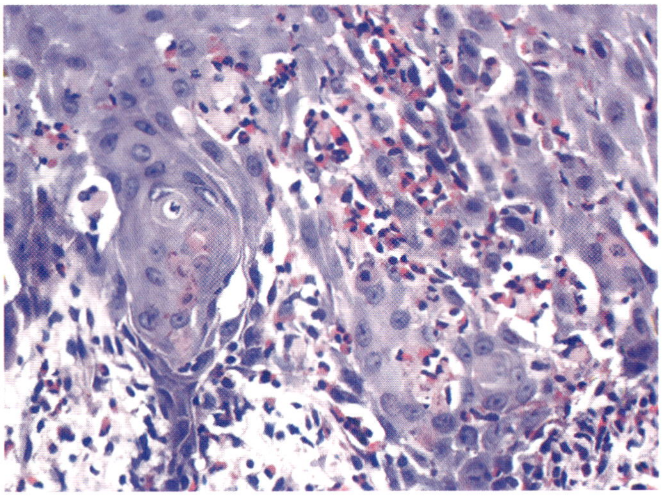

FIGURE 5.1.3.2

5.1.3: Incontinentia Pigmenti

5.1.3.1: Eosinophilic spongiosis and irregular hyperplasia of the epidermis (vesicular stage), dermis with mild chronic inflammatory infiltrate (*Low power view*)

5.1.3.2: Spongiosis with eosinophils (*High power view*)

5.1.3.3: Scattered dyskeratotic cells (*High power view*)

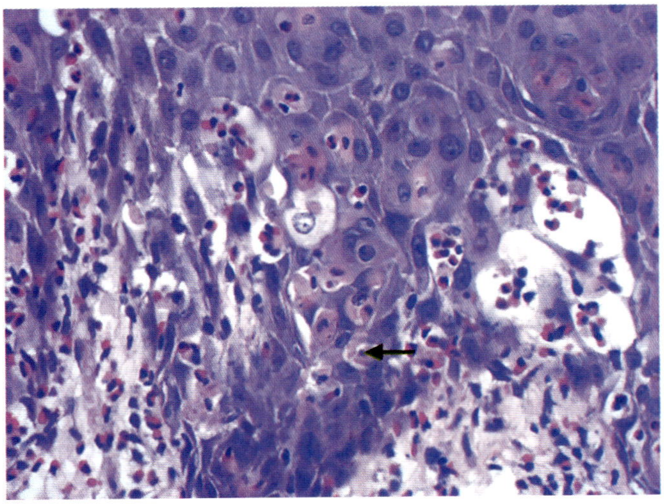

FIGURE 5.1.3.3

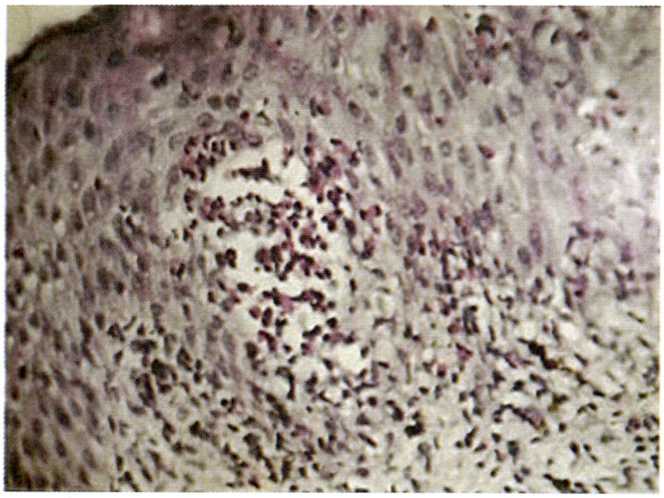

FIGURE 5.1.3.4

5.1.3.4: Another case with eosinophilic spongiosis (*Low power view*)

5.1.3.5: Epidermis shows irregular hyperplasia and whorls of squamous cells (Verrucous stage) (*Low power view*)

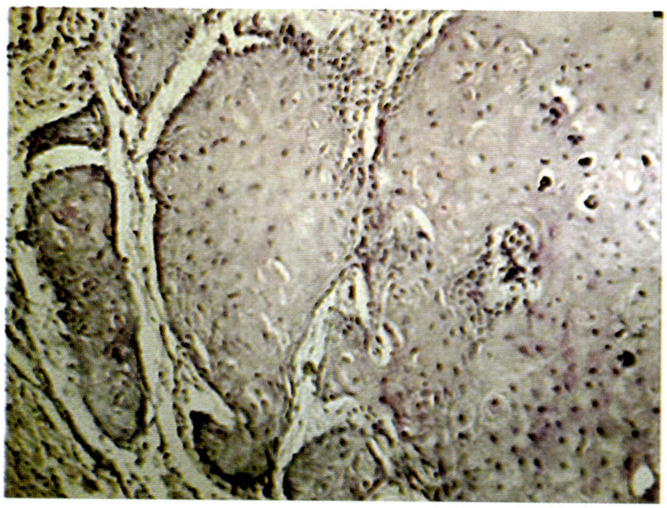

FIGURE 5.1.3.5

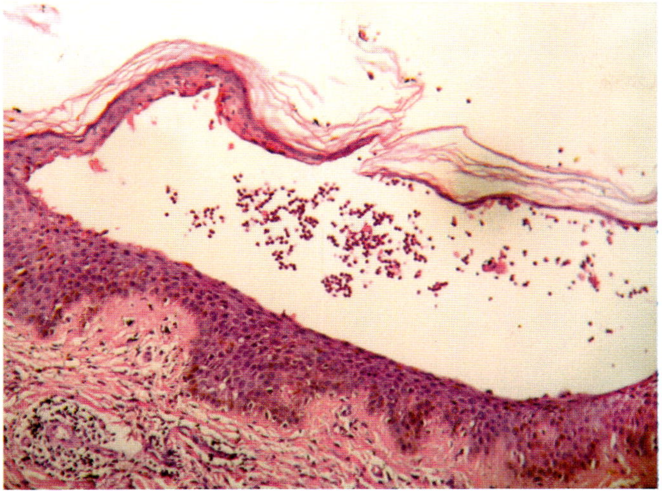

FIGURE 5.2.1.1

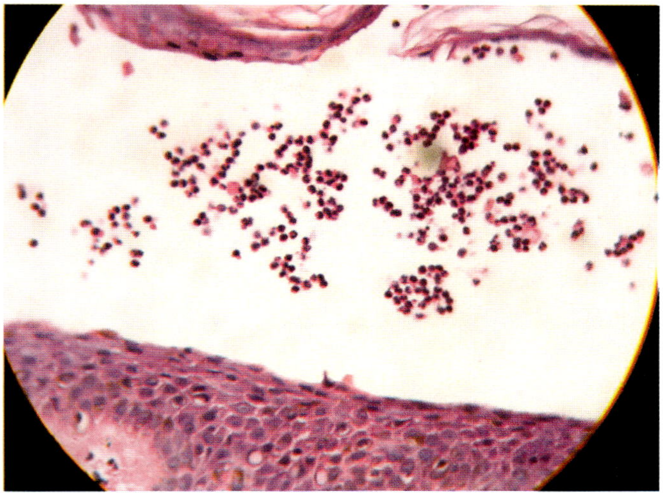

FIGURE 5.2.1.2

5.2: SPONGIOSIS WITH NEUTROPHILS

5.2.1: Acute Generalized Exanthematous Pustulosis

5.2.1.1: Subcorneal and intraepidermal collections of neutrophils (*Low power view*)

5.2.1.2: Mild spongiosis and neutrophils in the blister cavity (*High power view*)

5.2.1.3: Upper dermal perivascular inflammatory infiltrate of lymphocytes, neutrophils and a few eosinophils (*High power view*)

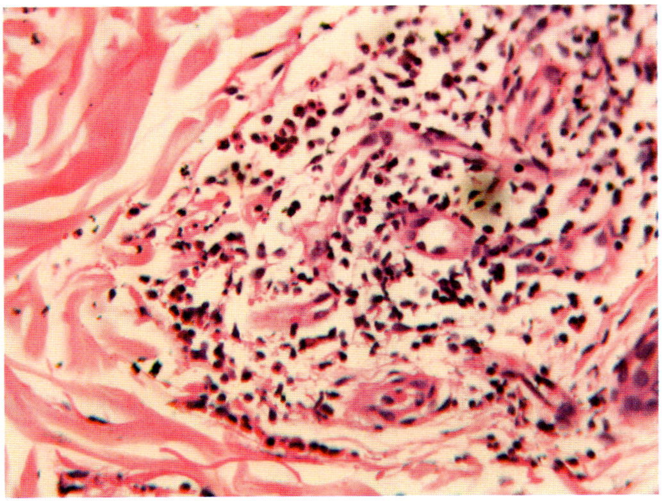

FIGURE 5.2.1.3

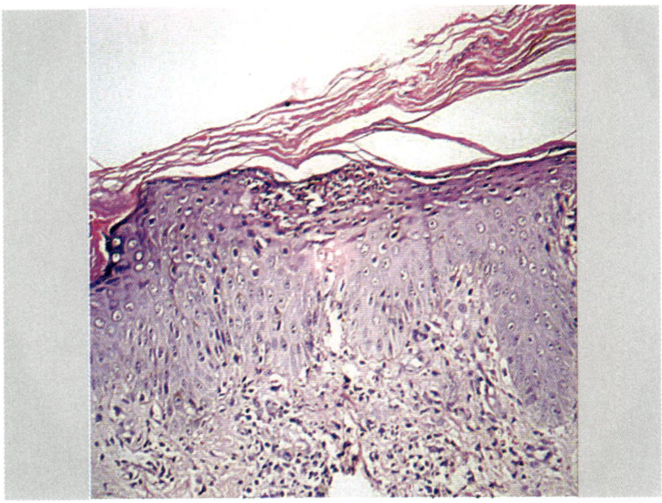

FIGURE 5.2.2.1

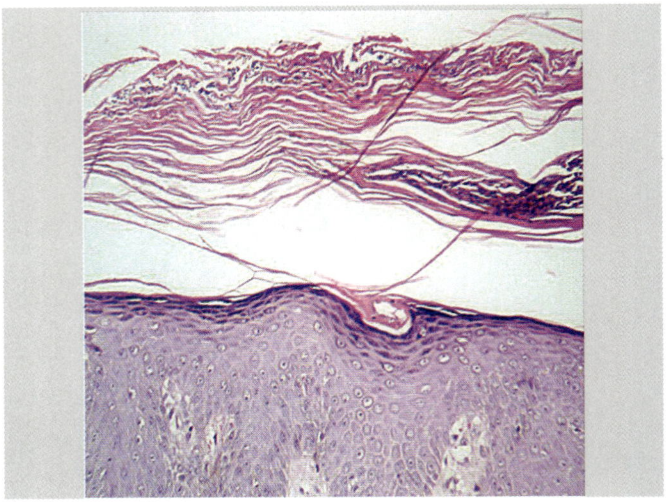

FIGURE 5.2.2.2

5.2.2: Dermatophytosis and Candidiasis

5.2.2.1: Spongiosis and subcorneal collection of neutrophils, mixed dermal infiltrate (*Low power view*)

5.2.2.2: Hyperkeratosis with fungal elements (*Low power view*)

5.2.2.3: Pseudohyphae (2–4 μm) in stratum corneum, pseudohyphae branch at 90° (*High power view*)

5.2.2.4: Spores (3–6 μm) seen in stratum corneum (*High power view*)

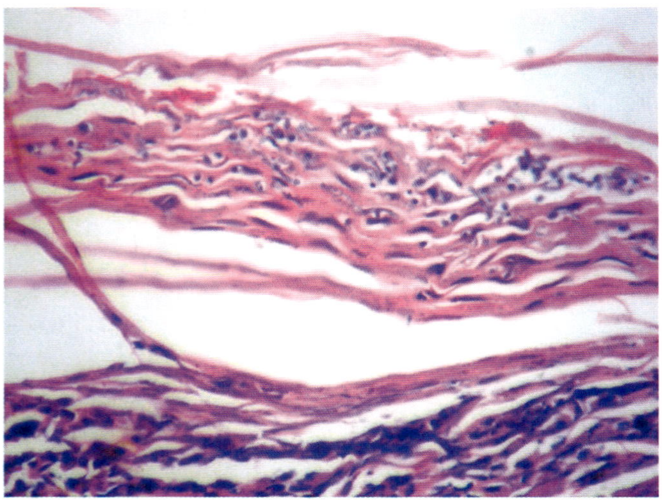

FIGURE 5.2.2.3

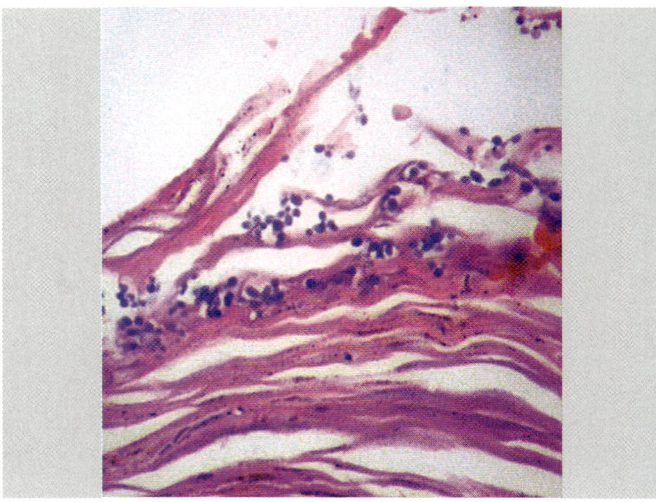

FIGURE 5.2.2.4

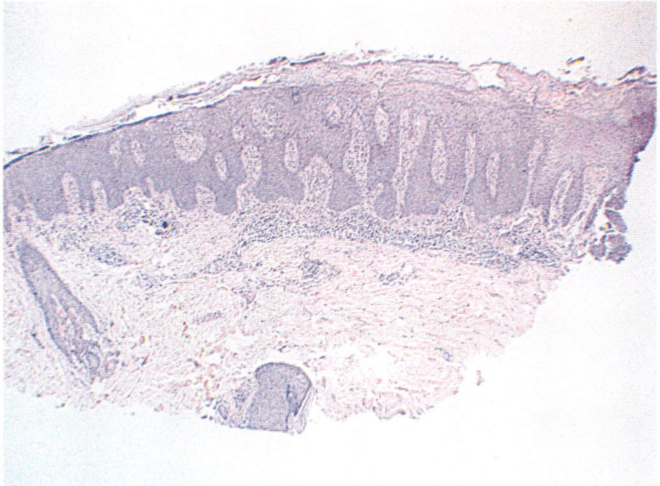

FIGURE 5.3.1.1

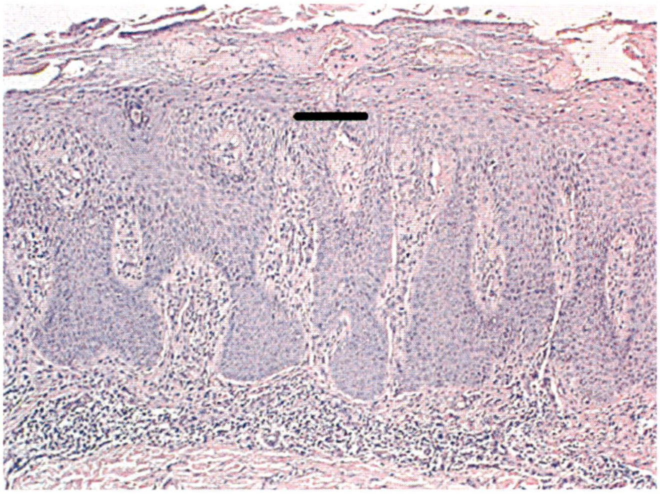

FIGURE 5.3.1.2

5.3: OTHER SPONGIOTIC DISORDERS

5.3.1: Nummular Dermatitis

5.3.1.1: Irregular hyperplasia and superficial perivascular inflammatory infiltrate (*Scanner view*)

5.3.1.2: Spongiosis with exocytosis (subacute dermatitis) (*Low power view*)

5.3.1.3: Parakeratosis with accumulation of plasma (scale-crust formation) (*High power view*)

5.3.1.4: Perivascular lymphocytic infiltrate (*High power view*)

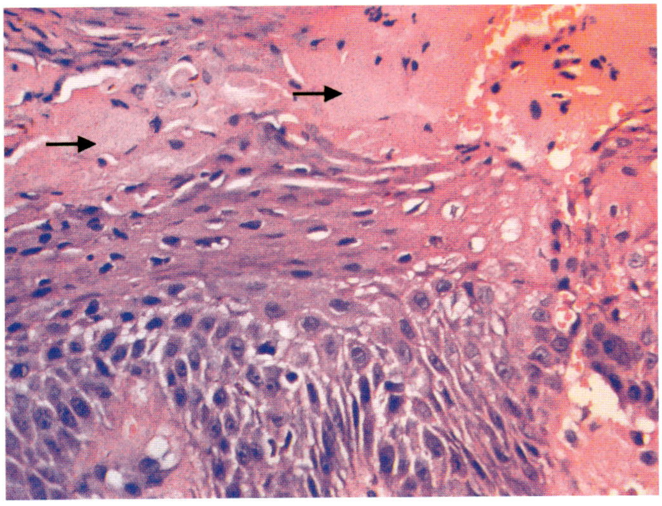

FIGURE 5.3.1.3

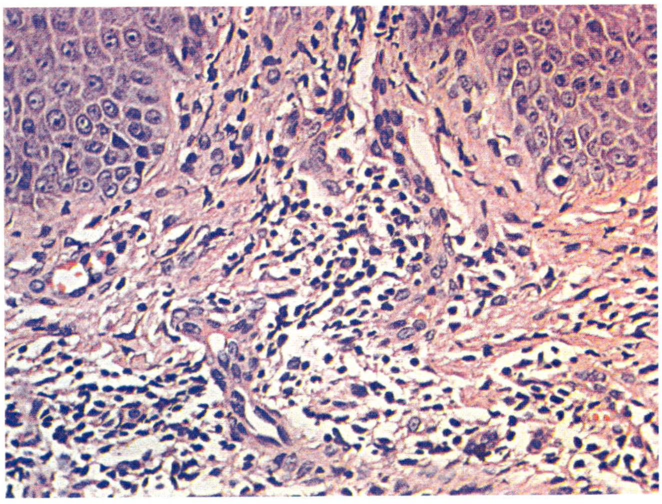

FIGURE 5.3.1.4

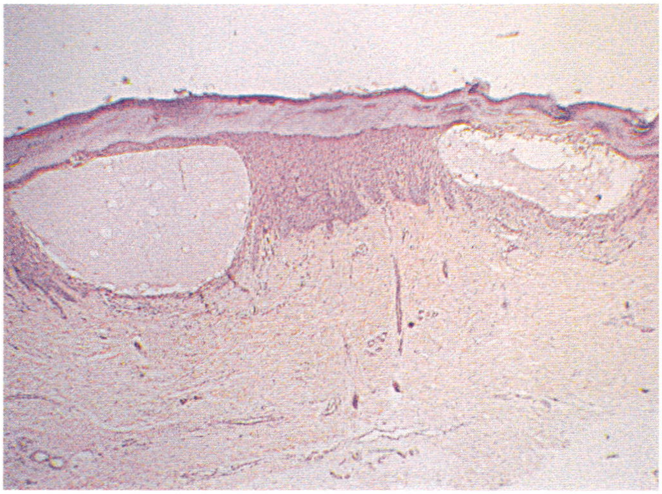

FIGURE 5.3.2.1

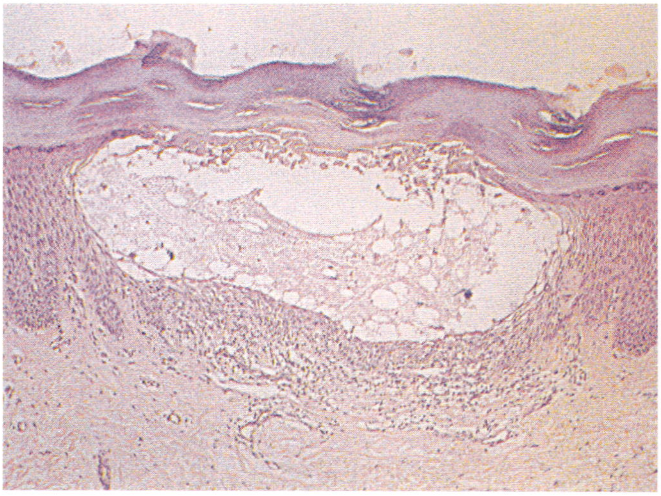

FIGURE 5.3.2.2

5.3.2: Dyshidrosiform Dermatitis (Pompholyx)

5.3.2.1: Hyperkeratosis with marked spongiosis leading to intraepidermal vesicles (acute dermatitis) (*Scanner view*)

5.3.2.2: Marked hyperkeratosis indicating palmar skin (*Low power view*)

5.3.2.3: Spongiotic vesicle with fibrin (*High power view*)

5.3.2.4: Marked spongiosis (*High power view*)

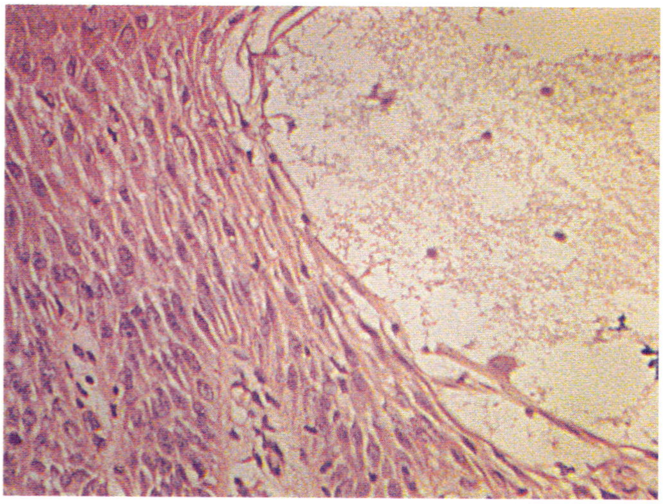

FIGURE 5.3.2.3

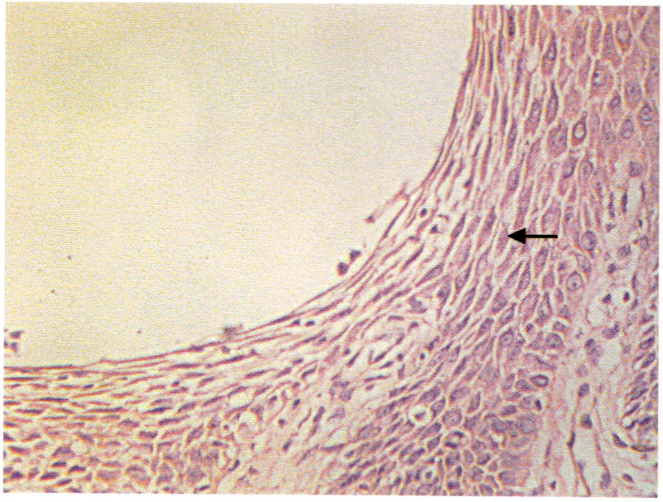

FIGURE 5.3.2.4

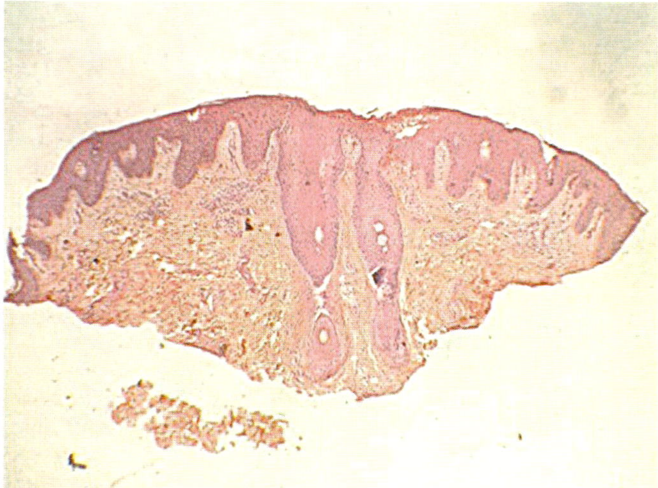

FIGURE 5.3.3.1

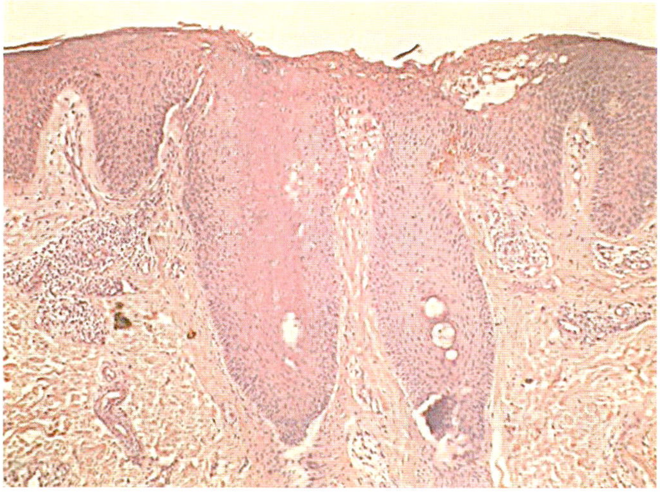

FIGURE 5.3.3.2

5.3.3: Seborrheic Dermatitis

5.3.3.1: Epidermal hyperplasia with regular elongation of rete ridge (*Scanner view*)

5.3.3.2: Parakeratotic mounds overlying follicular ostium (*Low power view*)

5.3.3.3: Another case with involvement mainly of follicular infundibulum (*Low power view*)

5.3.3.4: Parakeratosis and spongiosis centered at follicle (*High power view*)

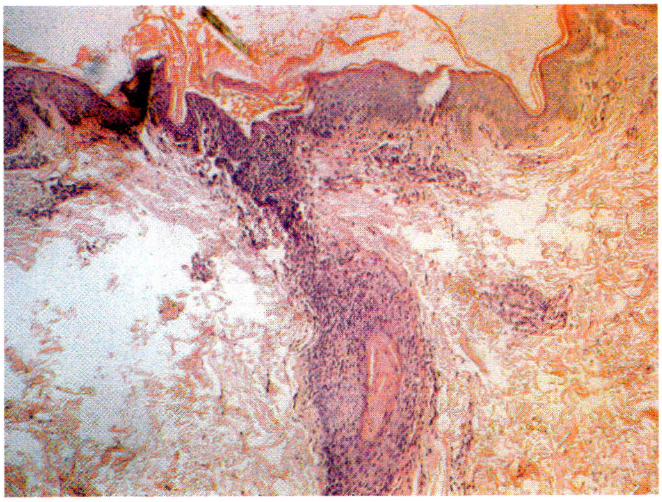

FIGURE 5.3.3.3

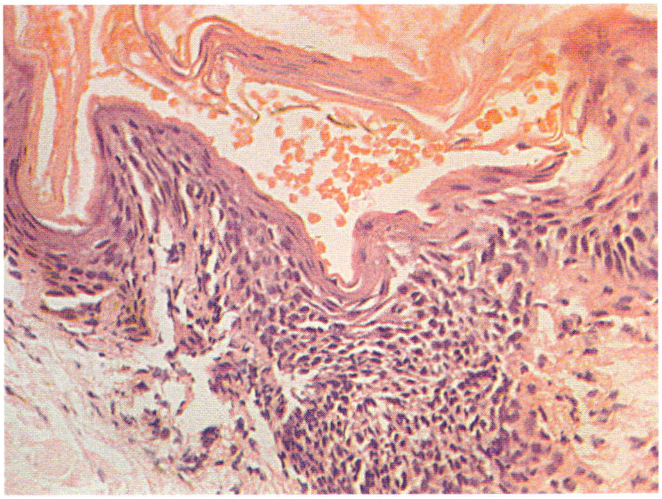

FIGURE 5.3.3.4

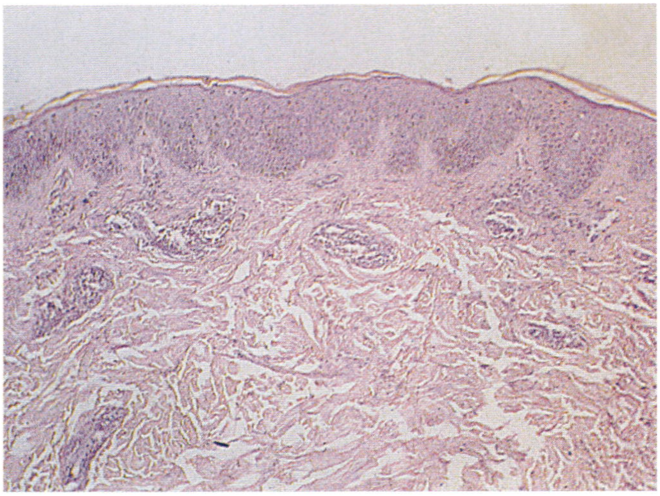

FIGURE 5.3.4.1

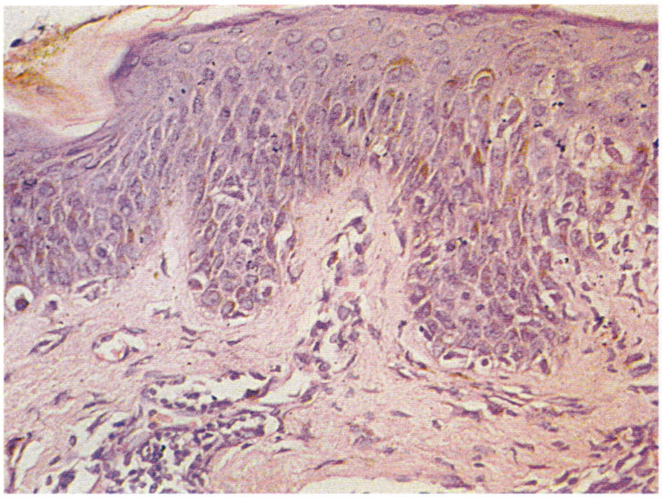

FIGURE 5.3.4.2

5.3.4: Atopic Dermatitis

5.3.4.1: Hyperplasia with elongation of rete ridges (may be focal parakeratosis) (*Low power view*)

5.3.4.2: Mild spongiosis, dilated capillaries and perivascular lymphocytes (occasional eosinophil) in the dermis (*High power view*)

5.3.4.3: Increased volume of the epidermis with not much of psoriasiform elongation of rete ridges (*High power view*)

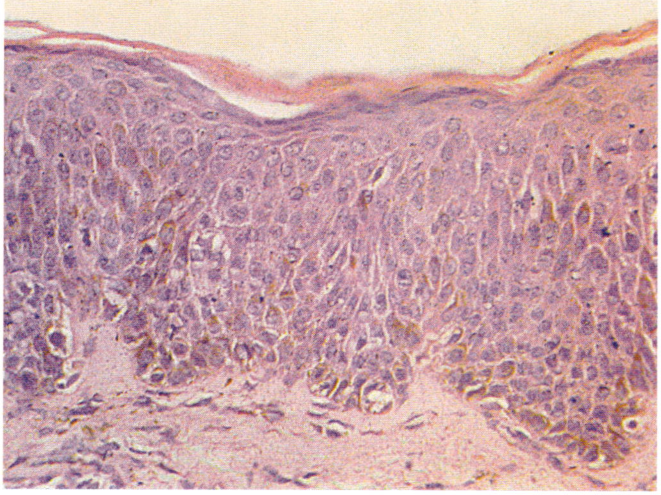

FIGURE 5.3.4.3

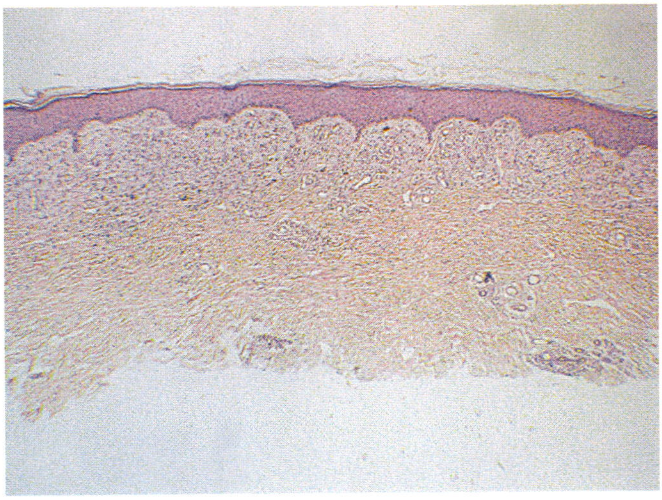

FIGURE 5.3.5.1

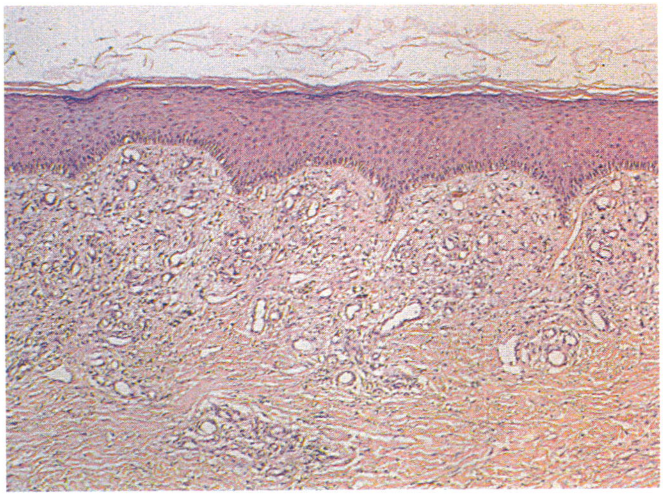

FIGURE 5.3.5.2

5.3.5: Stasis Dermatitis

5.3.5.1: The spongiosis is usually mild, may be associated with focal parakeratosis or scale crust (*Scanner view*)

5.3.5.2: Proliferation of small blood vessels in the papillary dermis (*Low power view*)

5.3.5.3: Minimum spongiosis (*High power view*)

5.3.5.4: Blood vessels and hemosiderin pigment in the dermis (*High power view*)

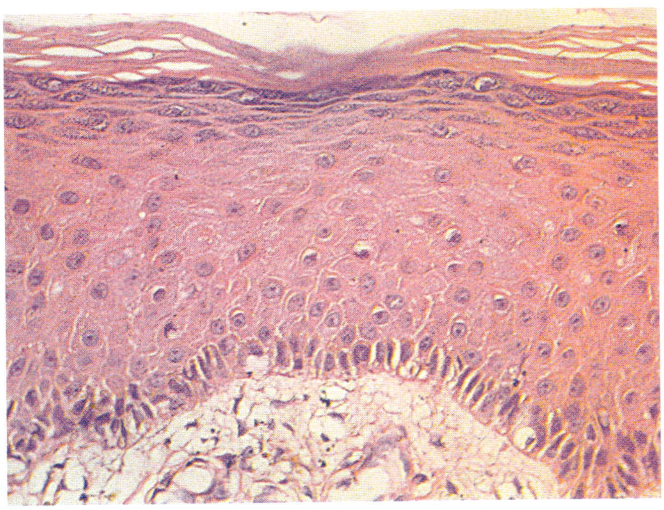

FIGURE 5.3.5.3

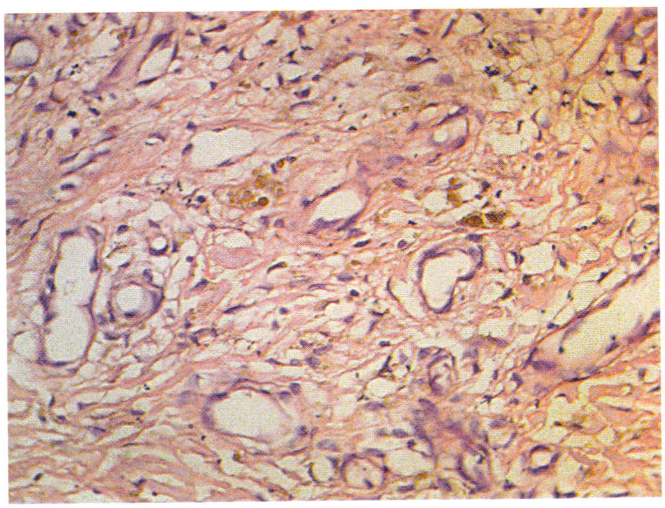

FIGURE 5.3.5.4

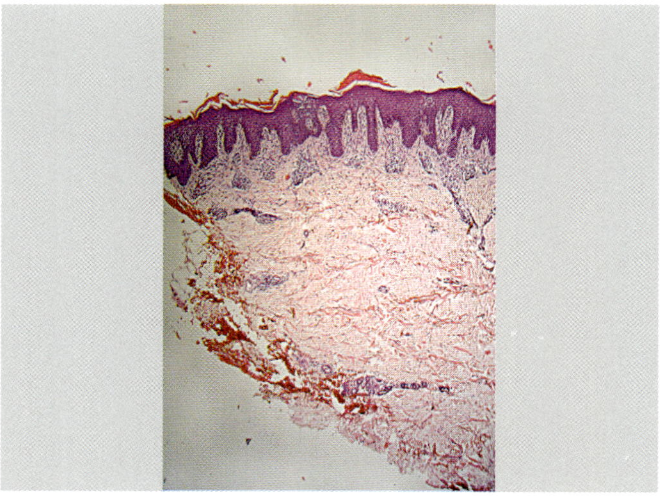

FIGURE 5.3.6.1

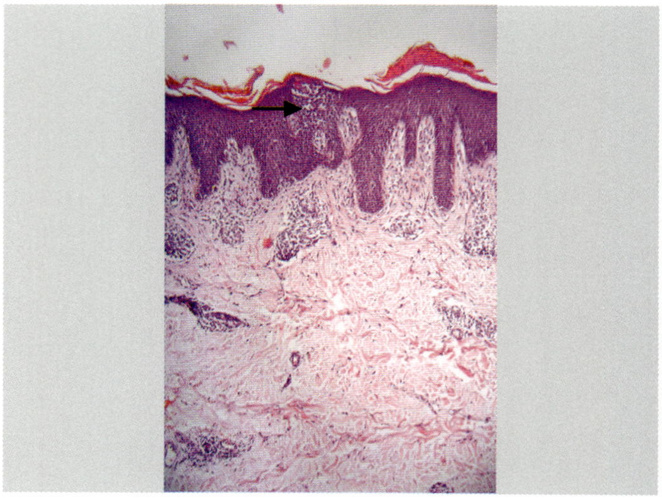

FIGURE 5.3.6.2

5.3.6: Pityriasis Rosea

5.3.6.1: Superficial perivascular infiltrate of lymphocytes, spongiosis and focal parakeratosis (*Scanner view*)

5.3.6.2: Hyperplasia of epidermis and focal spongiosis with exocytosis (*Low power view*)

5.3.6.3: Mounds of parakeratosis, diminished granular cell layer and extravasated erythrocyte (*High power view*)

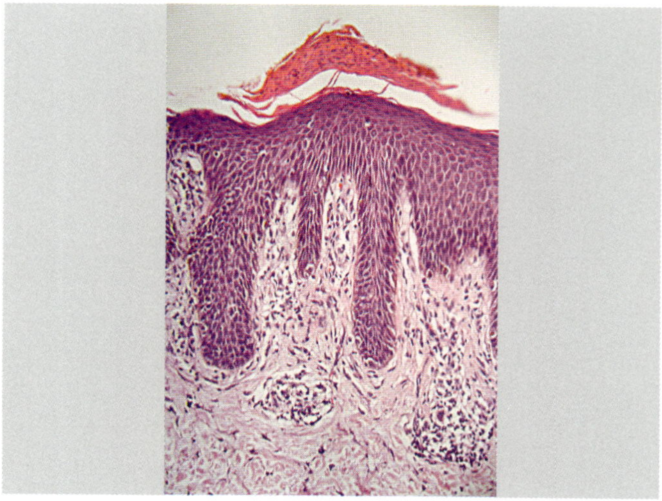

FIGURE 5.3.6.3

DIFFERENTIAL DIAGNOSIS

1. Eosinophilic spongiosis
   a. Pemphigus group
   b. Bullous pemphigoid and variants
   C. Atopic dermatitis
   d. Eosinophilic folliculitis (Ofuji's disease)
   e. Drug reactions
2. Neutrophilic spongiosis
   a. Pustular psoriasis
   b. Reiter's syndrome
   c. IgA pemphigus
   d. Palmoplantar pustulosis
   e. Glucagonoma syndrome
   f. Infantile acropustulosis
3. Other spongiotic disorders
   a. Miliaria
   b. Infundibulofolliculitis
   c. Autoeczematization
   d. Spongiotic drug reactions
   e. Autoimmune progesterone dermatitis
   f. Pruritic urticarial papules and plaques of pregnancy
   g. Blaschko dermatitis
   h. Grover's disease (spongiotic variant)
   i. Pityriasis alba
   j. Lichen striatus
   k. Erythroderma
   l. Polymorphic light eruption

DIAGNOSTIC PEARLS

1. Miliaria shows spongiosis, intraepidermal edema centered on the acrosyringium and lymphocytic infiltrate.
2. In infundibulofolliculitis, there is focal parakeratosis, follicular spongiosis with exocytosis of lymphocyte and mild inflammatory infiltrate in dermis.
3. Pityriasis rosea: Other features include small spongiotic vesicles and lymphocytic exocytosis similar to Pautrier microabscesses, dyskeratotic cells in epidermis.
4. Irritant contact dermatitis shows ballooning degeneration of keratinocytes, necrosis and presence of neutrophils.
5. Pityriasis alba shows mild epidermal spongiosis and focal parakeratosis.

Vesiculobullous Disorders

6

Chapter Outline

6.1: Subcorneal-intraepidermal Blisters
6.2: Suprabasal Blisters
6.3: Subepidermal Blisters with Minimum Inflammation
6.4: Subepidermal Blisters with Eosinophils
6.5: Subepidermal Blisters with Neutrophils

Pradeep Mahajan, Nathan Lee, Jerad Gardner, Smita Ghate, Atul Dongre, Uday Khopkar, Mohamad Buraik, Nandakumar Gopinath

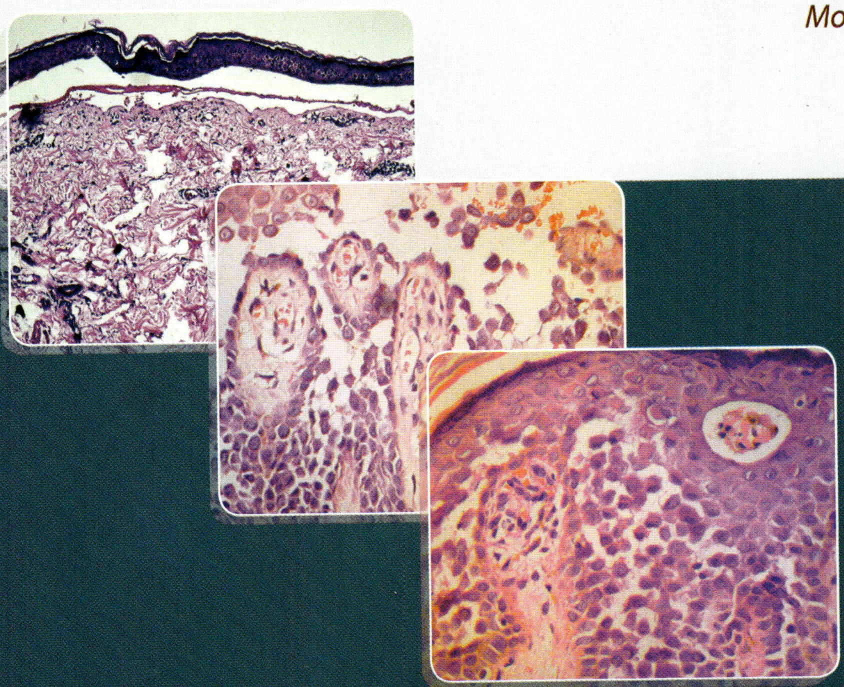

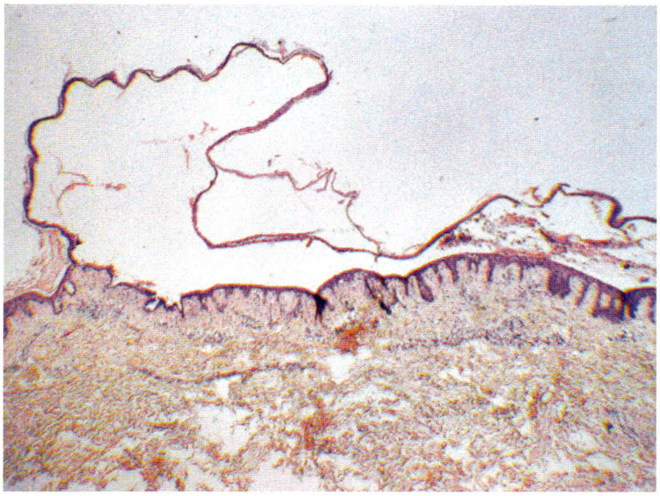

FIGURE 6.1.1.1

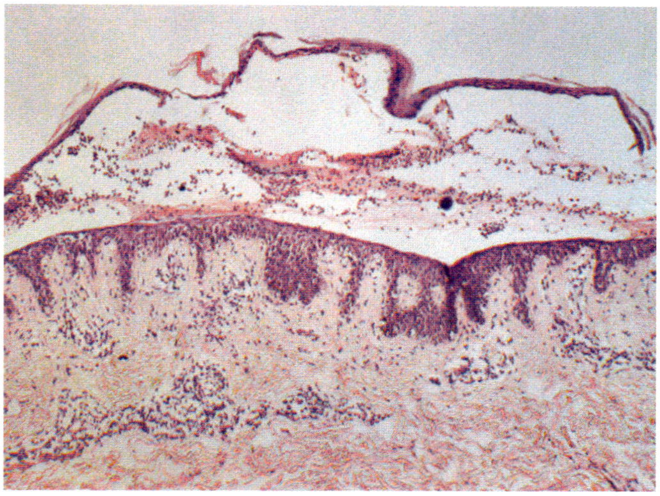

FIGURE 6.1.1.2

6.1: SUBCORNEAL-INTRAEPIDERMAL BLISTERS

6.1.1: Pemphigus Foliaceous

6.1.1.1: Subcorneal blister (*Scanner view*)

6.1.1.2: Fibrin and inflammatory infiltrate in the blister cavity (*Low power view*)

6.1.1.3: Acantholytic cells near the roof of the cavity (*High power view*)

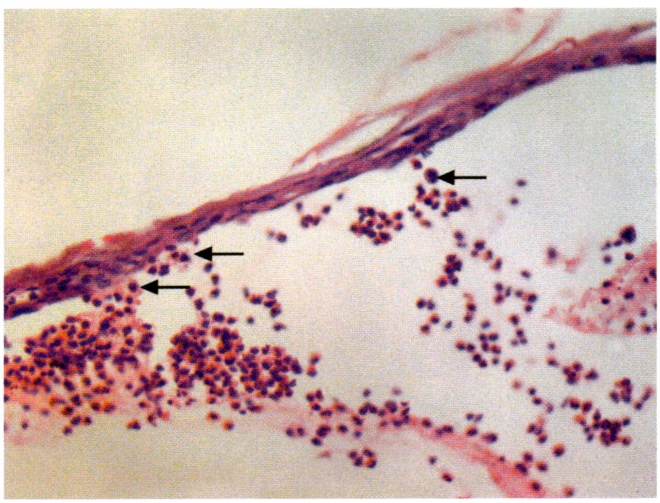

FIGURE 6.1.1.3

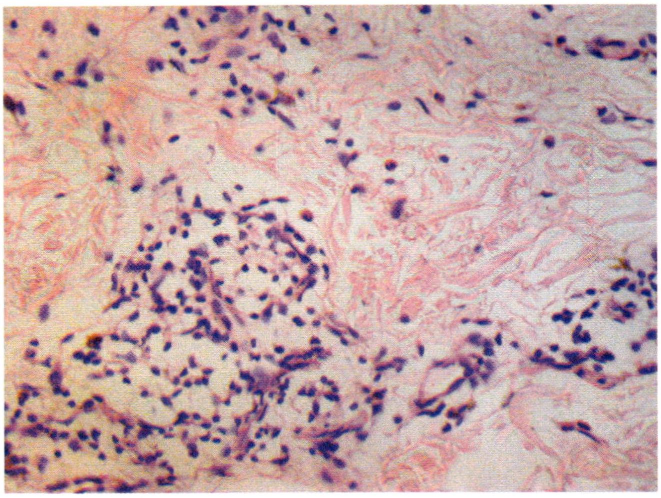

FIGURE 6 .1.1.4

6.1.1.4: Perivascular infiltrate with a few eosinophils in the dermis (*High power view*)

6.1.1.5: Floor of the blister with multiple epidermal layers (*High power view*)

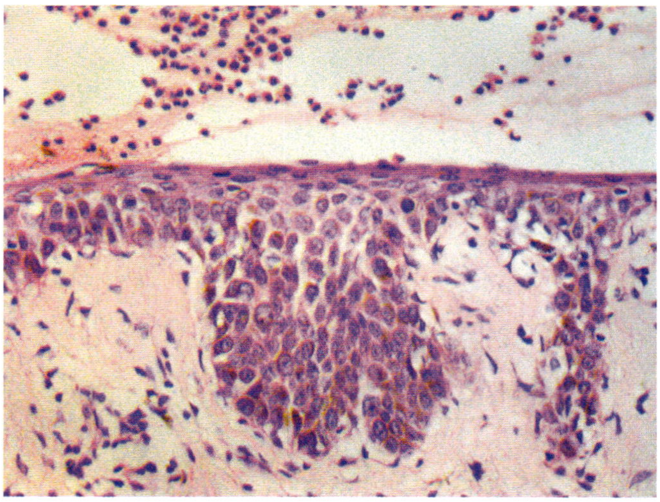

FIGURE 6 .1.1.5

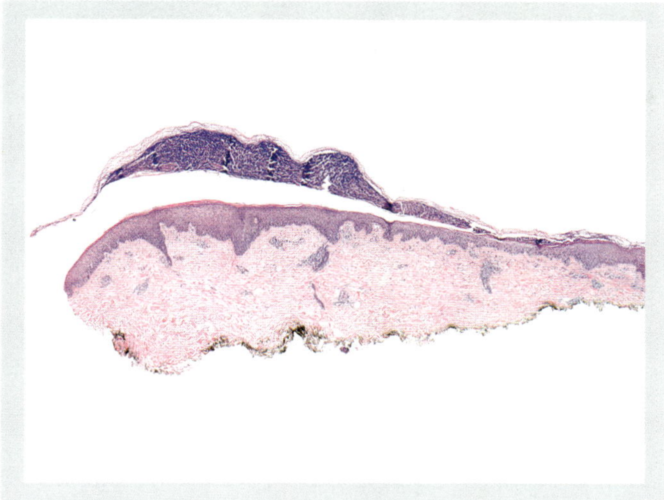

FIGURE 6.1.2.1

6.1.2: Subcorneal Pustular Dermatoses

6.1.2.1: The subcorneal pustule, normally does not lead to depression of the underlying epidermis (*Scanner view*)

6.1.2.2: Subcorneal neutrophils but no spongiform pustules involving upper epidermal layers or increased mitosis of basal cells as in pustular psoriasis (*High power view*)

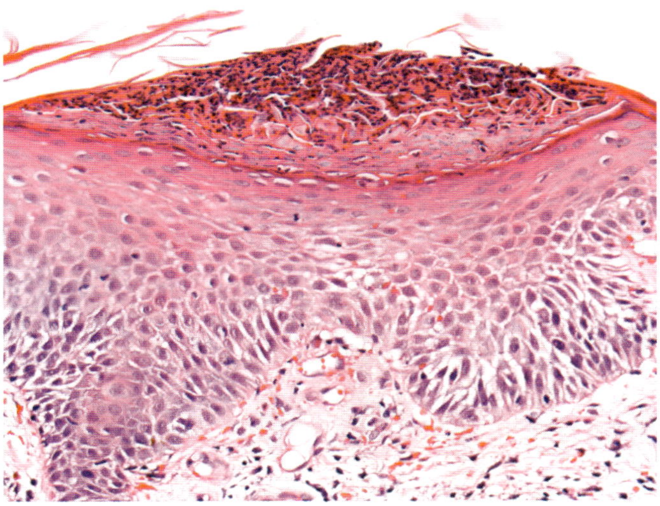

FIGURE 6.1.2.2

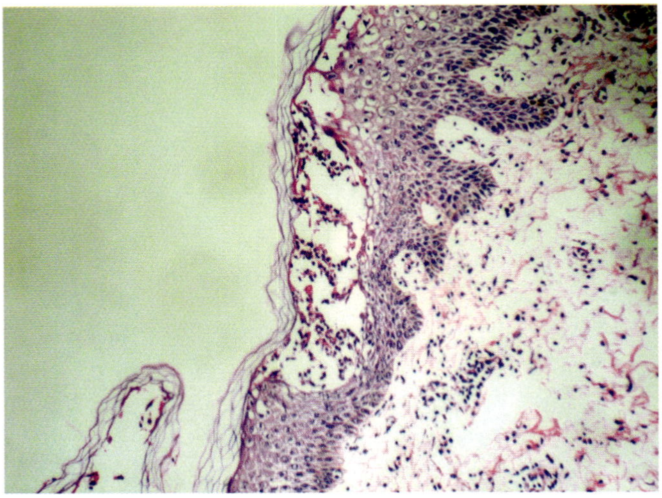

FIGURE 6.1.3.1

6.1.3: IgA Pemphigus

6.1.3.1: Subcorneal pustules with variable intraepidermal extension. Mild mixed inflammatory cell infiltrate in dermis (*Low power view*)

6.1.3.2: Subcorneal neutrophils, acantholytic cells and mild spongiosis in the epidermis (*High power view*)

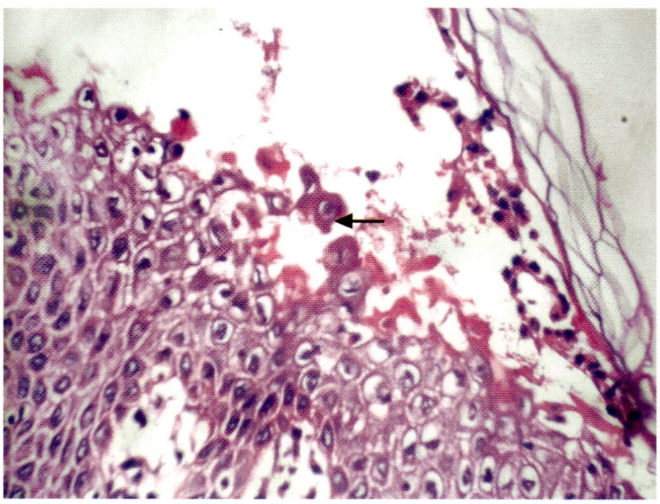

FIGURE 6.1.3.2

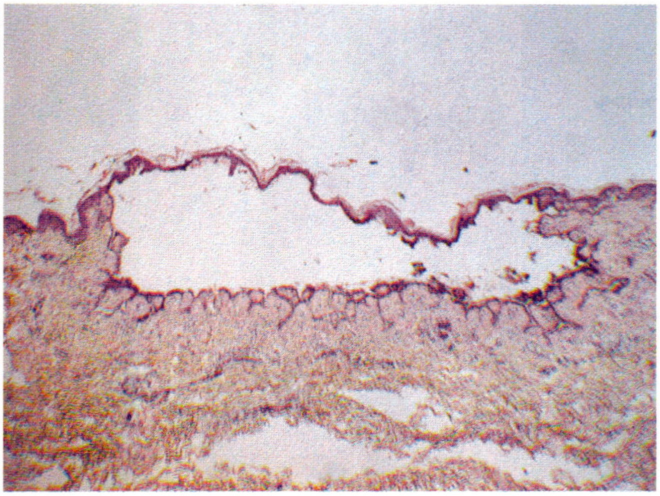

FIGURE 6.2.1.1

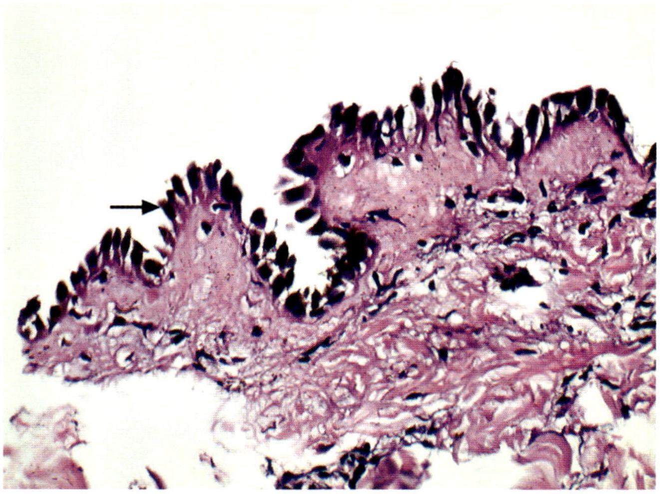

FIGURE 6.2.1.2

6.2: SUPRABASAL BLISTERS

6.2.1: Pemphigus Vulgaris

6.2.1.1: Suprabasal bulla with mild, superficial inflammatory infiltrate in the dermis composed of a few eosinophils (*Scanner view*)

6.2.1.2: Floor of the blister has single layer of basal cells separated from each other but attached to the dermis giving a 'tombstone appearance' (*High power view*)

6.2.1.3: The roof with multiple layers of epidermis and a few acantholytic cells (*High power view*)

6.2.1.4: Shows acantholytic cells and villi (villi are dermal papillae lined by single layer of basal cells cut across) (*High power view*)

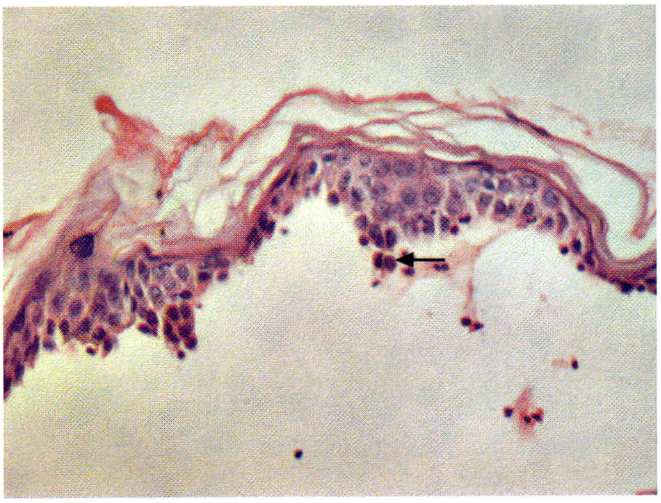

FIGURE 6.2.1.3

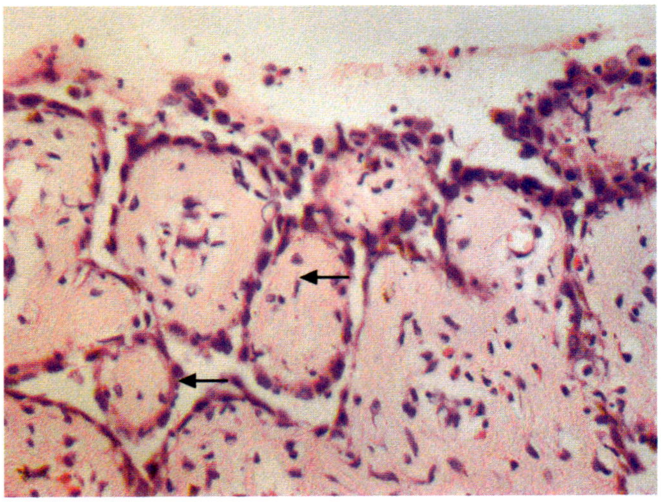

FIGURE 6.2.1.4

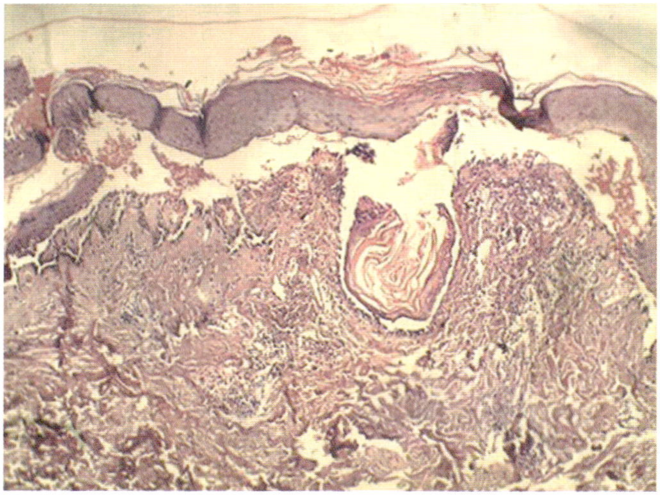

FIGURE 6.2.1.5

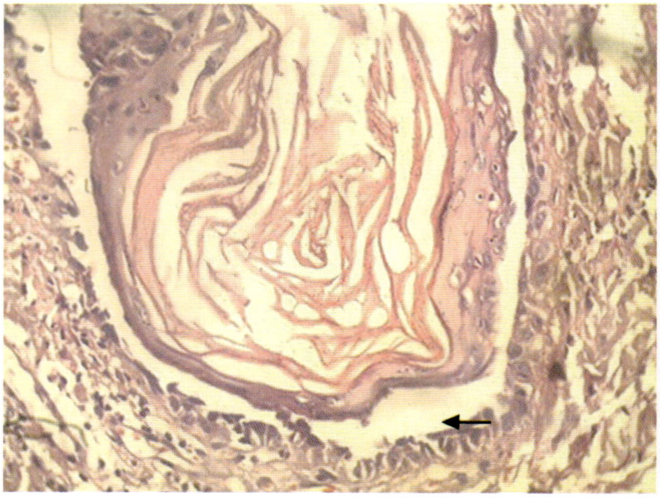

FIGURE 6.2.1.6

6.2.1.5: Suprabasal cleavage extends to the follicular epithelium (*Low power view*)

6.2.1.6: Closer view of hair cleavage (*High power view*)

6.2.1.7: Early suprabasal separation at the sides of the blister (shoulders). Blister cavity contains a few acantholytic cells, fibrin and eosinophils, and neutrophils (*Scanner view*)

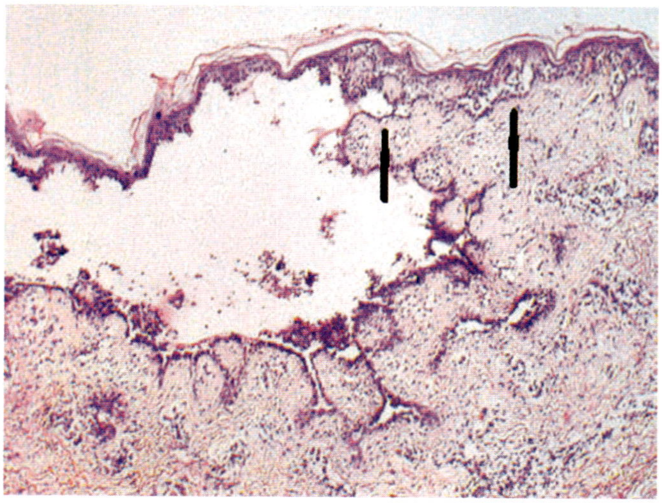

FIGURE 6.2.1.7

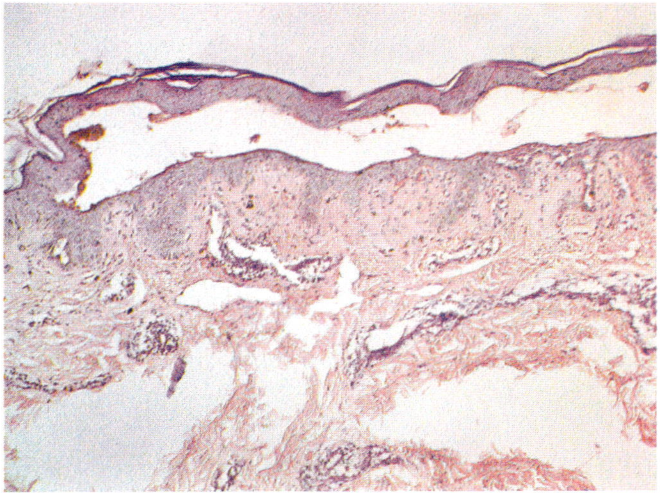

FIGURE 6.2.1.8

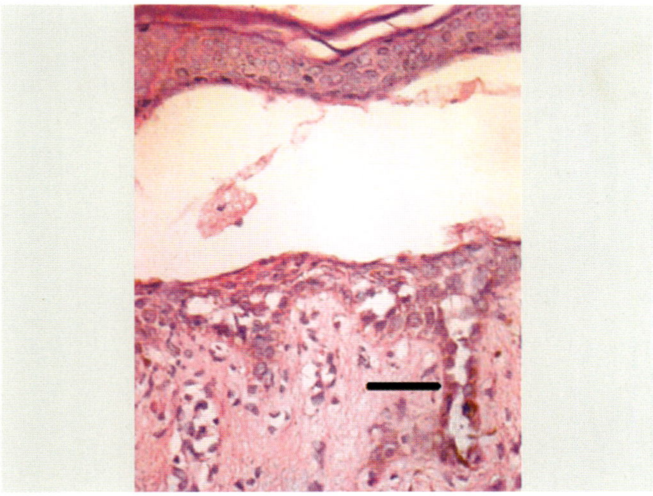

FIGURE 6.2.1.9

6.2.1.8: Old lesion of pemphigus with regeneration of the floor of the blister showing multiple layers of the epidermis (*Scanner view*)

6.2.1.9: Suprabasal cleavage still evident in the epidermis in the floor of the blister (*High power view*)

6.2.1.10: Mucosal pemphigus vulgaris-suprabasal cleavage, villi formation (*Low power view*)

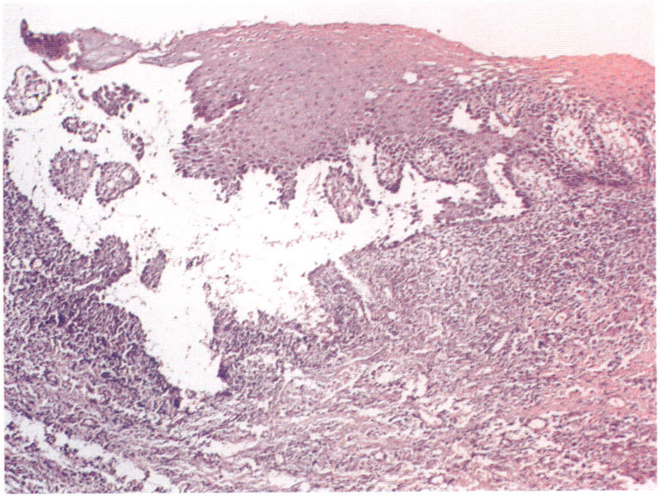

FIGURE 6.2.1.10

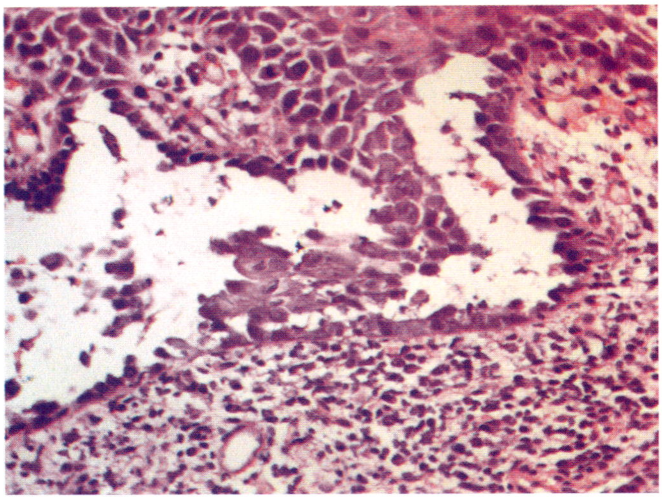

FIGURE 6.2.1.11

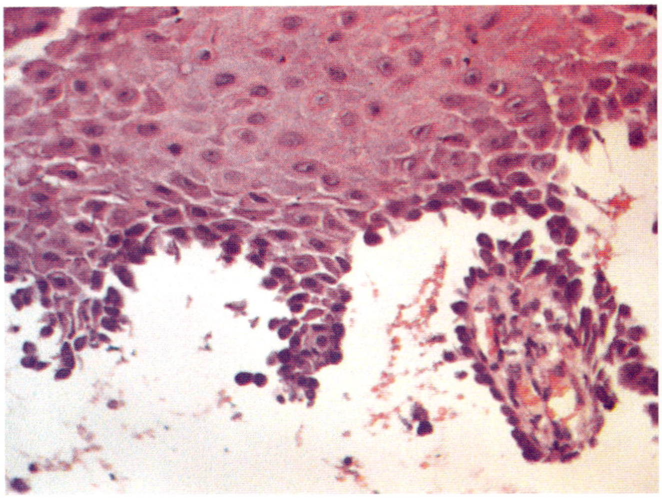

FIGURE 6.2.1.12

6.2.1.11: Floor of the blister has single layer of basal cells, acantholytic cells (*High power view*)

6.2.1.12: Multiple layers of the epithelium in the roof, acantholytic cells, villi formation (*High power view*)

6.2.1.13: Direct immunofluorescence (DIF) shows a fish-net pattern of IgG deposition (*Direct immunofluorescence*)

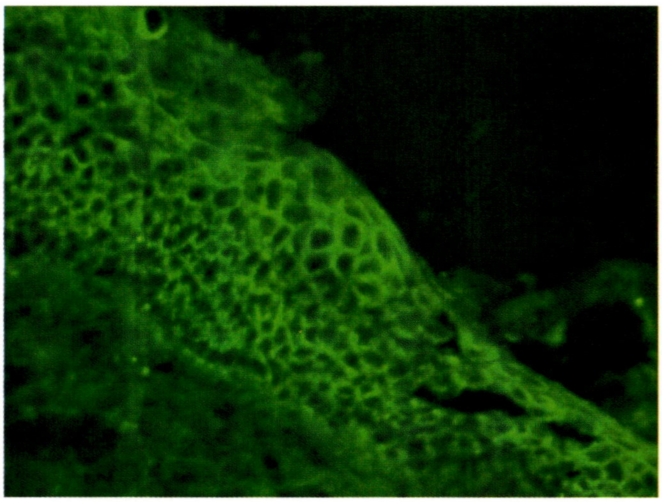

FIGURE 6.2.1.13

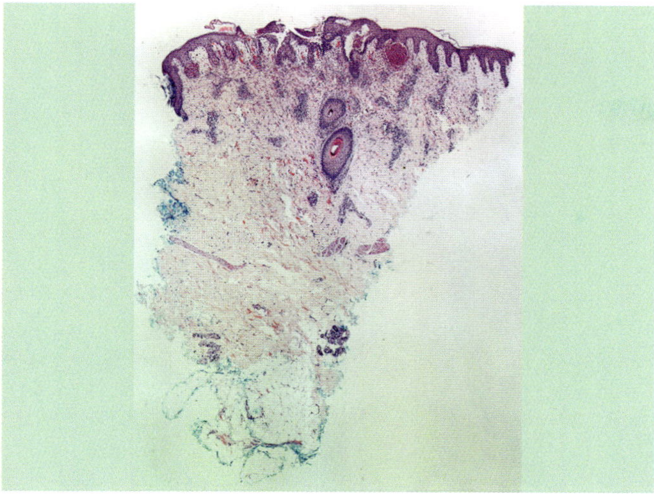

FIGURE 6.2.2.1

6.2.2: Pemphigus Vegetans

6.2.2.1: Pseudoepitheliomatous hyperplasia (often much more pronounced than seen in this example). Upper dermis has infiltrate of lymphocytes and eosinophils (*Scanner view*)

6.2.2.2: Aggregates of eosinophils (eosinophilic microabscesses) within the epidermis and follicular units are common histologic clues. Acantholysis is usually focal so that only a few acantholytic cells and small suprabasal lacunae may be present (*Low power view*)

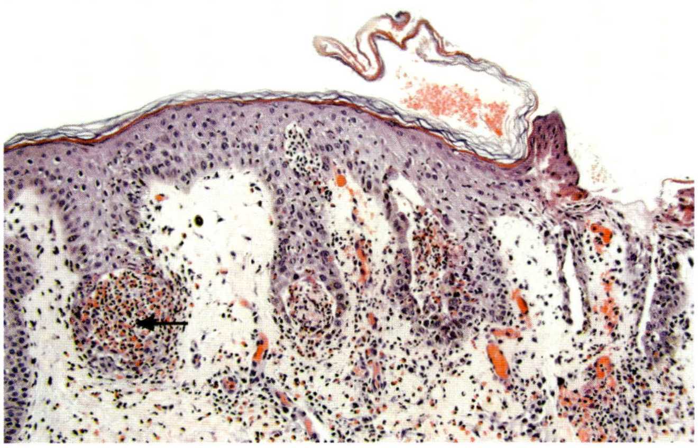

FIGURE 6.2.2.2

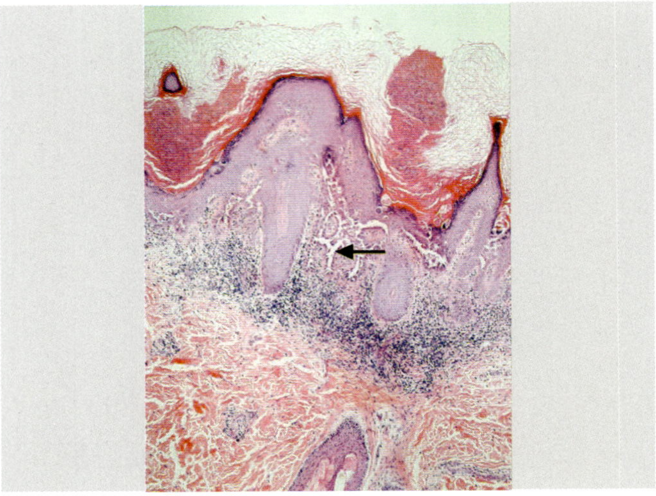

FIGURE 6.2.3.1

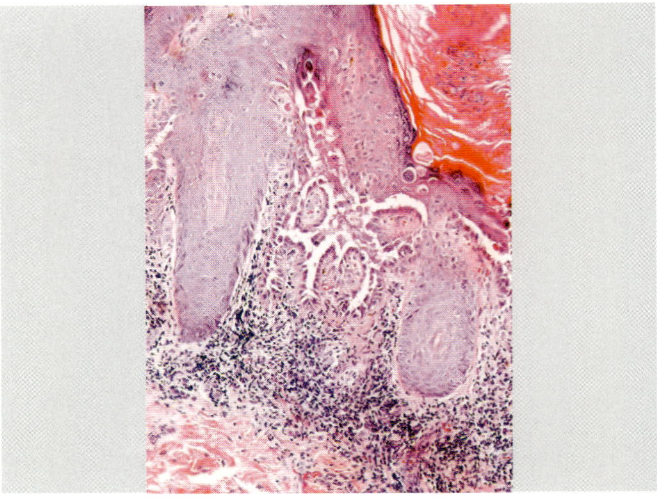

FIGURE 6.2.3.2

6.2.3: Darier's Disease

6.2.3.1: Papillomatosis with suprabasilar clefting and villi formation (*Scanner view*)

6.2.3.2: A few acantholytic cells in the cleft and dyskeratotic cells in the form of corps ronds in the upper epidermis (*Low power view*)

6.2.3.3: Closer view of the same (*High power view*)

6.2.3.4: Another view of dyskeratotic cells in the form of corps ronds and grains and acantholytic cells (*High power view*)

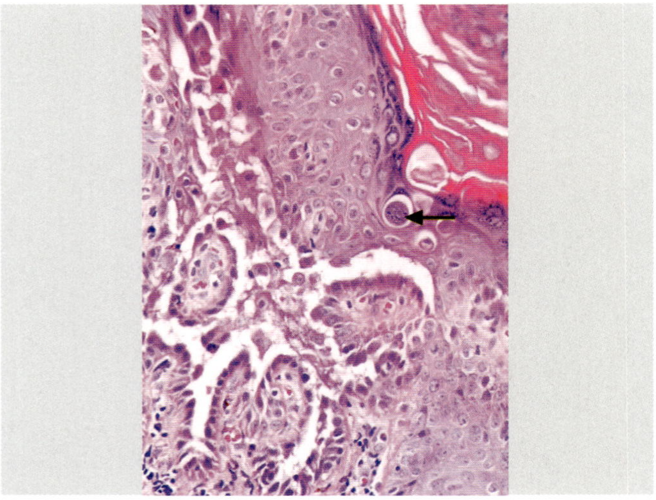

FIGURE 6.2.3.3

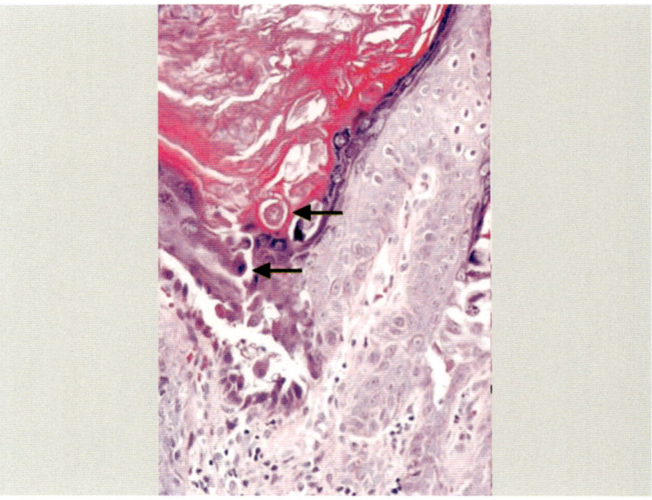

FIGURE 6.2.3.4

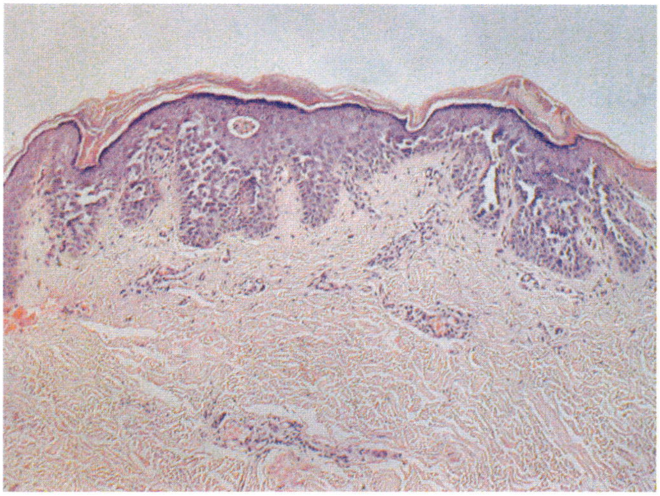

FIGURE 6.2.4.1

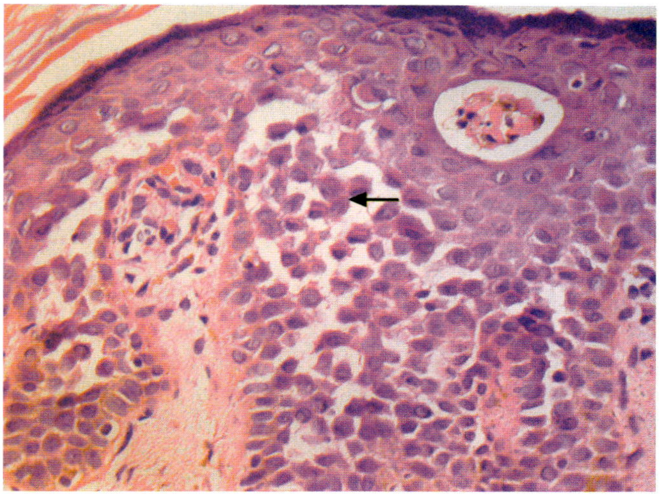

FIGURE 6.2.4.2

6.2.4: Familial Benign Pemphigus (Hailey Hailey Disease)

6.2.4.1: Suprabasal cleft with acantholytic cells (*Low power view*)

6.2.4.2: Extensive acantholysis involving many layers of the epidermis giving an appearance of 'dilapidated brick wall' (*High power view*)

6.2.4.3: Another section with acantholytic cells lining the cavity and within the cavity (*Low power view*)

6.2.4.4: Suprabasal separation, villi formation and widespread acantholysis (*High power view*)

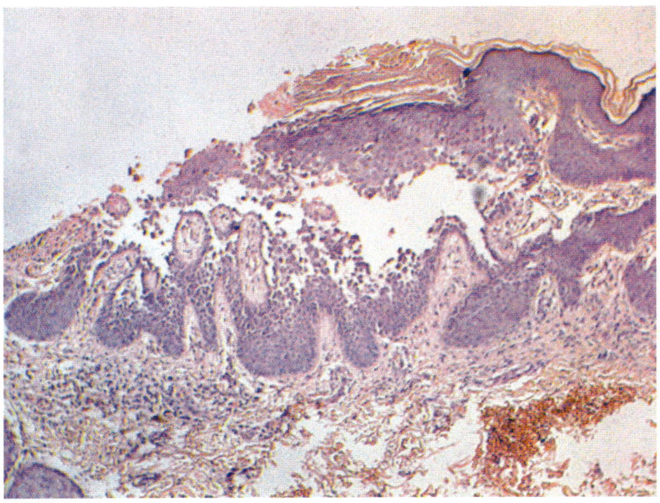

FIGURE 6.2.4.3

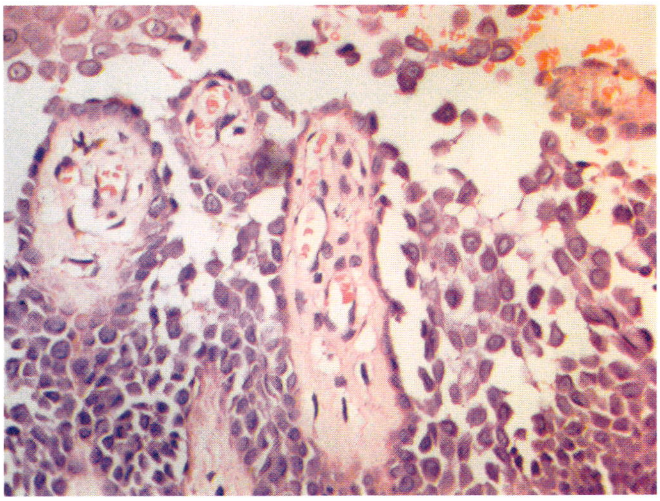

FIGURE 6.2.4.4

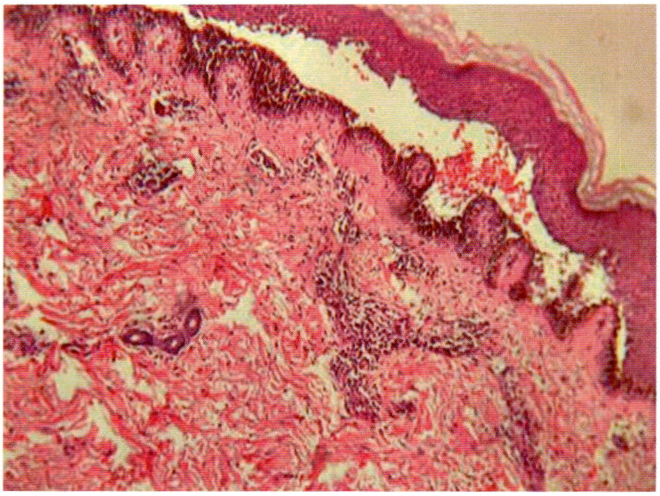

FIGURE 6.2.5.1

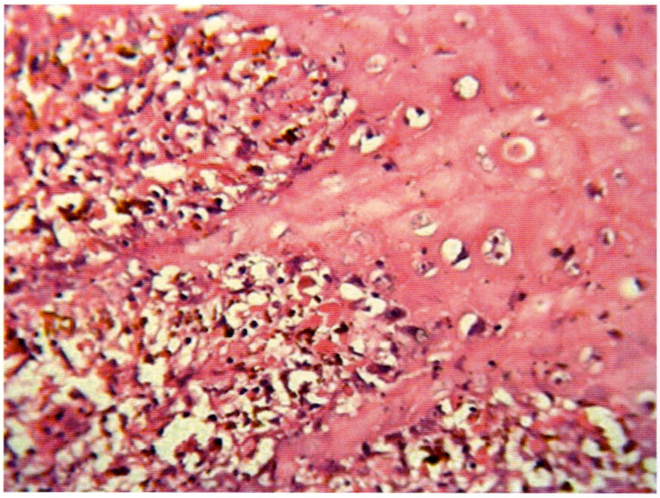

FIGURE 6.2.5.2

6.2.5: Paraneoplastic Pemphigus (PNP)

6.2.5.1: Acantholysis, suprabasal cleft, tombstone appearance (pemphigus like features) (*Low power view*)

6.2.5.2: Lichenoid dermatitis with necrotic keratinocytes (EM like features) (*High power view*)

6.2.5.3: DIF—staining with IgG—fishnet pattern like pemphigus (*Direct immunofluorescence*)

6.2.5.4: DIF—staining with C3—linear DEJ positivity of PNP (*Direct immunofluorescence*)

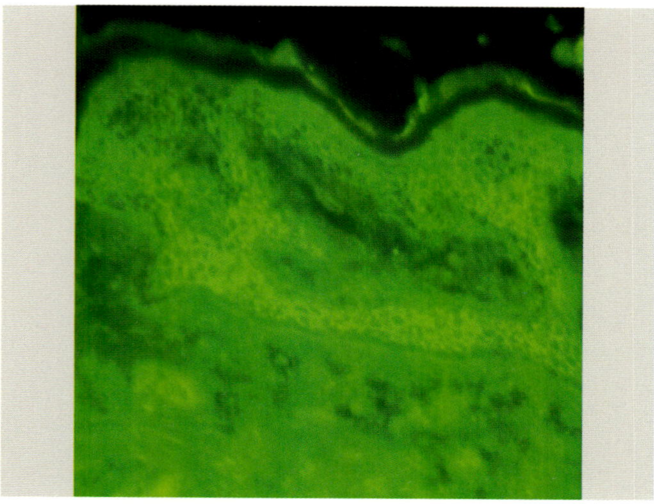

FIGURE 6.2.5.3

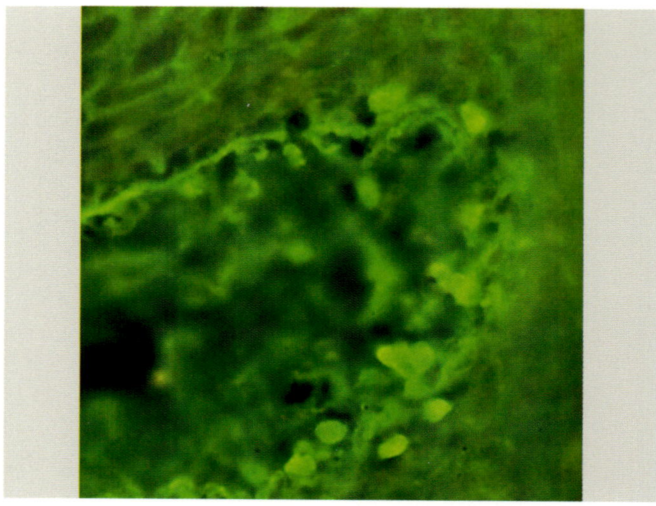

FIGURE 6.2.5.4

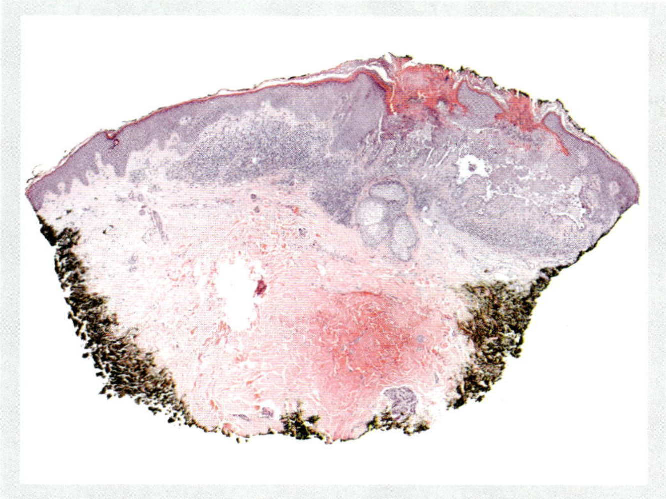

FIGURE 6.2.6.1

6.2.6: Grover's Disease

6.2.6.1: Acantholysis with dyskeratosis (corps ronds and grains). Intraepidermal vesicle formation may be seen. There is typically a mixed inflammatory infiltrate in the superficial dermis beneath the lesion, and eosinophils are often present (*Scanner view*)

6.2.6.2: The changes in Grover's disease are usually limited to a few rete ridges. Histologic mimics include other acantholytic and/or dyskeratotic diseases: Darier's disease, Hailey-Hailey disease, warty dyskeratoma, spongiotic dermatoses and pemphigus vulgaris (*Low power view*)

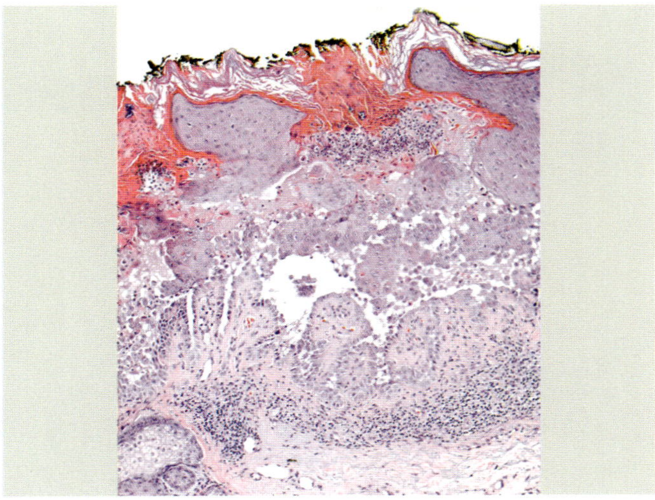

FIGURE 6.2.6.2

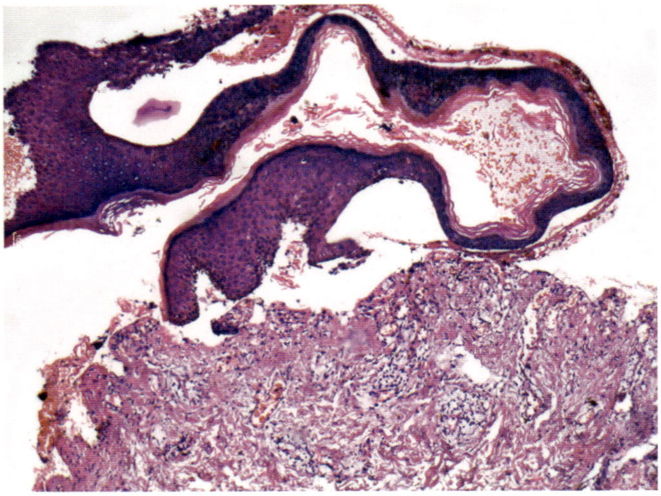

FIGURE 6.3.1.1

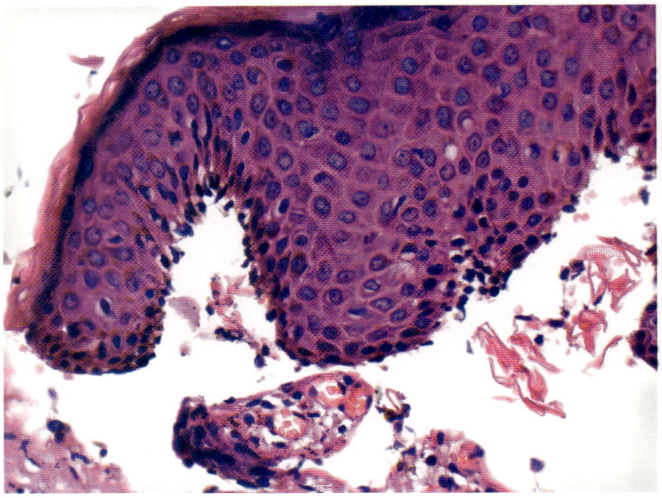

FIGURE 6.3.1.2

6.3: SUBEPIDERMAL BLISTERS WITH MINIMUM INFLAMMATION

6.3.1: Epidermolysis Bullosa

6.3.1.1: Epidermolysis bullosa simplex on light microscopy appears cell-poor subepidermal blister as the separation is very low in the epidermis (*Low power view*)

6.3.1.2: Fragments of basal keratinocytes are seen with H & E stain (when stained with PAS basement membrane is seen at the floor) (*High power view*)

6.3.1.3: The junctional forms also show subepidermal, cell-poor blister (*Low power view*)

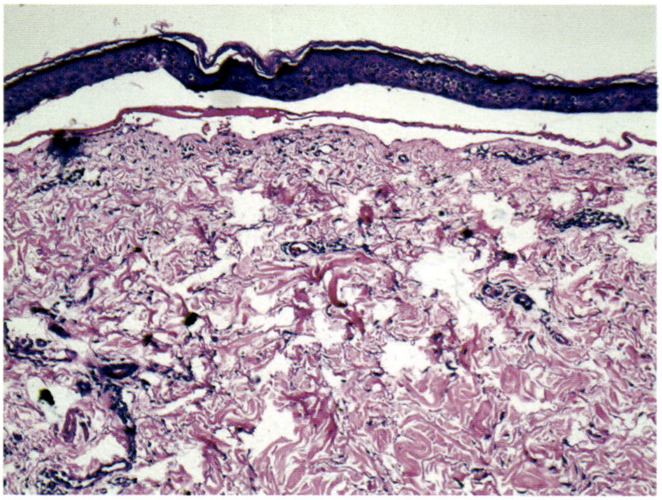

FIGURE 6.3.1.3

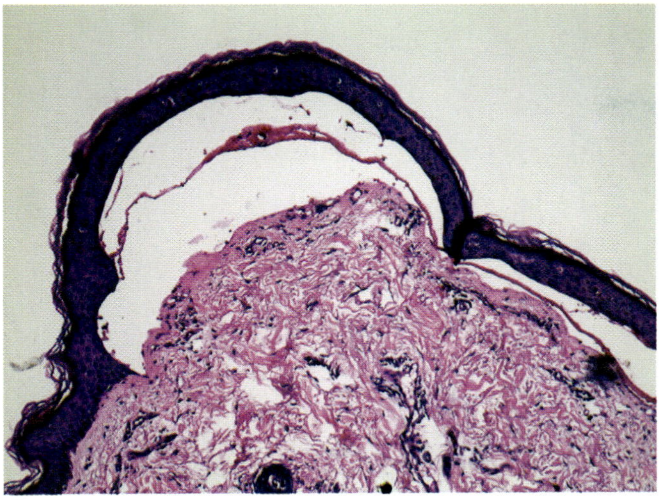

FIGURE 6.3.1.4

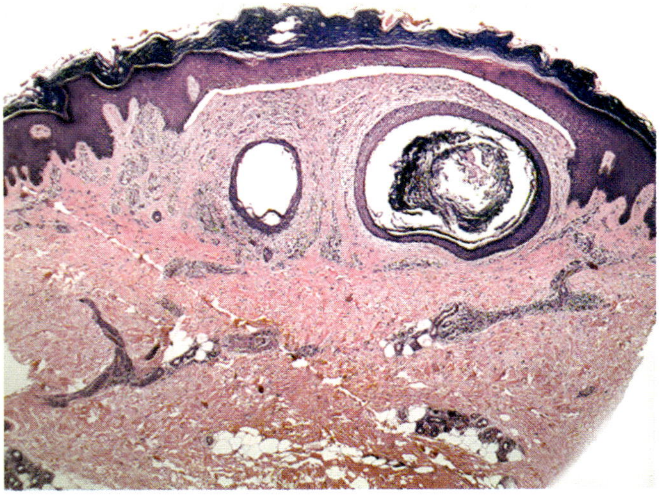

FIGURE 6.3.1.5

6.3.1.4: Another view stained with H & E (when stained with PAS basement membrane usually shows a split) (*Low power view*)

6.3.1.5: Dystrophic (dermolytic) forms of epidermolysis bullosa again show cell poor, subepidermal blister (*Scanner view*)

6.3.1.6: Dermal fibrosis and milia formation (when stained with PAS basement membrane in the roof of the blister) (*Low power view*)

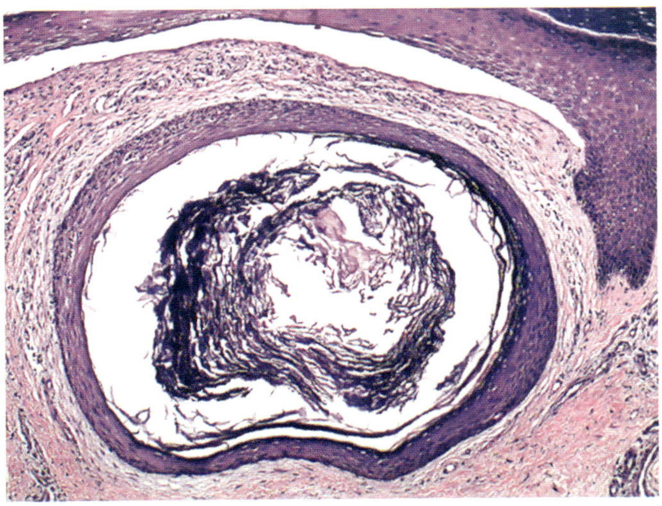

FIGURE 6.3.1.6

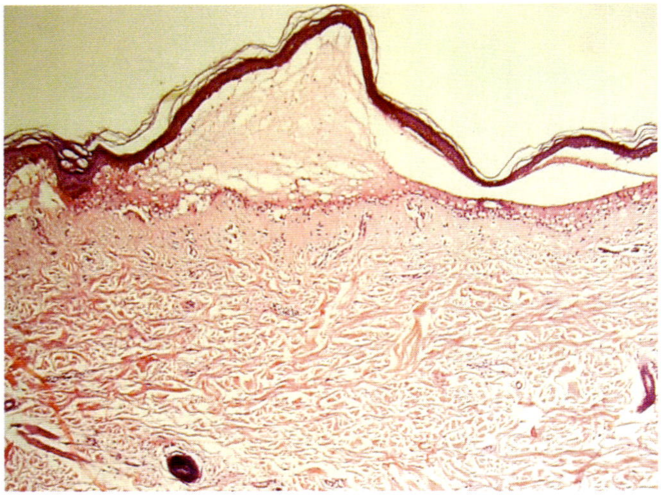

FIGURE 6.3.2.1

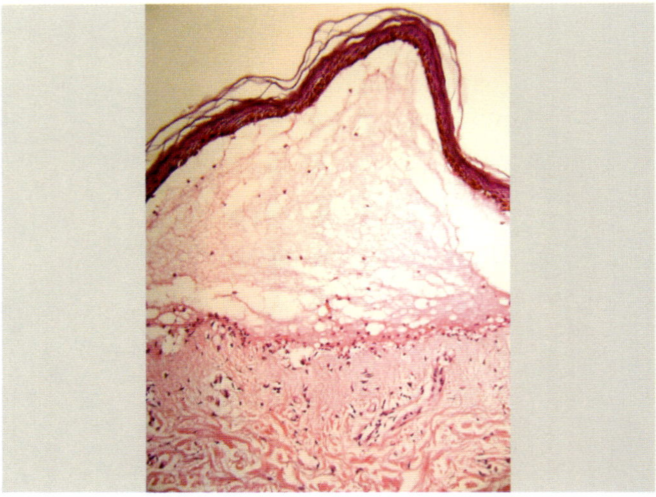

FIGURE 6.3.2.2

6.3.2: Epidermolysis Bullosa Acquisita

6.3.2.1: Subepidermal bulla with blister cavity containing fibrin and a few inflammatory cells (*Scanner view*)

6.3.2.2: Superficial perivascular lymphocytes and neutrophils (*Low power view*)

6.3.2.3: Dermal fragments seen attached to the epidermis (*High power view*)

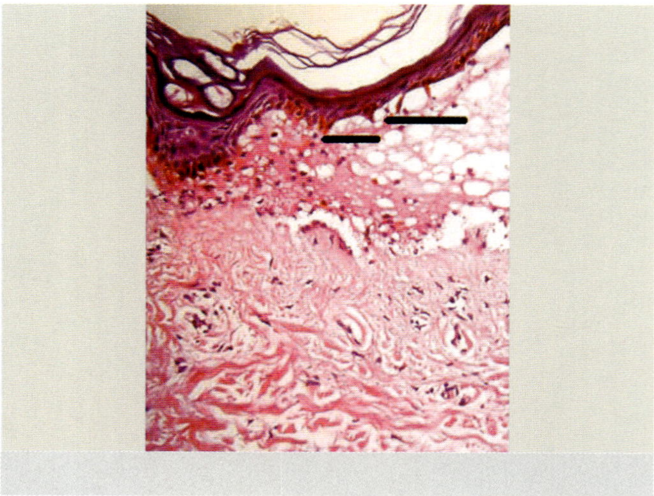

FIGURE 6.3.2.3

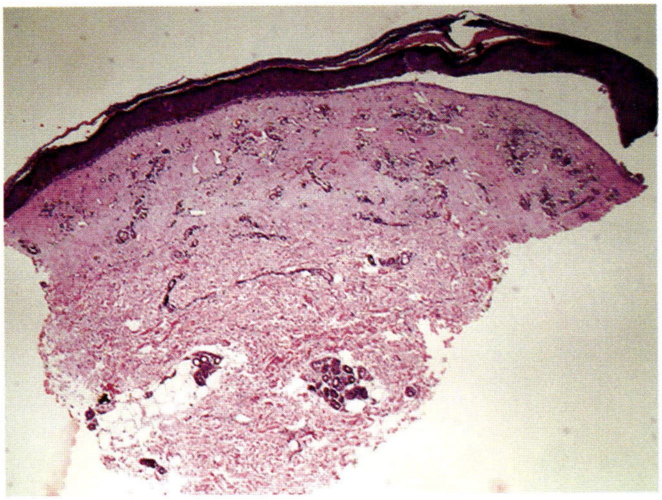

FIGURE 6.3.2.4

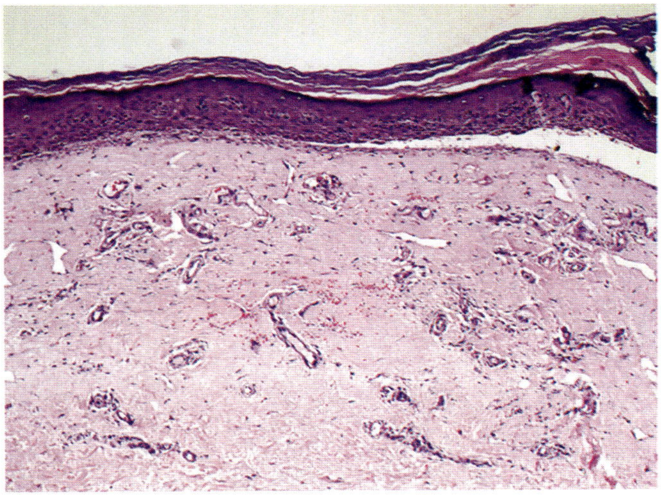

FIGURE 6.3.2.5

6.3.2.4: Another case with subepidermal separation with sparse inflammation (*Scanner view*)

6.3.2.5: Older lesions show dilated capillaries and dermal fibrosis (*Low power view*)

6.3.2.6: Difficult to differentiate from cell poor bullous pemphigoid by routine microscopy or PAS stain or DIF (split-skin immunofluorescence is helpful) (*High power view*)

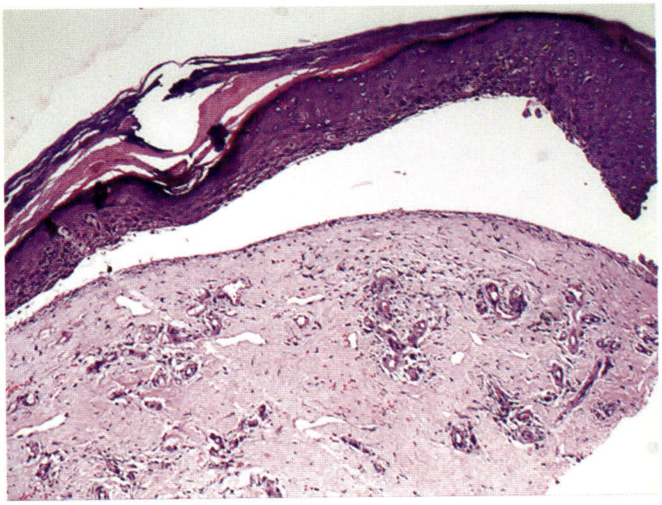

FIGURE 6.3.2.6

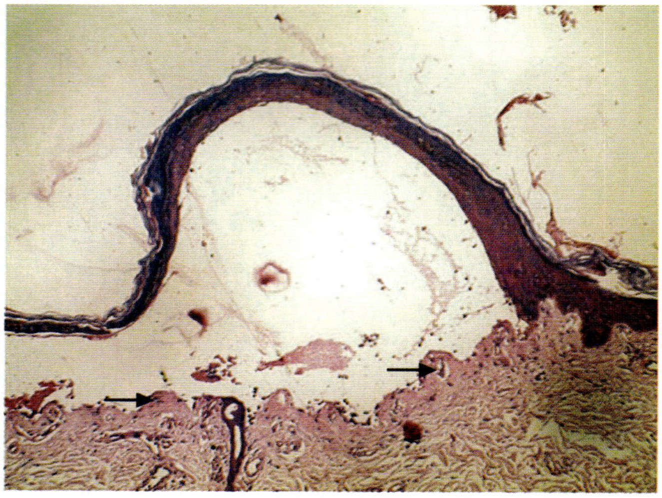

FIGURE 6.3.3.1

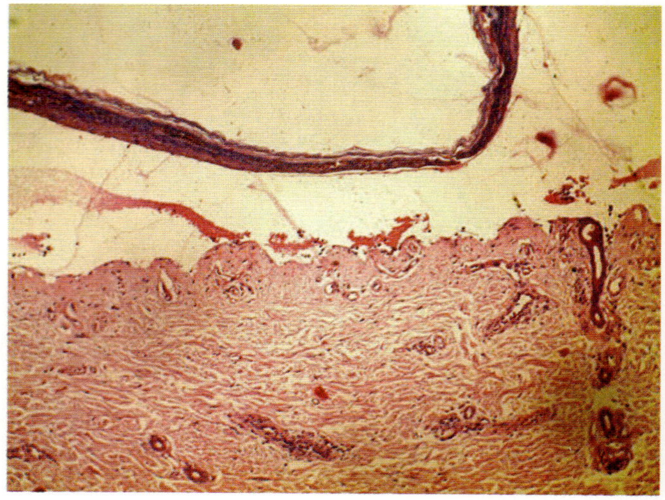

FIGURE 6.3.3.2

6.3.3: Porphyria Cutanea Tarda

6.3.3.1: Subepidermal blister showing preserved dermal papillae in the floor of the lesion referred to as festooning (*Scanner view*)

6.3.3.2: No inflammatory infiltrate (*Scanner view*)

6.3.3.3: PAS positive hyaline material in the walls of vessels in the upper dermis (*Scanner view*)

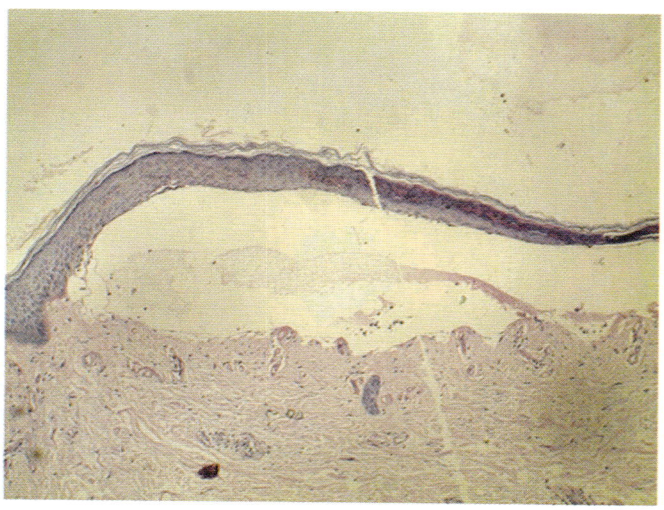

FIGURE 6.3.3.3

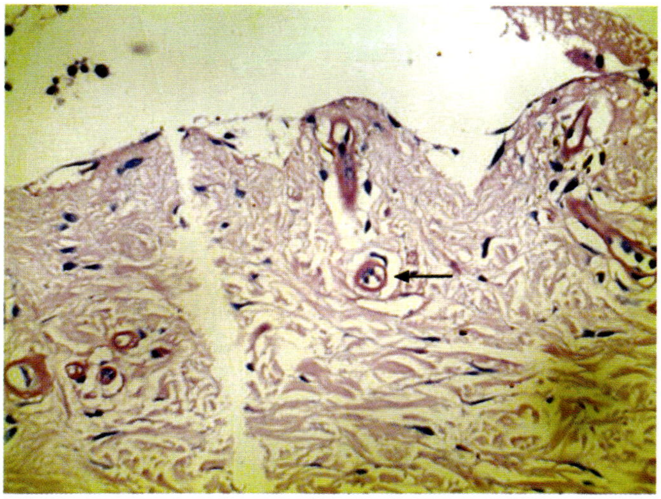

FIGURE 6.3.3.4

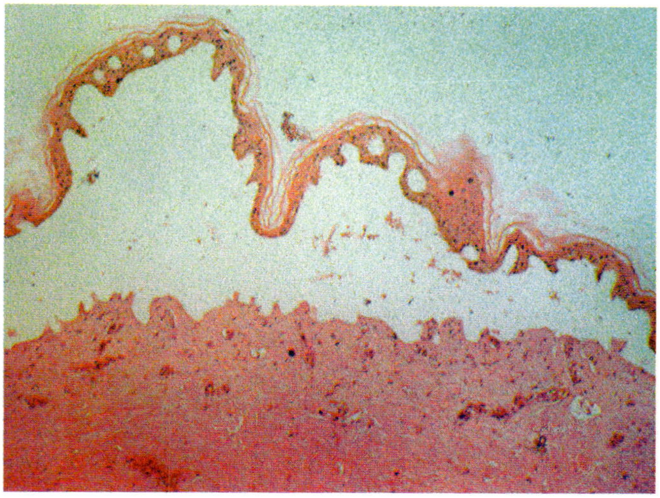

FIGURE 6.3.3.5

6.3.3.4: Higher magnification of PAS stain, the basement membrane may also show staining (*High power view*)

6.3.3.5: Another case, routine H & E stain, epidermal changes coinciding with dermal festooning (*Scanner view*)

6.3.3.6: Closer view of festooning (*High power view*)

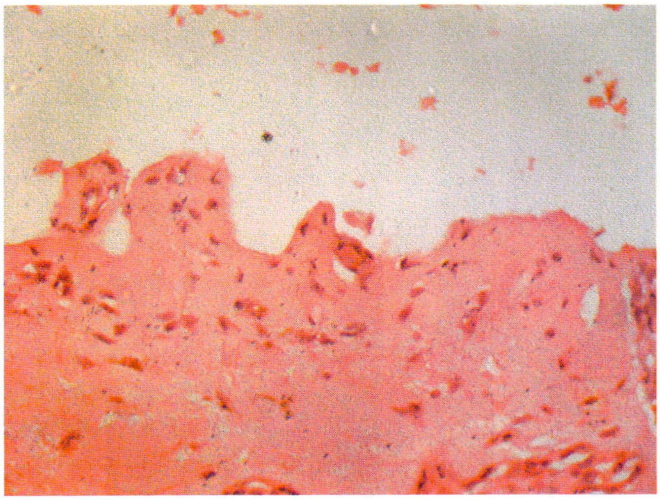

FIGURE 6.3.3.6

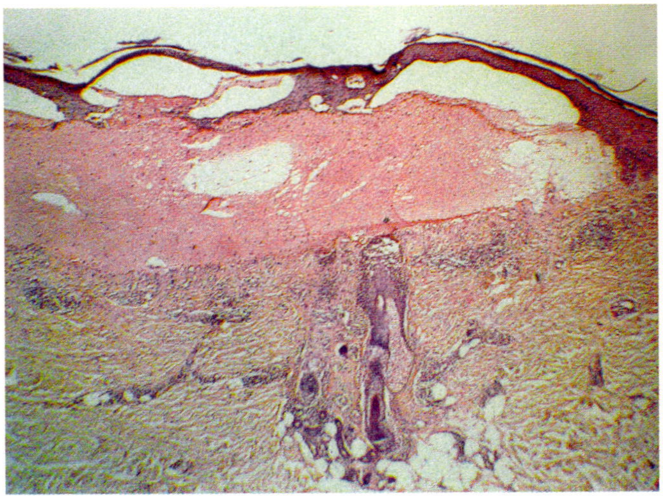

FIGURE 6.4.1.1

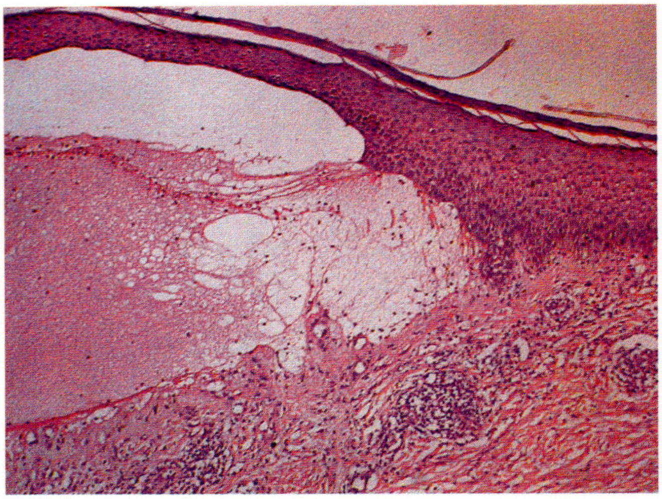

FIGURE 6.4.1.2

6.4: SUBEPIDERMAL BLISTERS WITH EOSINOPHILS

6.4.1: Bullous Pemphigoid

6.4.1.1: Unilocular subepidermal blister with fibrin and inflammatory infiltrate (*Scanner view*)

6.4.1.2: Moderately dense infiltrate in bullae with an erythematous base clinically (cell rich) (*Low power view*)

6.4.1.3: Roof of the blister with all the epidermal layers including pigmented basal cell layer (*High power view*)

6.4.1.4: The dermis is in the floor (*High power view*)

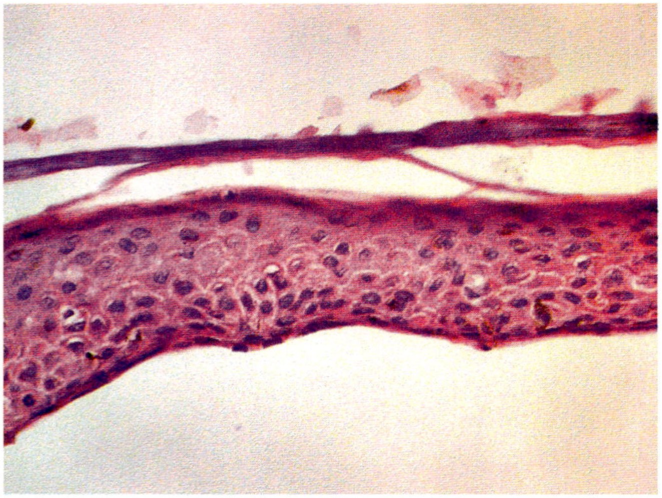

FIGURE 6.4.1.3

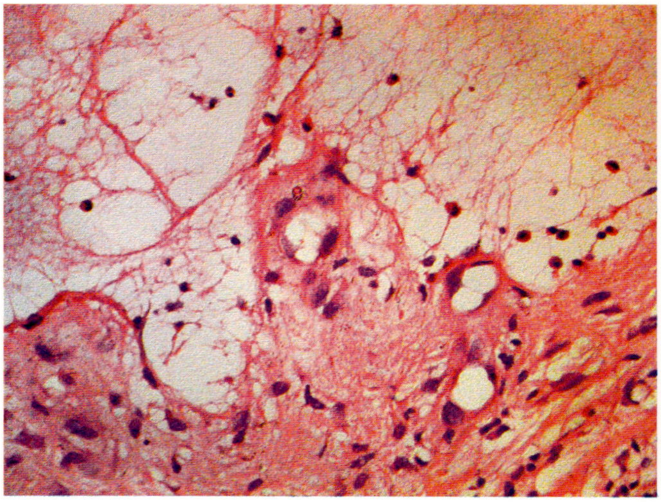

FIGURE 6.4.1.4

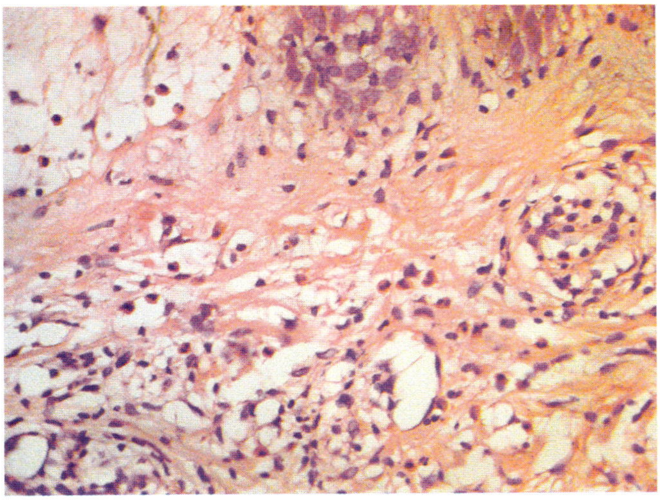

FIGURE 6.4.1.5

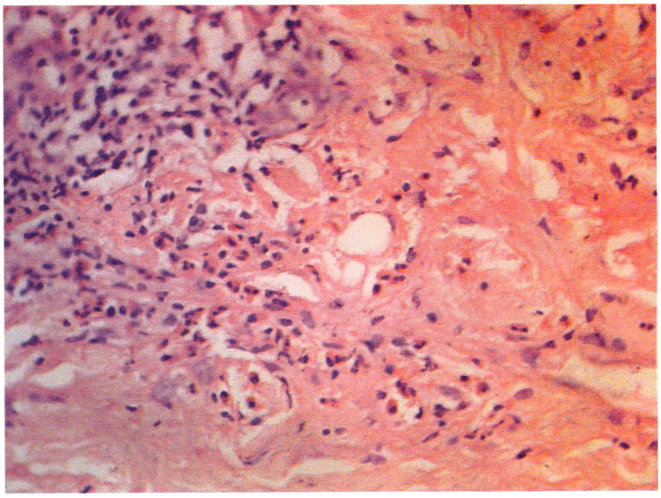

FIGURE 6.4.1.6

6.4.1.5: In addition to eosinophils, there are some neutrophils and lymphocytes (*High power view*)

6.4.1.6: Eosinophils predominate both in the blister cavity and in the dermis (*High power view*)

6.4.1.7: DIF showing IgG and/or C3 deposits at the dermoepidermal junction (*Direct immunofluorescence*)

6.4.1.8: Biopsy from a bulla on clinically normal appearing skin shows only sparse dermal infiltrate (cell poor) (*Scanner view*)

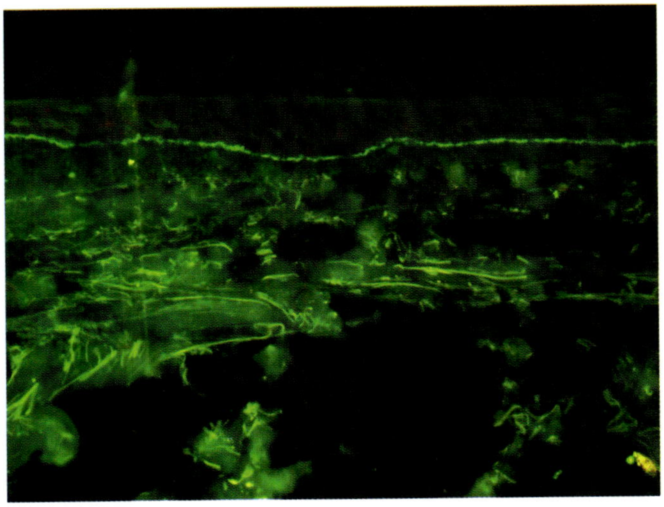

FIGURE 6.4.1.7

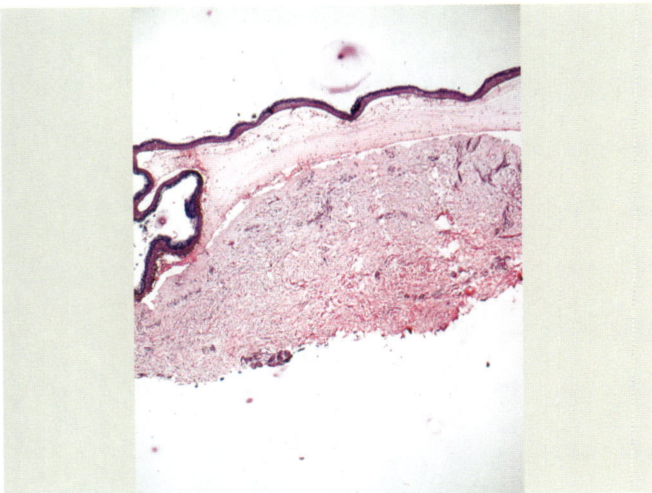

FIGURE 6.4.1.8

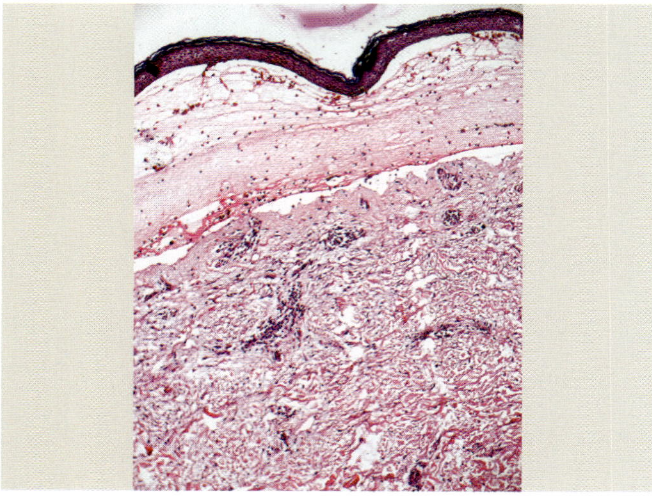

FIGURE 6.4.1.9

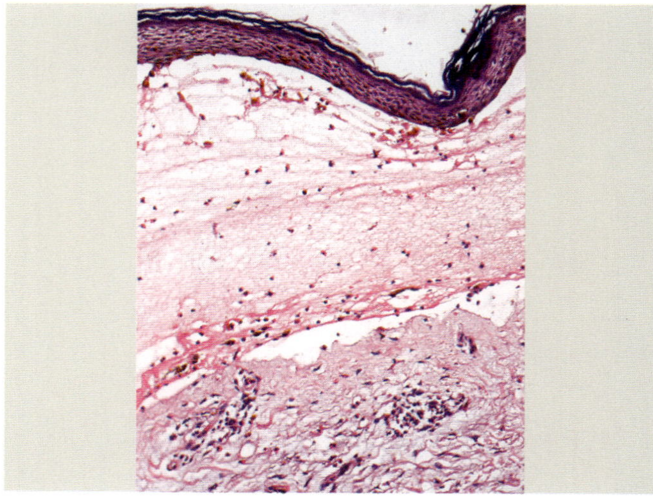

FIGURE 6.4.1.10

6.4.1.9: Closer view of minimum inflammatory infiltrate (*Low power view*)

6.4.1.10: Still eosinophils predominate (*Low power view*)

6.4.1.11: Eosinophilic spongiosis seen in the clinically erythematous skin surrounding the blister or an urticarial lesion, eosinophils line the basement membrane and a few individual eosinophils extend to the epidermis (*High power view*)

6.4.1.12: Older lesion of bullous pemphigoid with regeneration of the floor of the blister (*Scanner view*)

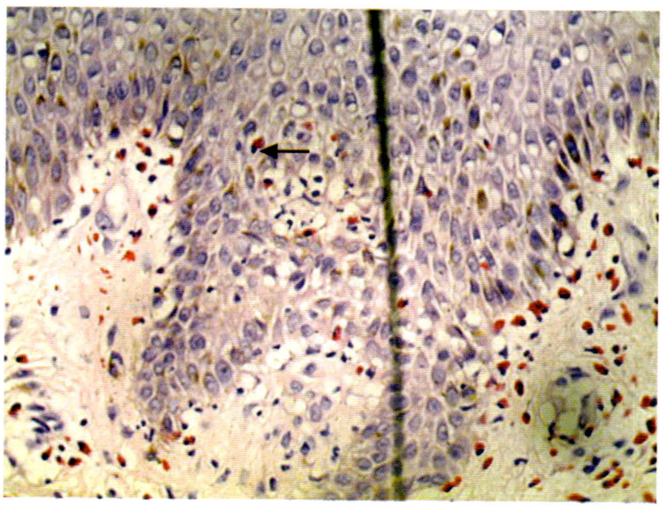

FIGURE 6.4.1.11

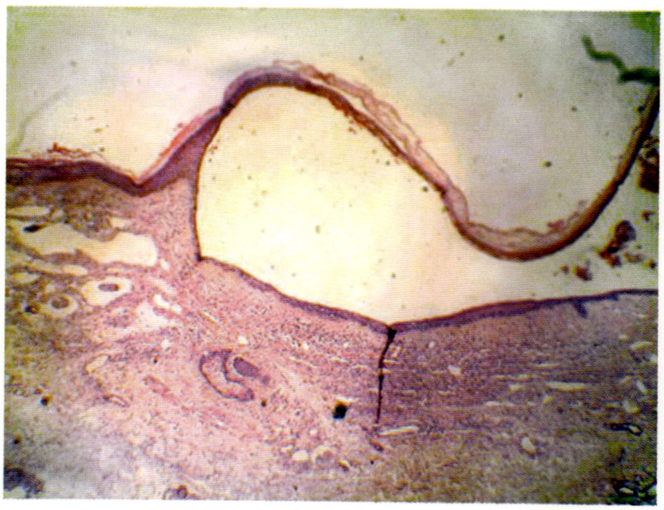

FIGURE 6.4.1.12

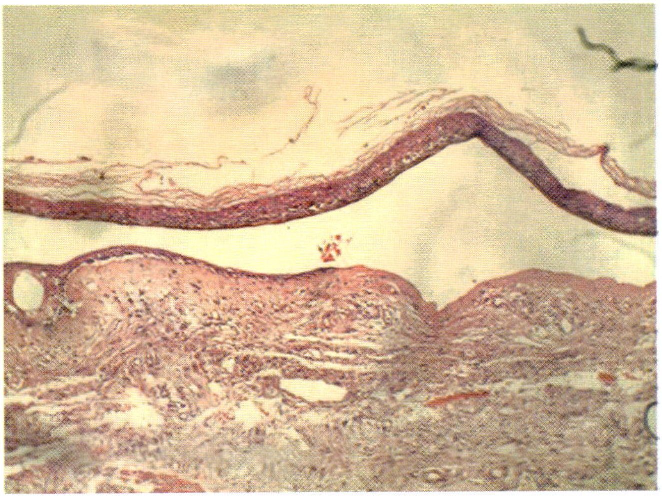

FIGURE 6.4.1.13

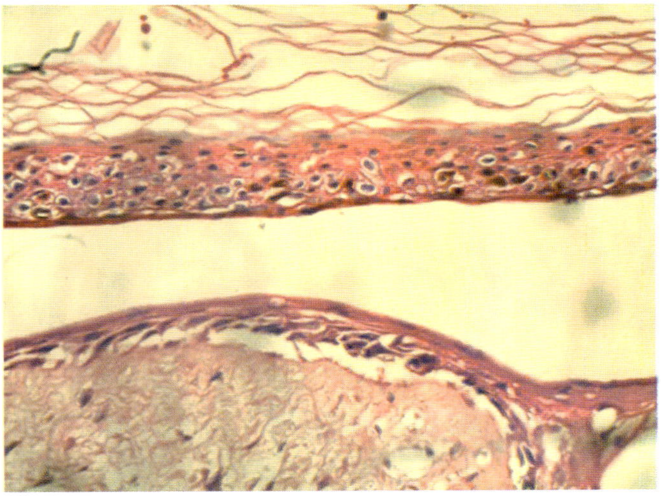

FIGURE 6.4.1.14

6.4.1.13: Regeneration starts from the shoulders (sides of the blister) (*Scanner view*)

6.4.1.14: Roof with entire epidermis, including pigmented basal cell layer and floor has few regenerated layers of epidermis (*High power view*)

6.4.1.15: At the center of the blister regeneration is not evident and only the dermis is in the floor (*High power view*)

6.4.1.16: Early lesions of mucous membrane (cicatricial) pemphigoid can be histologically similar to bullous pemphigoid and are characterized by a subepidermal blister with underlying mixed inflammation, as seen in this vulvar biopsy. Later lesions have a subepidermal blister with underlying dermal scar and eosinophils (*Scanner view*)

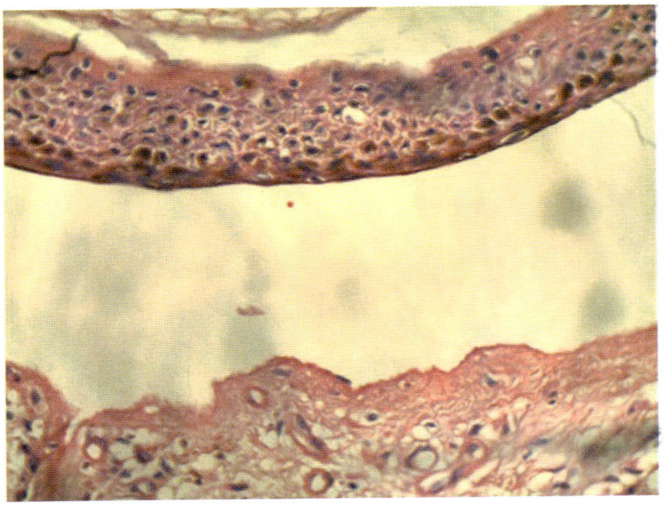

FIGURE 6.4.1.15

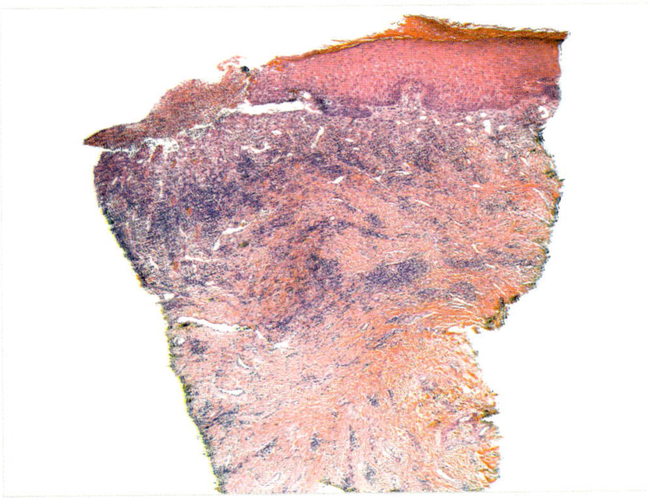

FIGURE 6.4.1.16

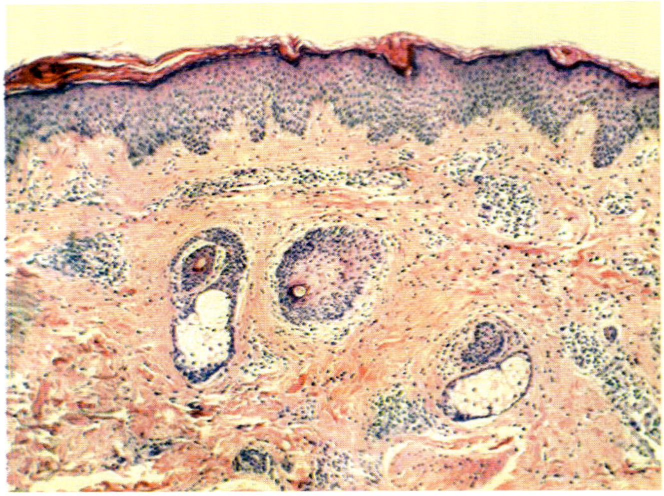

FIGURE 6.4.1.17

6.4.1.17: Early urticarial lesions of herpes gestationis show papillary edema and predominantly perivascular infiltrate (*Low power view*)

6.4.1.18: Infiltrate composed of many eosinophils with lymphocytes and histiocytes (*High power view*)

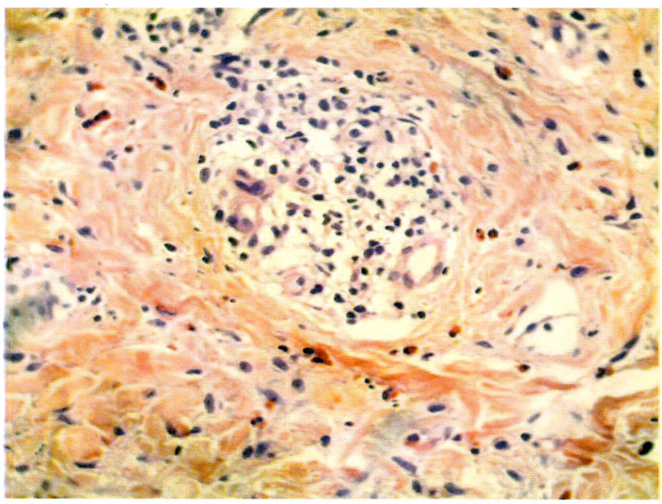

FIGURE 6.4.1.18

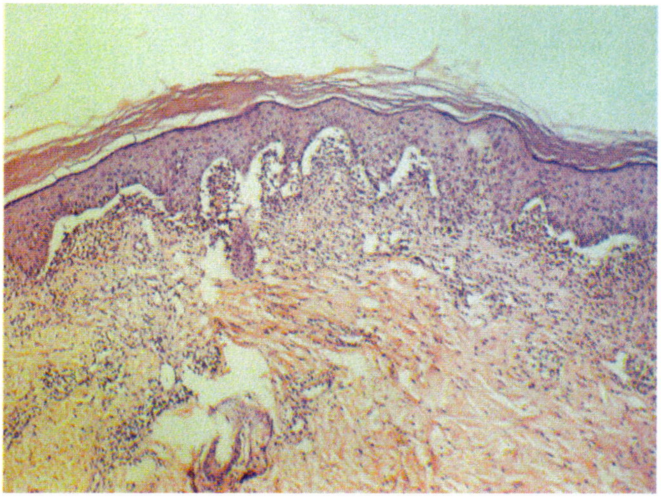

FIGURE 6.5.1.1

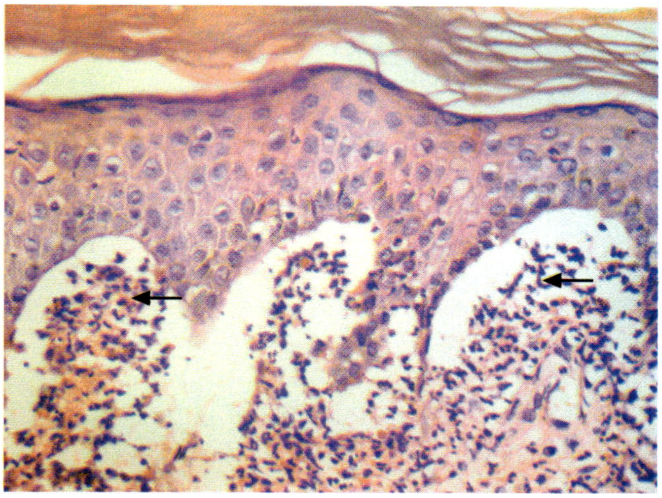

FIGURE 6.5.1.2

6.5: SUBEPIDERMAL BLISTERS WITH NEUTROPHILS

6.5.1: Dermatitis Herpetiformis

6.5.1.1: Early lesions show collections of neutrophils at the tips of dermal papillae with mutlilocular subepidermal cleavage (*Scanner view*)

6.5.1.2: Closer view of papillary microabscesses (*High power view*)

6.5.1.3: Intraepidermal neutrophils and a few eosinophils may be present (*High power view*)

6.5.1.4: Fibrin in the dermal papillae (*Low power view*)

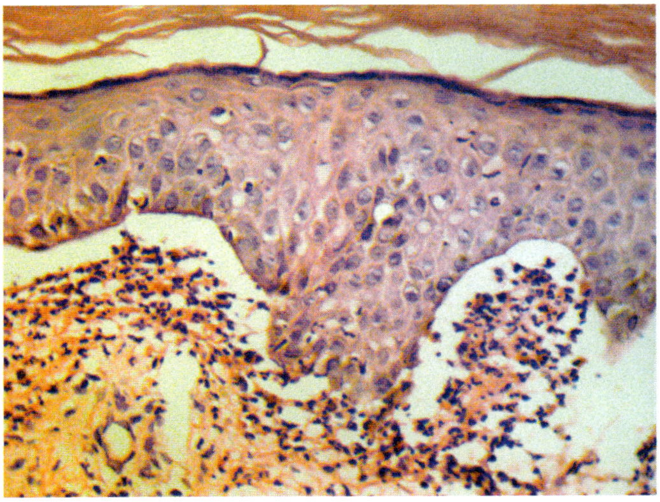

FIGURE 6.5.1.3

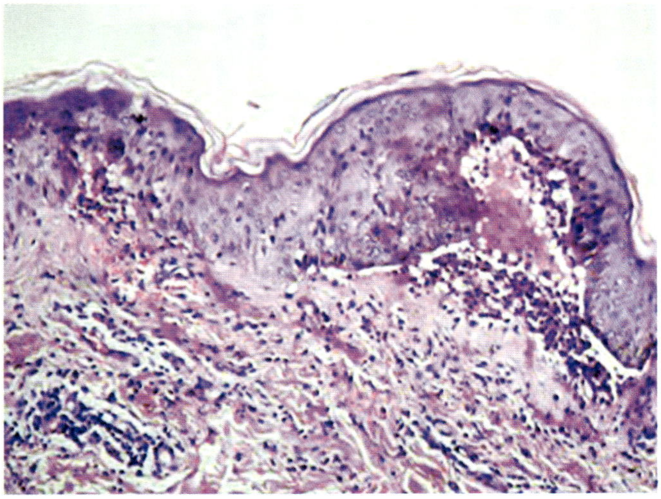

FIGURE 6.5.1.4

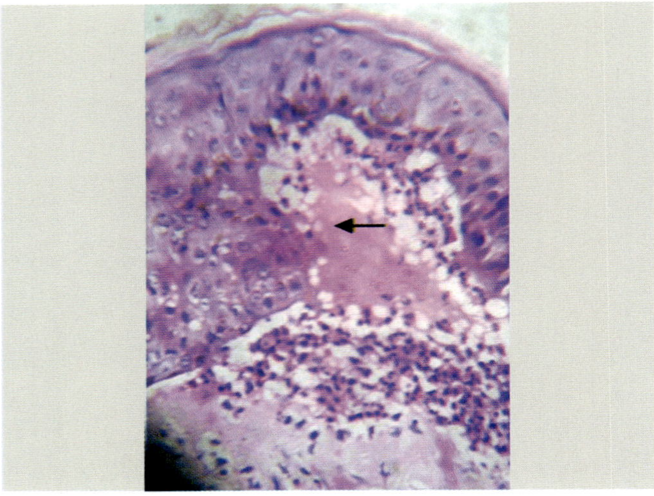

FIGURE 6.5.1.5

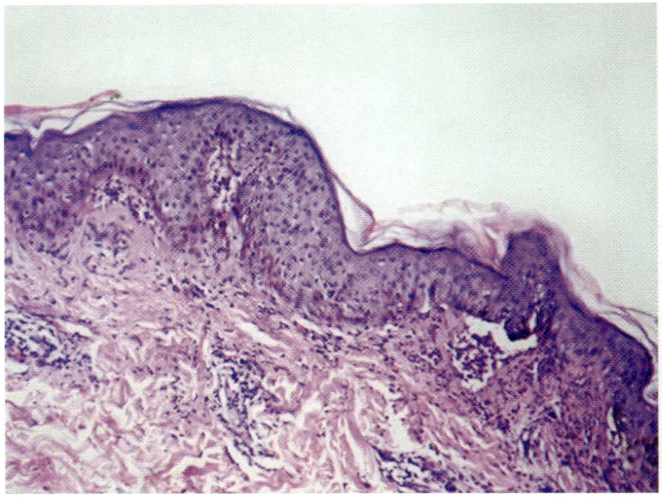

FIGURE 6.5.1.6

6.5.1.5: Subepidermal separation with fibrin (*High power view*)

6.5.1.6: Perivascular infiltrate of lymphocytes and a variable number of neutrophils and eosinophils in the dermis (*Low power view*)

6.5.1.7: Tips of rete ridges do not show infiltrate (*High power view*)

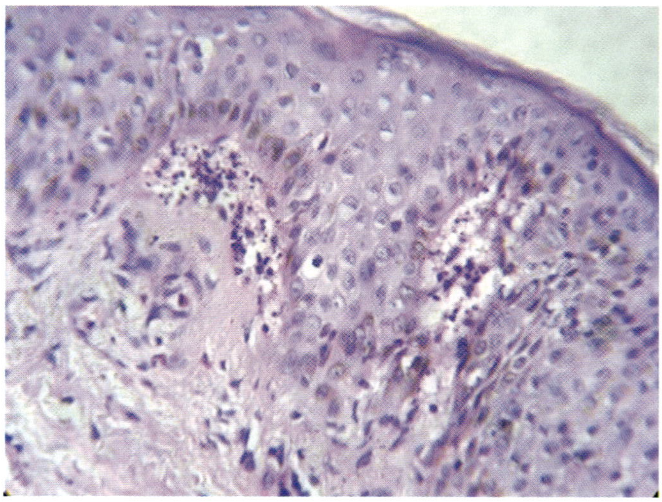

FIGURE 6.5.1.7

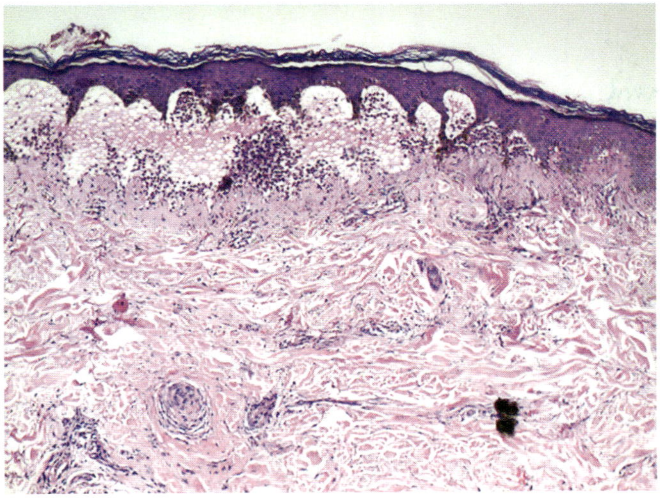

FIGURE 6.5.1.8

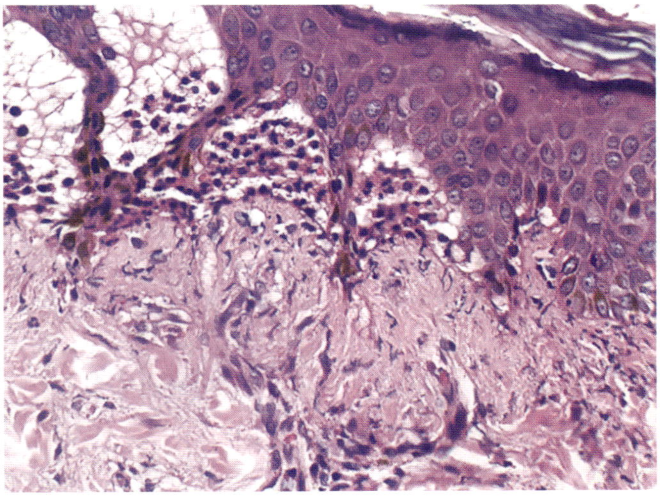

FIGURE 6.5.1.9

6.5.1.8: Clinically vesicular and older lesion shows subepidermal vesiculation with the formation of a unilocular blister (*Scanner view*)

6.5.1.9: High power view of vesicle containing fibrin, many neutrophils and an occasional eosinophil (*High power view*)

6.5.1.10: DIF showing granular IgA deposits in the dermal papilla (*Direct immunofluorescence*)

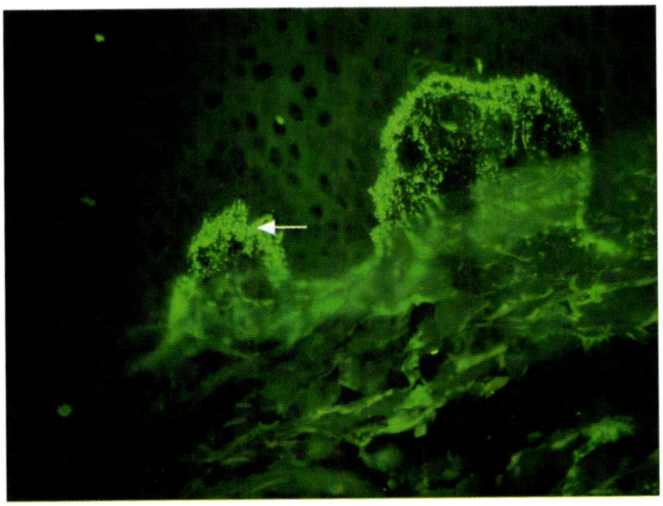

FIGURE 6.5.1.10

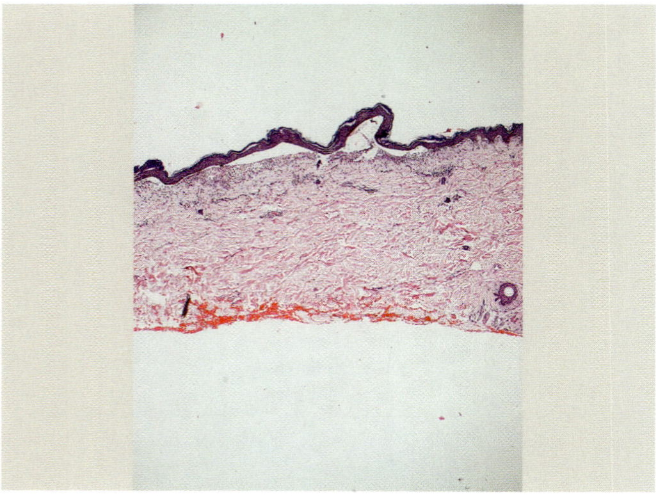

FIGURE 6.5.2.1

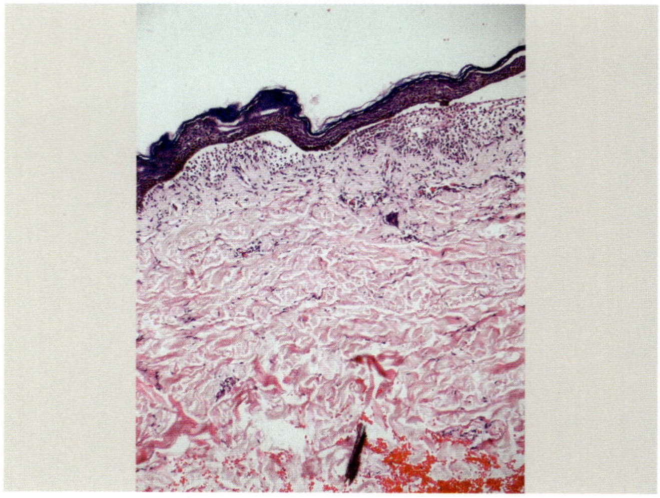

FIGURE 6.5.2.2

6.5.2: Linear IgA Bullous Disease

6.5.2.1: Unilocular subepidermal blister (*Scanner view*)

6.5.2.2: Papillary microabscess at the shoulders (*Scanner view*)

6.5.2.3: Neutrophils extend from the papillae to below the tips of rete ridges (*Low power view*)

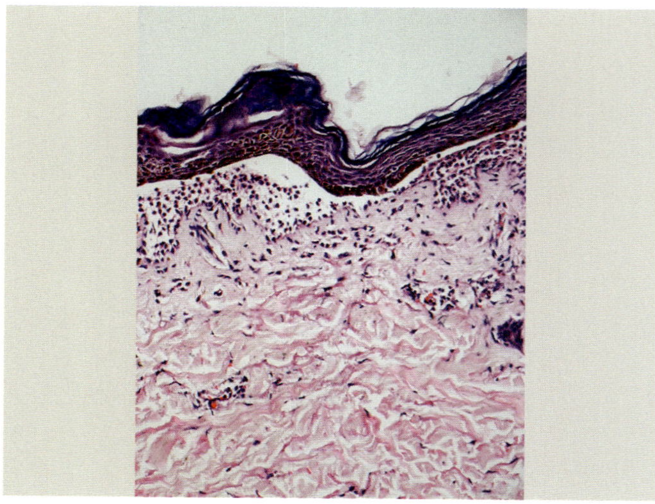

FIGURE 6.5.2.3

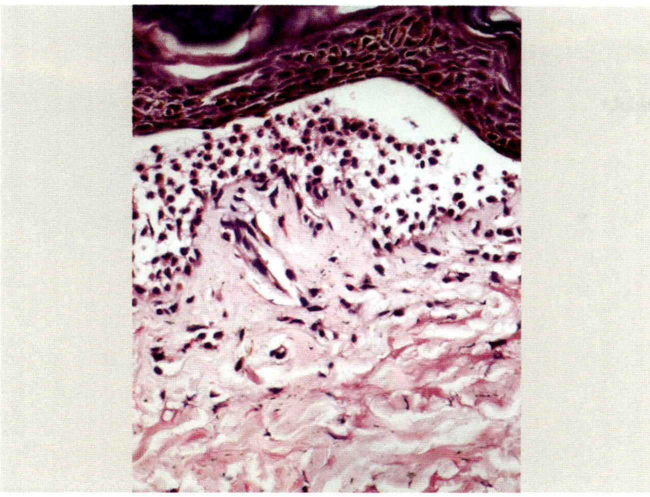

FIGURE 6.5.2.4

6.5.2.4: Neutrophils are the predominant cells in the infiltrate (*High power view*)

6.5.2.5: DIF showing linear IgA deposits at the dermo-epidermal junction (*Direct immunofluorescence*)

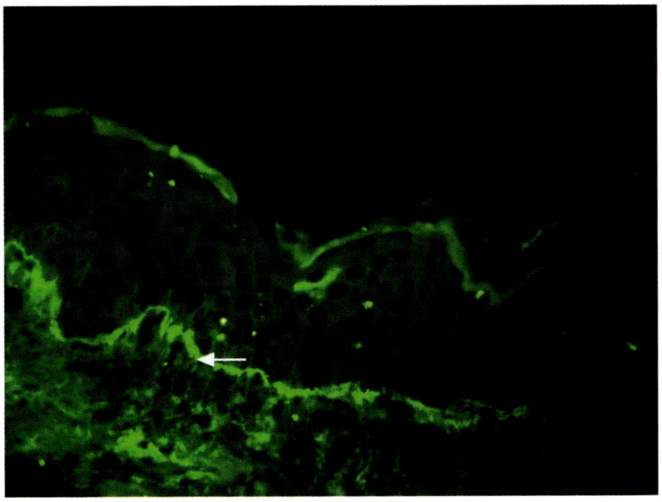

FIGURE 6.5.2.5

OTHER DISEASES SHOWING EPIDERMAL BLISTERS

1. Impetigo
2. Staphylococcal scalded skin syndrome
3. Infantile acropustulosis
4. Erythema toxicum neonatorum
5. Transient neonatal pustular melanosis
6. Incontinentia pigmenti (first stage)
7. Acute generalized exanthematous pustulosis
8. Miliaria
9. Spongiotic blisters
10. Arthropod-borne diseases
11. Viral blisters
12. Friction blister
13. Acantholytic solar keratosis

OTHER DISEASES SHOWING SUBEPIDERMAL BLISTERS

1. Erythema multiforme
2. Fixed drug eruptions
3. Toxic epidermal necrolysis
4. Bullous drug reactions
5. Lichen sclerosus et atrophicus
6. Lichen planus pemphigoides
7. Insect bite reactions
8. Bullous vasculitis
9. Bullous lupus erythematosus
10. Bullous leprosy
11. Sweet's syndrome
12. Bullous mastocytosis
13. Suction blisters

DIAGNOSTIC PEARLS

1. Impetigo vs pemphigus foliaceus—acantholysis is not prominent, and gram-positive cocci can be demonstrated in impetigo in contrast to pemphigus foliaceus.
2. Staphylococcal scalded skin syndrome—only sparse inflammatory infiltrate in the upper dermis, no organisms, difficult to get intact blister.
3. Histopathological findings in pemphigus erythematosus are similar to pemphigus foliaceus.
4. Spongiform pustules and mitotic figures are usually absent in subcorneal pustular dermatosis, unlike pustular psoriasis.
5. It is difficult to differentiate drug-associated pemphigus vulgaris from idiopathic cases on histology.
6. Paraneoplastic pemphigus shows features of erythema multiforme (lichenoid tissue reaction) and pemphigus vulgaris histologically.
7. Darier's disease has more dyskeratotic cells than pemphigus vulgaris and limited acantholysis as compared to Hailey-Hailey disease.
8. Acantholytic solar keratosis shows epithelial dysplasia in addition to suprabasal separation and solar elastotic changes.
9. Miliaria crystalina has vesicles related to sweat ducts usually situated below the stratum corneum.
10. Ballooning degeneration, secondary acantholysis, multinucleated keratinocytes and inclusion bodies are common features of viral blisters.
11. Bullous lichen planus will not show eosinophilic infiltrate as against lichen planus pemphigoides.

7

Granulomatous Tissue Reaction

Chapter Outline

7.1: Tuberculoid Granulomas
7.2: Leprosy
7.3: Suppurative Granulomas
7.4: Other Granulomas

Uday Khopkar, V Ramesh, Sudhir Arora, Col Deep Kumar Raman, Pradeep Mahajan, KC Nischal, M Ramam, Nathan Lee, Jerad Gardner, Gp Capt Sandeep Arora, Col Aradhana Sood

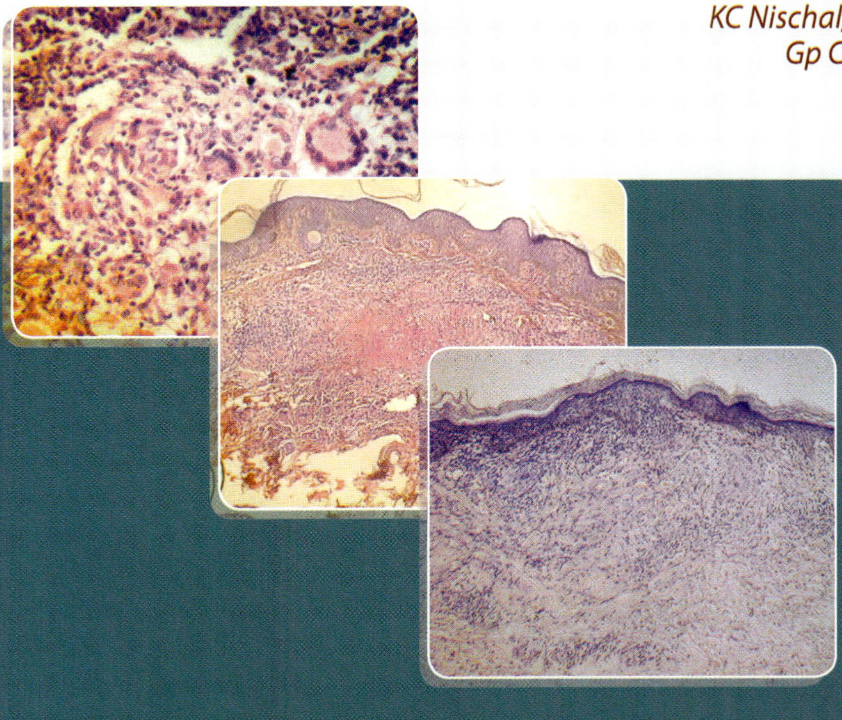

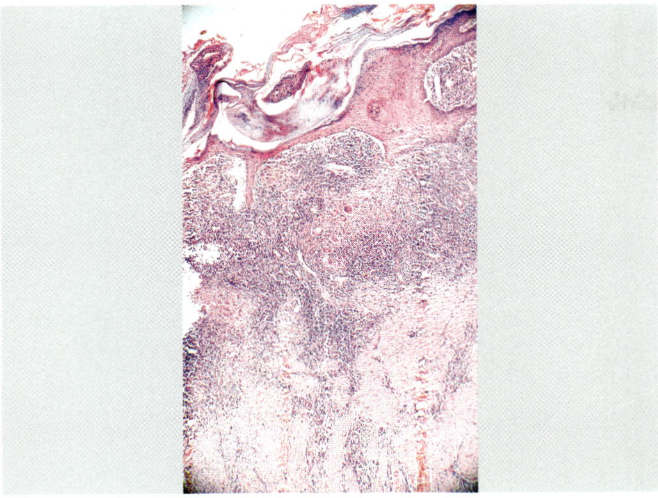

FIGURE 7.1.1.1

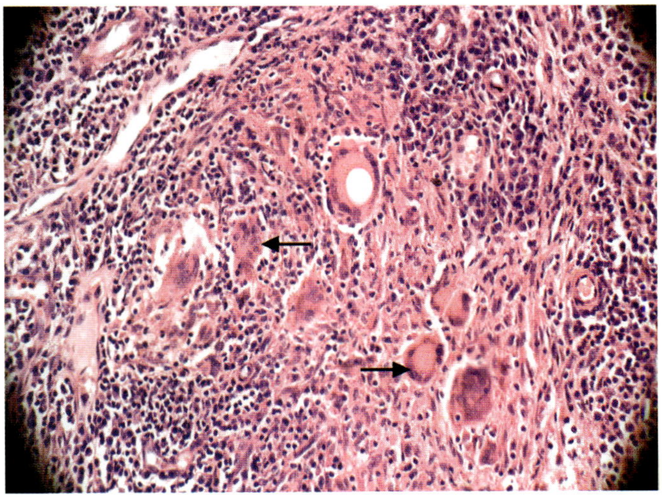

FIGURE 7.1.1.2

7.1: TUBERCULOID GRANULOMAS

7.1.1: Tuberculosis

7.1.1.1: Lupus vulgaris—tuberculoid granulomas with a mantle of lymphocytes in the upper and mid dermis, granulomas confluent, epidermis hyperplastic (*Scanner view*)

7.1.1.2: Closer view of granuloma with multinucleated giant cells both Langhans and foreign body type (*Low power view*)

7.1.1.3: Scrofuloderma—epidermis atrophic and ulcerated, dermis shows granulomas, often with caseation and admixture of neutrophils (*Scanner view*)

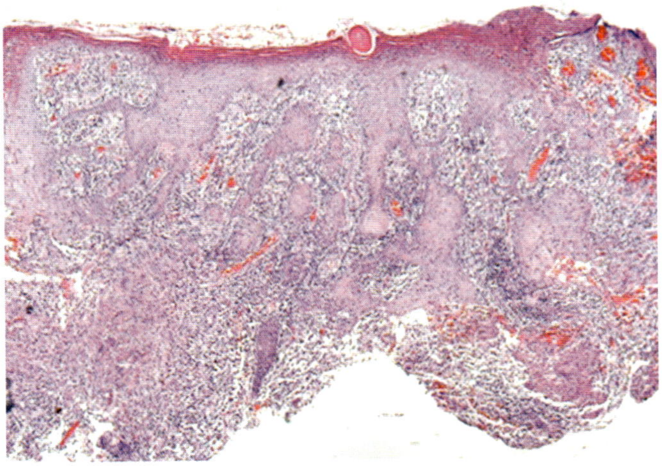

FIGURE 7.1.1.3

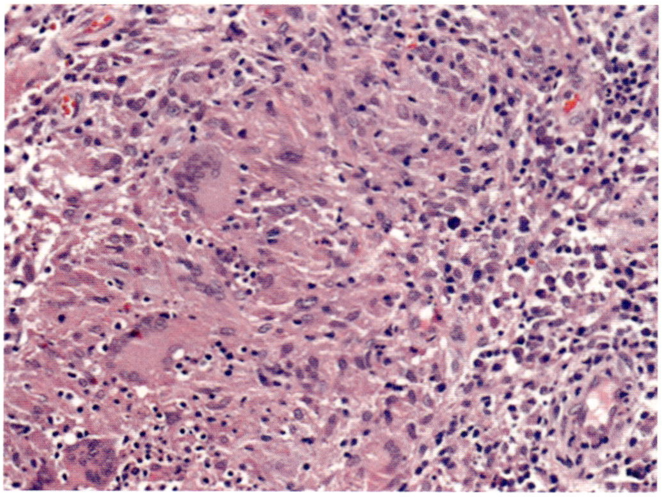

FIGURE 7.1.1.4

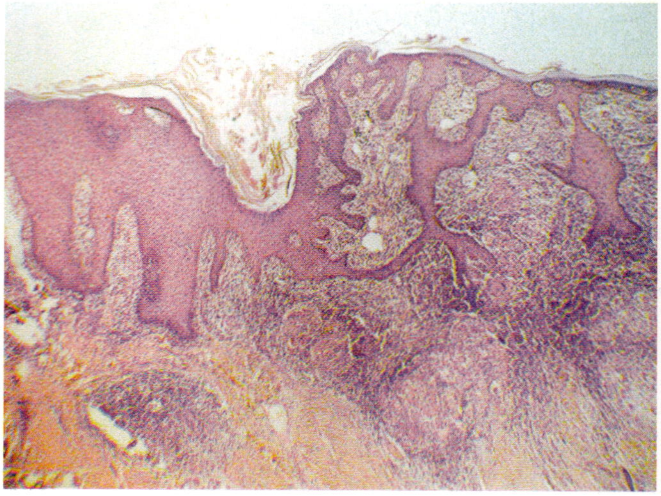

FIGURE 7.1.1.5

7.1.1.4: Granulomas with giant cells both Langhans as well as foreign body type and a few lymphocytes (*High power view*)

7.1.1.5: Tuberculosis verrucosa cutis (TVC)—hyperkeratosis and pseudoepitheliomatous hyperplasia of the epidermis (*Scanner view*)

7.1.1.6: Granulomas with giant cells in the mid-dermis (TVC may show caseation or acid-fast bacilli) (*High power view*)

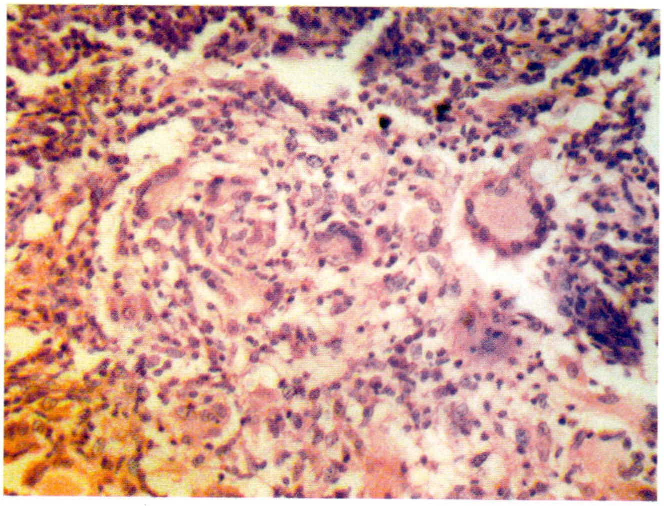

FIGURE 7.1.1.6

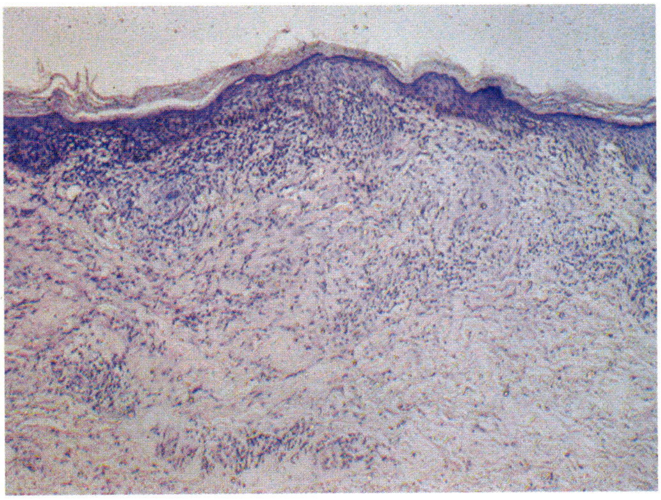

FIGURE 7.1.1.7

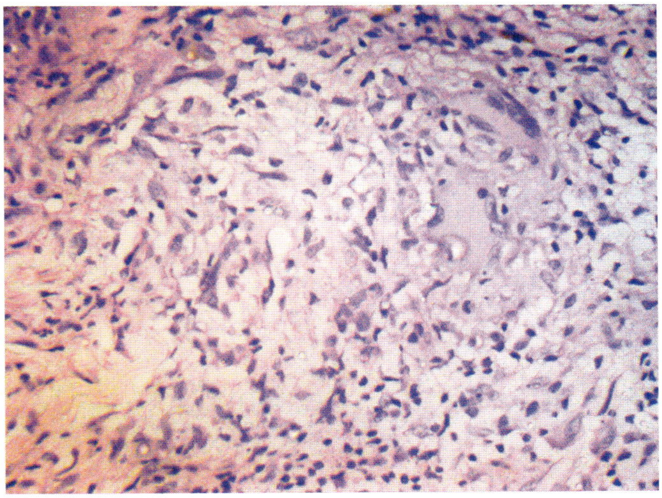

FIGURE 7.1.1.8

7.1.1.7: Lichenoid—granulomatous reaction as a part of cutaneous tuberculosis, section showing lichenoid reaction (*Low power view*)

7.1.1.8: Granulomas with multinucleated giant cells on higher magnification (*High power view*)

7.1.1.9: Caseation necrosis in cutaneous tuberculosis (*Scanner view*)

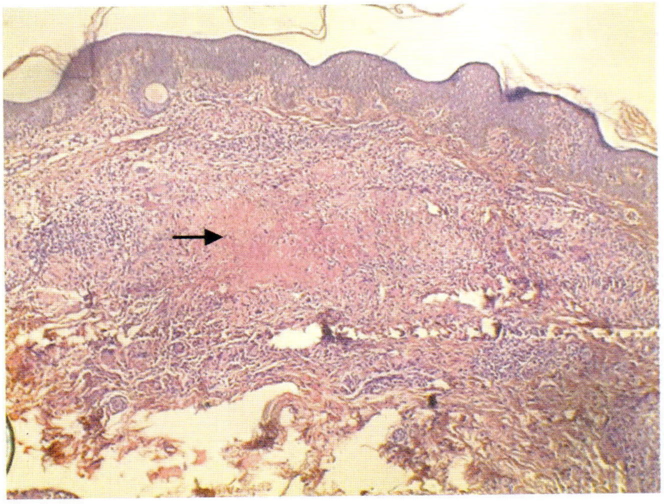

FIGURE 7.1.1.9

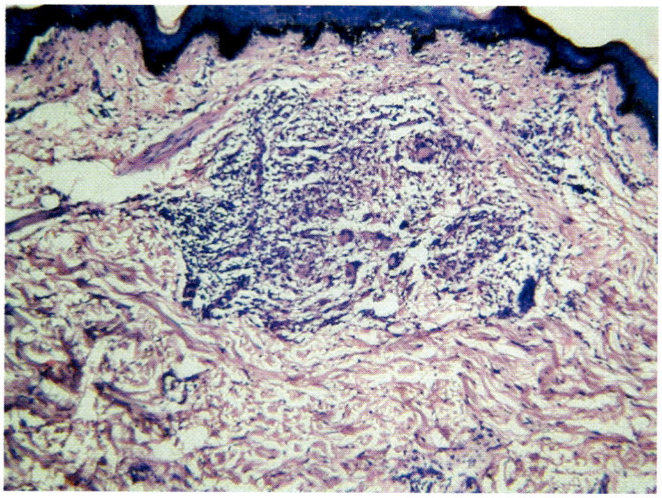

FIGURE 7.1.2.1

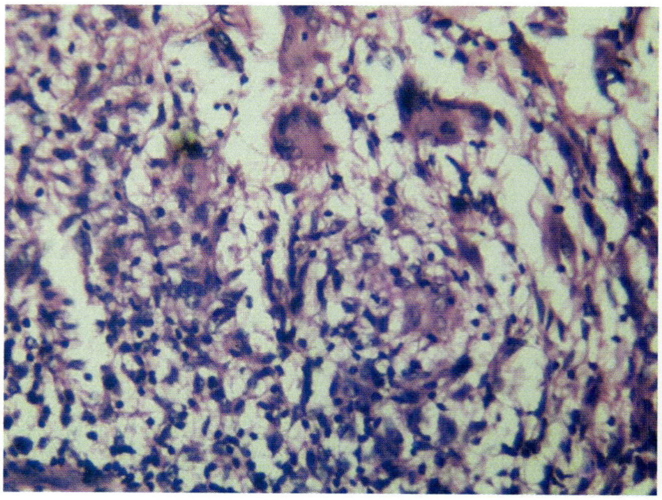

FIGURE 7.1.2.2

7.1.2: Tuberculids

7.1.2.1: Lichen scrofulosorum—perifollicular infiltrate in the upper dermis (*Scanner view*)

7.1.2.2: Non-caseating tuberculoid granulomas with multinucleated giant cells (*Low power view*)

7.1.2.3: Papulonecrotic tuberculid—wedge-shaped area of infiltrate and necrosis, surrounding area has chronic inflammatory cells and granulomas (*Scanner view*)

7.1.2.4: Vasculitis with fibrinoid necrosis and neutrophilic infiltrate (*Low power view*)

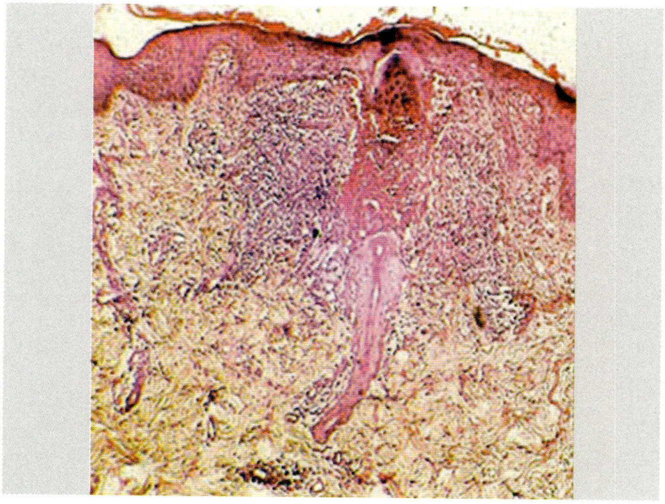

FIGURE 7.1.2.3

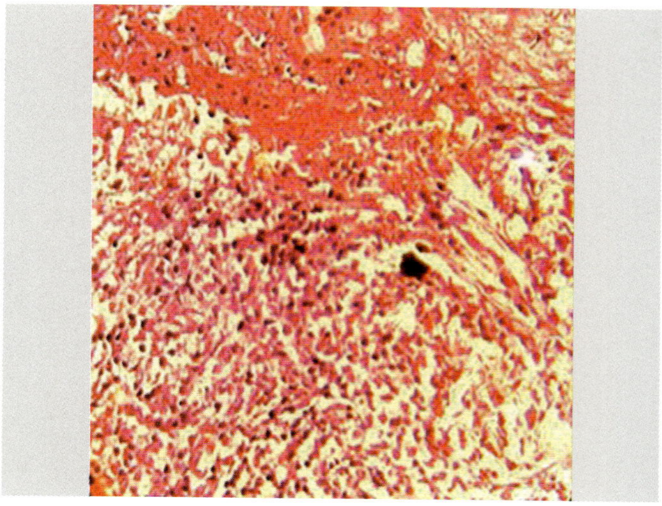

FIGURE 7.1.2.4

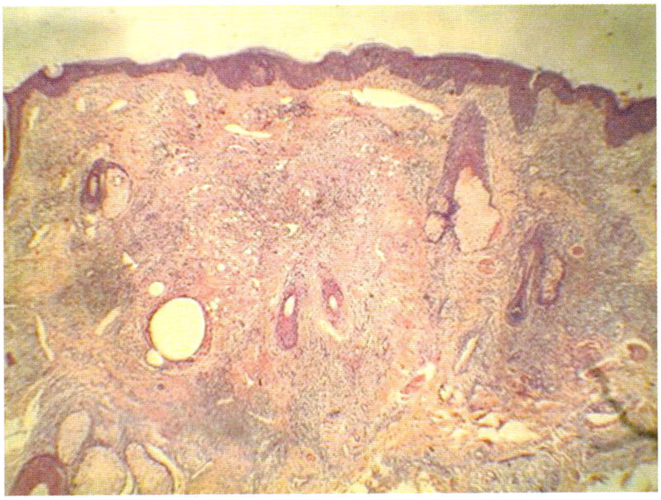

FIGURE 7.1.3.1

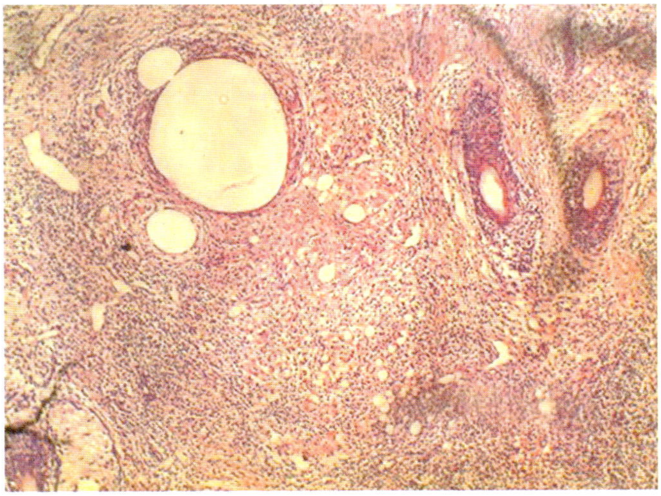

FIGURE 7.1.3.2

7.1.3: Leishmaniasis

7.1.3.1: Marked dermal infiltrate (*Scanner view*)

7.1.3.2: Infiltrate composed of lymphocytes, histiocytes, plasma cells, and sometimes a few eosinophils (*Low power view*)

7.1.3.3: Epithelioid cell granulomas (*High power view*)

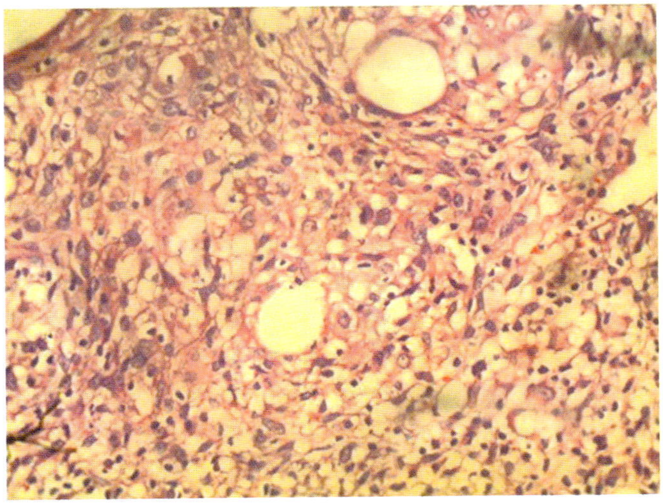

FIGURE 7.1.3.3

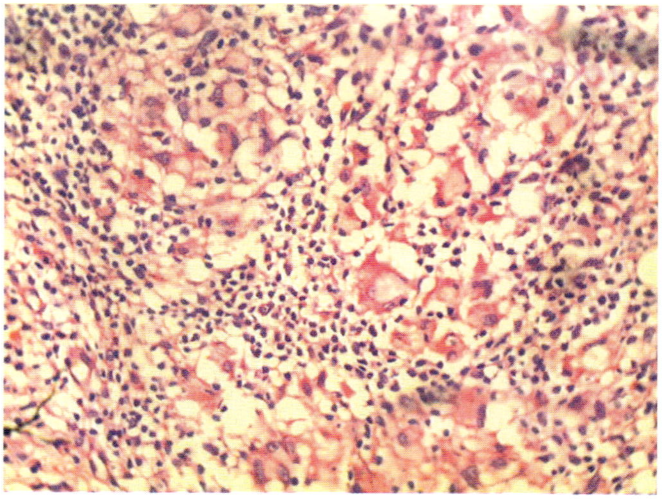

FIGURE 7.1.3.4

7.1.3.4: Tuberculoid granulomas with giant cells but no necrosis (*High power view*)

7.1.3.5: Shows organisms in the macrophages in sections stained with the Giemsa stain (Leishman–Donovan bodies) (*Oil immersion view*)

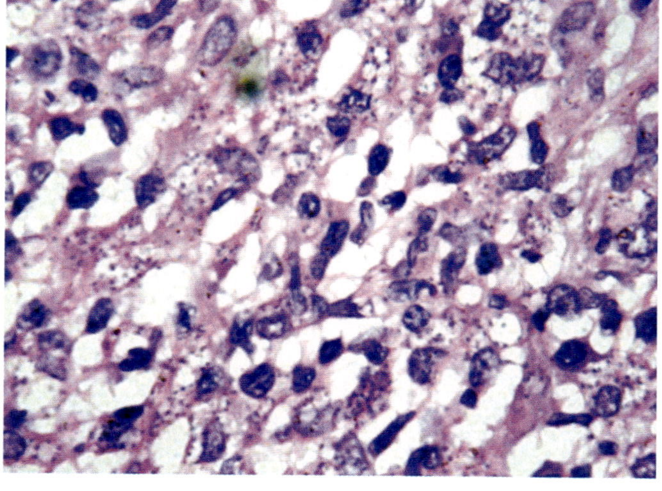

FIGURE 7.1.3.5

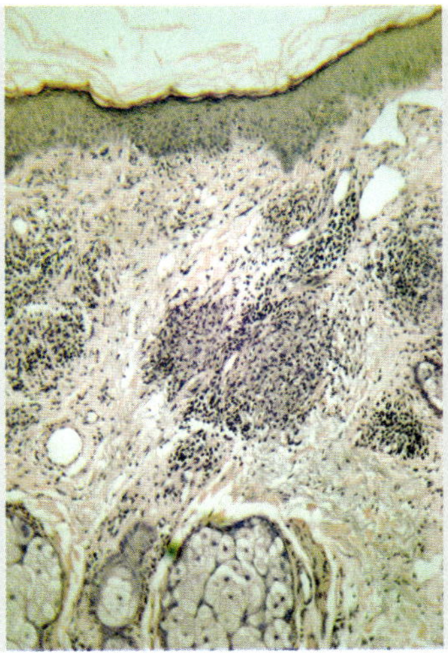

FIGURE 7.1.4.1

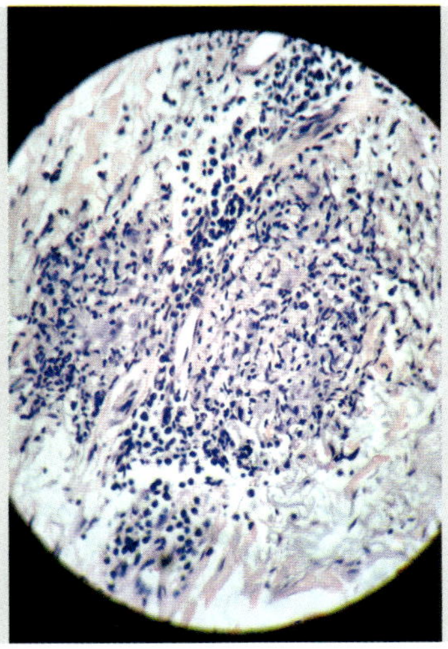

FIGURE 7.1.4.2

7.1.4: Granulomatous Rosacea

7.1.4.1: Dilated capillaries and perifollicular inflammatory infiltrate in the dermis (*Low power view*)

7.1.4.2: Epithelioid histiocytes and giant cells forming tuberculoid granulomas (*High power view*)

7.1.4.3: Another case with perifollicular granuloma (*Low power view*)

7.1.4.4: Closer view of epithelioid cell granuloma (*High power view*)

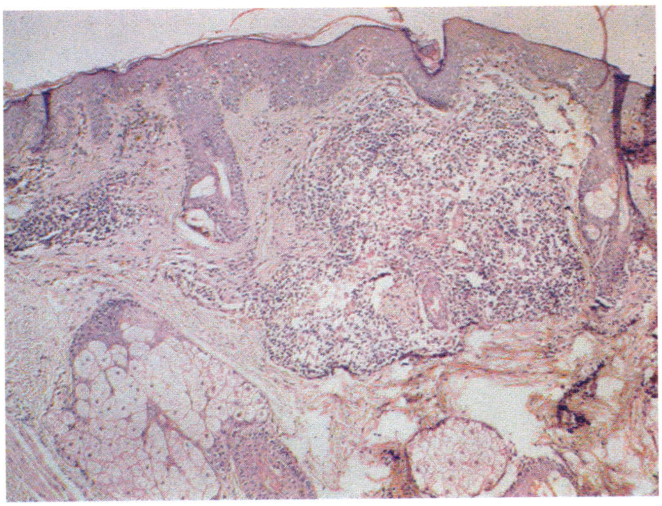

FIGURE 7.1.4.3

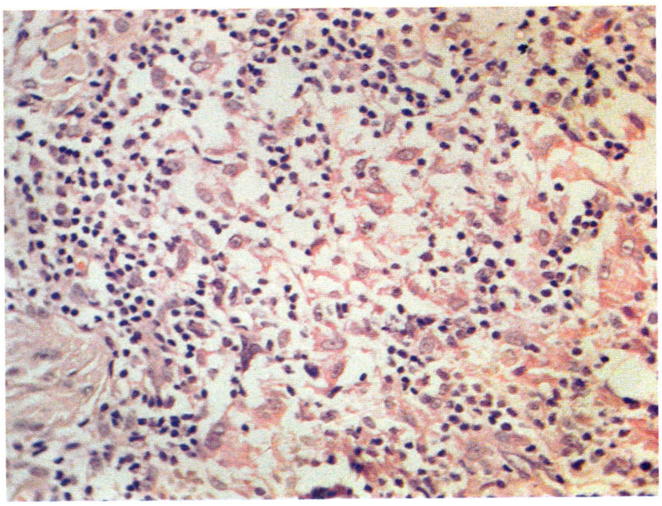

FIGURE 7.1.4.4

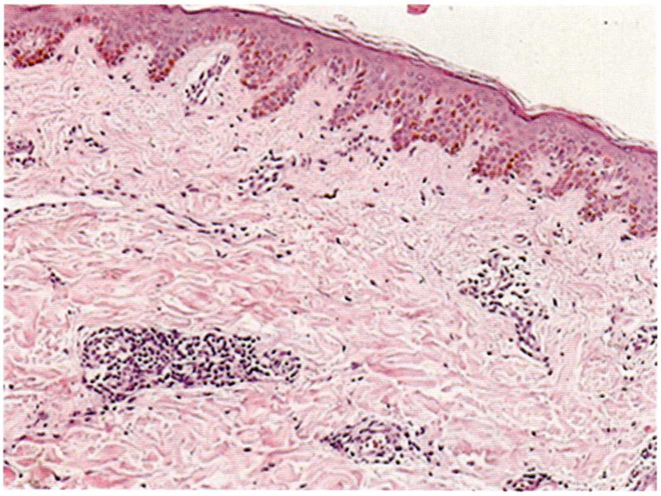

FIGURE 7.2.1.1

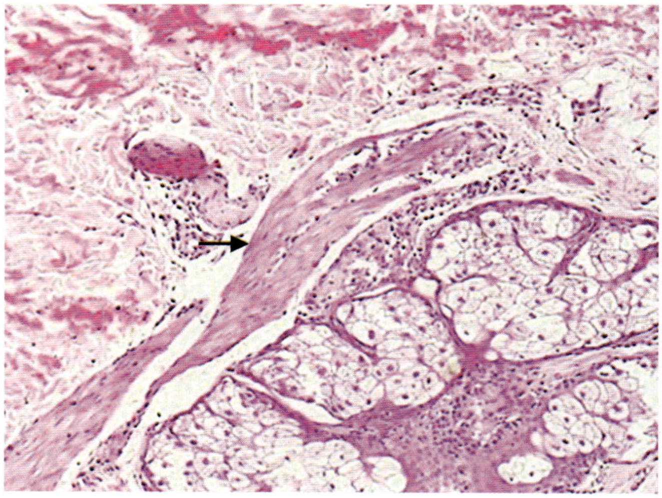

FIGURE 7.2.1.2

7.2: LEPROSY

7.2.1: Hansen's Disease—Indeterminate

7.2.1.1: Lymphohistiocytic infiltrate around blood vessels, granulomas are not seen, (Presence of lymphocytes in epidermis may be a sign of early leprosy but difficult to confirm Hansen's disease with only that feature) (*Low power view*)

7.2.1.2: Lymphohistiocytic infiltrate around arrector pilorum (*High power view*)

7.2.1.3: Lymphohistiocytic infiltrate around nerves (*High power view*)

7.2.1.4: Lymphohistiocytic infiltrate around sweat glands, identification of leprosy bacillus is helpful in the diagnosis (*High power view*)

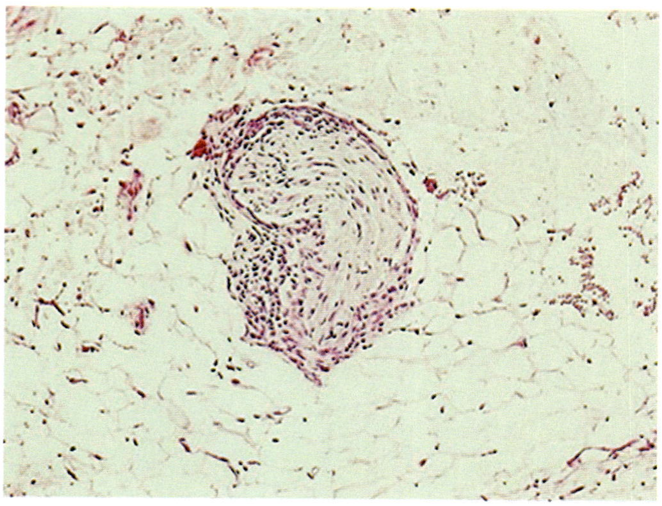

FIGURE 7.2.1.3

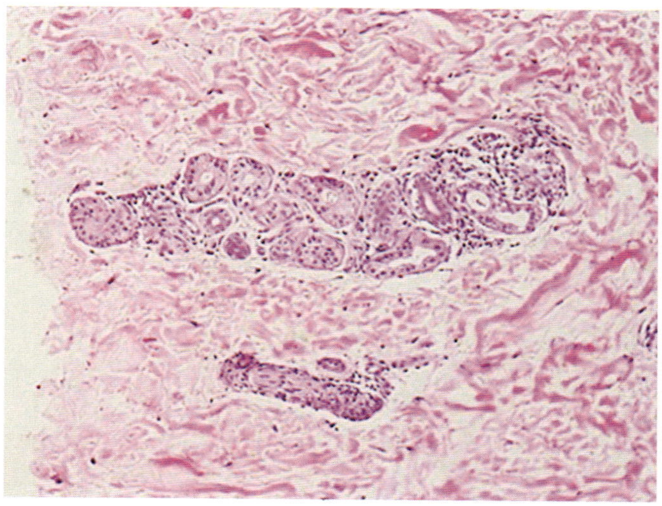

FIGURE 7.2.1.4

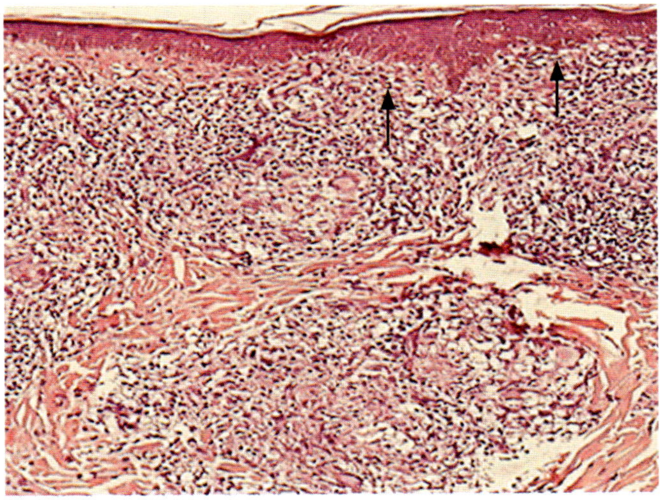

FIGURE 7.2.2.1

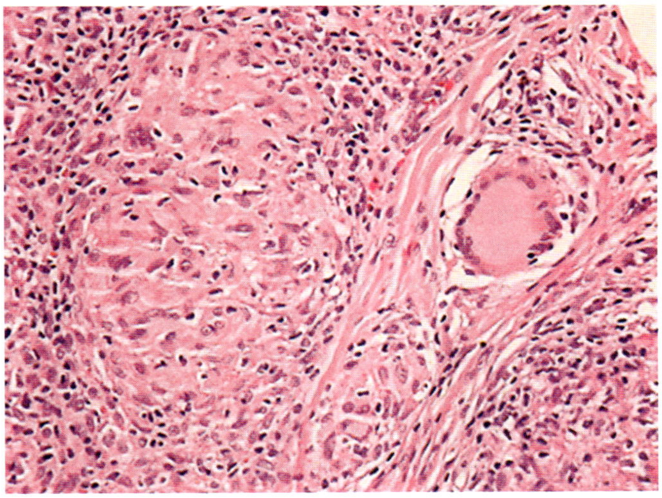

FIGURE 7.2.2.2

7.2.2: Hansen's Disease—Tuberculoid (TT)

7.2.2.1: Multiple focal epithelioid granulomas with a peripheral rim of lymphocyte almost touching the epidermis (*Low power view*)

7.2.2.2: Granulomas with multinucleated giant cells—Langhans type (*High power view*)

7.2.2.3: Granulomas may extend to deep dermis and subcutis (*High power view*)

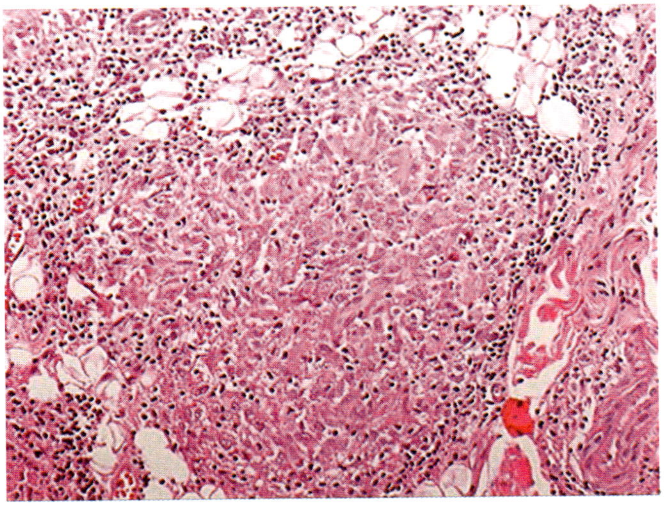

FIGURE 7.2.2.3

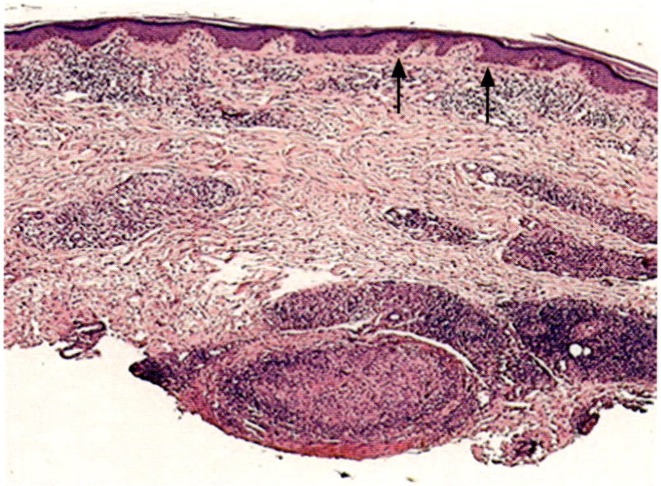

FIGURE 7.2.3.1

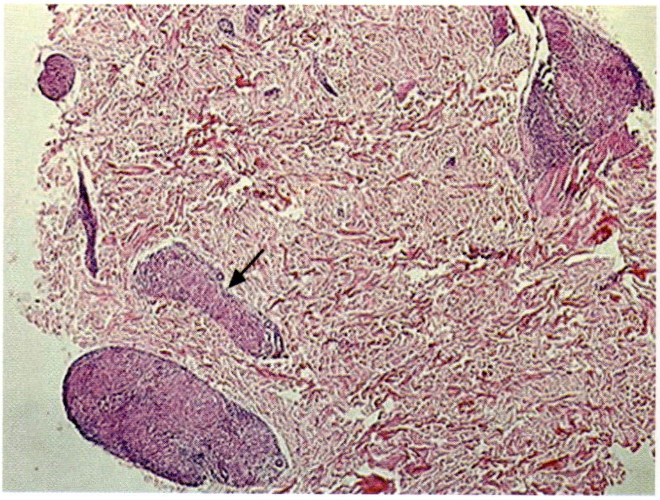

FIGURE 7.2.3.2

7.2.3: Hansen's Disease—Borderline Tuberculoid

7.2.3.1: Uninvolved epidermis with grenz zone and well-formed epithelioid cell granulomas in the dermis (*Scanner view*)

7.2.3.2: Oblong granulomas along the neurovascular bundle and around the adnexal structures (*Low power view*)

7.2.3.3: Granulomas around the nerve, lymphocytes abundant around the granulomas (Bacilli sparse) (*High power view*)

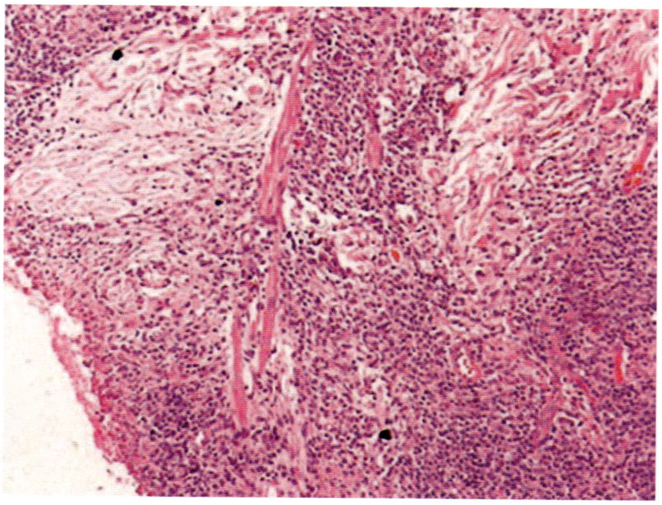

FIGURE 7.2.3.3

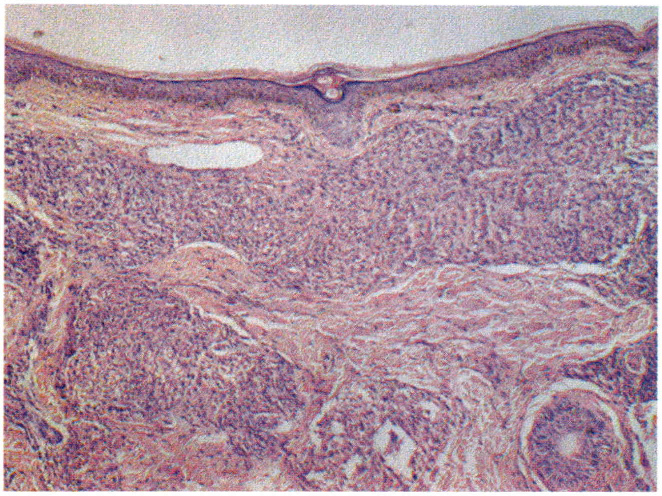

FIGURE 7.2.4.1

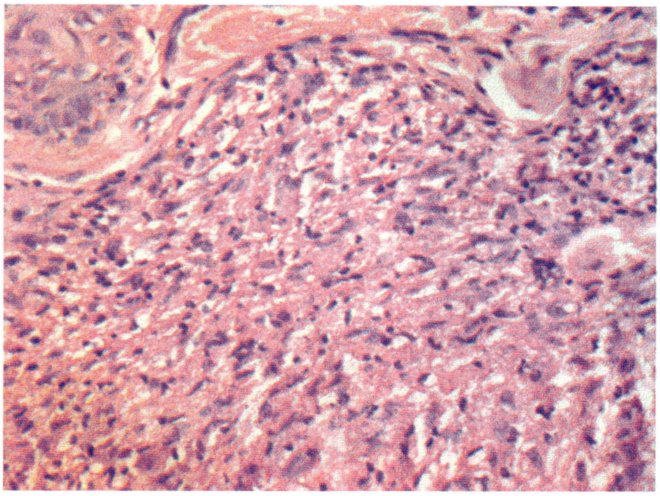

FIGURE 7.2.4.2

7.2.4: Hansen's Disease—Borderline Lepromatous

7.2.4.1: Atrophic epidermis, grenz zone, lymphohistiocytic infiltration in the dermis (*Low power view*)

7.2.4.2: Epithelioid cell granulomas but no giant cells (*High power view*)

7.2.4.3: Periadnexal infiltrate, a few macrophages show foamy cytoplasm (*High power view*)

7.2.4.4: Infiltrate involving neurovascular bundles (multiple bacilli but no globi) (*Low power view*)

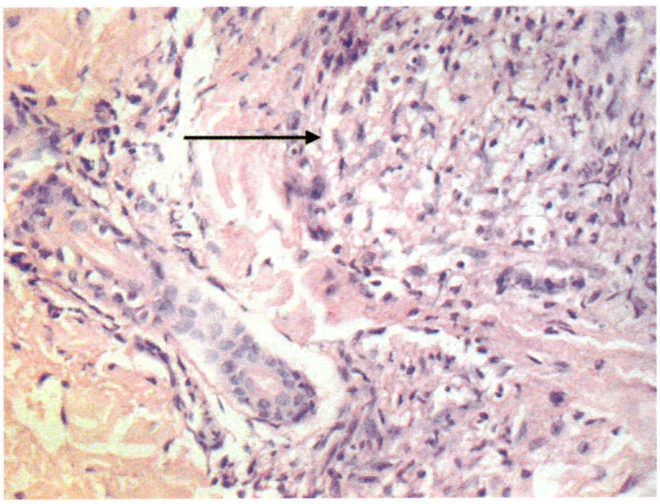

FIGURE 7.2.4.3

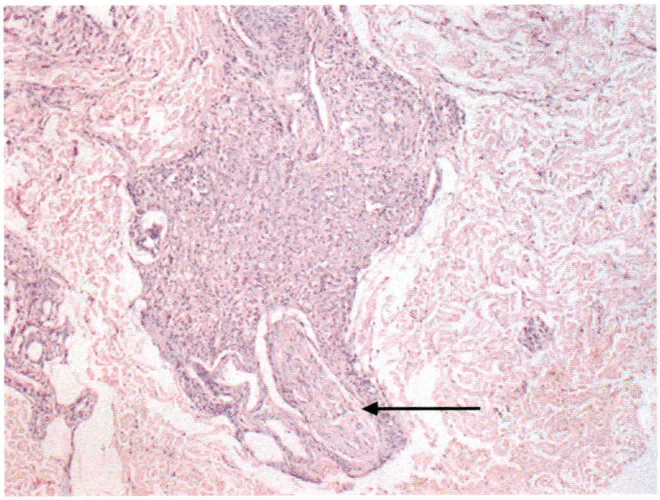

FIGURE 7.2.4.4

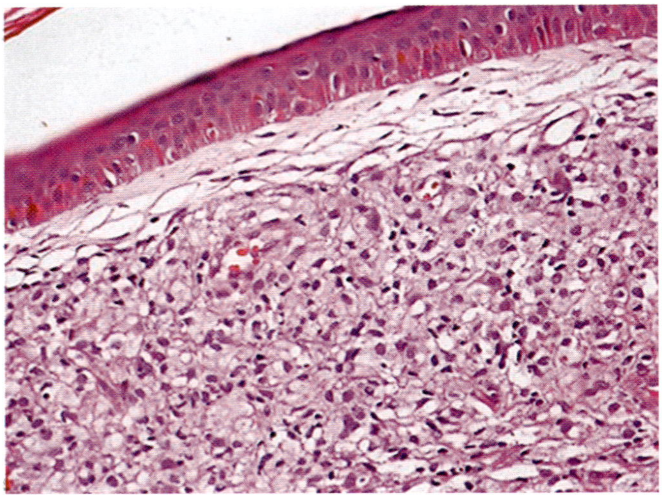

FIGURE 7.2.5.1

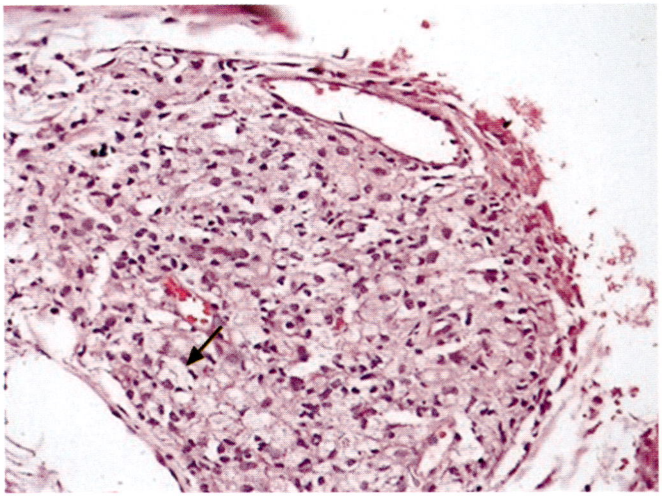

FIGURE 7.2.5.2

7.2.5: Hansen's Disease—Lepromatous (LL)

7.2.5.1: Atrophic epidermis with grenz zone and sheets of foamy histiocytes in the dermis below. There is sparsity of lymphocytes (*Low power view*)

7.2.5.2: Perivascular foamy histiocytic, less number of lymphocytes (*High power view*)

7.2.5.3: Periadnexal foamy histiocytic collection with the involvement of arrector pili muscle bundle (*Low power view*)

7.2.5.4: Modified Ziehl-Neelsen stain shows numerous globi of easily identifiable lepra bacilli (BI=5 or 6) (*Oil immersion view*)

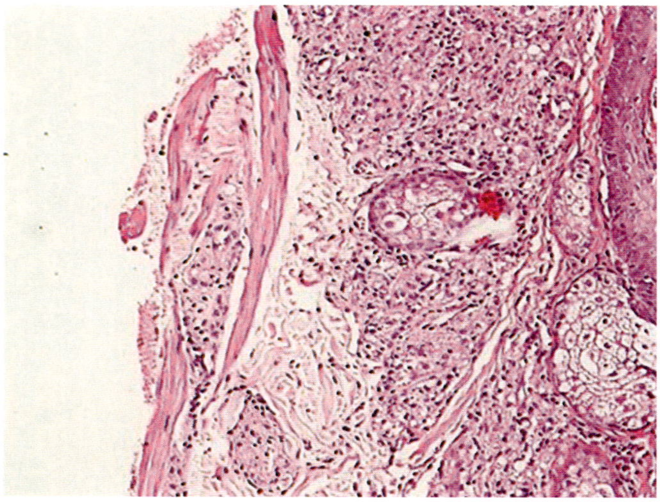

FIGURE 7.2.5.3

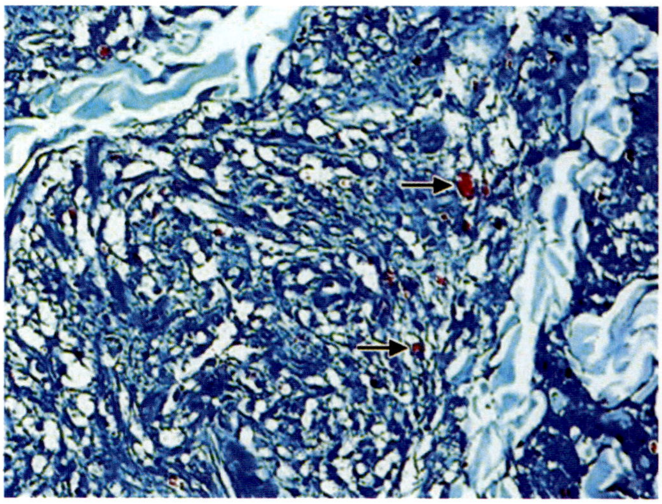

FIGURE 7.2.5.4

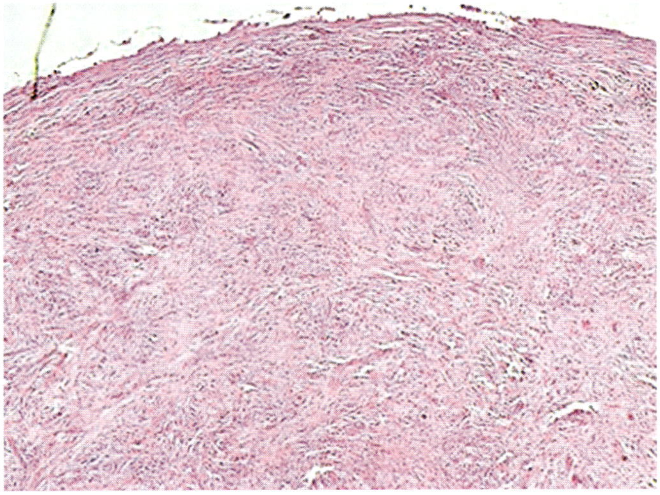

FIGURE 7.2.6.1

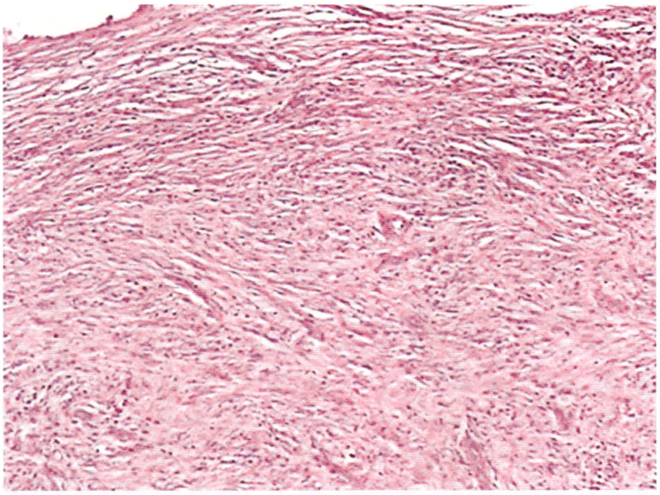

FIGURE 7.2.6.2

7.2.6: Histoid Leprosy

7.2.6.1: A dense and diffuse collection of spindle-shaped macrophages in the dermis (*Scanner view*)

7.2.6.2: Arranged in storiform pattern (*Low power view*)

7.2.6.3: A few foamy histiocytes in between (*Low power view*)

7.2.6.4: Modified Ziehl-Neelsen stain reveals heavy bacillary load with clumps of longer bacilli (so no confusion with spindle cell tumors like dermatofibroma) (*Oil immersion view*)

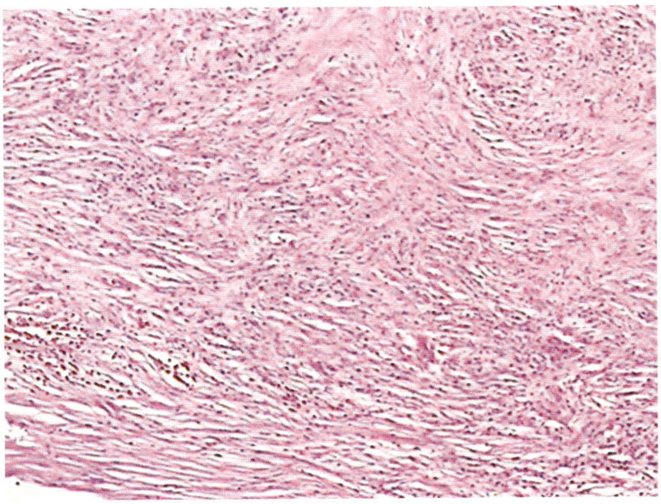

FIGURE 7.2.6.3

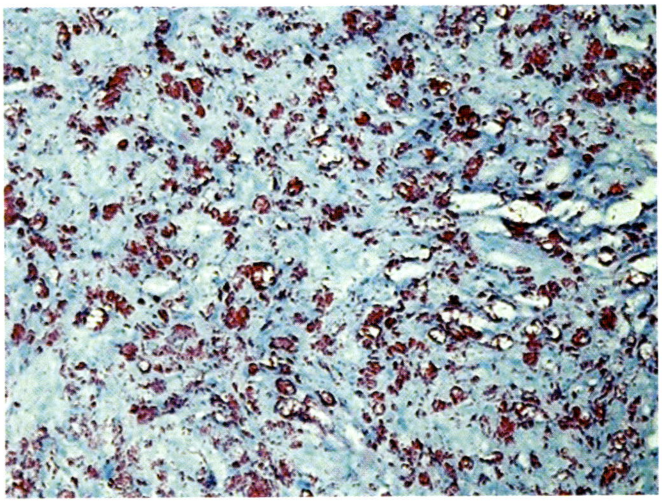

FIGURE 7.2.6.4

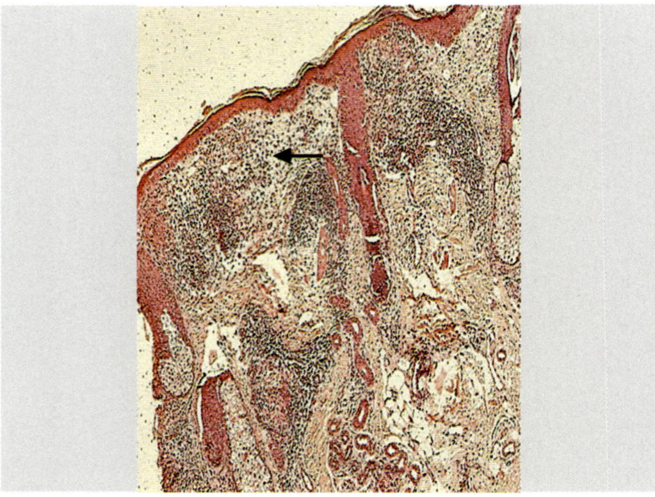

FIGURE 7.2.7.1

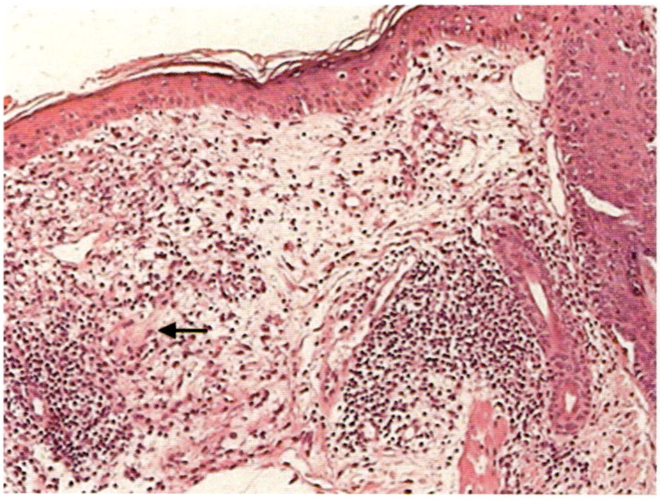

FIGURE 7.2.7.2

7.2.7: Hansen's Disease—Type 1 Lepra Reaction

7.2.7.1: Dermal edema with an increase in number of lymphocytes (*Scanner view*)

7.2.7.2: Edema in and around the epithelioid cell granulomas (*Low power view*)

7.2.7.3: Closer view of dermal edema, dispersed granuloma, perivascular lymphocytes (*Low power view*)

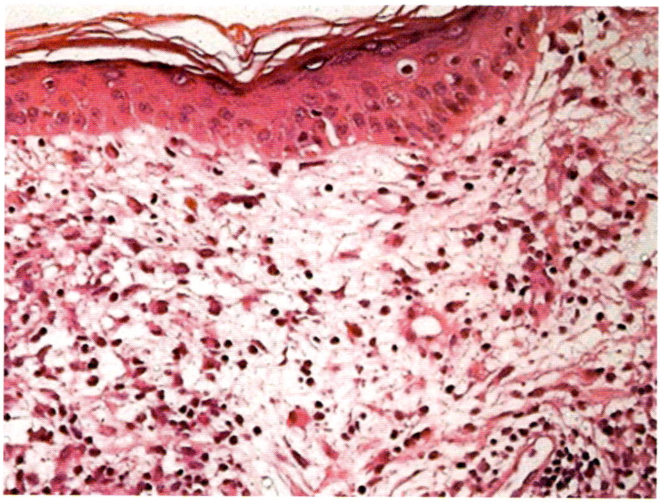

FIGURE 7.2.7.3

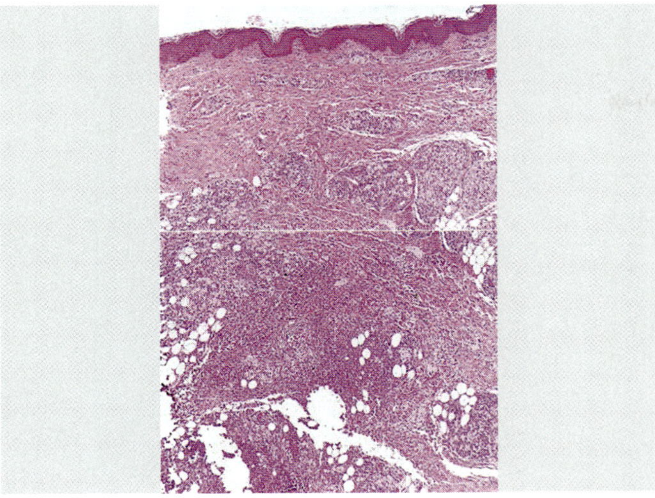

FIGURE 7.2.8.1

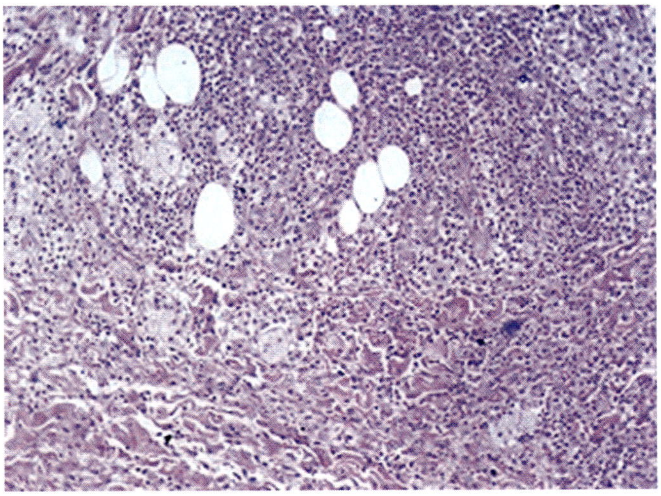

FIGURE 7.2.8.2

7.2.8: Erythema Nodosum Leprosum (ENL)

7.2.8.1: Edema of the papillary dermis and a mixed dermal infiltrate (*Scanner view*)

7.2.8.2: Involvement of the subcutis, with lobular panniculitis (*Low power view*)

7.2.8.3: Perivascular neutrophils and collection of foamy macrophages (*High power view*)

7.2.8.4: Modified Ziehl-Neelsen stain shows fragmented lepra bacilli (*Oil immersion view*)

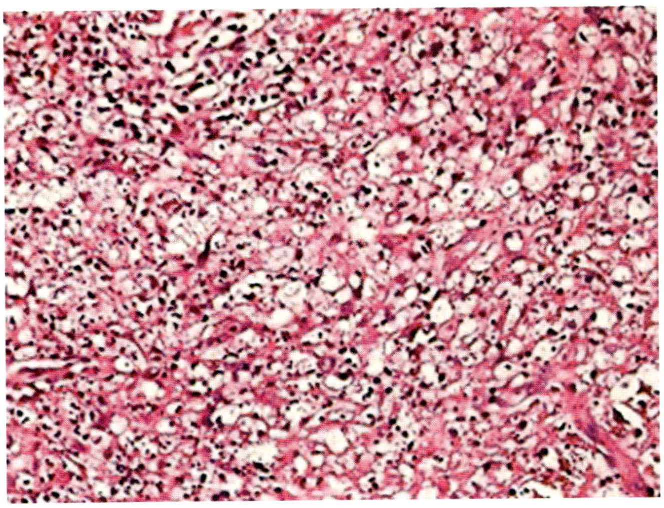

FIGURE 7.2.8.3

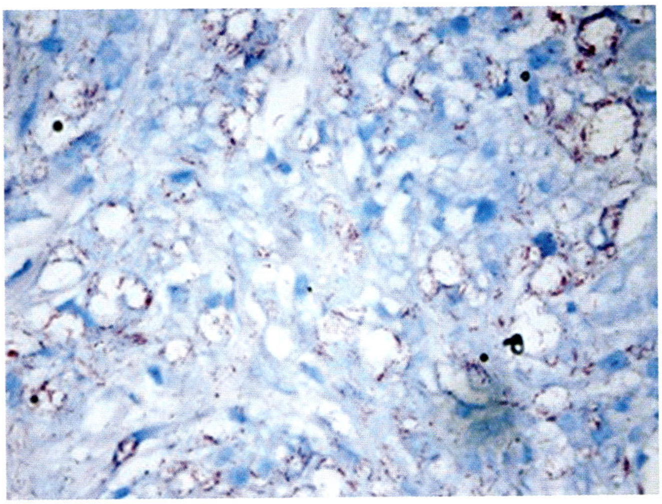

FIGURE 7.2.8.4

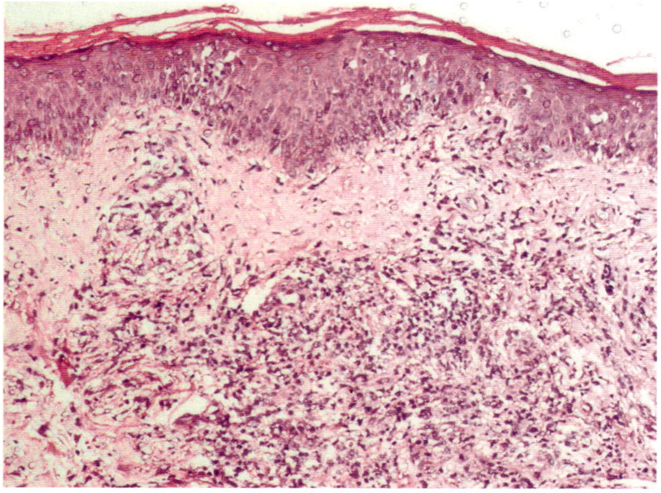

FIGURE 7.2.9.1

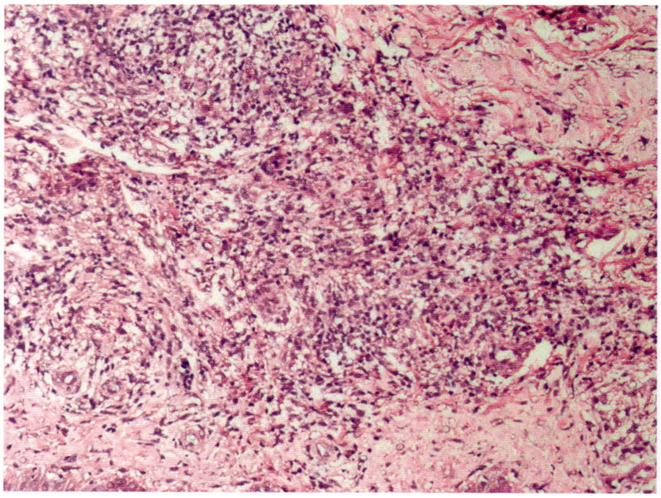

FIGURE 7.2.9.2

7.2.9: Hansen's Disease—Midborderline (BB)

7.2.9.1: Poorly formed granulomas with plump and immature epithelioid cells (*Low power view*)

7.2.9.2: Granulomas showing edema. Lymphocytes usually less in number, no giant cells (*High power view*)

7.2.9.3: Nerve involvement (AFB positive) (*High power view*)

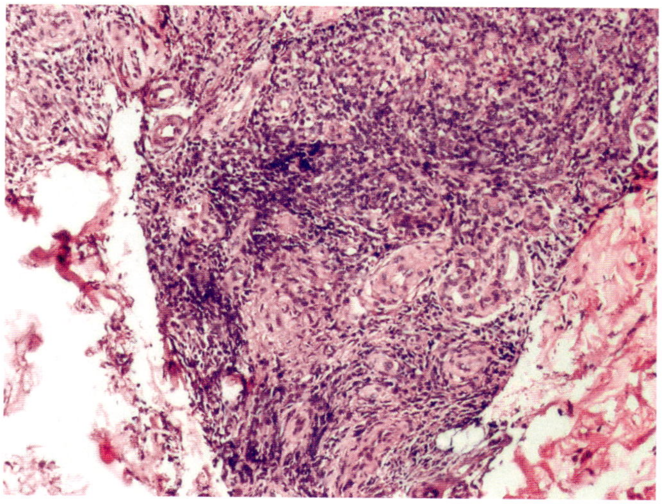

FIGURE 7.2.9.3

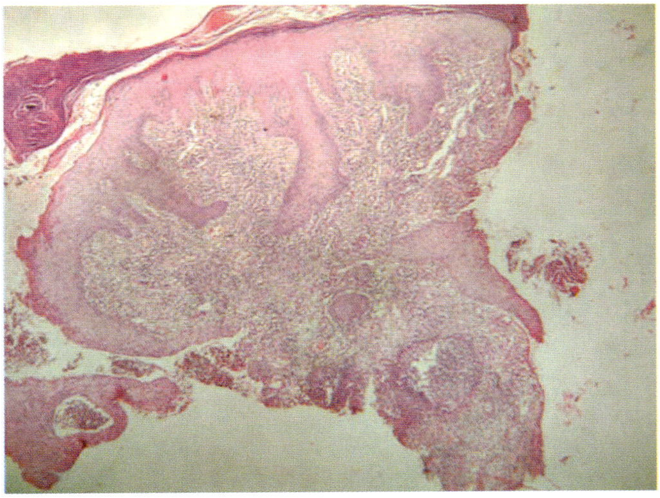

FIGURE 7.3.1.1

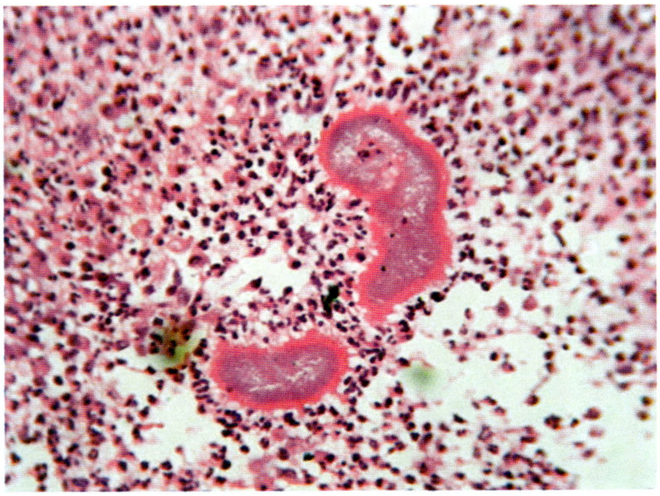

FIGURE 7.3.1.2

7.3: SUPPURATIVE GRANULOMAS

7.3.1: Actinomycetoma

7.3.1.1: Epidermis hyperplastic, dense mixed infiltrate in the dermis (*Scanner view*)

7.3.1.2: Granules are found in the center of zones of suppuration (*Low power view*)

7.3.1.3: Grains are composed of filamentous bacteria, higher magnification shows a pink eosinophilic material around the grain (Splendore-Hoeppli phenomenon) (*High power view*)

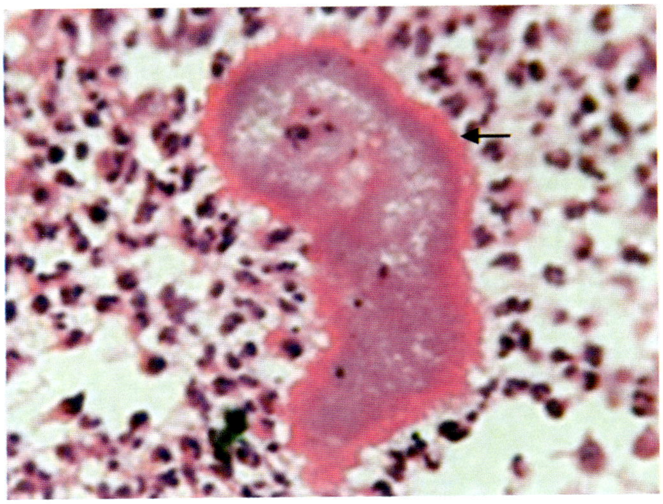

FIGURE 7.3.1.3

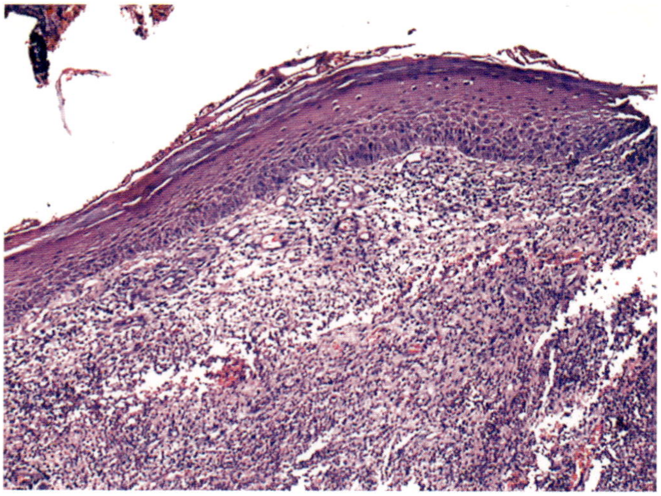

FIGURE 7.3.1.4

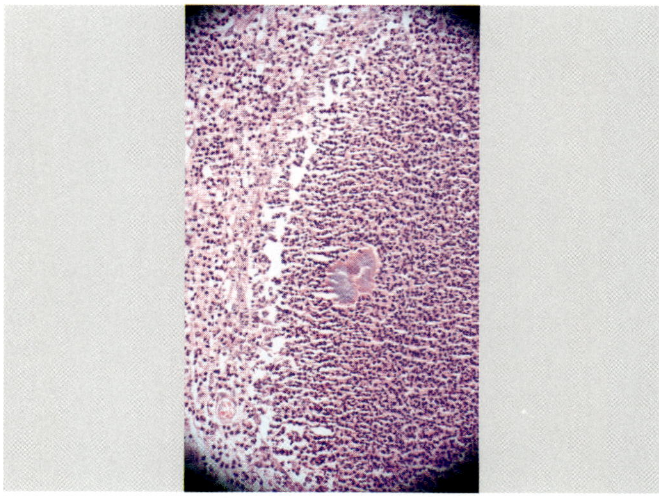

FIGURE 7.3.1.5

7.3.1.4: Another case with mixed inflammatory infiltrate and histiocytes with granuloma (*Scanner view*)

7.3.1.5: Suppurative granuloma of nocardiosis with dense neutrophilic infiltrate (*Low power view*)

7.3.1.6: Higher magnification showing grains of nocardia (*High power view*)

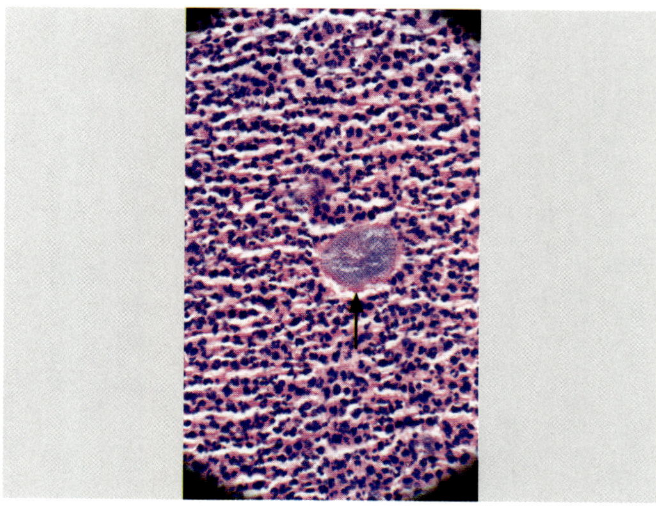

FIGURE 7.3.1.6

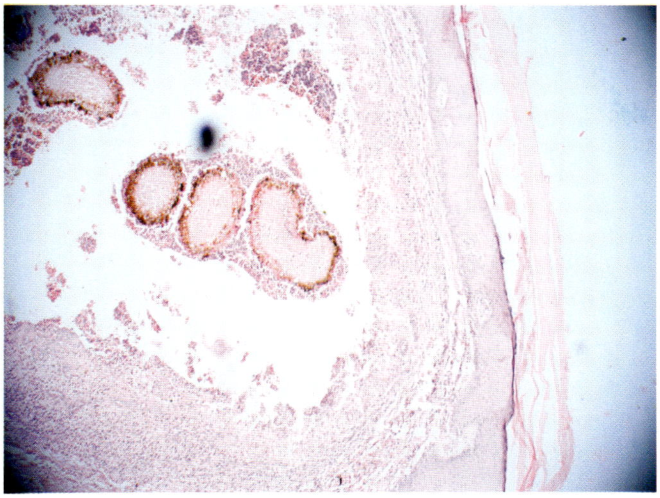

FIGURE 7.3.2.1

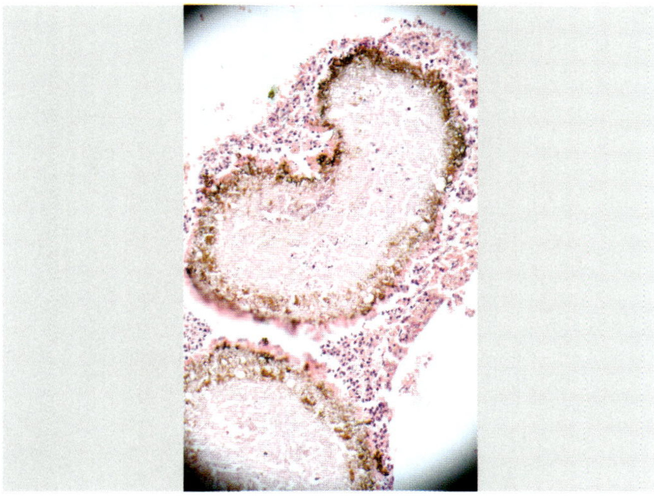

FIGURE 7.3.2.2

7.3.2: Eumycetoma

7.3.2.1: Epidermal hyperplasia at one end, mixed infiltrate in the dermis and granulomas with fungal colonies in neutrophilic abscesses (*Low power view*)

7.3.2.2: High magnification showing the yellow brown fungal hyphae (*High power view*)

7.3.2.3: Filamentous fungi with broad septate hyphae (*Oil immersion view*)

7.3.2.4: Another case with fungal colony—H & E stain (*High power view*)

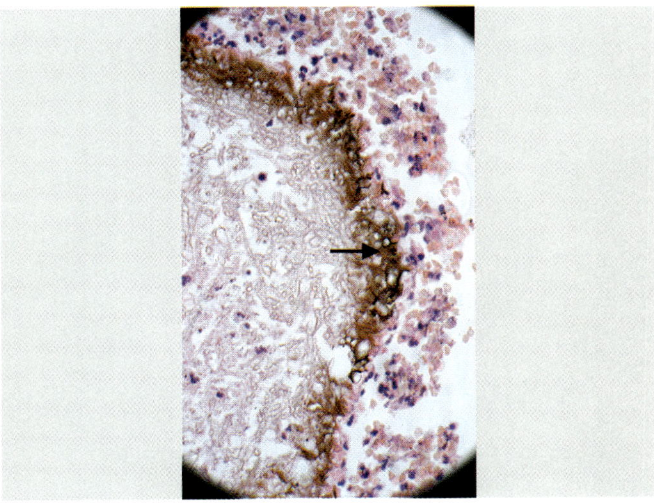

FIGURE 7.3.2.3

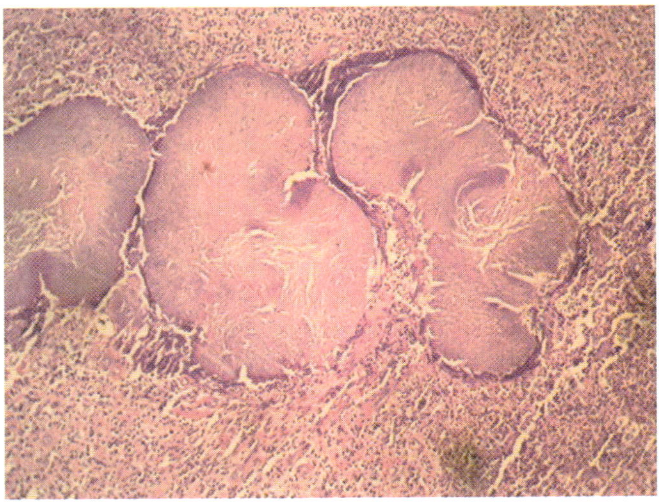

FIGURE 7.3.2.4

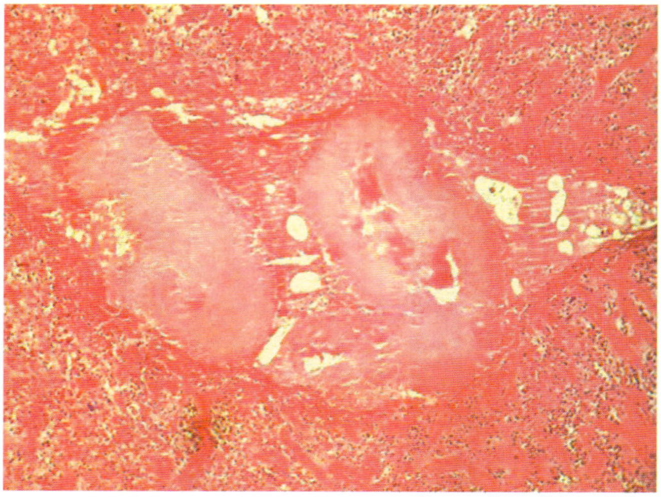

FIGURE 7.3.2.5

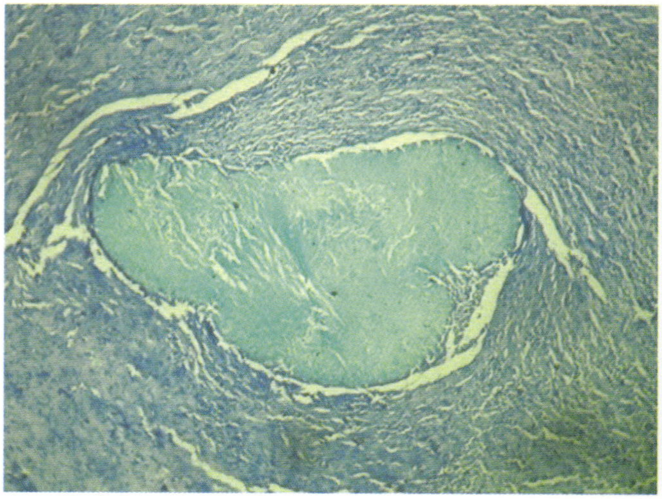

FIGURE 7.3.2.6

7.3.2.5: Gram stain—negative (*High power view*)
7.3.2.6: Acid-fast bacilli (AFB) stain—negative (*High power view*)
7.3.2.7: Periodic acid-Schiff (PAS) stain—positive (*High power view*)
7.3.2.8: Silver methenamine stain—positive (*High power view*)

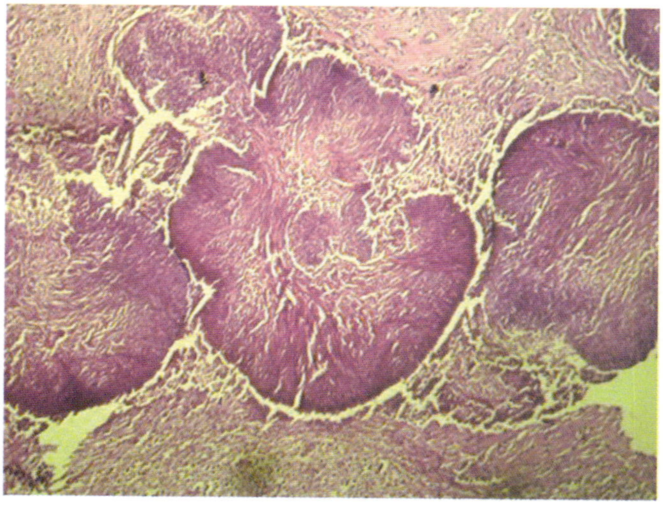

FIGURE 7.3.2.7

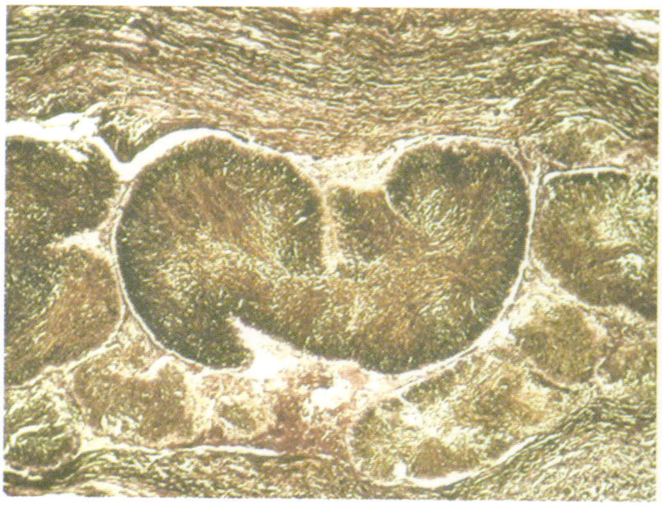

FIGURE 7.3.2.8

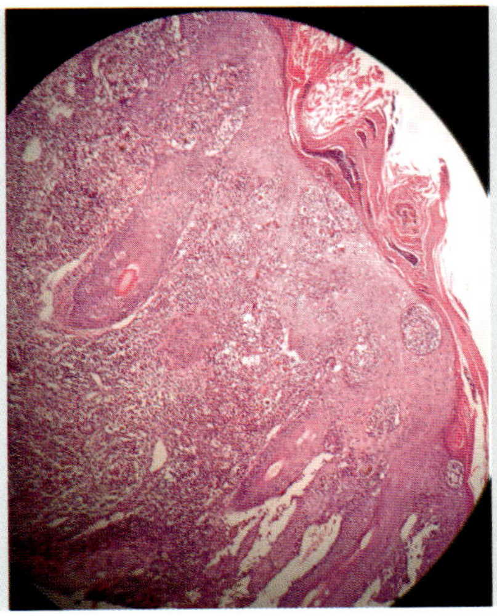

FIGURE 7.3.3.1

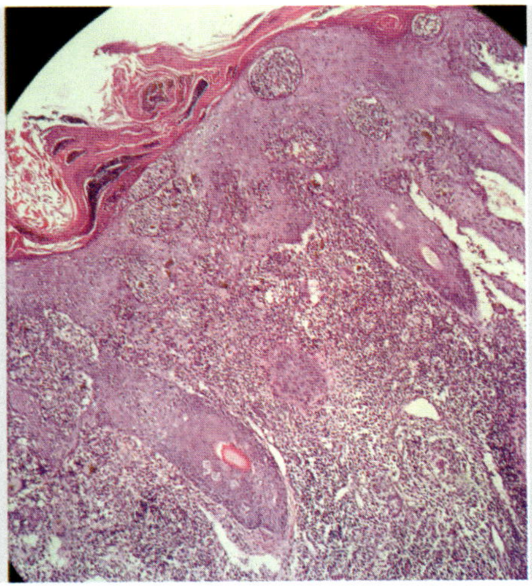

FIGURE 7.3.3.2

7.3.3: Chromomycosis

7.3.3.1: Hyperkeratosis, pseudoepitheliomatous hyperplasia, and mixed infiltrate with granulomas in the upper and mid-dermis (*Scanner view*)

7.3.3.2: Intraepidermal microabscesses and a few eosinophils in the upper dermis (*Low power view*)

7.3.3.3: The fungus is seen with H & E stain also as round, thick-walled golden brown sclerotic bodies (copper penny bodies) either in giant cells or lying free in the dermis (*High power view*)

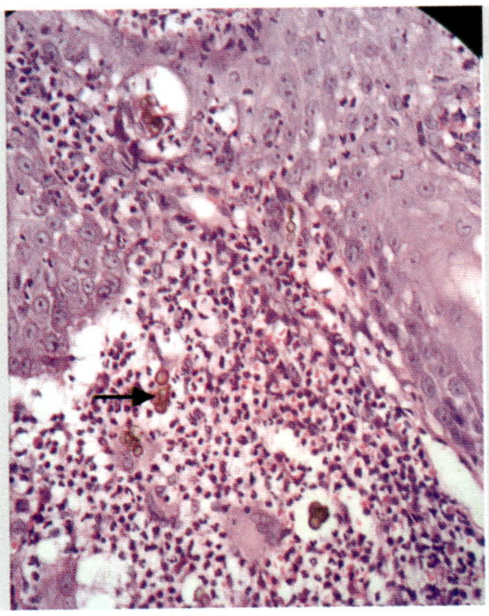

FIGURE 7.3.3.3

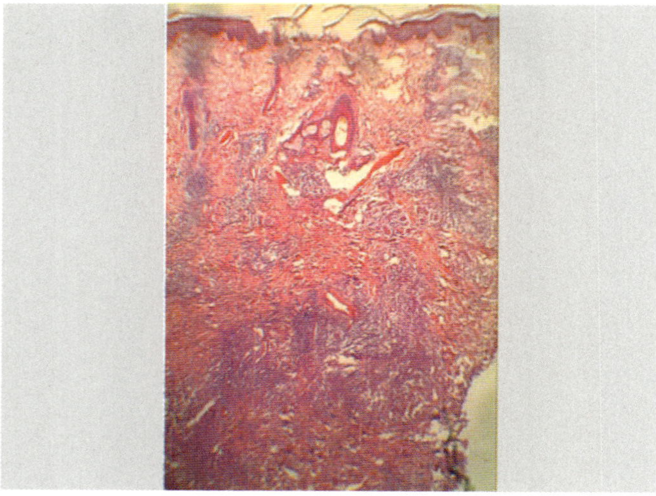

FIGURE 7.3.4.1

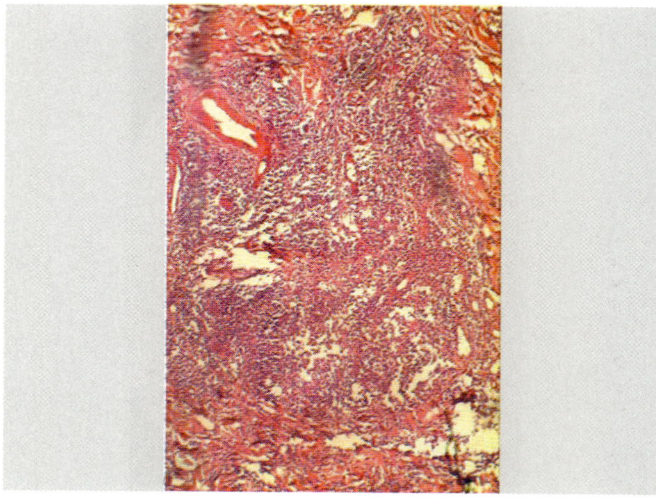

FIGURE 7.3.4.2

7.3.4: Cryptococcosis

7.3.4.1: Granulomatous infiltration extending to deep dermis, the epidermis shows ulceration (*Scanner view*)

7.3.4.2: Dense neutrophilic infiltrate is seen in the dermis (*Low power view*)

7.3.4.3: H & E stain showing Yeast forms (*High power view*)

7.3.4.4: PAS positive organisms (*High power view*)

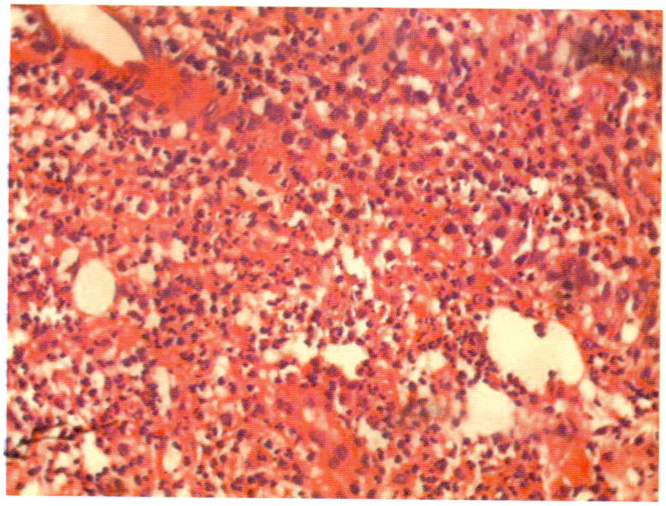

FIGURE 7.3.4.3

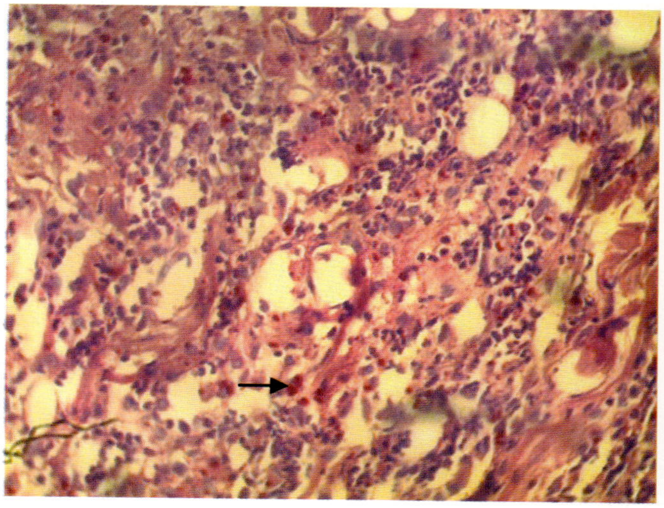

FIGURE 7.3.4.4

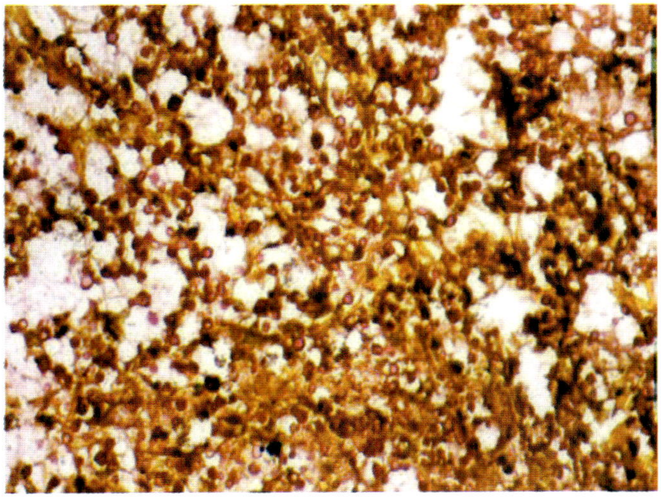

FIGURE 7.3.4.5

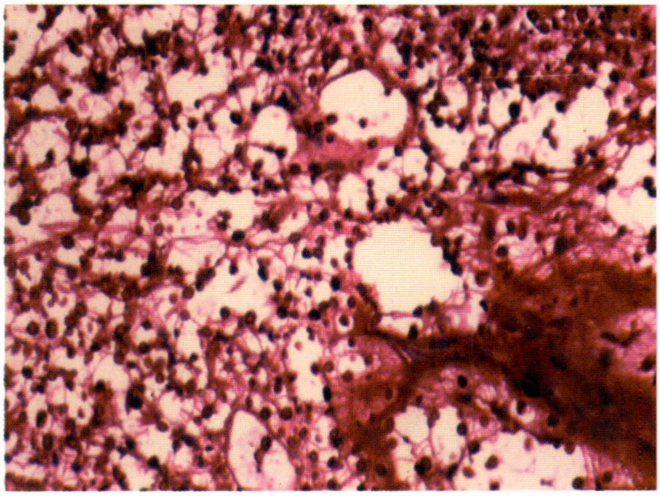

FIGURE 7.3.4.6

7.3.4.5: Silver methenamine stain positive (*High power view*)

7.3.4.6: Mucicarmine stain delineating the fungus better (mucinous capsule) (*High power view*)

7.3.4.7: India ink preparation—the particles of ink pigment do not enter the capsule that surrounds the spherical yeast cell, resulting in a zone of clearance or 'halo' around the cells (*Oil immersion view*)

7.3.4.8: Culture growth—Sabouraud dextrose agar showing creamy colonies

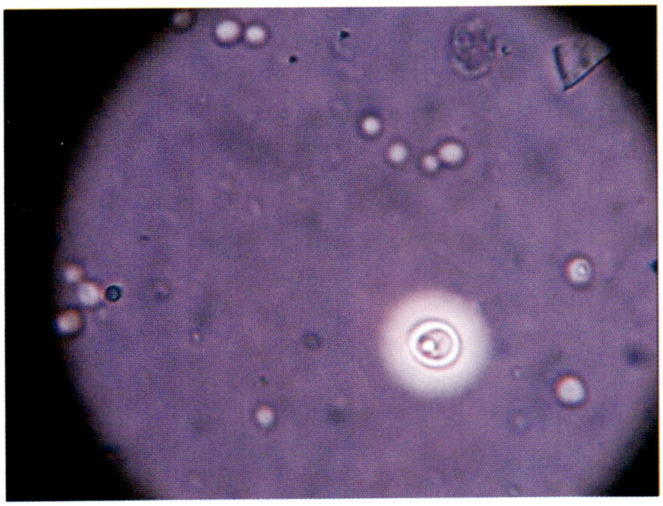

FIGURE 7.3.4.7

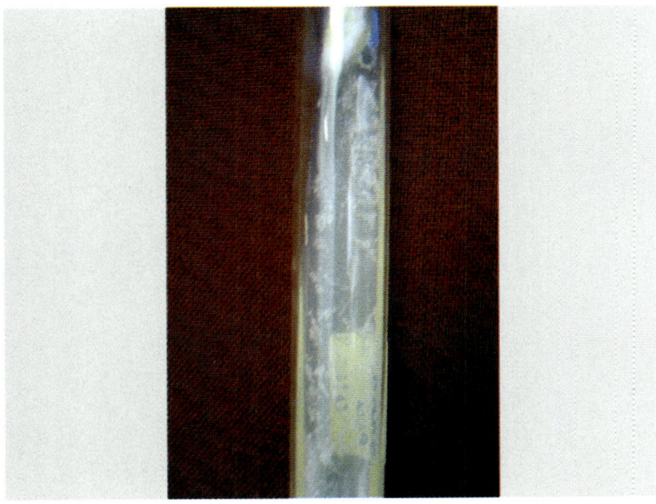

FIGURE 7.3.4.8

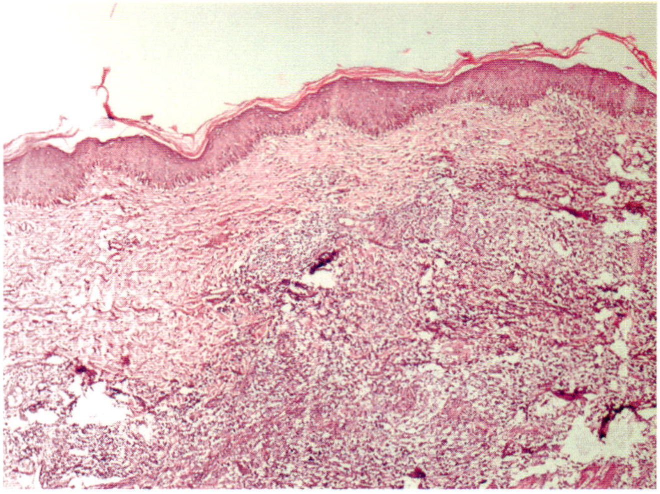

FIGURE 7.3.5.1

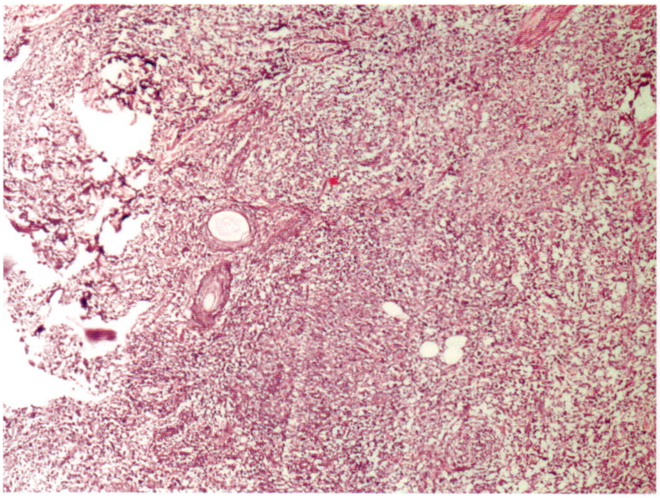

FIGURE 7.3.5.2

7.3.5: Histoplasmosis

7.3.5.1: Granulomatous infiltrate in dermis (*Scanner view*)

7.3.5.2: Inflammatory infiltrate composed of lymphocytes, histiocytes and plasma cells (*Low power view*)

7.3.5.3: On higher magnification yeast forms of histoplasma are seen intracellulary within the histiocytes and extracellularly (*High power view*)

7.3.5.4: Another case with clear halo around the spores. The spores are thick-walled with single nucleus (*Oil immersion view*)

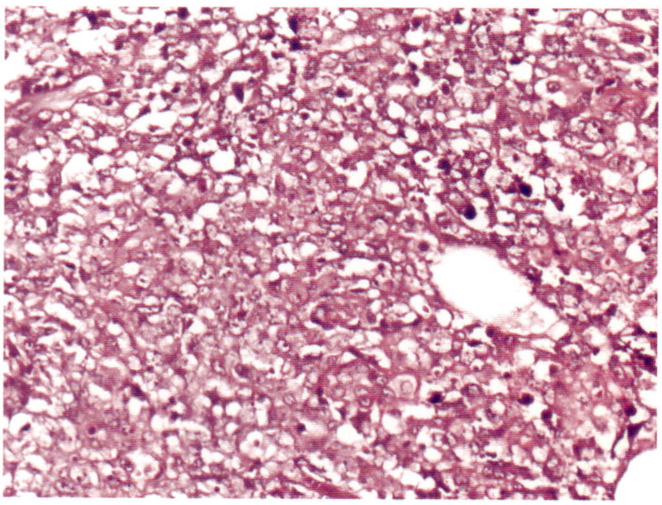

FIGURE 7.3.5.3

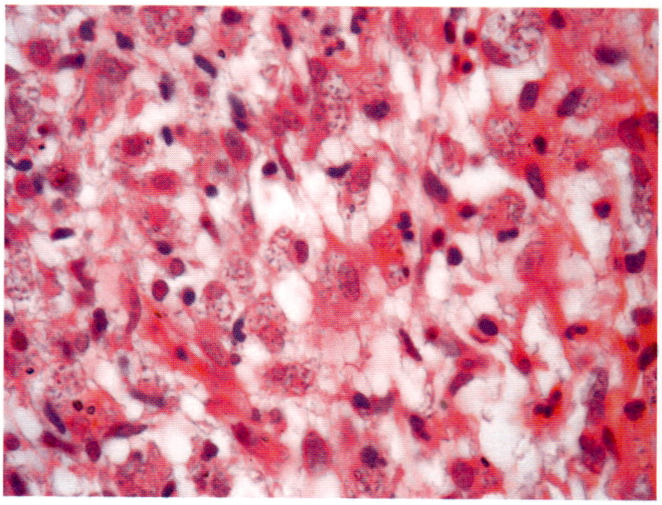

FIGURE 7.3.5.4

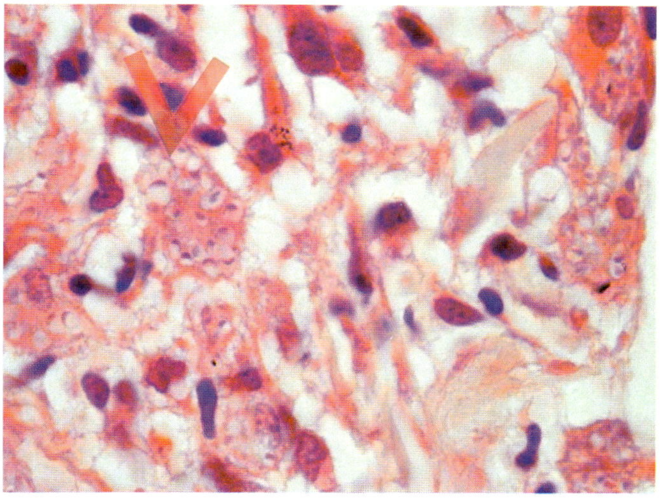

FIGURE 7.3.5.5

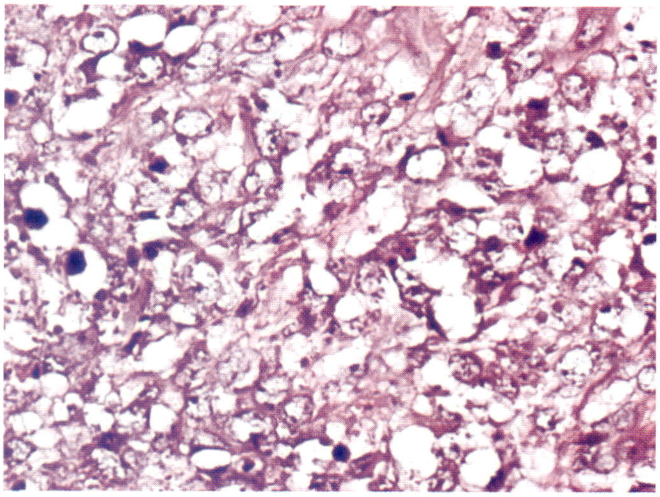

FIGURE 7.3.5.6

7.3.5.5: Histoplasma spores seen within giant cells (*Oil immersion view*)
7.3.5.6: PAS stain showing intracellular spores of histoplasma (*High power view*)
7.3.5.7: Another case with PAS stain demonstrating organisms (*High power view*)

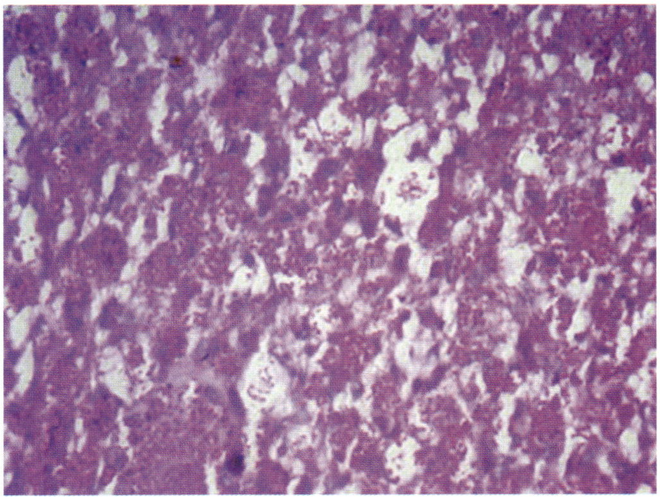

FIGURE 7.3.5.7

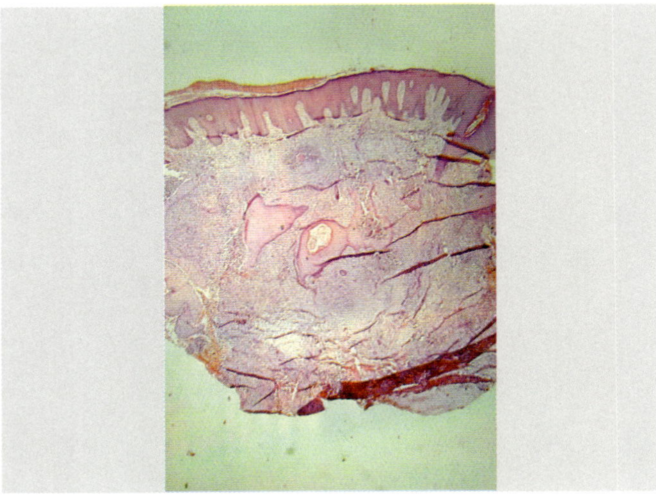

FIGURE 7.3.6.1

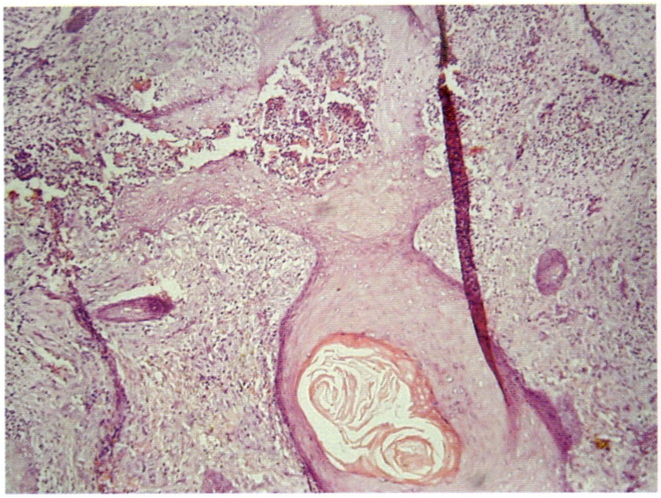

FIGURE 7.3.6.2

7.3.6: Phaeohyphomycosis

7.3.6.1: Scanner view shows deep dermal inflammation (*Scanner view*)

7.3.6.2: The inflammation is mixed granulomatous and suppurative (*Low power view*)

7.3.6.3: Closer view of neutrophils, granuloma and giant cells (*High power view*)

7.3.6.4: Fungal hyphae—thin and septate highlighted in Grocott's methenamine silver (GMS) stain (*Oil immersion view*)

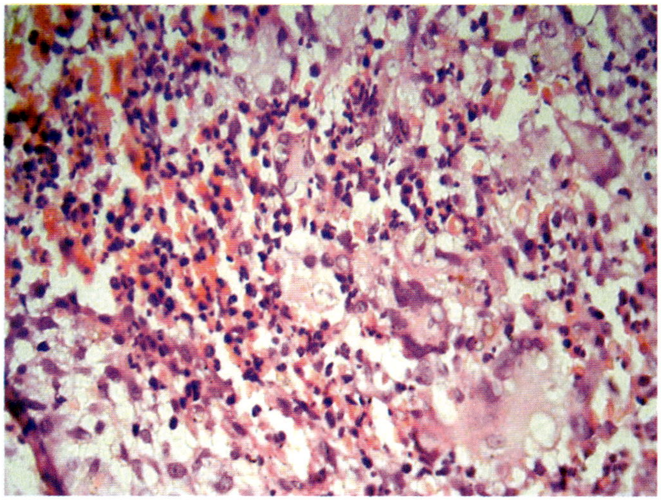

FIGURE 7.3.6.3

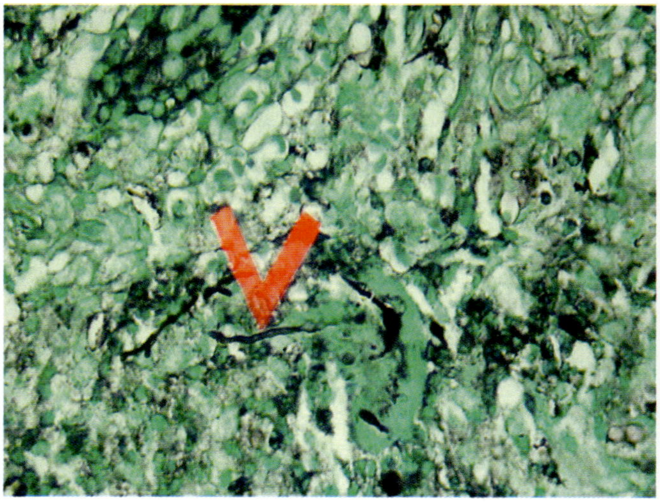

FIGURE 7.3.6.4

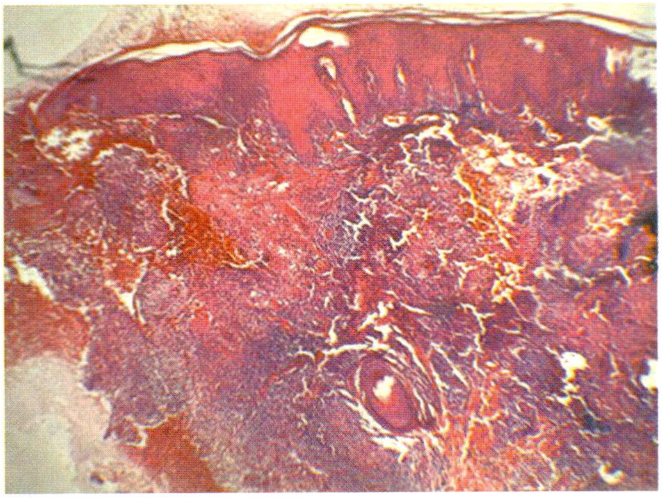

FIGURE 7.3.7.1

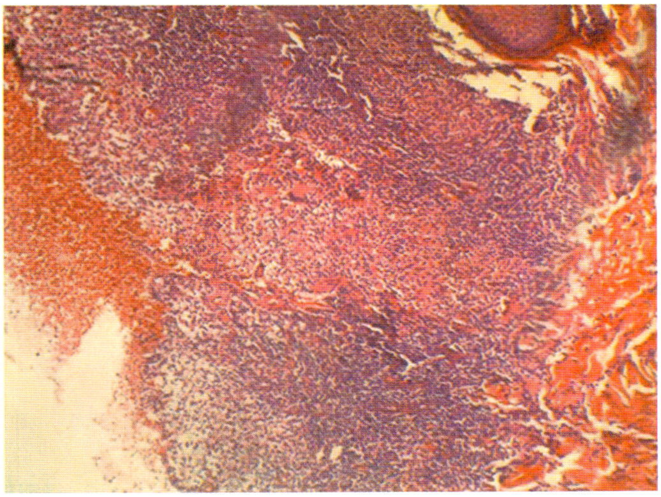

FIGURE 7.3.7.2

7.3.7: Sporotrichosis

7.3.7.1: Prominent pseudoepitheliomatous hyperplasia with some overlying hyperkeratosis (*Scanner view*)

7.3.7.2: Suppurative granulomas in the upper dermis (*Low power view*)

7.3.7.3: Intense neutrophilic infiltrate with giant cells seen (*High power view*)

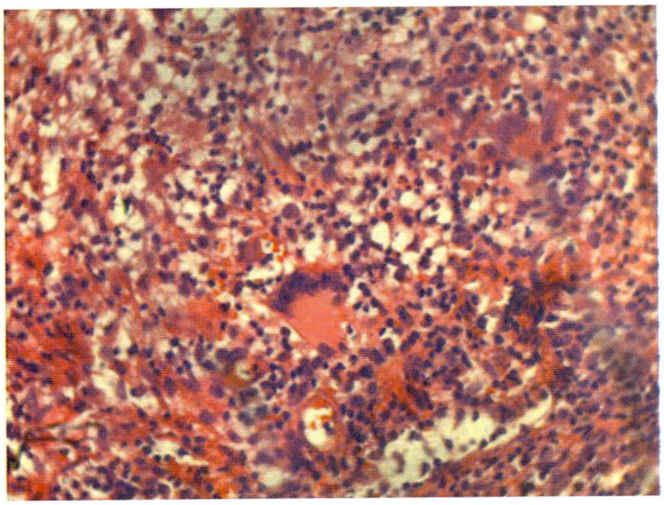

FIGURE 7.3.7.3

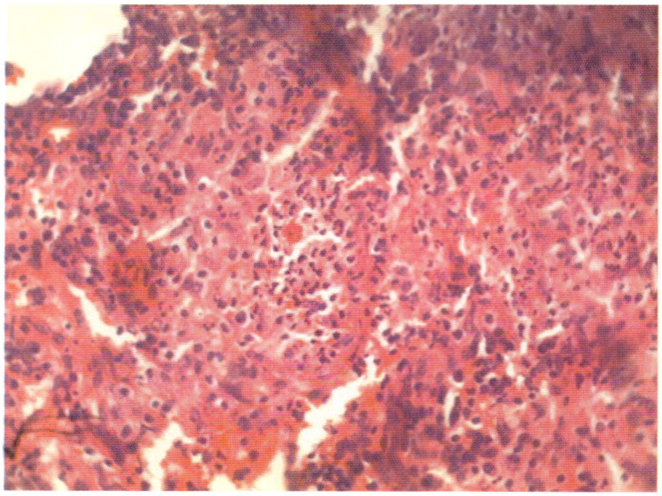

FIGURE 7.3.7.4

7.3.7.4: Organism seen in the midst of neutrophils (*High power view*)

7.3.7.5: Sporothrix asteroid which is a yeast form—blastospore surrounded by an eosinophilic, hyaline material and ray-like processes from the core (*Oil immersion view*)

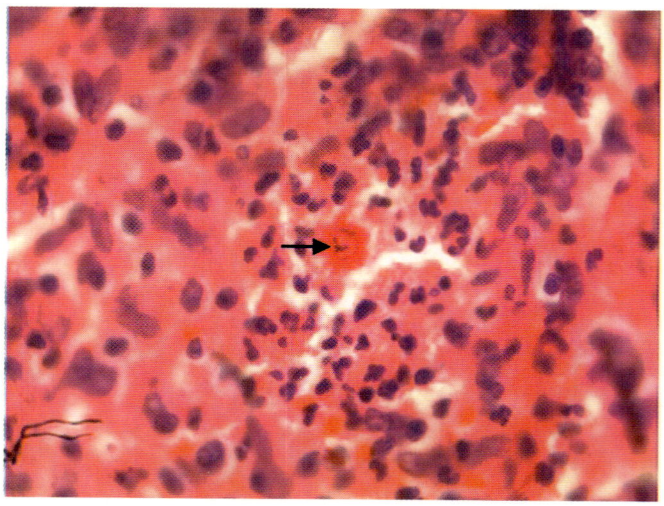

FIGURE 7.3.7.5

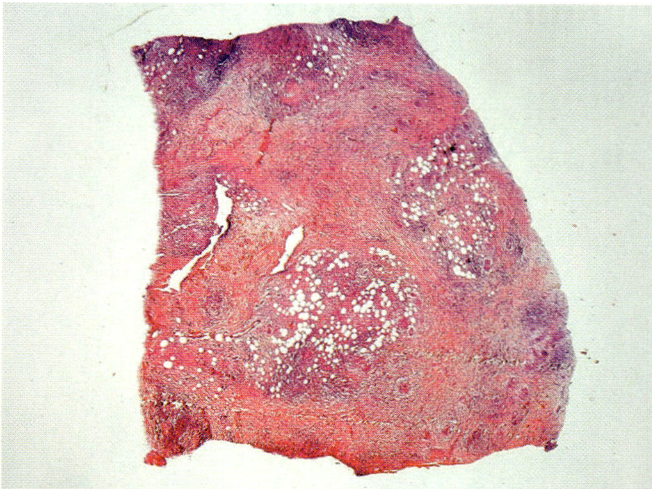

FIGURE 7.3.8.1

7.3.8: Subcutaneous Zygomycosis

7.3.8.1: Dense granulomatous infiltrate in deep dermis and subcutaneous fat (*Scanner view*)

7.3.8.2: Infiltration of histiocytes and giant cells seen around the subcutaneous fat (*Low power view*)

7.3.8.3: Thick-walled fungal hyphae seen as oval or ring-like structures on cross section along with granuloma, giant cells and eosinophils (*High power view*)

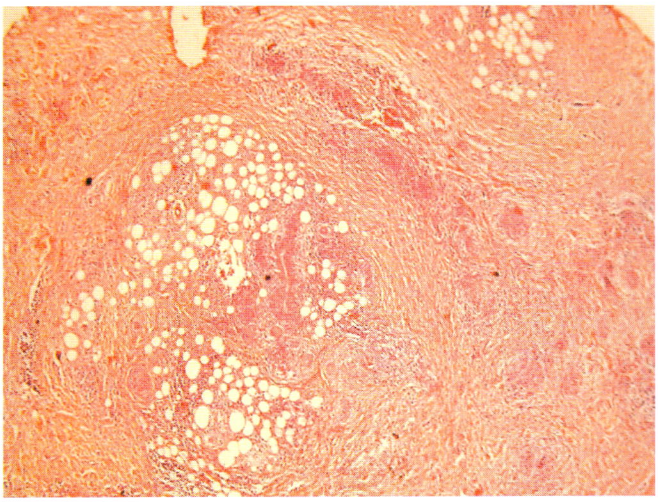

FIGURE 7.3.8.2

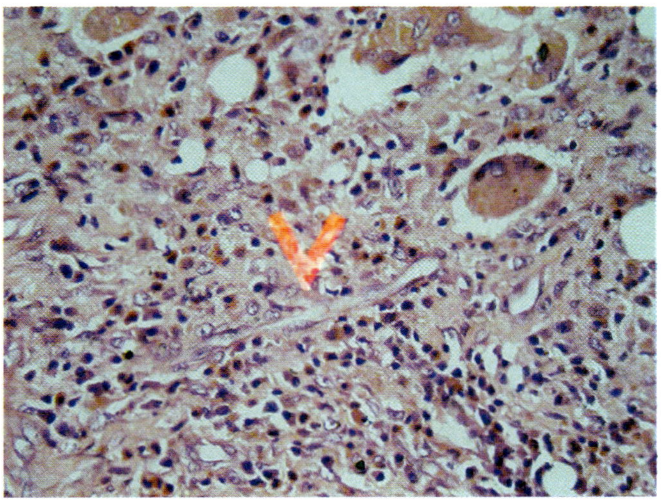

FIGURE 7.3.8.3

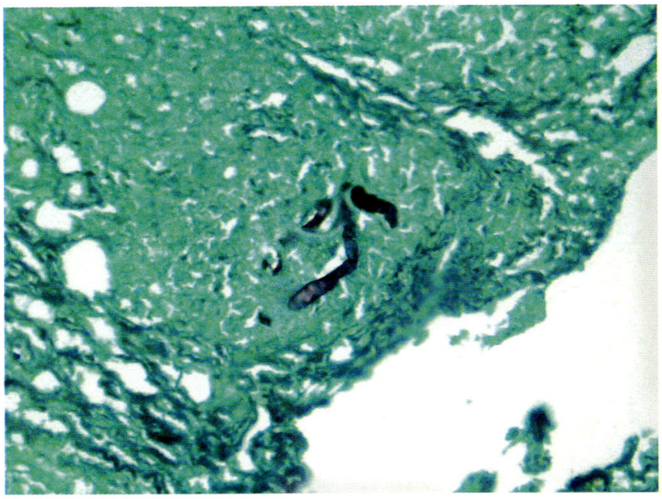

FIGURE 7.3.8.4

7.3.8.4: Aseptate hyphae branching at irregular angles and intervals seen in GMS stain (*Oil immersion view*)

7.3.8.5: Long twisted and collapsed hyphae seen in PAS stain (*High power view*)

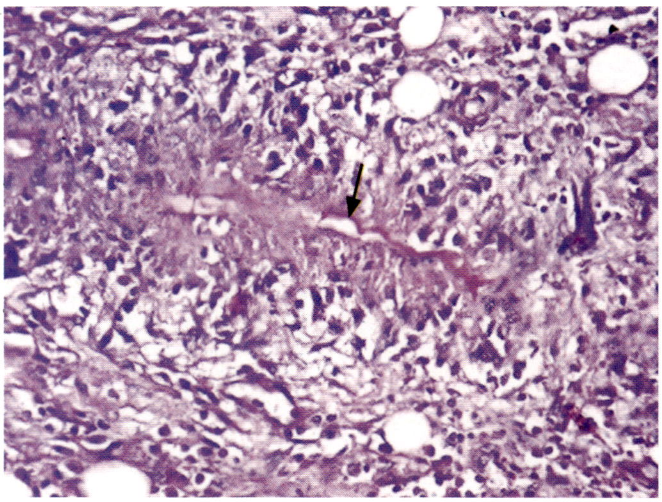

FIGURE 7.3.8.5

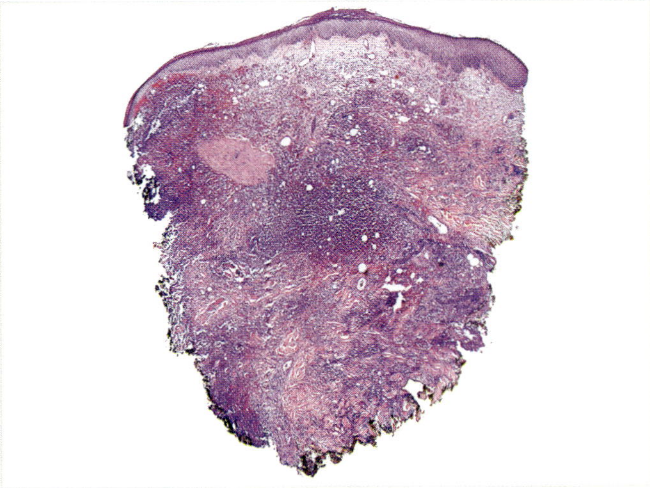

FIGURE 7.3.9.1

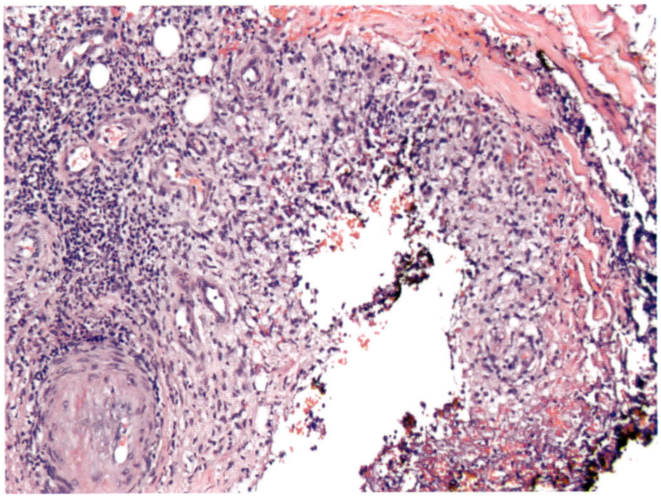

FIGURE 7.3.9.2

7.3.9: Non-tuberculous Mycobacterial Infections

7.3.9.1: *Mycobacterium chelonae*—granulomatous dermatitis (*Scanner view*)

7.3.9.2: Epithelioid cell granuloma (*Low power view*)

7.3.9.3: Dermal neutrophil abscess (*High power view*)

7.3.9.4: AFB positive (*Oil immersion view*)

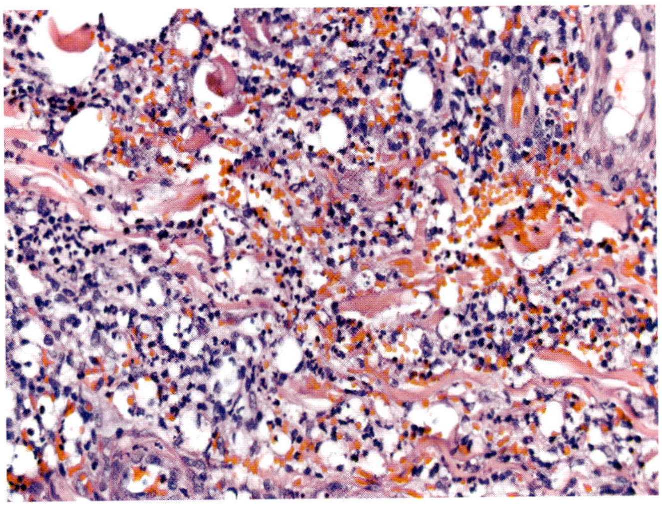

FIGURE 7.3.9.3

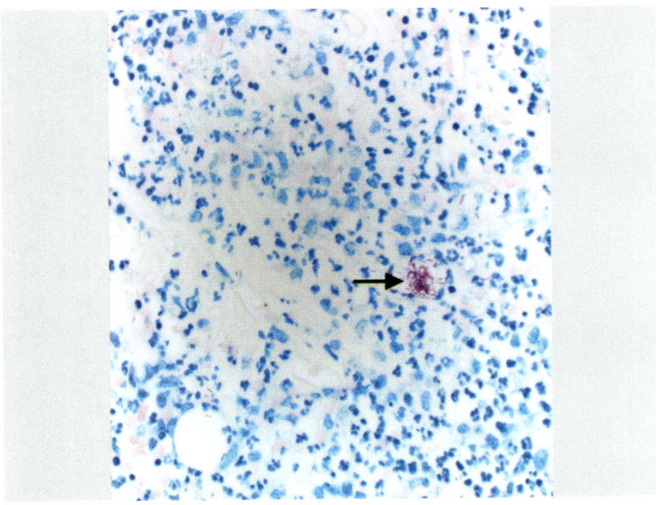

FIGURE 7.3.9.4

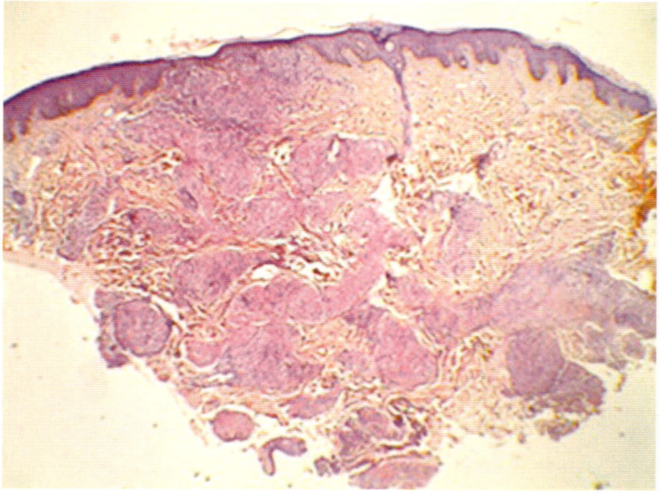

FIGURE 7.4.1.1

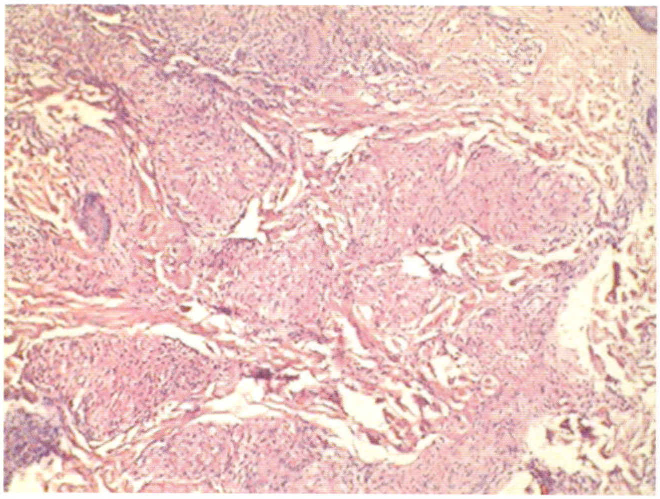

FIGURE 7.4.1.2

7.4: OTHER GRANULOMAS

7.4.1: Sarcoidosis

7.4.1.1: Discrete, round collections of epithelioid histiocytes (*Scanner view*)

7.4.1.2: Low power view of granulomas (*Low power view*)

7.4.1.3: Paucity of surrounding lymphocytes and plasma cells (naked granulomas) (*High power view*)

7.4.1.4: Lymphocytes are usually not seen within the granuloma (*High power view*)

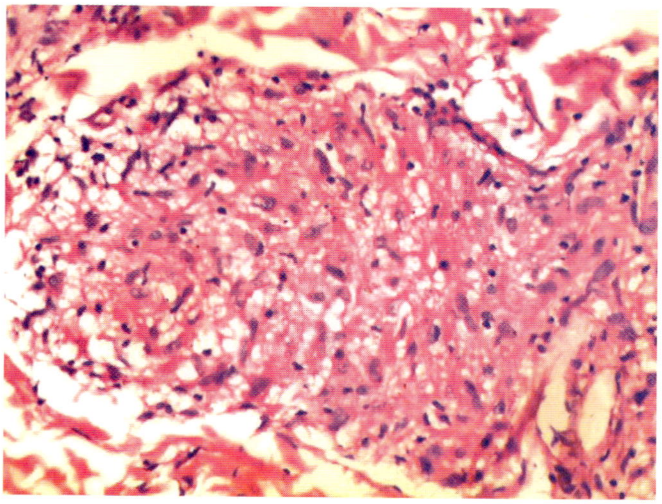

FIGURE 7.4.1.3

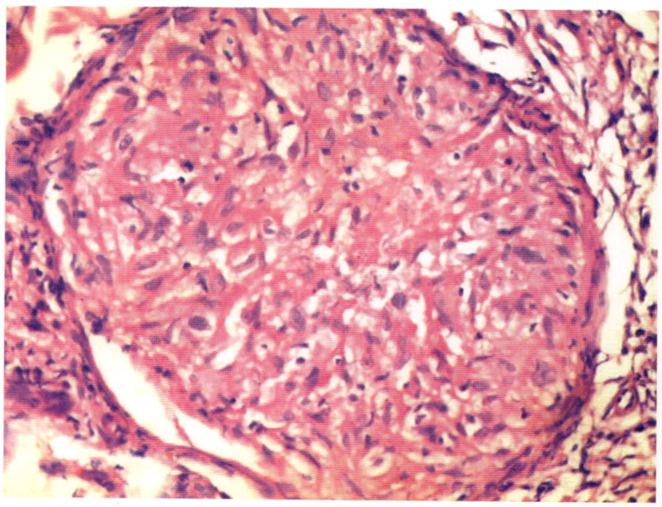

FIGURE 7.4.1.4

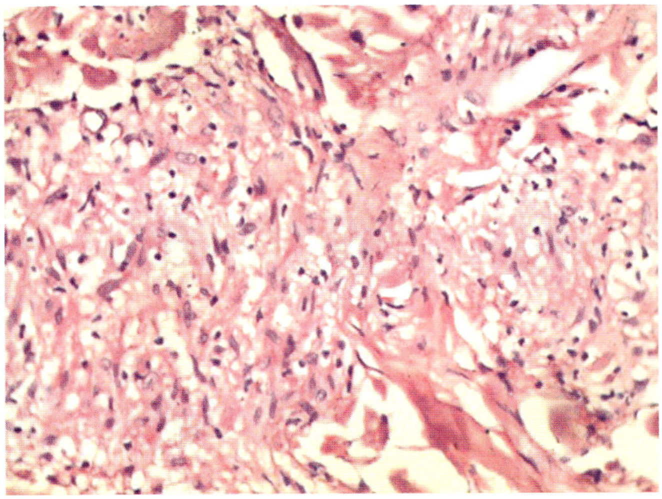

FIGURE 7.4.1.5

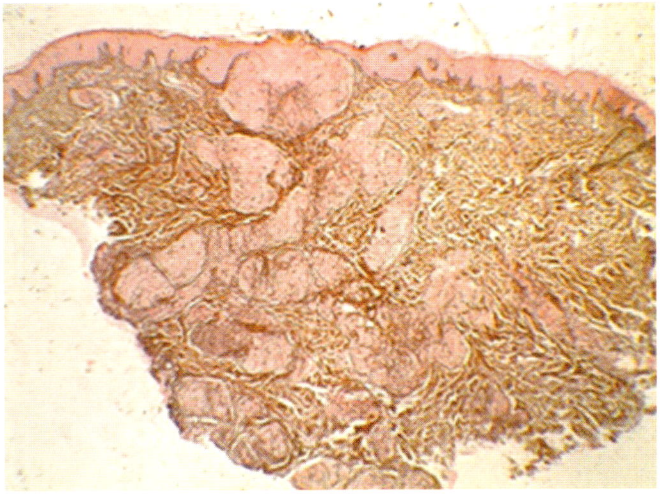

FIGURE 7.4.1.6

7.4.1.5: Noncaseating granulomas lie in close proximity but not confluent like tuberculosis (*High power view*)

7.4.1.6: Reticulin stain (*Scanner view*)

7.4.1.7: Fine reticulin fiber network encircles the granulomas (*Low power view*)

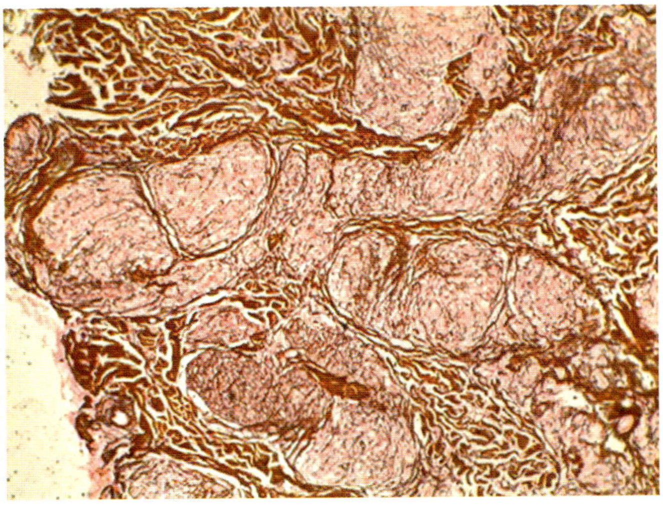

FIGURE 7.4.1.7

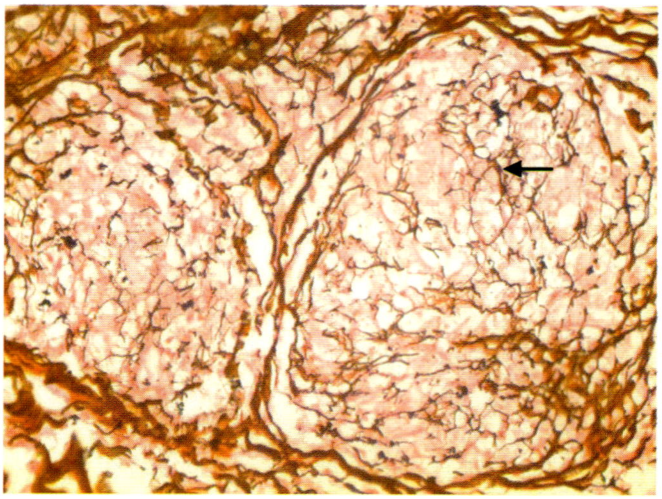

FIGURE 7.4.1.8

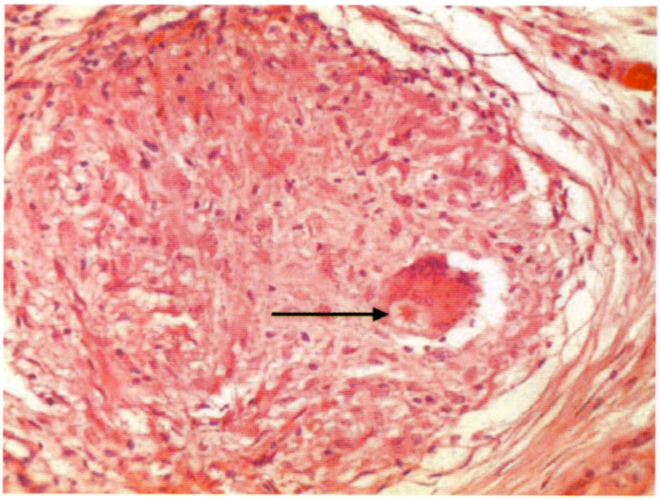

FIGURE 7.4.1.9

7.4.1.8: Reticulin fibers penetrate the granulomas (*High power view*)

7.4.1.9: Asteroid body (Central core and radiating spicules) in giant cell (*High power view*)

7.4.1.10: Schaumann bodies (*Scanner view*)

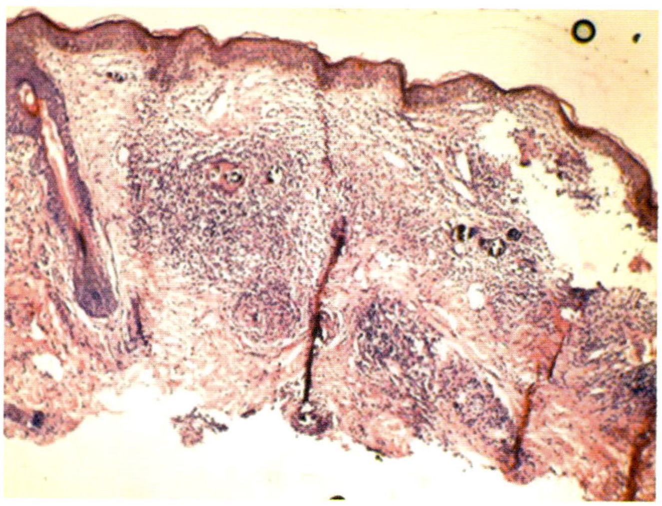

FIGURE 7.4.1.10

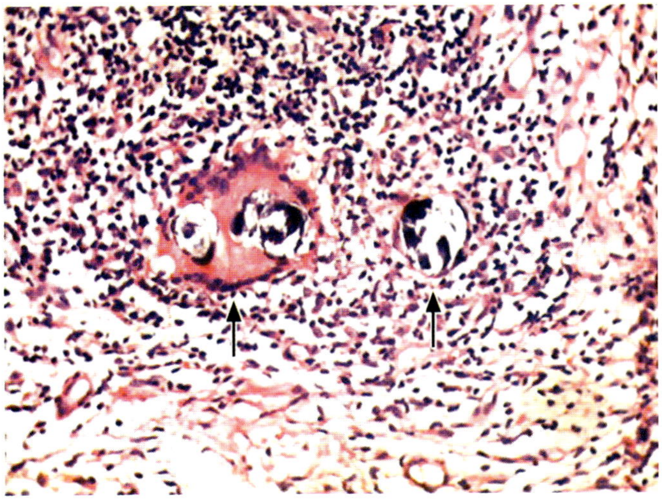

FIGURE 7.4.1.11

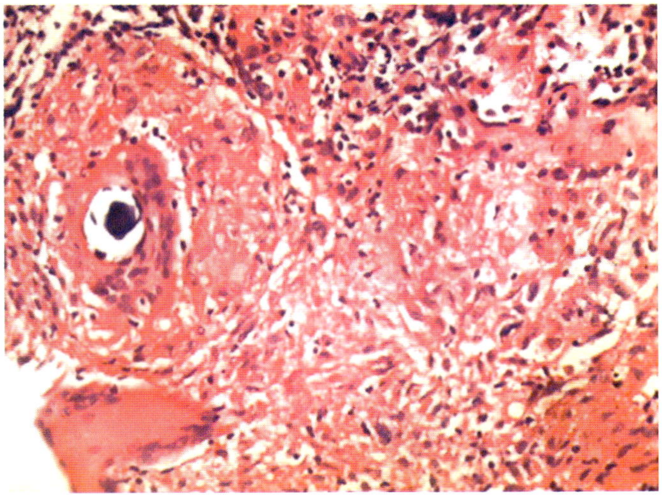

FIGURE 7.4.1.12

7.4.1.11: Schaumann bodies—shell-like calcium-impregnated protein complexes (*High power view*)

7.4.1.12: Multinucleated giant cells (both langhans and foreign body type) (*High power view*)

7.4.1.13: Granuloma with Schaumann body, specific for sarcoid than tuberculosis, very uncommon in skin, usually found in lymph nodes (*High power view*)

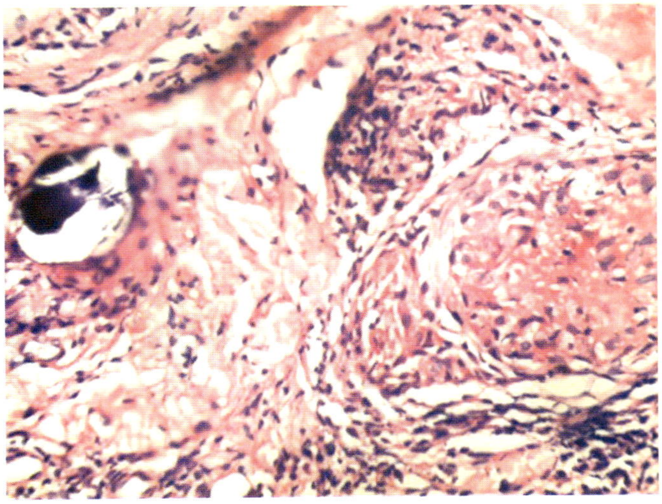

FIGURE 7.4.1.13

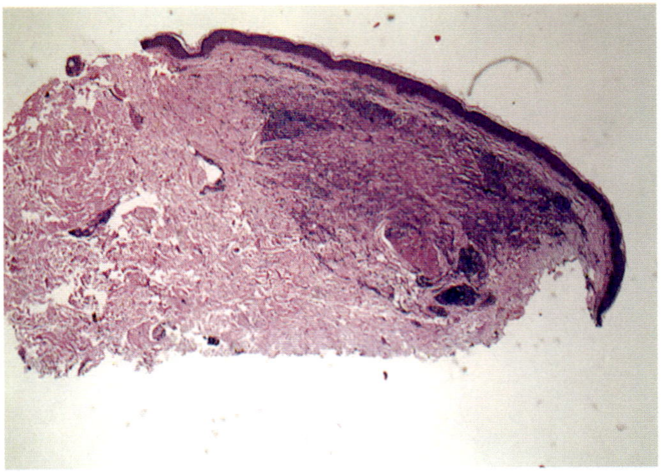

FIGURE 7.4.2.1.1

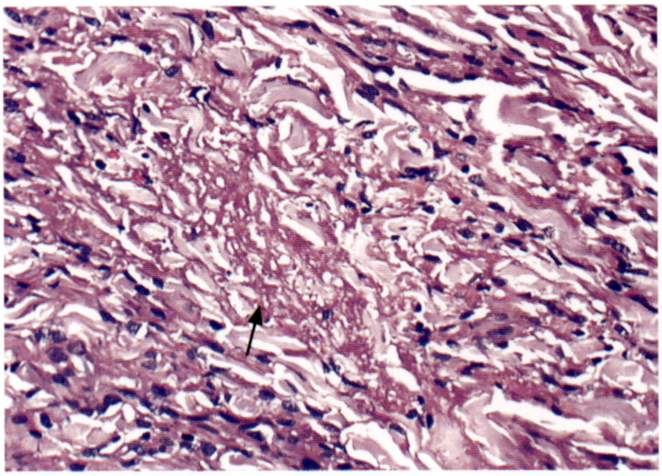

FIGURE 7.4.2.1.2

7.4.2: Palisading Granuloma

7.4.2.1: Granuloma Annulare

7.4.2.1.1: Focus of necrobiosis, surrounded by histiocytes and lymphocytes, in the superficial dermis. The dermis in between normal with no fibrosis (*Scanner view*)

7.4.2.1.2: Necrobiotic zone with palisading of lymphocytes and histiocytes (*High power view*)

7.4.2.1.3: Multinucleated giant cells (*High power view*)

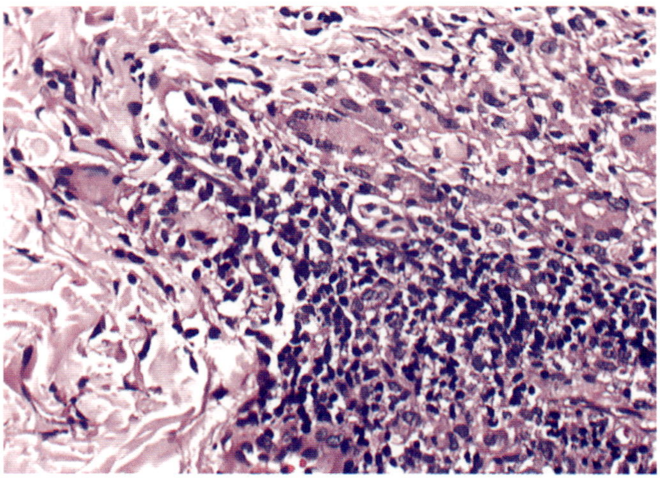

FIGURE 7.4.2.1.3

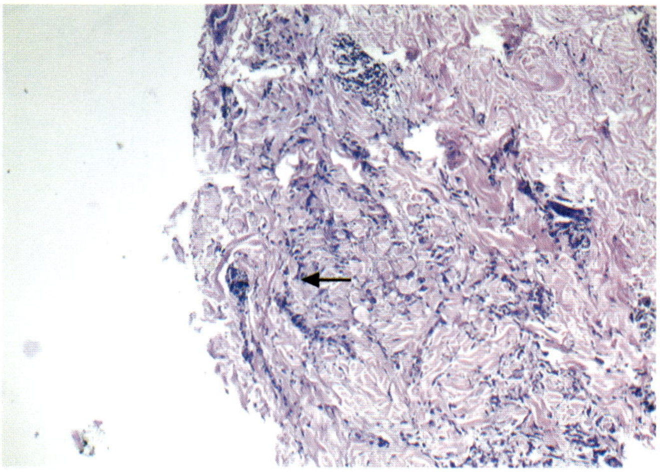

FIGURE 7.4.2.1.4

7.4.2.1.4: Interstitial granuloma annulare—the dermis is hypercellular referred to as busy dermis. Necrobiosis not prominent (*Low power view*)

7.4.2.1.5: Lymphohistiocytes in between collagen bundles. Increased interstitial mucin (*High power view*)

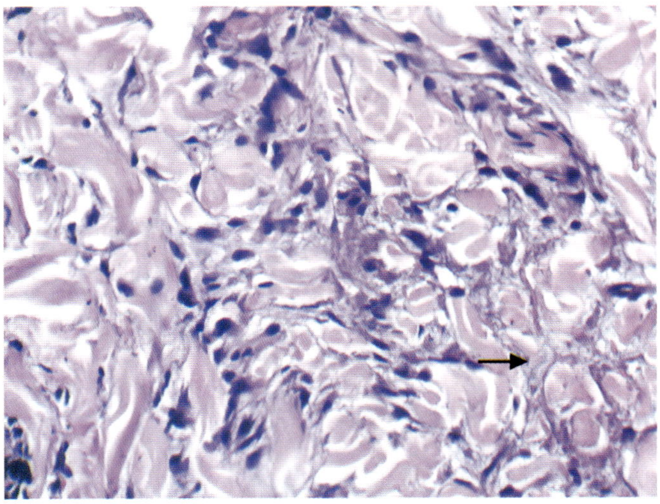

FIGURE 7.4.2.1.5

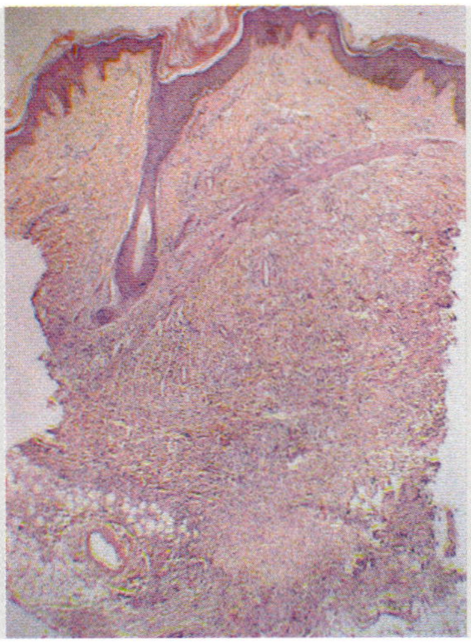

FIGURE 7.4.2.2.1

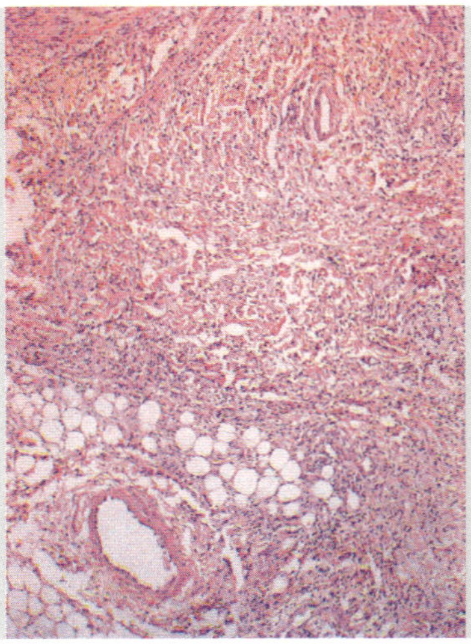

FIGURE 7.4.2.2.2

7.4.2.2: Necrobiosis Lipoidica

7.4.2.2.1: Deep dermis and subcutaneous tissue involvement (*Scanner view*)

7.4.2.2.2: Changes of partial necrobiosis and infiltrate in layers (*Low power view*)

7.4.2.2.3: Another case with lymphohistiocytes and giant cells (*High power view*)

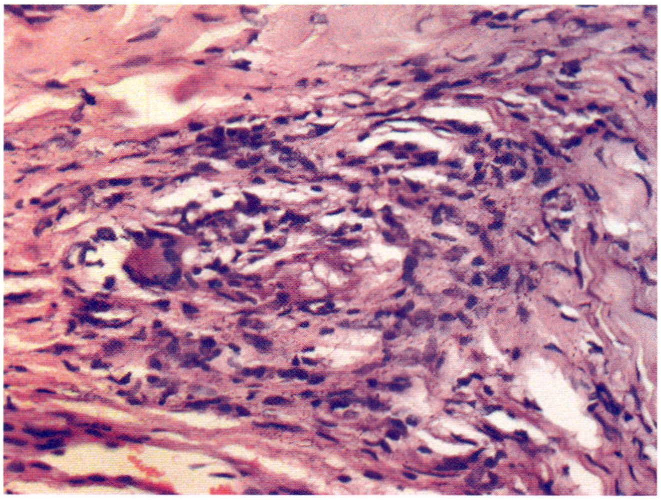

FIGURE 7.4.2.2.3

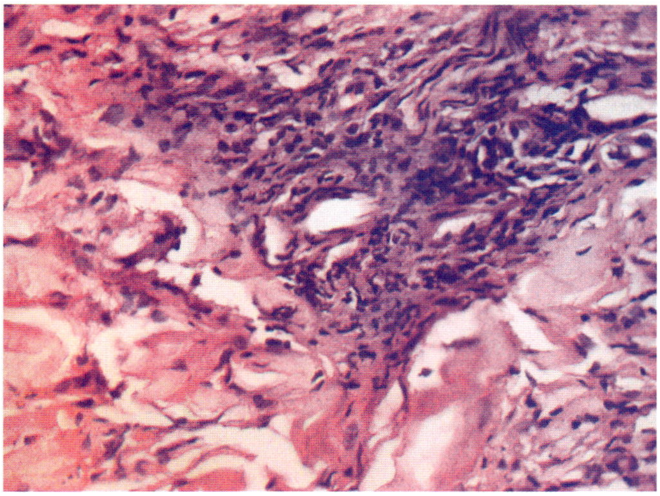

FIGURE 7.4.2.2.4

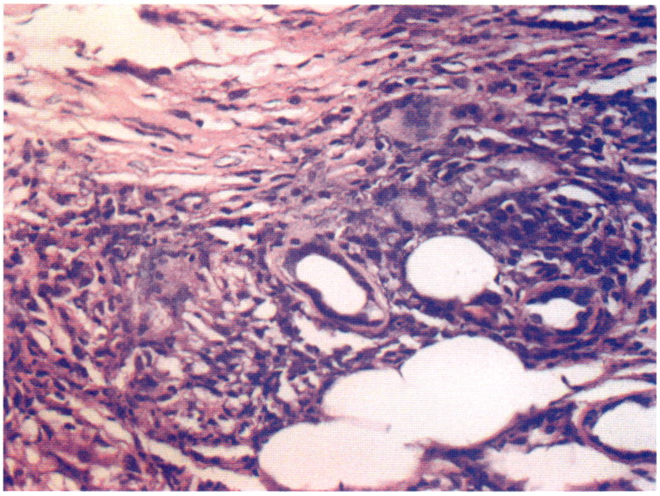

FIGURE 7.4.2.2.5

7.4.2.2.4: Perivascular lymphocytes and plasma cells (*High power view*)

7.4.2.2.5: Multiple giant cells, less prominent necrobiosis and mucin (*High power view*)

7.4.2.2.6: Dermal fibrosis (*High power view*)

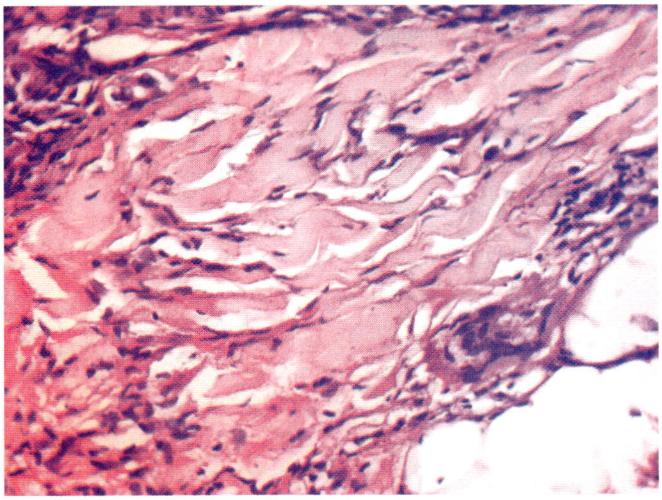

FIGURE 7.4.2.2.6

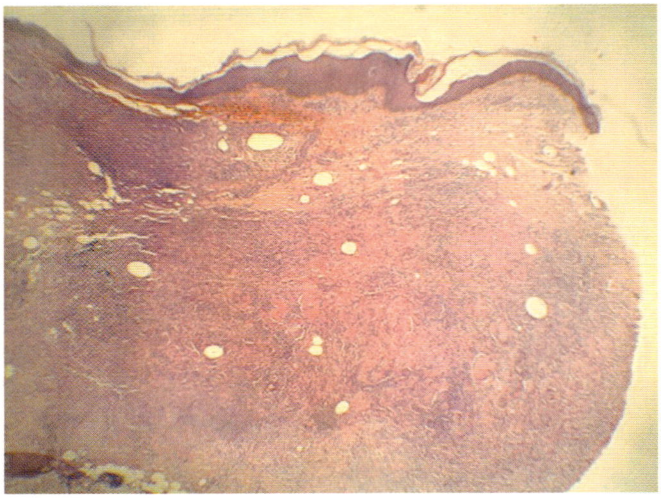

FIGURE 7.4.3.1

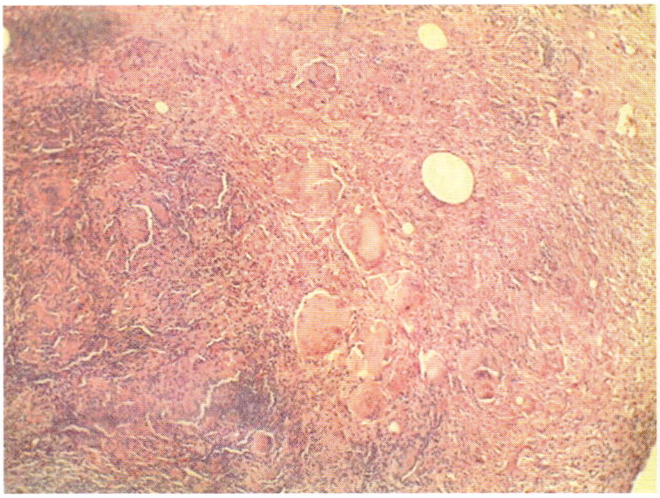

FIGURE 7.4.3.2

7.4.3: Foreign Body Granuloma

7.4.3.1: Dense inflammatory infiltrate in the dermis (*Scanner view*)

7.4.3.2: Multiple giant cells seen (*Low power view*)

7.4.3.3: Foreign body giant cells (*High power view*)

7.4.3.4: Refractile foreign body inside a multinucleate giant cell (*High power view*)

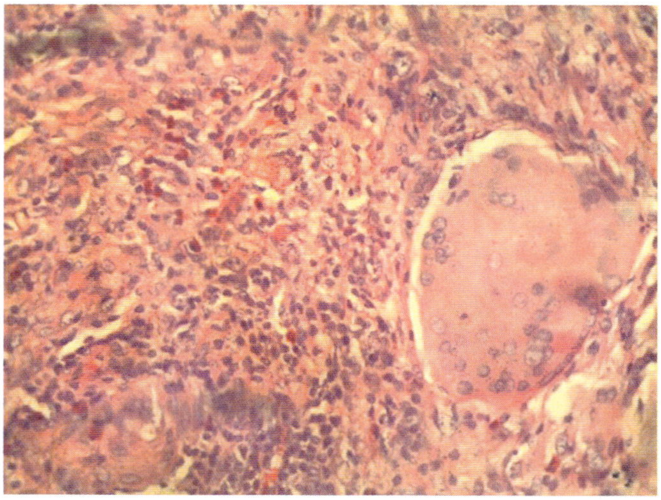

FIGURE 7.4.3.3

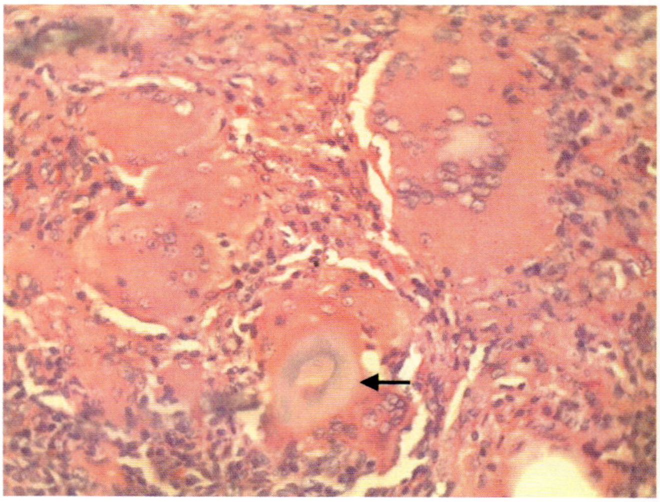

FIGURE 7.4.3.4

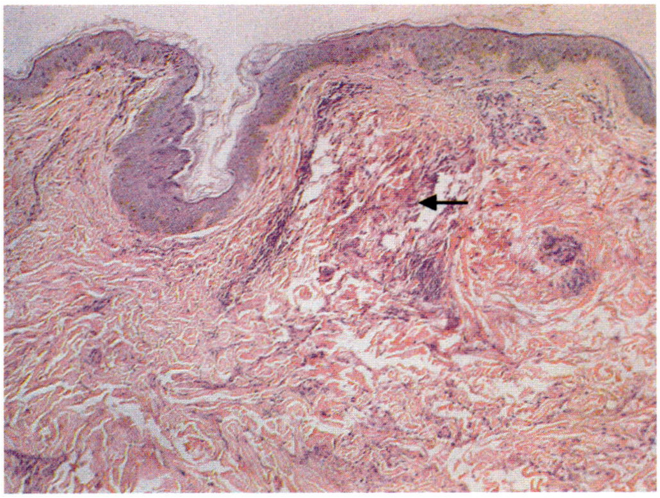

FIGURE 7.4.4.1.1

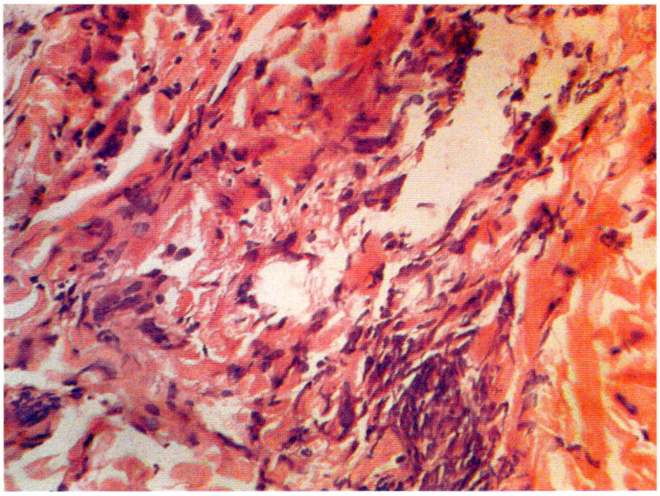

FIGURE 7.4.4.1.2

7.4.4: Miscellaneous Conditions with Granulomas

7.4.4.1: Actinic Granuloma

7.4.4.1.1: A zone of elastic degeneration with infiltrate (*Low power view*)

7.4.4.1.2: Lymphohistiocytes with attempt towards formation of multinucleated giant cells and degenerated material (*High power view*)

7.4.4.1.3: Another case with degraded elastin and giant cell reaction (*High power view*)

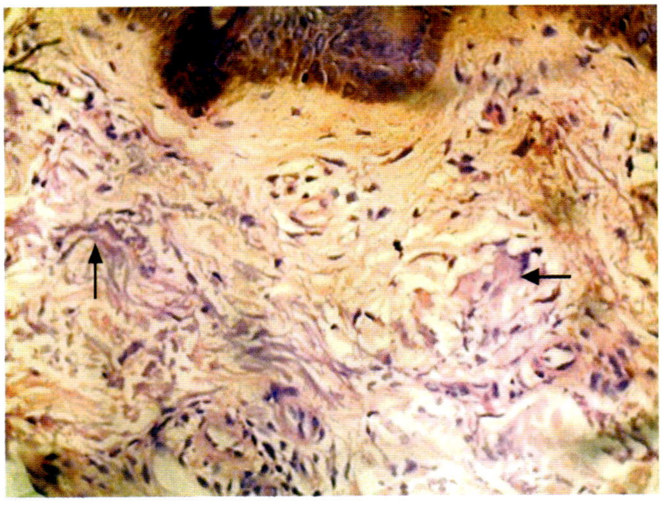

FIGURE 7.4.4.1.3

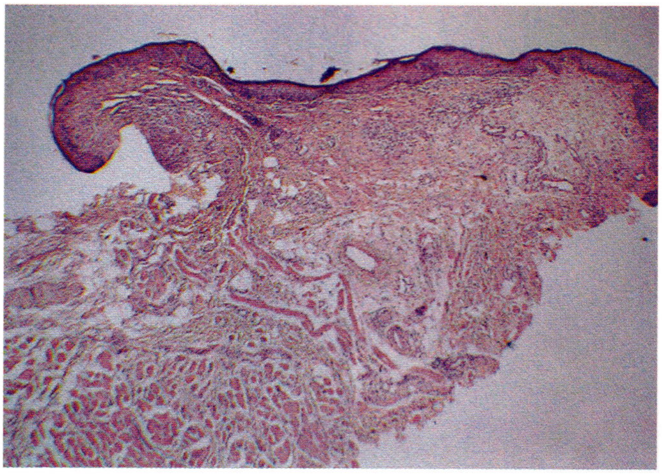

FIGURE 7.4.4.2.1

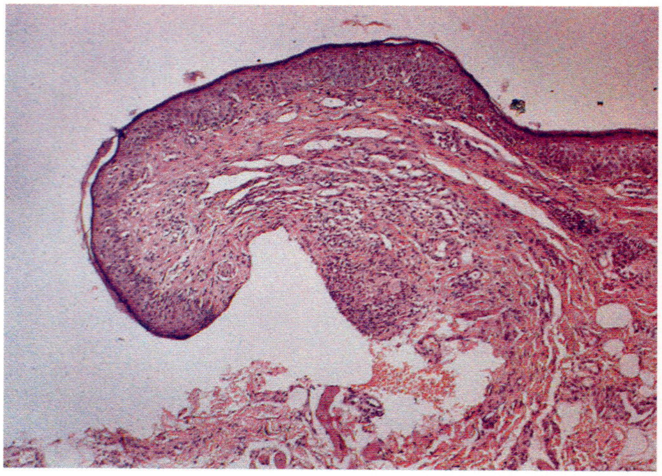

FIGURE 7.4.4.2.2

7.4.4.2: Cheilitis Granulomatosa

7.4.4.2.1: Mucosa of lip with superficial dermal infiltrate (*Scanner view*)

7.4.4.2.2: Dermal edema and granuloma (*Low power view*)

7.4.4.2.3: Granuloma with giant cells (*High power view*)

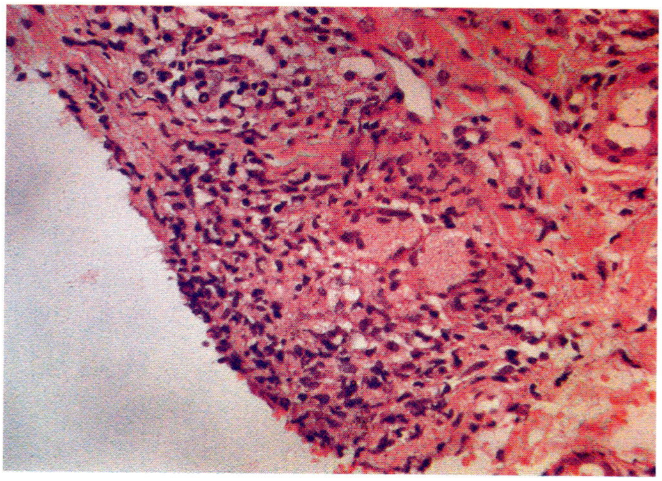

FIGURE 7.4.4.2.3

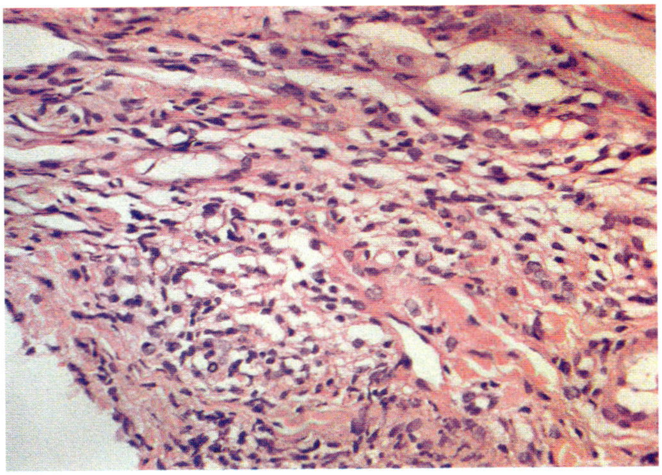

FIGURE 7.4.4.2.4

7.4.4.2.4: Perivascular lymphohistiocytes (*High power view*)

7.4.4.2.5: One of the patients who had gastrointestinal (GI) symptoms showed granulomas on colon biopsy (Crohn's disease) (*High power view*)

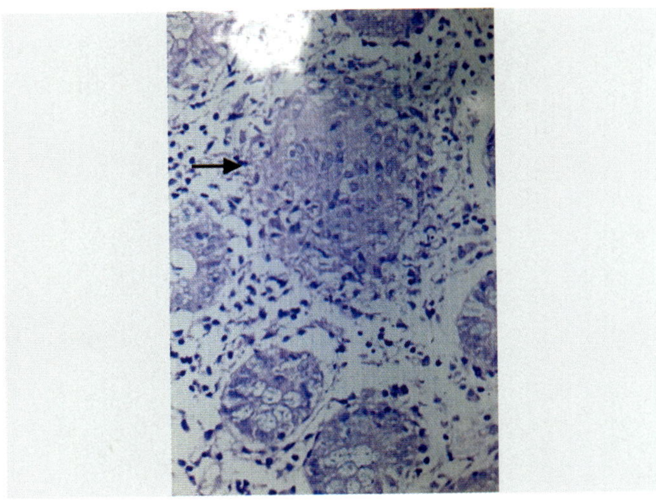

FIGURE 7.4.4.2.5

DIFFERENTIAL DIAGNOSIS

1. Rheumatic nodule
2. Necrobiotic xanthogranuloma
3. Palisaded neutrophilic and granulomatous dermatitis
4. Facial idiopathic granulomas with regressive evolution (FIGURE)

DIAGNOSTIC PEARLS

1. Presence of birefringent crystals on polarization in the granulomas can be seen in sarcoidosis in addition to foreign body granulomas.
2. Early lesions of granuloma annulare may not show palisading granulomas. There is macrophage infiltration between collagen bundles and increased mucin.
3. Subcutaneous palisaded granulomas with central fibrinoid necrosis lacking mucin is characteristic of rheumatoid nodules.
4. Fontana Masson stain is useful in identifying *Cryptococcus* in patients of AIDS infected with low virulence. *Cryptococcus* stains with little capsular material. It stains the organism black.
5. The yeast forms of histoplasma do not stain with Gram stain.
6. Asteroid bodies in sporotrichosis are extracellular as compared to sarcoidosis.
7. The use of an immunoperoxidase technique assists in making a specific diagnosis of histoplasmosis on paraffin-embedded material.

8

Vasculitis and Other Vascular Reaction Patterns

Chapter Outline

8.1: Leukocytoclastic Vasculitis
8.2: Urticarial Vasculitis
8.3: Polyarteritis Nodosa
8.4: Wegener's Granulomatosis (Necrotizing Vasculitis with Granulomatosis)
8.5: Churg-Strauss Disease
8.6: Granuloma Faciale
8.7: Erythema Elevatum Diutinum
8.8: Behcet's Disease
8.9: Sweet's Syndrome
8.10: Pyoderma Gangrenosum
8.11: Livedoid Vasculitis
8.12: Pigmented Purpuric Dermatoses

Uday Khopkar, Sujay Khandpur, Venkataram Mysore, Pradeep Mahajan, KC Nischal, Nathan Lee, Jerad Gardner

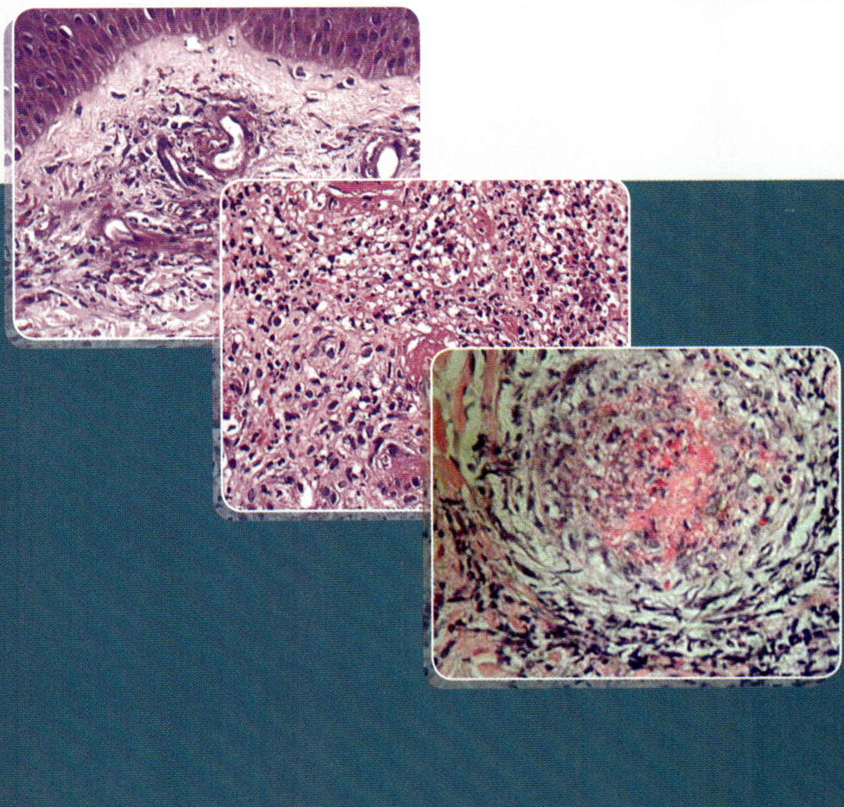

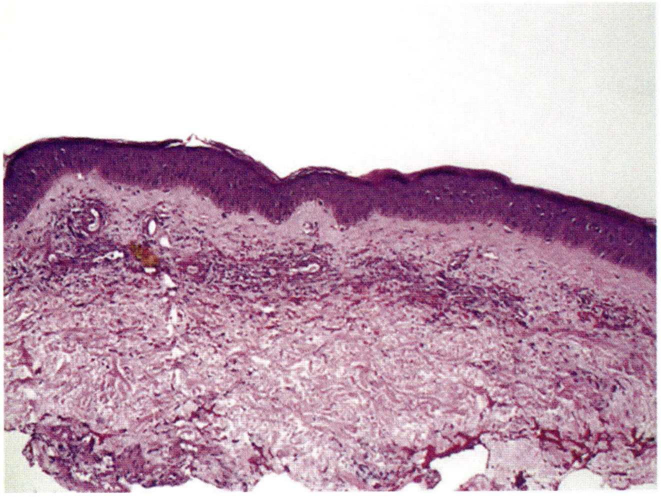

FIGURE 8.1.1

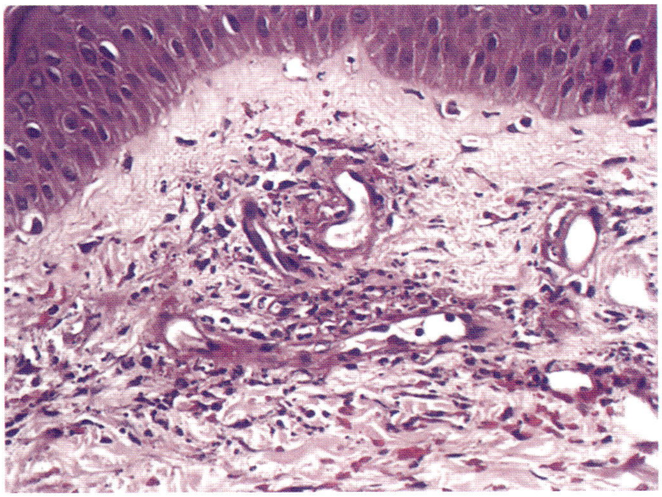

FIGURE 8.1.2

8.1: LEUKOCYTOCLASTIC VASCULITIS

8.1.1: Superficial perivascular infiltrate *(Scanner view)*

8.1.2: Endothelial cell thickening and neutrophilic infiltrate *(Low power view)*

8.1.3: Exudation of fibrin ('fibrinoid degeneration') extending outwards *(High power view)*

8.1.4: Case showing infiltration of vessel wall with neutrophils, neutrophils also undergo degeneration (leukocytoclasis) with the formation of nuclear dust *(High power view)*

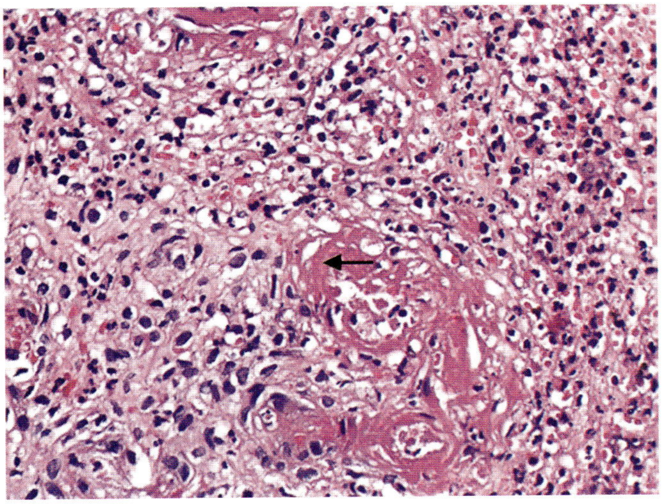

FIGURE 8.1.3

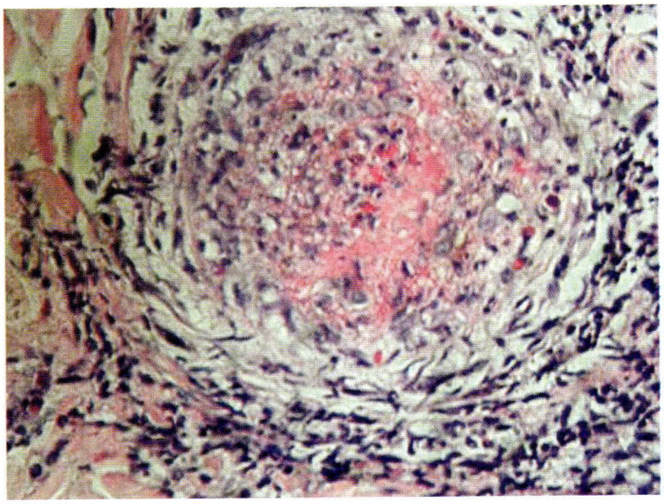

FIGURE 8.1.4

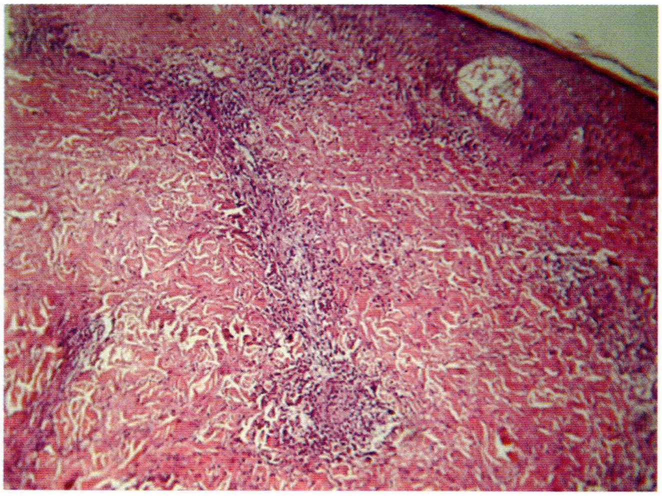

FIGURE 8.1.5

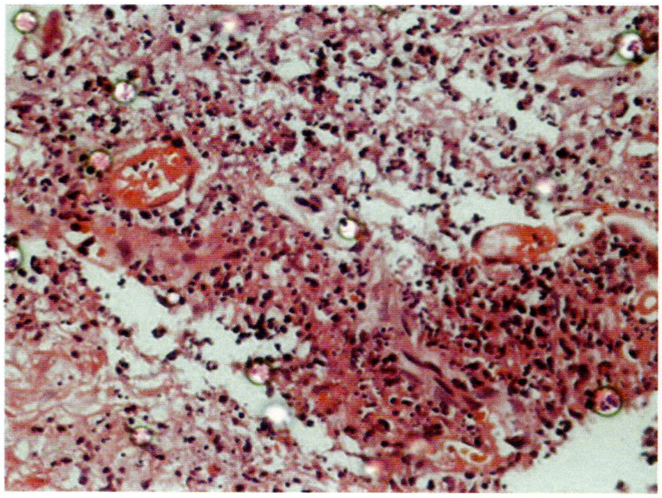

FIGURE 8.1.6

8.1.5: Another case with perivascular infiltrate *(Low power view)*

8.1.6: Fibrinoid necrosis, thrombosis of the vessels, nuclear dust (drug-induced vasculitis will have more number of eosinophils) *(High power view)*

8.1.7: Resolving lesions older than 24–48 hours show mild perivascular infiltrate of lymphocytes only *(High power view)*

8.1.8: Direct immunofluorescence showing granular staining of basement membrane zone with IgA, C3 and fibrinogen (leukocytoclastic vasculitis of Henoch-Schonlein type) *(High power view)*

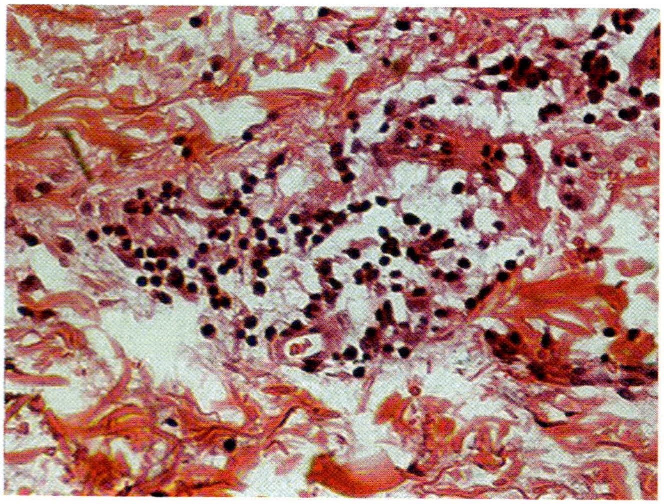

FIGURE 8.1.7

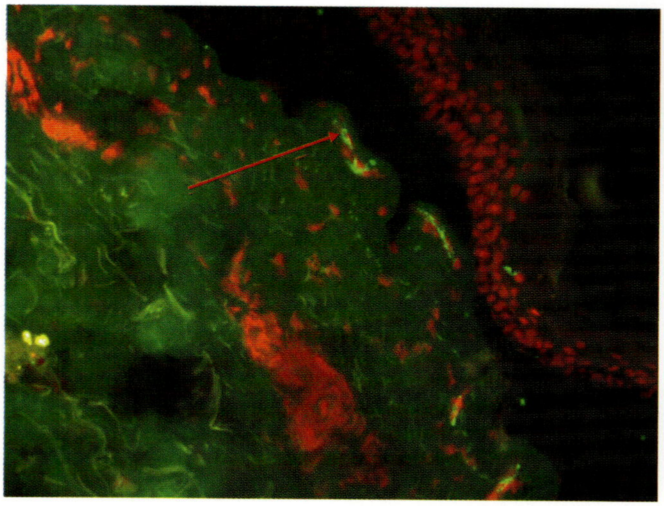

FIGURE 8.1.8

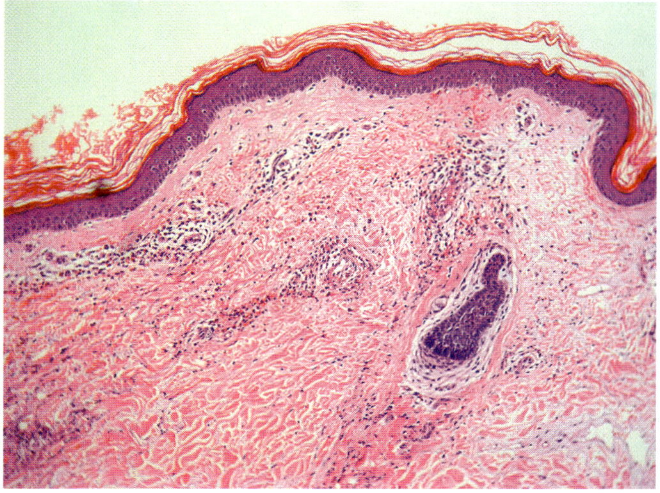

FIGURE 8.2.1

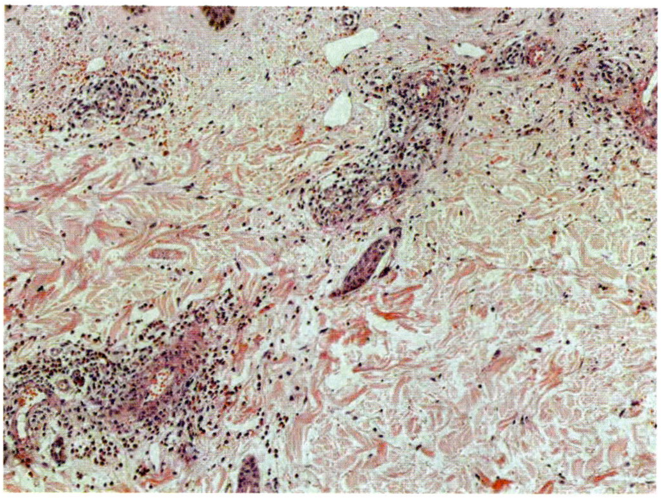

FIGURE 8.2.2

8.2: URTICARIAL VASCULITIS

8.2.1: The changes are similar to those seen in leukocytoclastic vasculitis with edema of the upper dermis *(Scanner view)*

8.2.2: Perivascular infiltrate *(Low power view)*

8.2.3: The inflammatory infiltrate is composed of neutrophils and a few eosinophils with endothelial cell swelling and fibrin deposition *(High power view)*

8.2.4: Nuclear dust in vessel wall and many eosinophils *(High power view)*

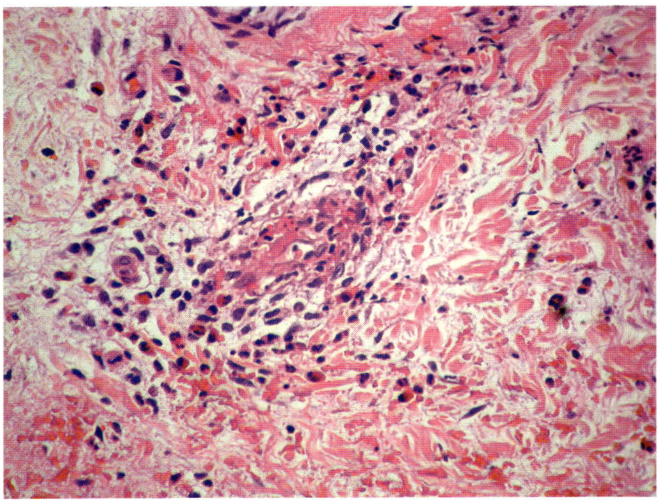

FIGURE 8.2.3

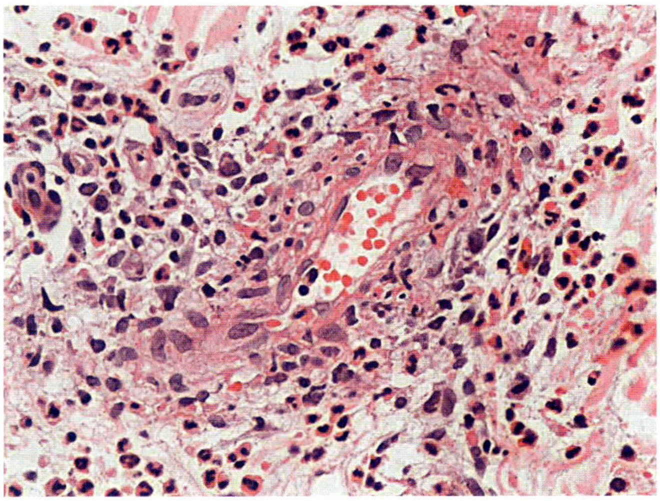

FIGURE 8.2.4

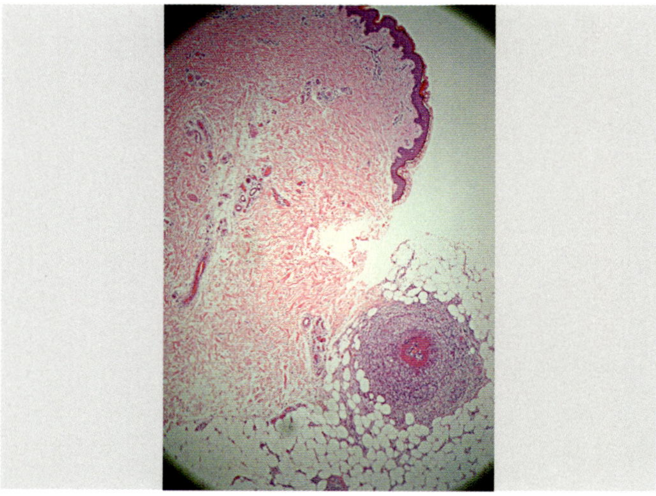

FIGURE 8.3.1

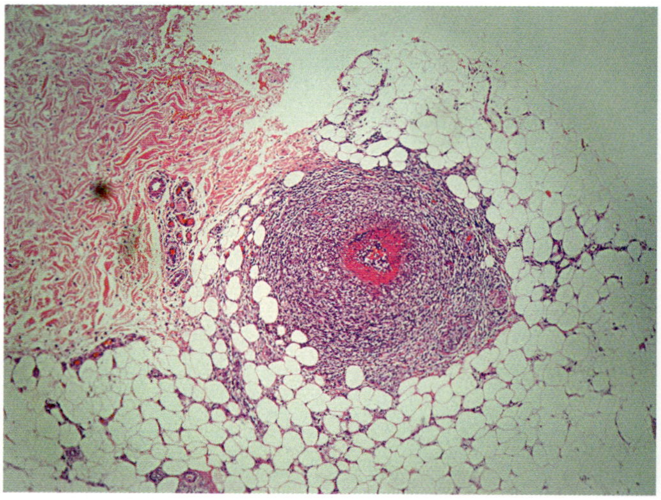

FIGURE 8.3.2

8.3: POLYARTERITIS NODOSA

8.3.1: Involvement of medium sized vessel in deep dermis and subcutis *(Scanner view)*

8.3.2: Closer view of the vessel in subcutis showing involvement *(Low power view)*

8.3.3: Marked thickening of vessel wall due to edema, infiltrate and fibrin deposition *(High power view)*

8.3.4: Infiltrate consists of neutrophils with some eosinophils and lymphocytes with intimal fibrosis leading to obliteration of the vessel *(High power view)*

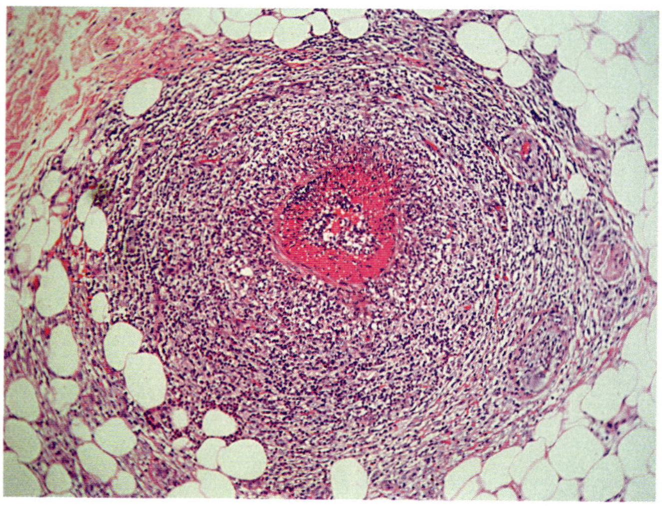

FIGURE 8.3.3

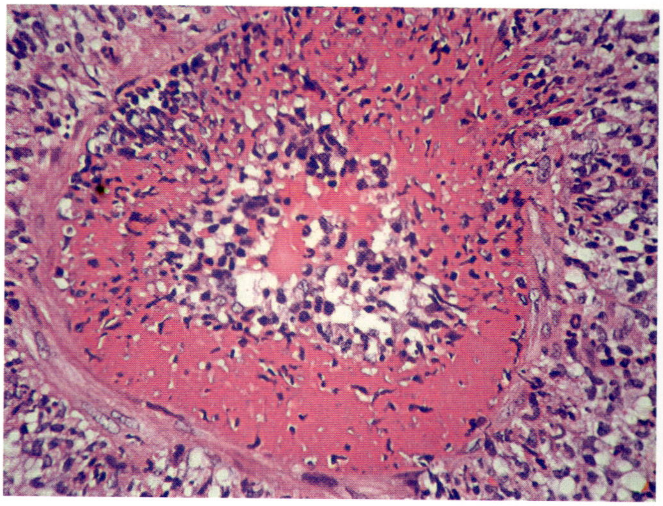

FIGURE 8.3.4

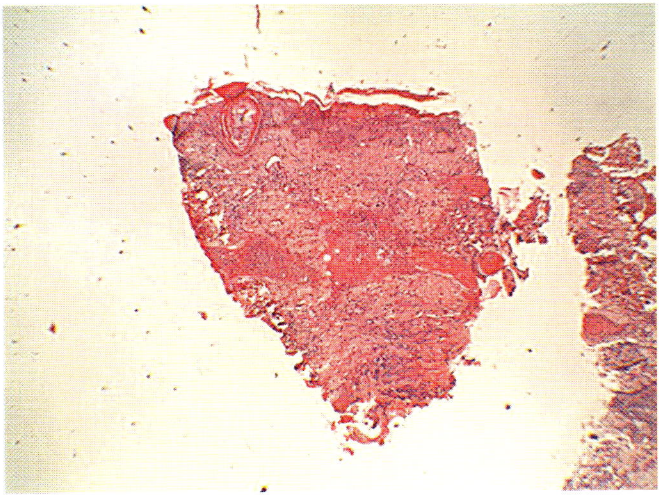

FIGURE 8.4.1

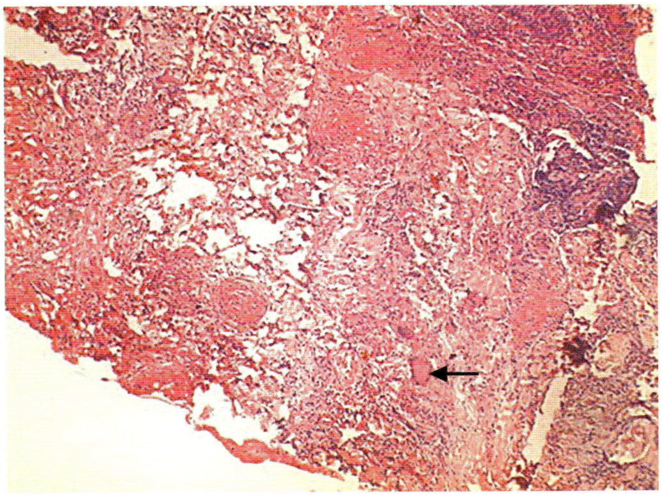

FIGURE 8.4.2

8.4: WEGENER'S GRANULOMATOSIS (NECROTIZING VASCULITIS WITH GRANULOMATOSIS)

8.4.1: Superficial and deep perivascular inflammatory infiltrate *(Scanner view)*

8.4.2: Vasculitis and giant cell in deep dermis *(Low power view)*

8.4.3: Vascular changes in the form of a necrotizing angiitis involving small and medium-sized dermal vessels *(High power view)*

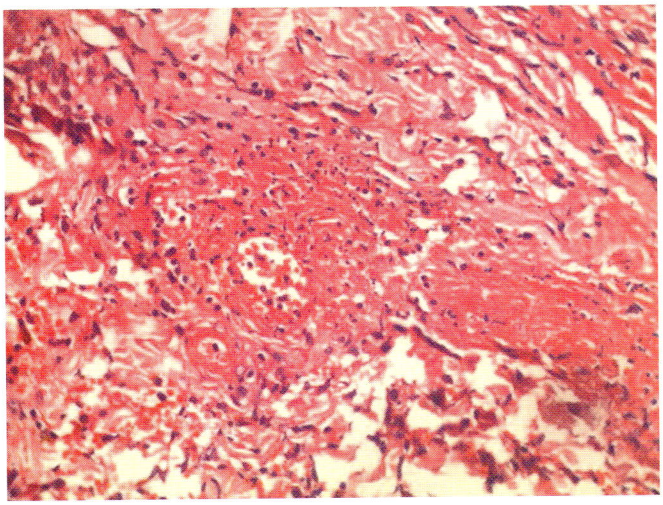

FIGURE 8.4.3

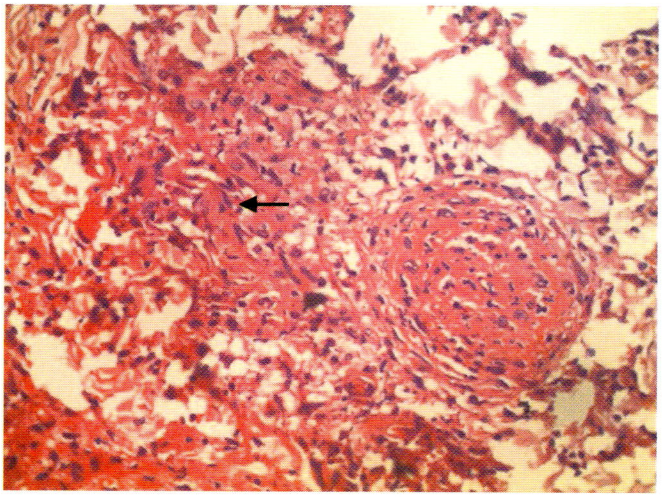

FIGURE 8.4.4

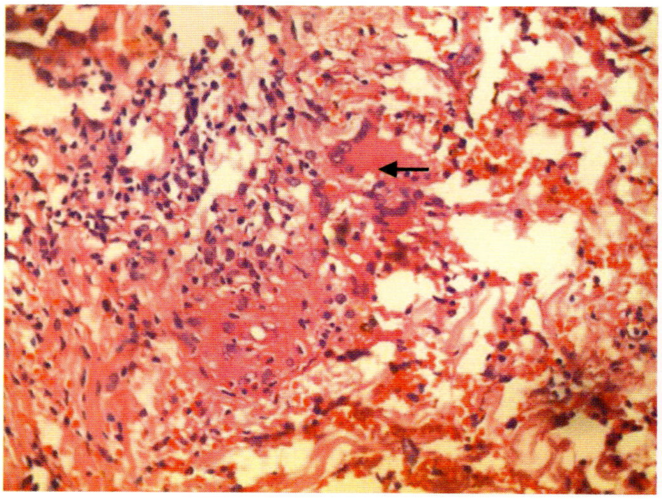

FIGURE 8.4.5

8.4.4: Fibrin around the vessel wall and obliteration of lumen by fibrin thrombus along with poorly formed granuloma around the vessel *(High power view)*

8.4.5: Granulomas with giant cells *(High power view)*

8.4.6: Another case with vascular changes and surrounding granuloma with giant cells *(High power view)*

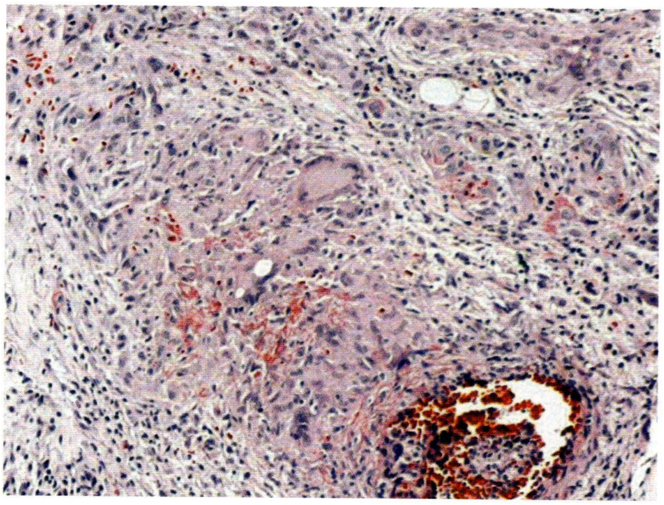

FIGURE 8.4.6

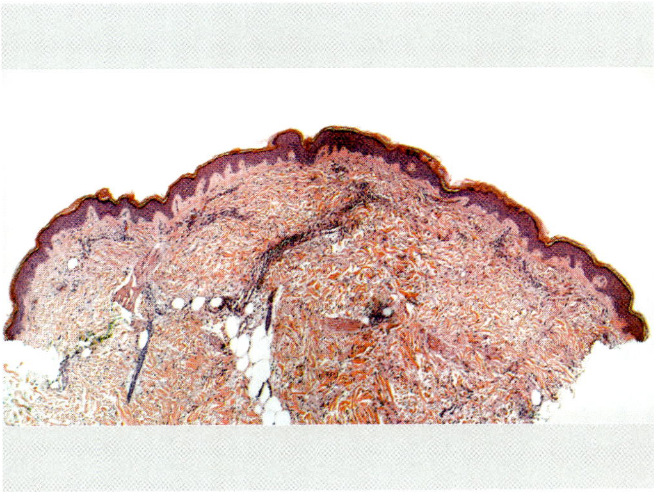

FIGURE 8.5.1

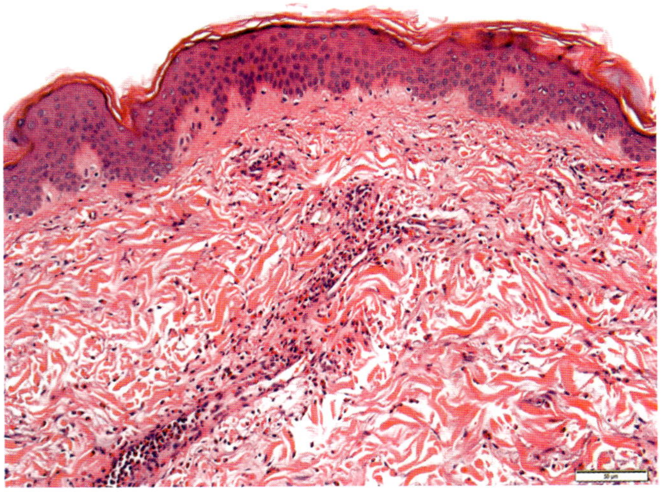

FIGURE 8.5.2

8.5: CHURG-STRAUSS DISEASE

8.5.1: Perivascular infiltrate in the upper dermis *(Scanner view)*

8.5.2: Small vessel involvement with infiltration by eosinophils *(Low power view)*

8.5.3: Closer view of infiltrate where eosinophils predominate, some neutrophils *(High power view)*

8.5.4: Extravascular granuloma *(High power view)*

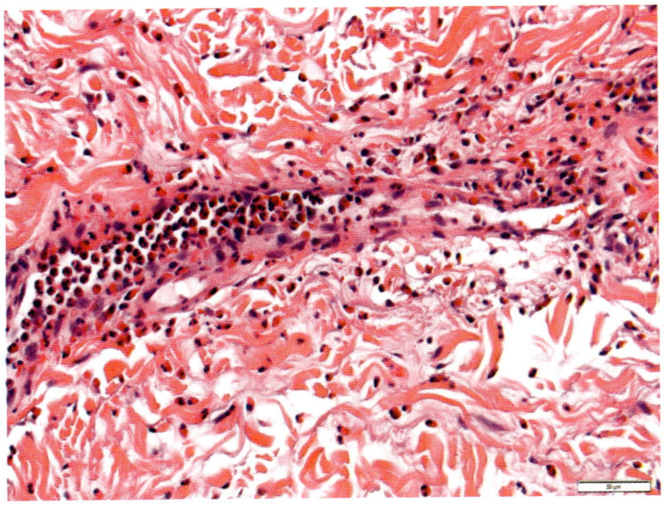

FIGURE 8.5.3

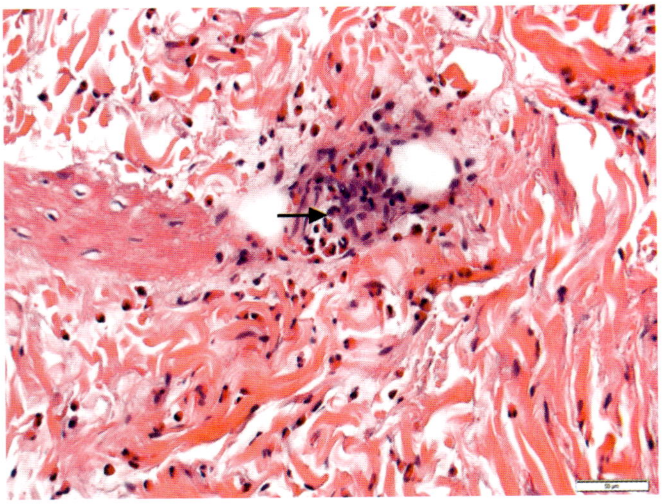

FIGURE 8.5.4

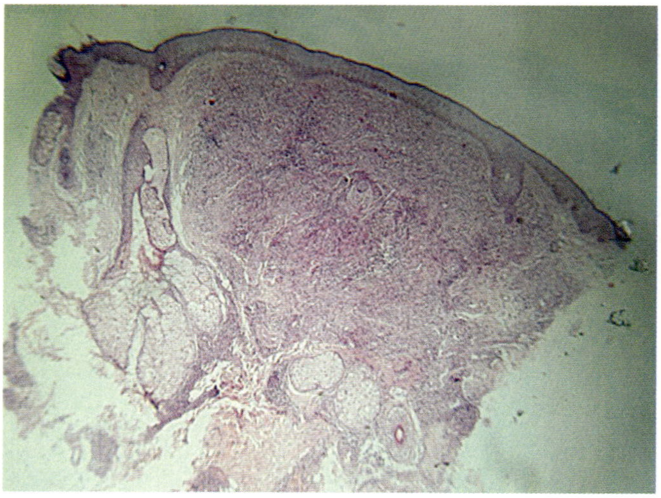

FIGURE 8.6.1

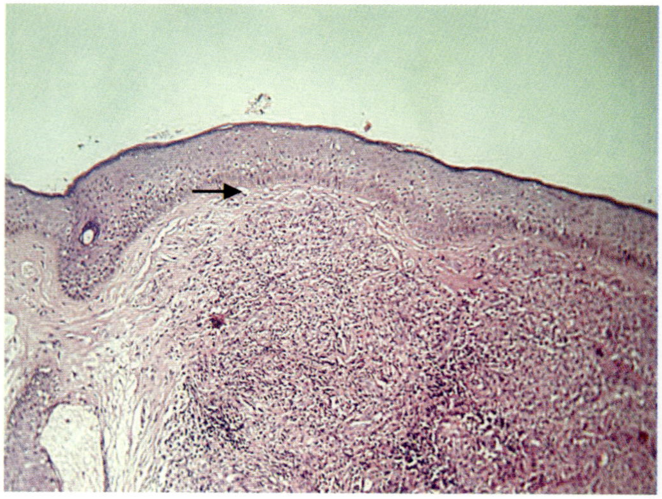

FIGURE 8.6.2

8.6: GRANULOMA FACIALE

8.6.1: Dense, polymorphous, inflammatory cell infiltrate in the dermis *(Scanner view)*

8.6.2: A narrow, uninvolved grenz zone beneath the epidermis *(Low power view)*

8.6.3: The infiltrate consists of eosinophils with neutrophils, lymphocytes, histiocytes and few plasma cells. Blood vessels show endothelial cell swelling, but no fibrin deposition *(High power view)*

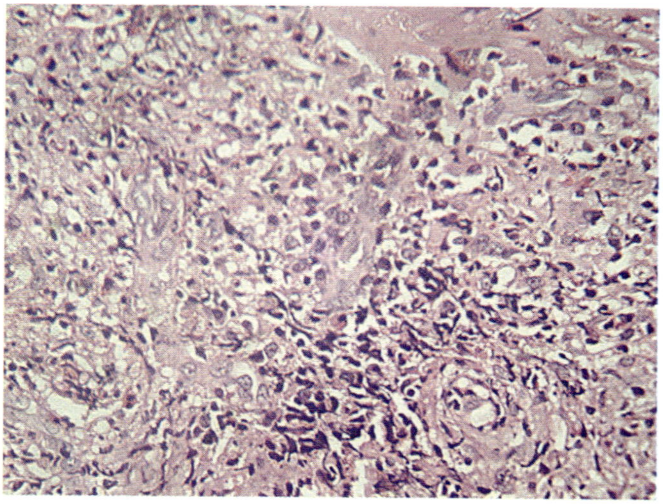

FIGURE 8.6.3

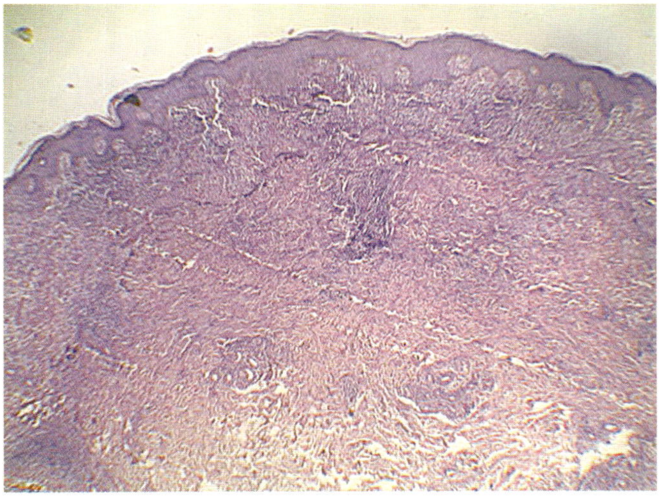

FIGURE 8.7.1

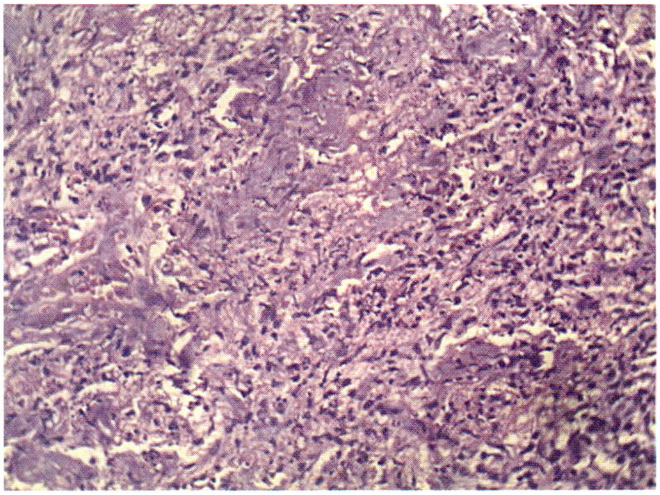

FIGURE 8.7.2

8.7: ERYTHEMA ELEVATUM DIUTINUM

8.7.1: Dense and diffuse infiltrate in the dermis. Epidermis unremarkable, no grenz zone *(Scanner view)*

8.7.2: Mixed inflammatory infiltrate with predominant neutrophils, less numbers of histiocytes and lymphocytes and only a few eosinophils *(High power view)*

8.7.3: Moderately dense perivascular infiltrate of neutrophils. Blood vessels show endothelial swelling. Nuclear dust is seen but extravasation of red blood cells is uncommon *(High power view)*

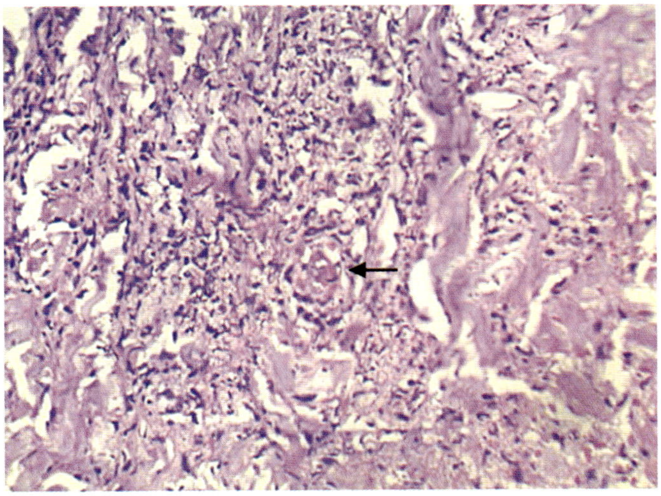

FIGURE 8.7.3

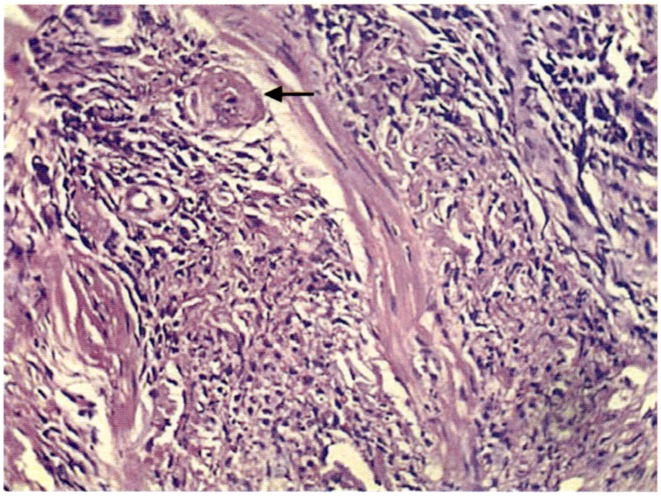

FIGURE 8.7.4

8.7.4: Fibrinoid deposition around the walls of small dermal blood vessels *(High power view)*

8.7.5: Late lesion showing dermal fibrosis and neutrophils *(High power view)*

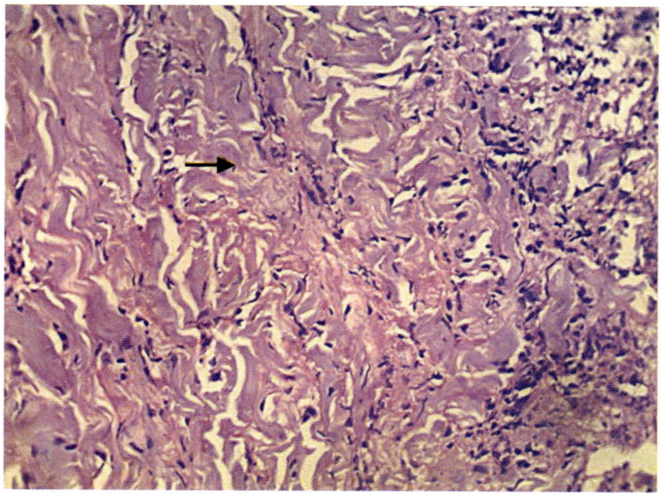

FIGURE 8.7.5

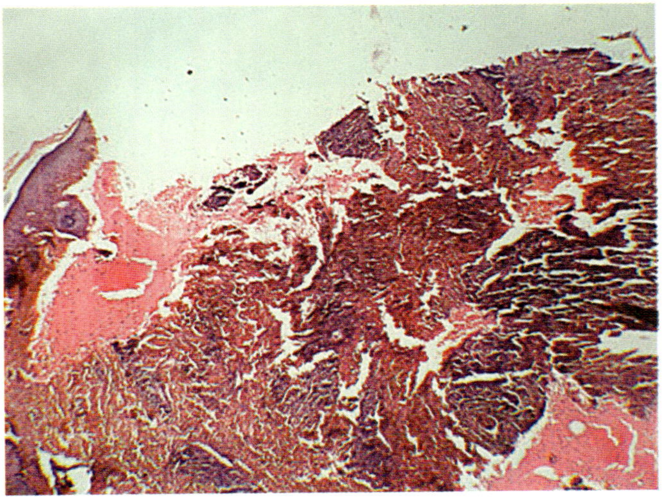

FIGURE 8.8.1

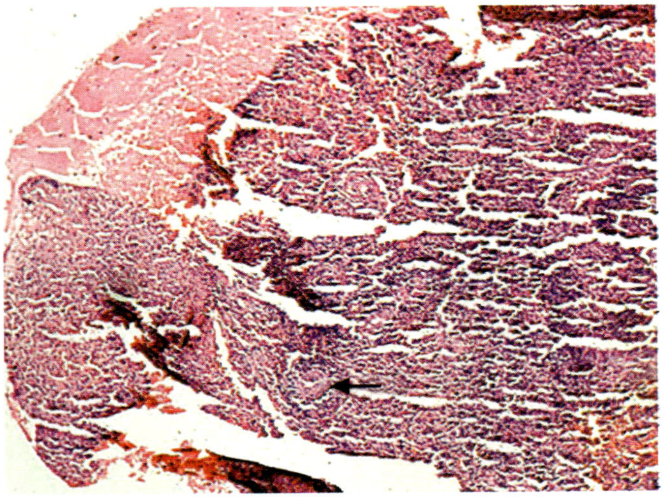

FIGURE 8.8.2

8.8: BEHCET'S DISEASE

8.8.1: Infiltrate of lymphocytes, macrophages, and neutrophils in the base of the ulcer *(Scanner view)*

8.8.2: The infiltrate around small vessels *(Low power view)*

8.8.3: Leukocytoclastic vasculitis with fibrinoid degeneration *(High power view)*

8.8.4: Also nuclear dust in vessel wall and endothelial cell swelling *(High power view)*

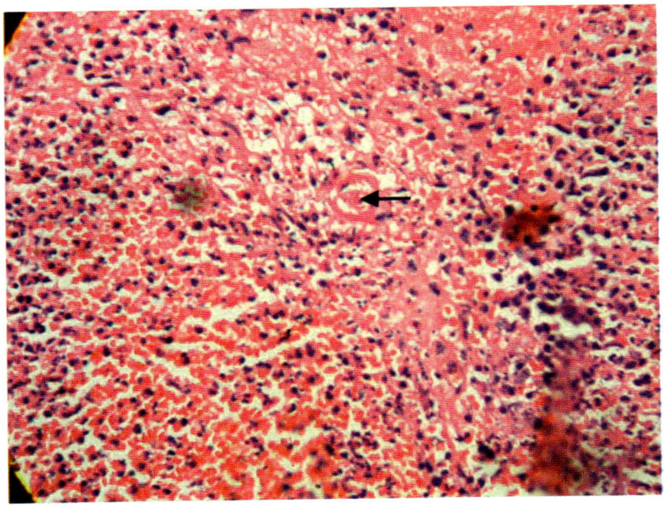

FIGURE 8.8.3

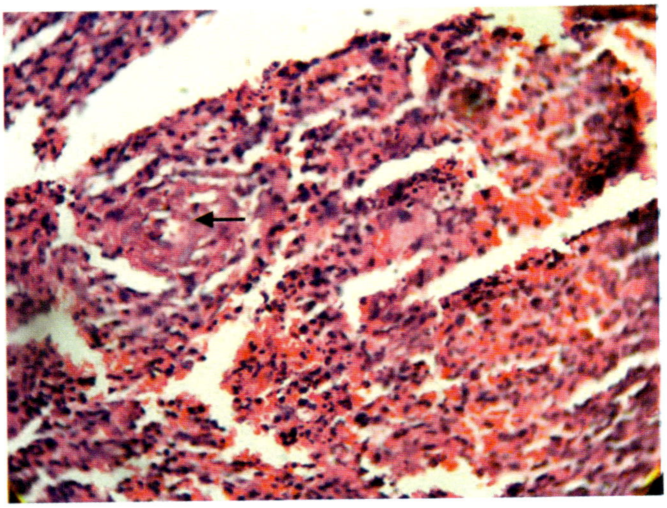

FIGURE 8.8.4

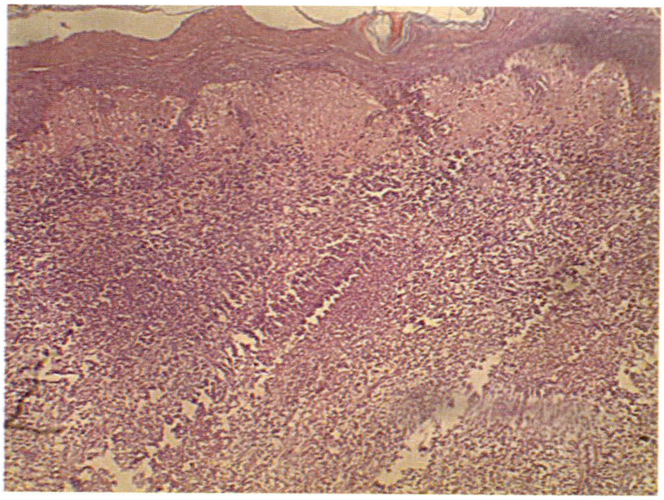

FIGURE 8.9.1

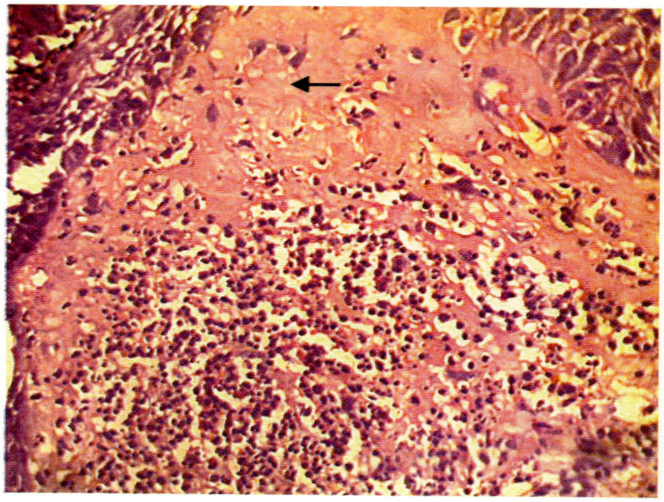

FIGURE 8.9.2

8.9: SWEET'S SYNDROME

8.9.1: Dense infiltrate of neutrophils in the upper half of the dermis. Neutrophils extend throughout the dermis and the subcutis *(Low power view)*

8.9.2: Papillary edema with neutrophils *(High power view)*

8.9.3: Dense infiltrate of neutrophils forming microabscess *(High power view)*

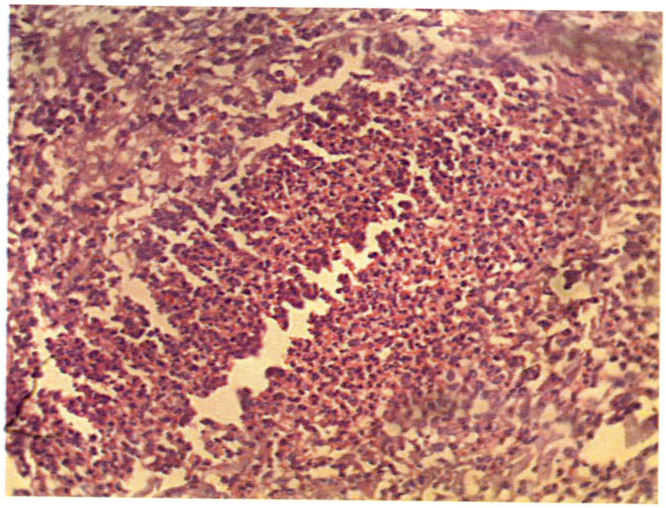

FIGURE 8.9.3

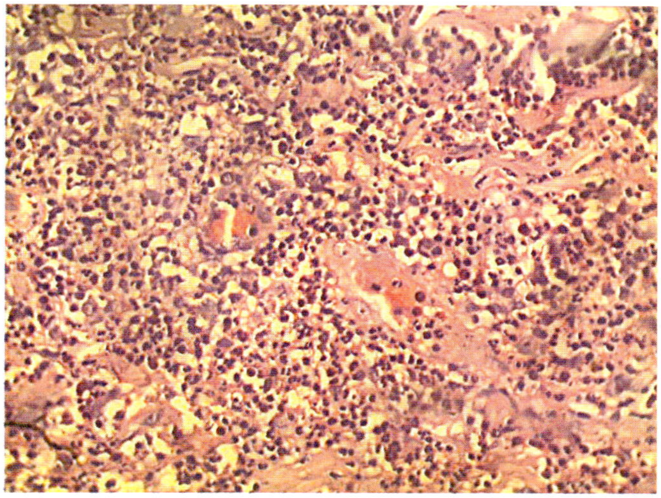

FIGURE 8.9.4

8.9.4: Leukocytoclasis with nuclear dust *(High power view)*

8.9.5: No vasculitis or fibrinoid extravasation *(High power view)*

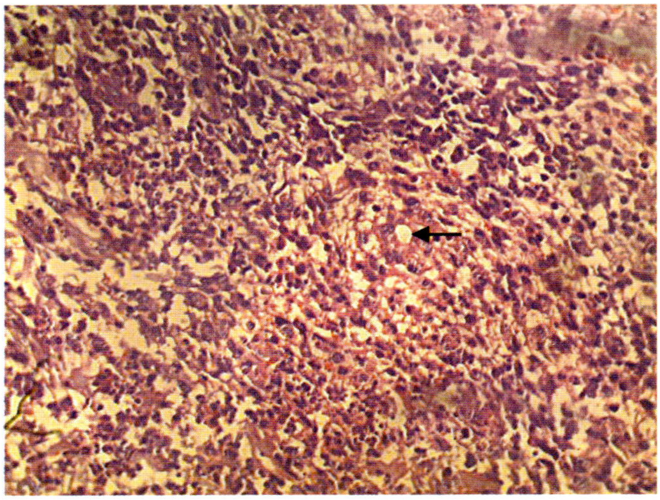

FIGURE 8.9.5

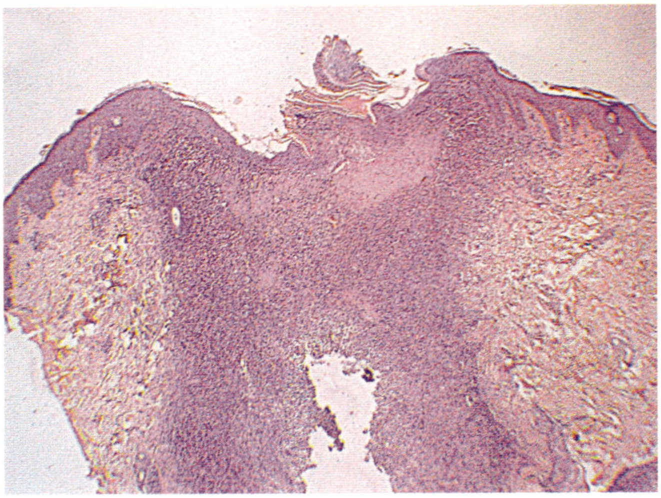

FIGURE 8.10.1

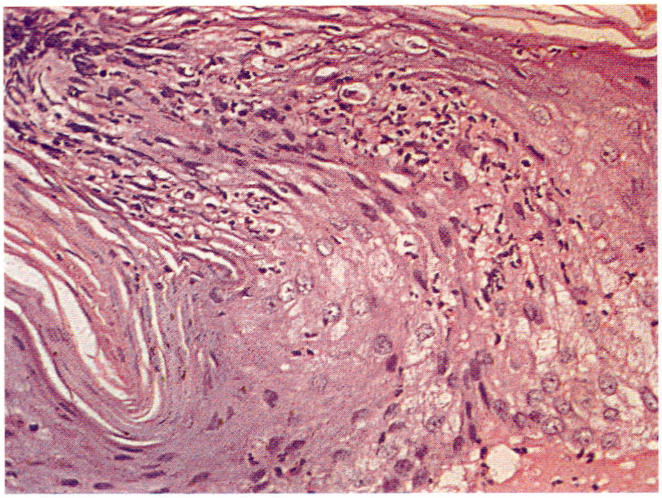

FIGURE 8.10.2

8.10: PYODERMA GANGRENOSUM

8.10.1: Perifollicular infiltrate *(Low power view)*

8.10.2: Intraepidermal neutrophils *(High power view)*

8.10.3: Neutrophilic microabscess in the dermis *(High power view)*

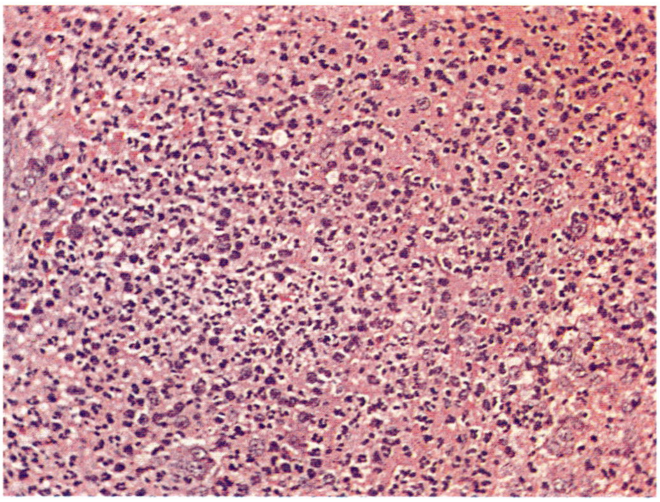

FIGURE 8.10.3

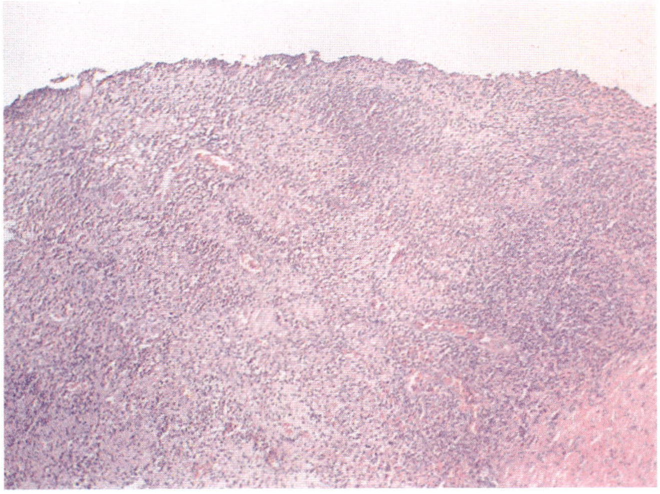

FIGURE 8.10.4

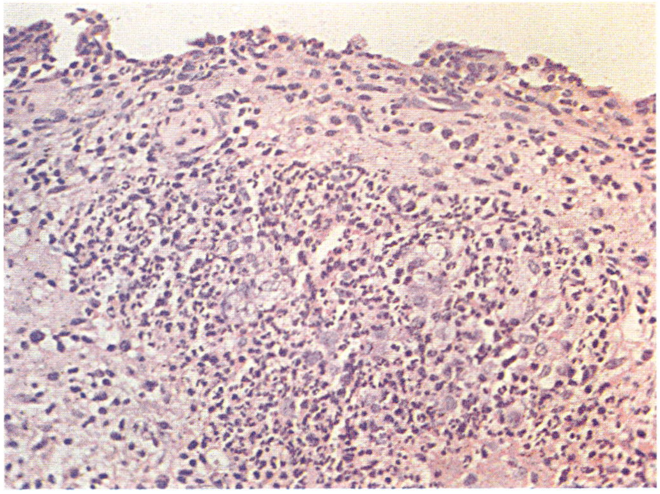

FIGURE 8.10.5

8.10.4: Case showing epidermal necrosis leading to an ulcer *(Low power view)*
8.10.5: Microabscesses at the base *(High power view)*
8.10.6: Lymphocytes around the blood vessels, but no vasculitis *(High power view)*

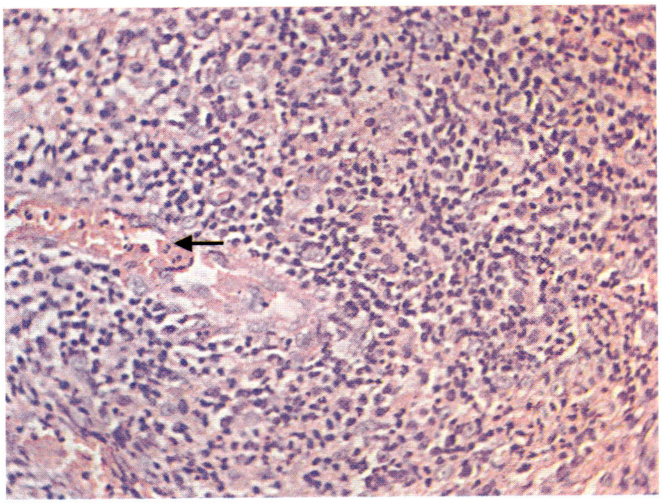

FIGURE 8.10.6

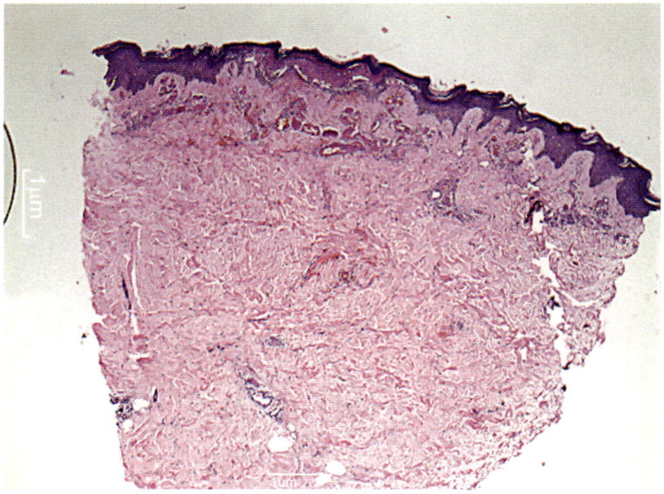

FIGURE 8.11.1

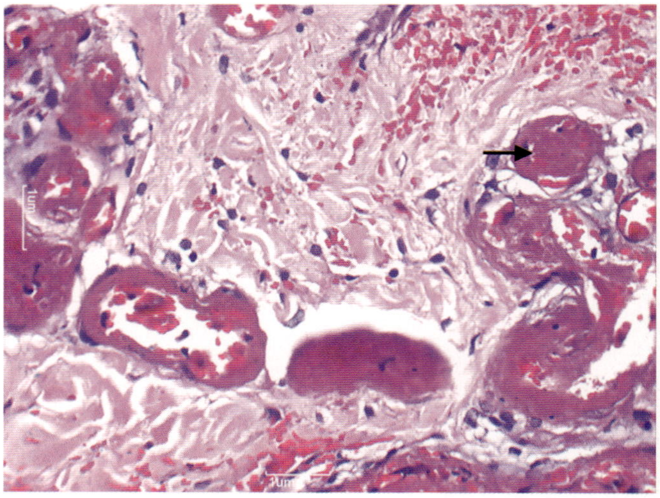

FIGURE 8.11.2

8.11: LIVEDOID VASCULITIS

8.11.1: Hyaline thrombi in the lumen of small vessels in the upper and mid-dermis *(Scanner view)*

8.11.2: Closer view of thrombi, fibrin deposition, and extravasated red cells in the upper dermis *(High power view)*

8.11.3: Another case with only sparse perivascular lymphocytic infiltrate, but there is no vasculitis *(Low power view)*

8.11.4: Fibrin deposition and thrombi *(High power view)*

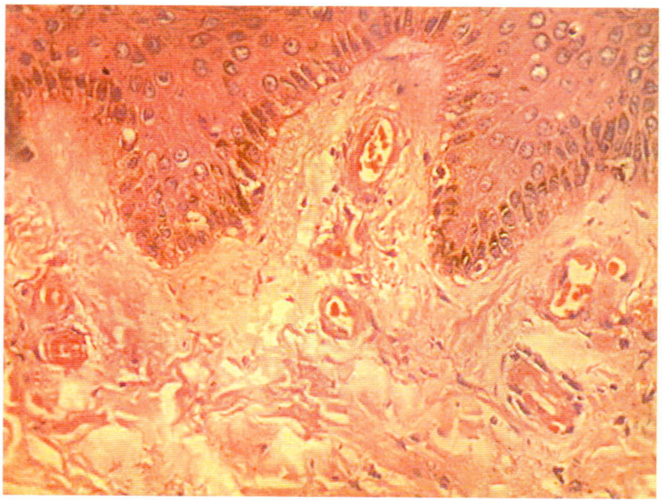

FIGURE 8.11.3

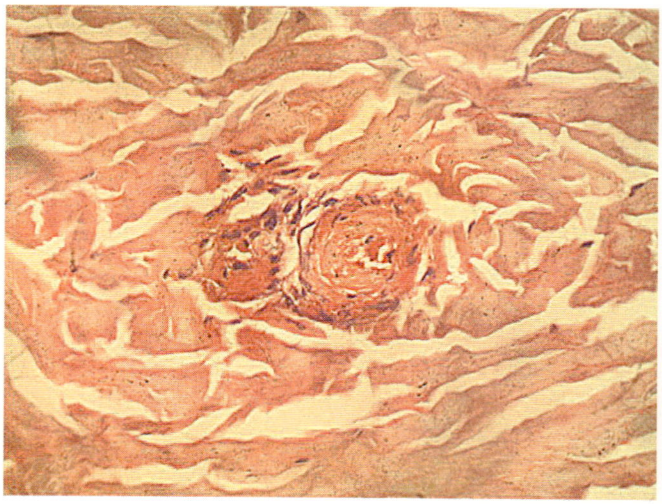

FIGURE 8.11.4

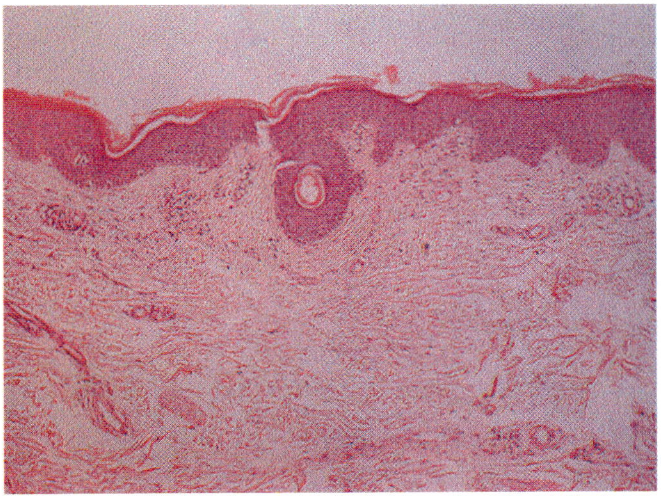

FIGURE 8.12.1

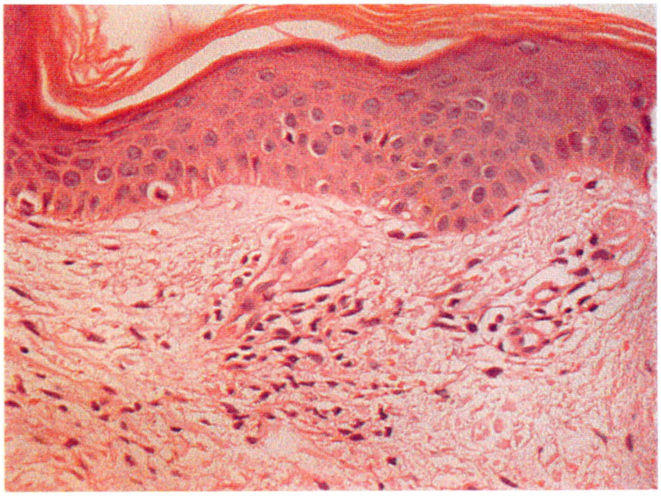

FIGURE 8.12.2

8.12: PIGMENTED PURPURIC DERMATOSES

8.12.1: Perivascular infiltrate of lymphocytes in the upper dermis *(Scanner view)*

8.12.2: Extravasation of red blood cells and lymphocytic vasculitis without fibrin deposition *(High power view)*

8.12.3: Hemosiderin in macrophages *(Low power view)*

8.12.4: Closer view of hemosiderin (X100) *(Oil immersion view)*

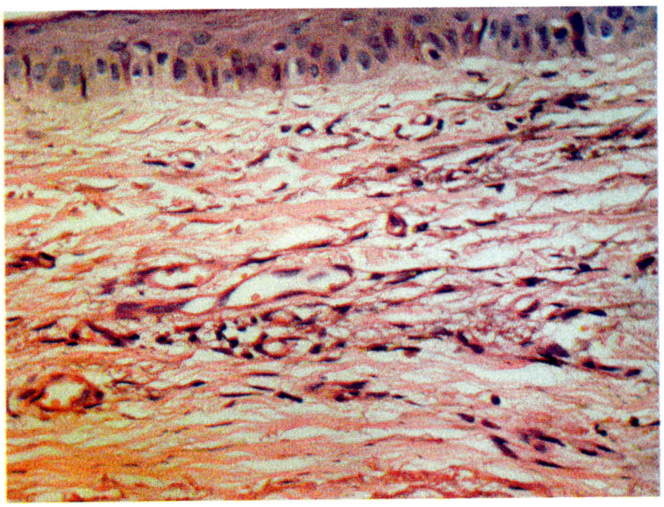

FIGURE 8.12.3

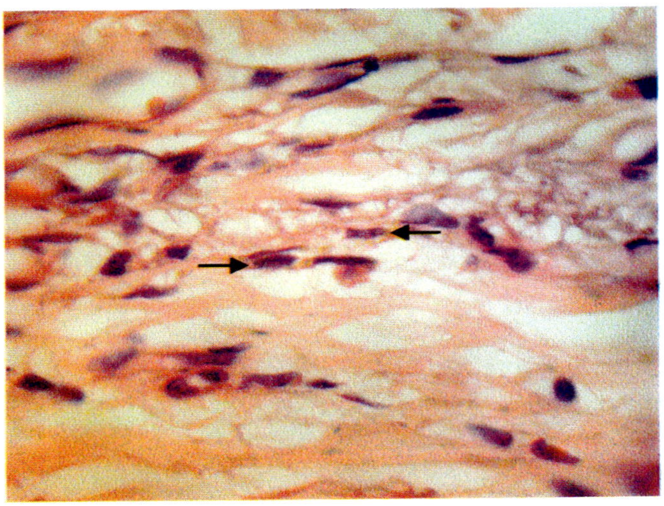

FIGURE 8.12.4

DIFFERENTIAL DIAGNOSIS

1. Purpuras
2. Cryoglobulinemia
3. Antiphospholipid antibody syndrome
4. Urticarias
5. Lymphomatoid granulomatosis
6. Lymphocytic vasculitis as seen in:
   a. Collagen vascular disease
   b. Pruritic urticarial papules and plaques of pregnancy (PUPPP)
   c. Gyrate and annular erythemas
   d. Pityriasis lichenoides
   e. Malignant atrophic papulosis (Degos)
   f. Rickettsial and viral infections

DIAGNOSTIC PEARLS

1. Leukocytoclastic vasculitis shows IgG deposits, polyarteritis nodosa IgM and Henoch-Schonlein purpura shows IgA deposition in vessel wall on direct immunofluorescence.
2. There is no grenz zone and eosinophils are less in number in erythema elevatum diutinum as against granuloma faciale.
3. Clonal T-lymphocytes may be seen in some cases of pigmented purpuric dermatosis (PPD) and there may be overlap of features between mycosis fungoides and PPD.
4. Cryoglobulinemia shows homogenous eosinophilic periodic acid-Schiff positive deposits in small vessels or ulcer base.

9

Disorders of Pigmentation

Chapter Outline

9.1: Vitiligo
9.2: Nevus Depigmentosus
9.3: Becker's Nevus
9.4: Melasma
9.5: Freckles
9.6: Dowling-Degos Disease
9.7: Patterned Hypermelanosis/Nevoid Hypermelanosis/Progressive Cribriform and Zosteriform Hyperpigmentation
9.8: Postinflammatory Hyperpigmentation

Pradeep Mahajan

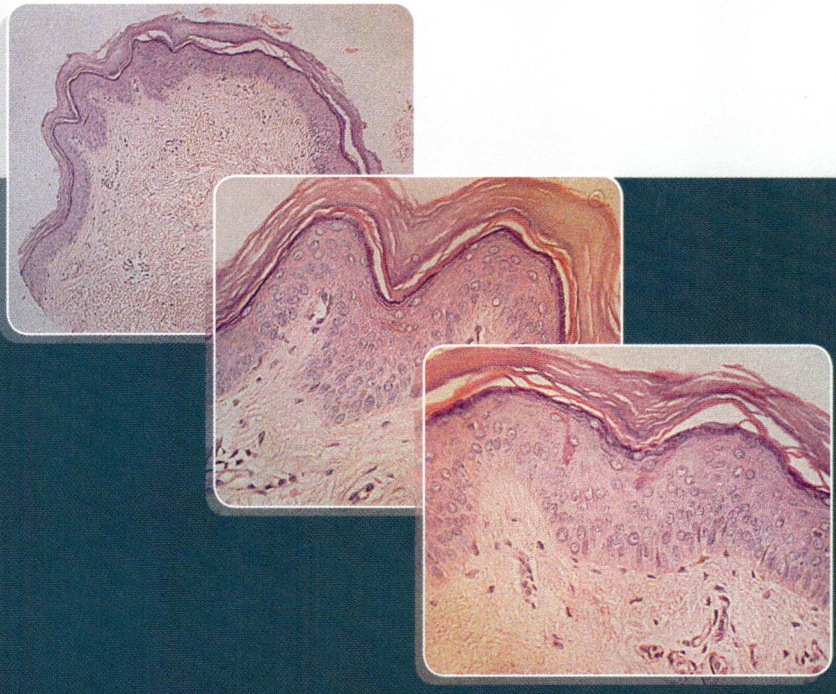

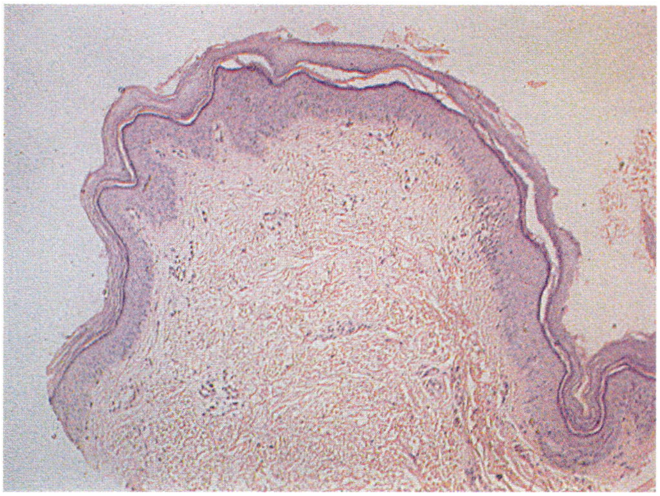

FIGURE 9.1.1

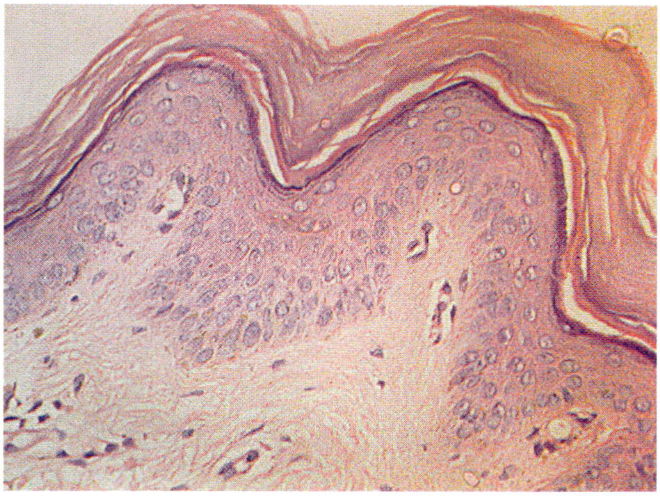

FIGURE 9.1.2

9.1: VITILIGO

9.1.1: Alteration of melanocytes and pigment at the dermal-epidermal junction *(Low power view)*

9.1.2: On H & E stain well-established lesions of vitiligo are totally devoid of melanocytes (can be confirmed by silver stains or dopa reaction) *(High power view)*

9.1.3: Total loss of melanin pigment *(High power view)*

9.1.4: Periphery of expanding lesions, which are hypopigmented rather than completely depigmented, still show a few melanocytes. Also, a few lymphocytes are seen surrounding the melanocyte there *(High power view)*

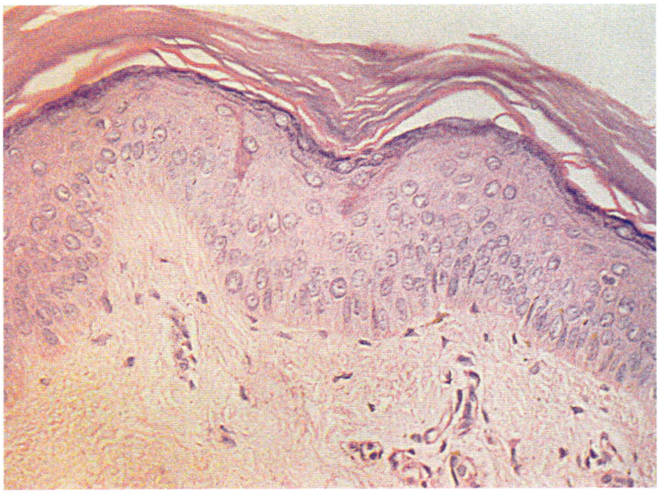

FIGURE 9.1.3

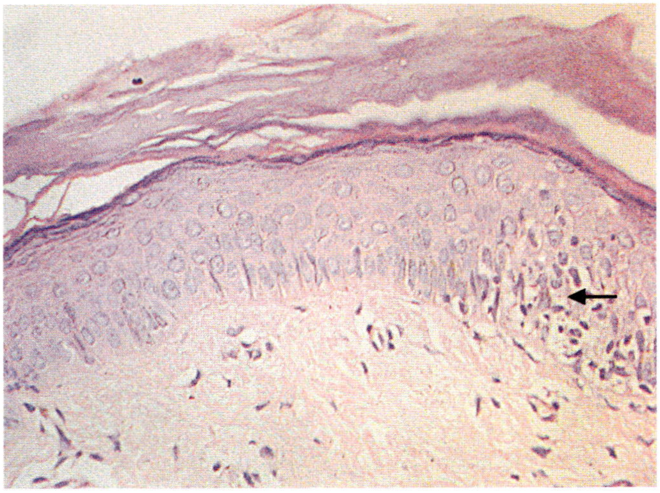

FIGURE 9.1.4

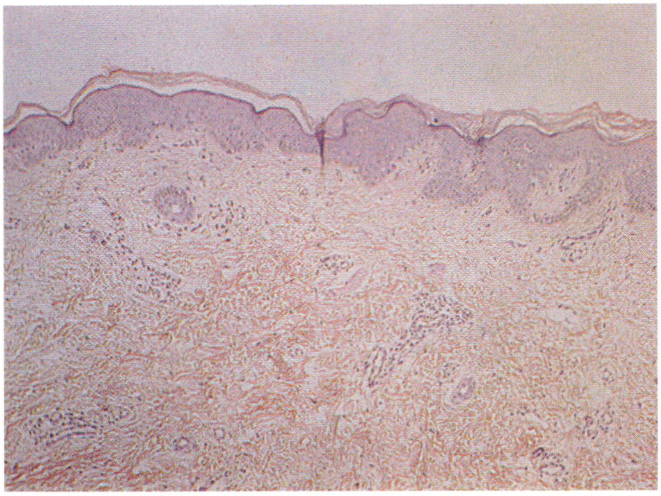

FIGURE 9.2.1

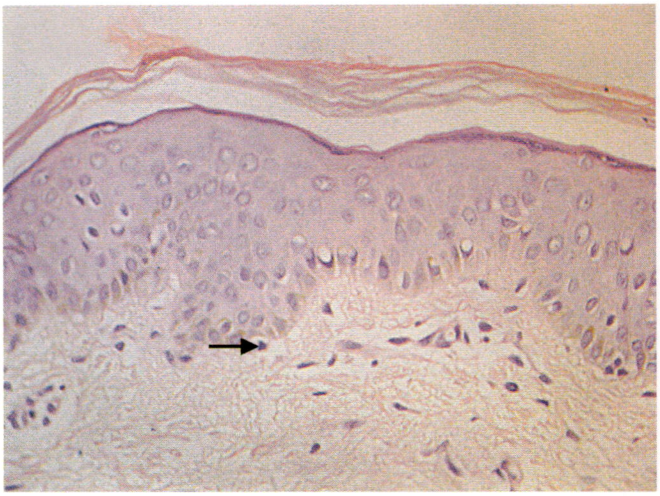

FIGURE 9.2.2

9.2: NEVUS DEPIGMENTOSUS

9.2.1: Affected area has reduced melanin pigment in the basal cell layer but not absent as in vitiligo *(Low power view)*

9.2.2: Melanocytes also reduced in number but not absent *(High power view)*

9.2.3: Pigment and melanocytes normal in surrounding skin *(High power view)*

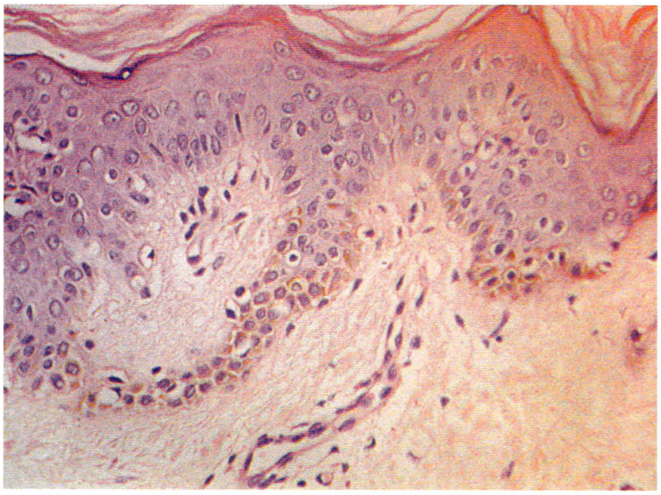

FIGURE 9.2.3

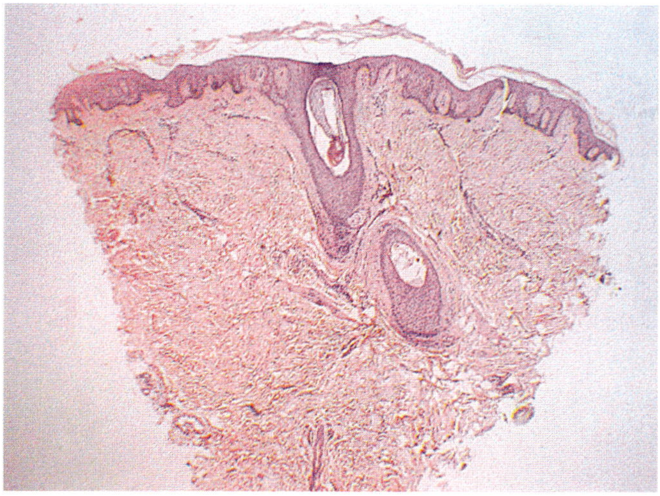

FIGURE 9.3.1

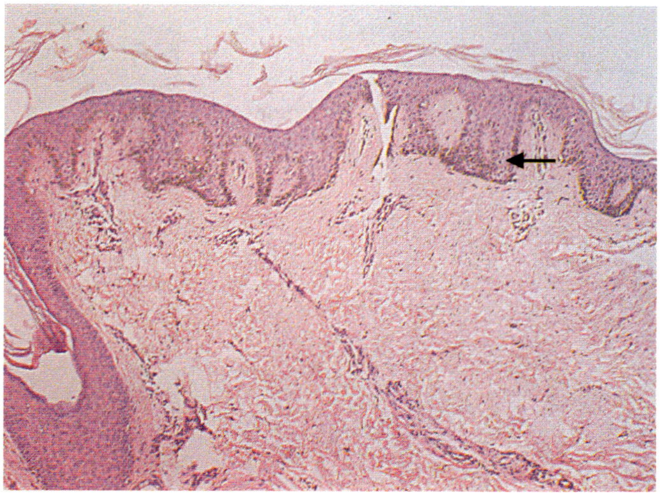

FIGURE 9.3.2

9.3: BECKER'S NEVUS

9.3.1: Epidermis shows hyperplasia (cases with associated hamartoma show increase in the number and size of hair follicles and sebaceous glands, and hypertrophy of the arrectores pilorum muscle) *(Scanner view)*

9.3.2: Rete ridges are broad and flat, towards dermis *(Low power view)*

9.3.3: Closer view showing flat rete ridges and hyperpigmentation of the basal layer. Mild melanocyte proliferation *(High power view)*

9.3.4: Hyperpigmentation of the basal layer and melanophages in the dermis *(High power view)*

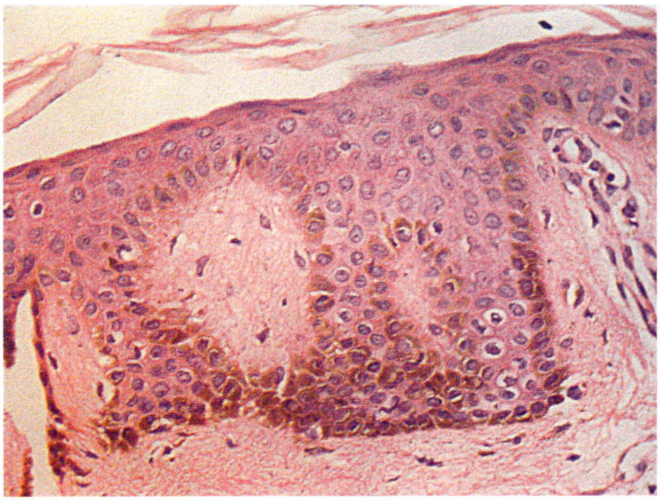

FIGURE 9.3.3

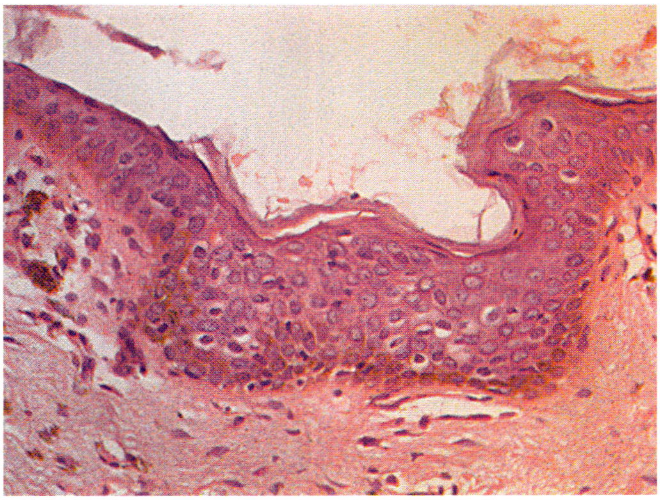

FIGURE 9.3.4

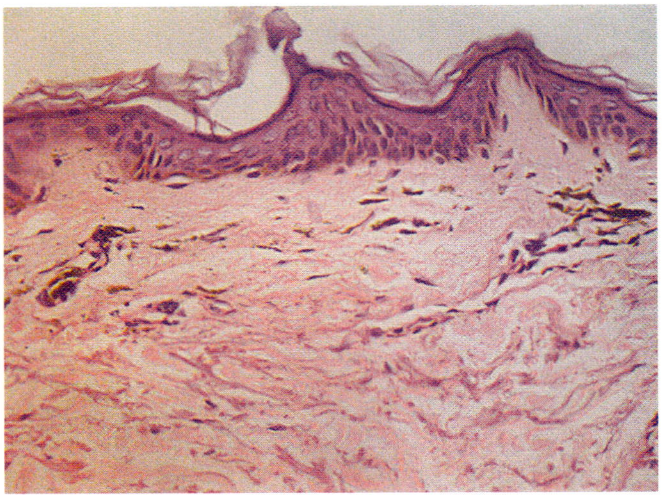

FIGURE 9.4.1

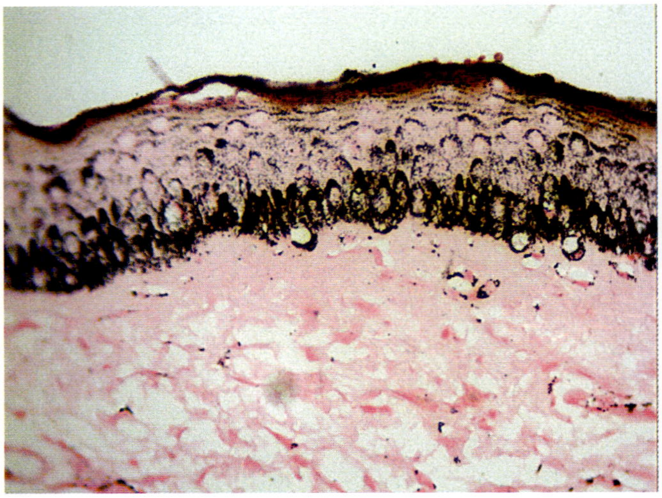

FIGURE 9.4.2

9.4: MELASMA

9.4.1: Increased melanin in the epidermis, particularly in the basal cell layer *(Low power view)*

9.4.2: Above the keratinocyte nuclei melanin is seen as a cap (Masson's fontana stain highlighting the feature) *(High power view)—Image contributed by Meeta Mantri*

9.4.3: Mild pigment incontinence and solar changes *(Low power view)*

9.4.4: Dilated capillaries, stellate fibroblasts, elastin changes (all features of solar damage seen with H & E stain but would be better appreciated in Verhoeff-van Gieson stained sections) and pigment incontinence *(Low power view)*

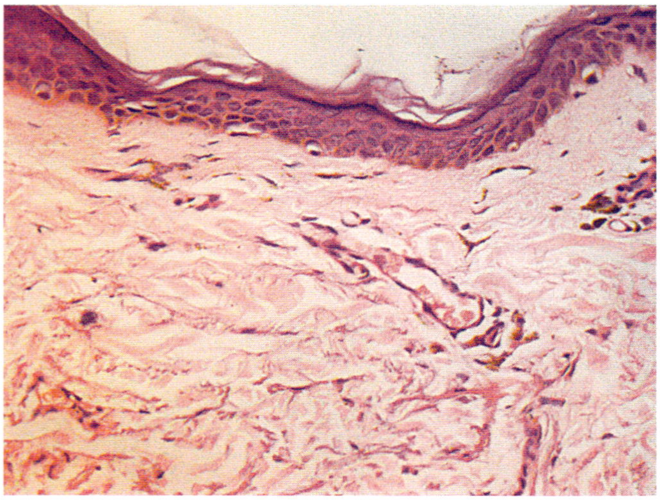

FIGURE 9.4.3

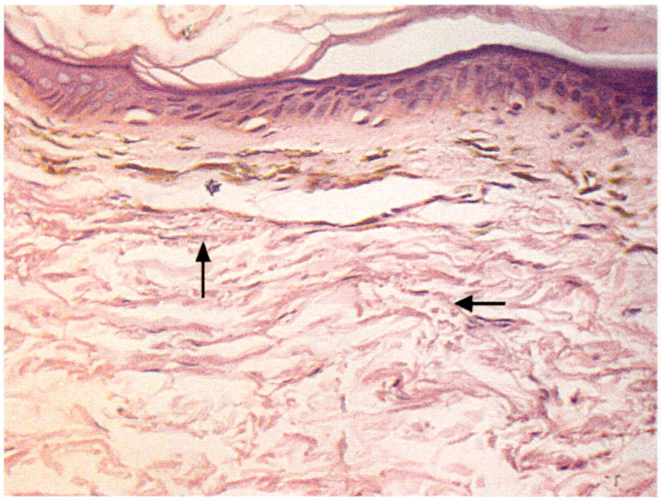

FIGURE 9.4.4

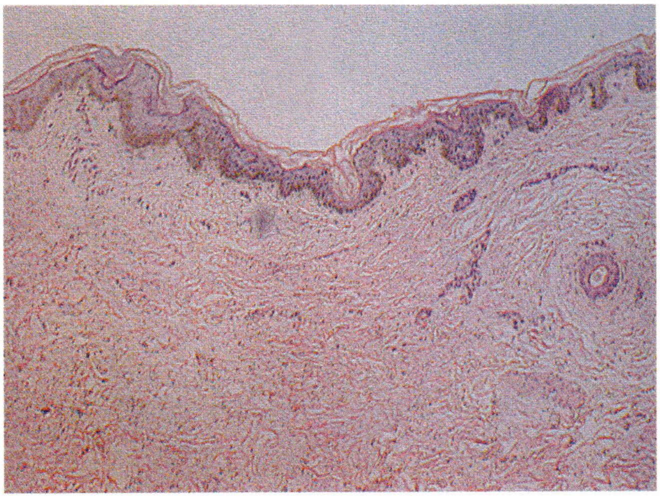

FIGURE 9.5.1

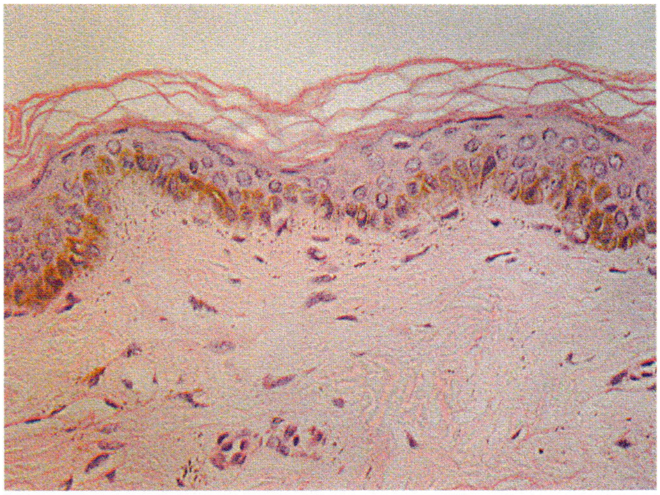

FIGURE 9.5.2

9.5: FRECKLES

9.5.1: Increased pigmentation of the basal cell layer *(Scanner view)*

9.5.2: Numbers of melanocytes normal, no pigment incontinence *(Low power view)*

9.5.3: Markedly increased pigment in the basal cells (distinct difference exists in the pigment of lesional area and surrounding normal skin) *(Low power view)*

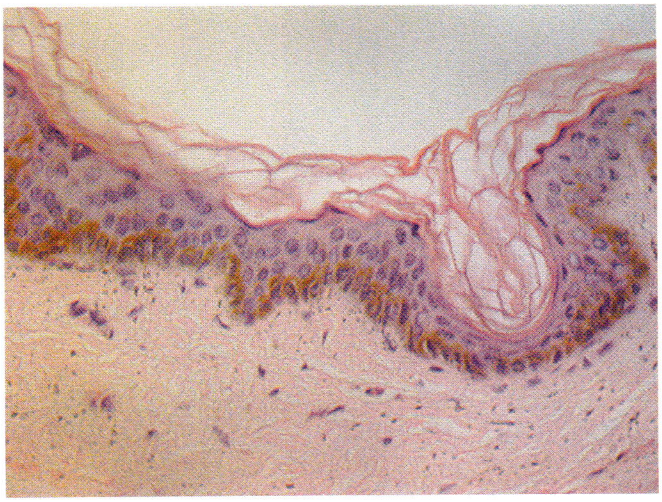

FIGURE 9.5.3

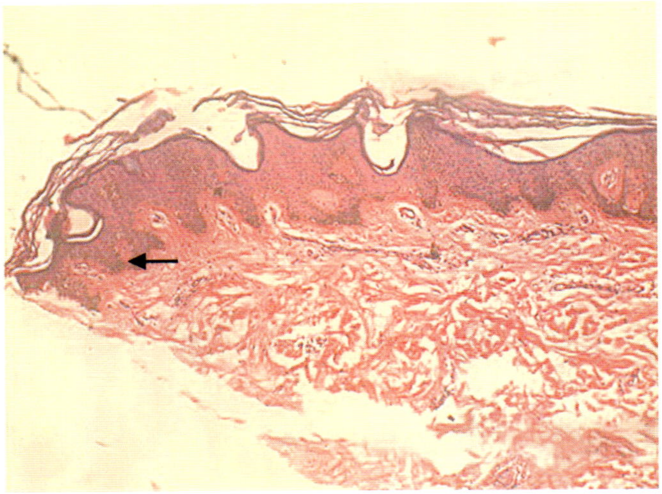

FIGURE 9.6.1

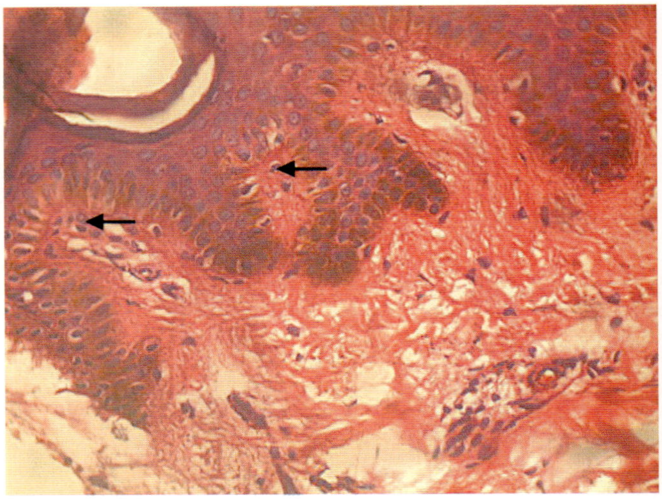

FIGURE 9.6.2

9.6: DOWLING-DEGOS DISEASE

9.6.1: Digitated elongations of the hyperpigmented rete ridges, mild papillomatosis *(Scanner view)*

9.6.2: Pigmentation of the basal cell layer of the suprapapillary epithelium not accentuated *(Low power view)*

9.6.3: Another case with thin, branching heavily pigmented downward proliferations of epidermis *(Low power view)*

9.6.4: Small horn cysts and comedo like lesions are seen *(Low power view)*

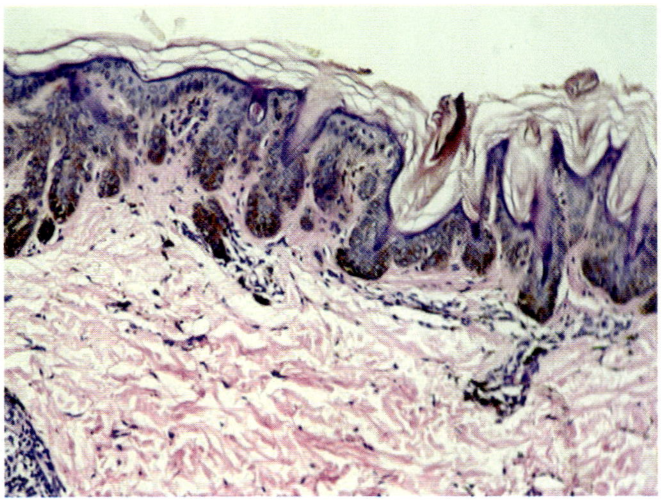

FIGURE 9.6.3

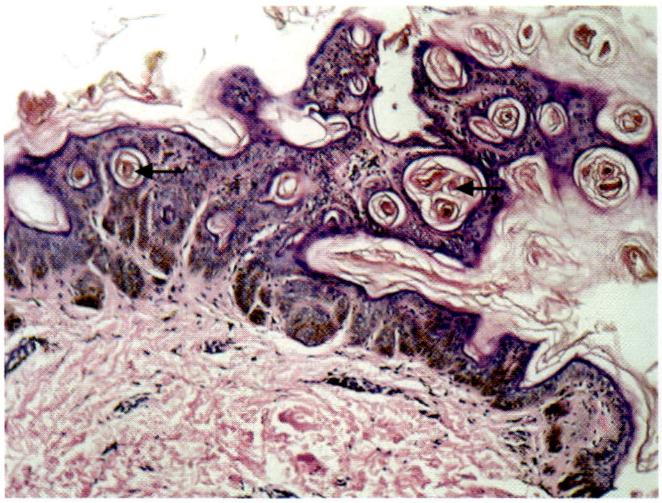

FIGURE 9.6.4

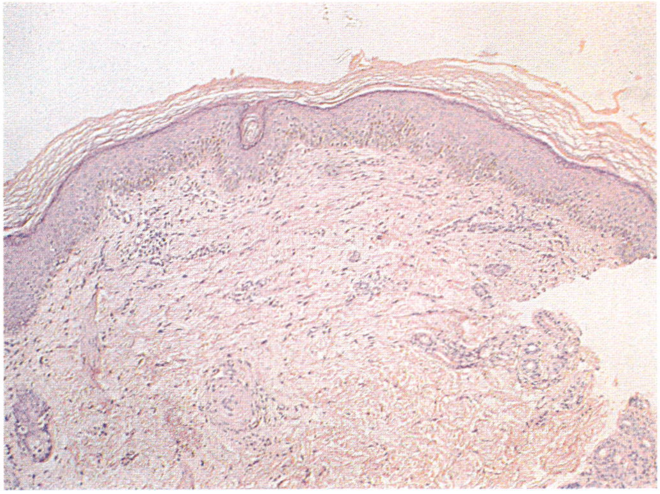

FIGURE 9.7.1

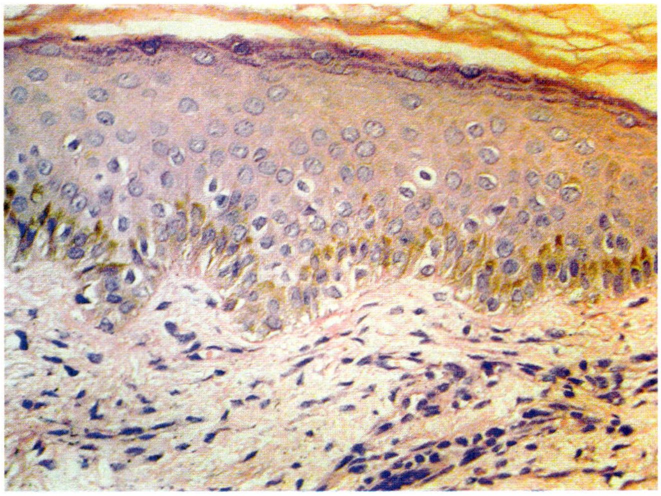

FIGURE 9.7.2

9.7: PATTERNED HYPERMELANOSIS/NEVOID HYPERMELANOSIS/PROGRESSIVE CRIBRIFORM AND ZOSTERIFORM HYPERPIGMENTATION

9.7.1: Increase in melanin pigment in the basal cell layer *(Low power view)*

9.7.2: Closer view of pigment, normal number of melanocytes in the basal cell layer *(High power view)*

9.7.3: Pigment incontinence is mild or absent *(High power view)*

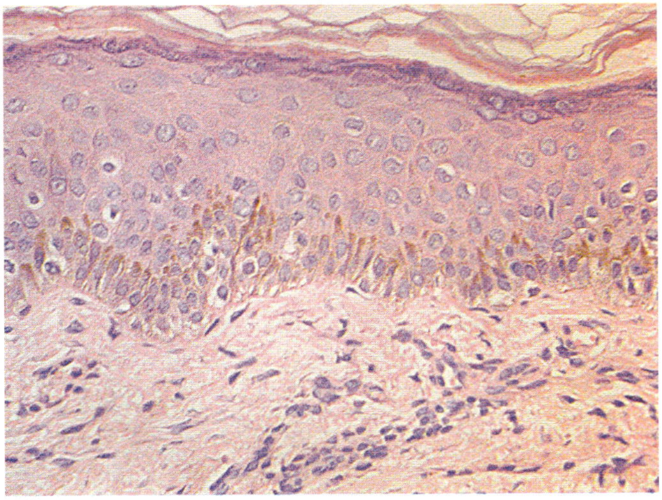

FIGURE 9.7.3

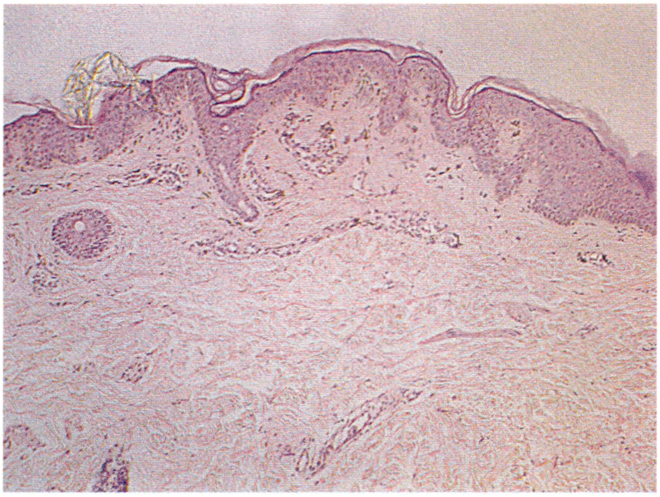

FIGURE 9.8.1

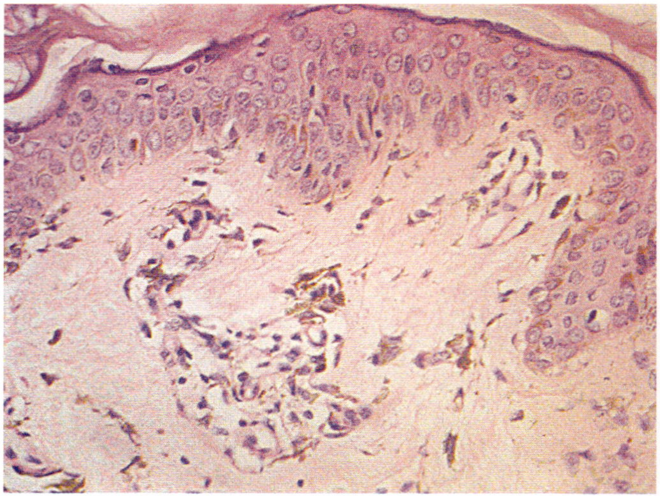

FIGURE 9.8.2

9.8: POSTINFLAMMATORY HYPERPIGMENTATION

9.8.1: Dermal infiltrate and pigment incontinence, epidermis unremarkable *(Scanner view)*

9.8.2: Prominent melanin incontinence with mild increase of melanin pigment in the basal cell layer *(Low power view)*

9.8.3: Lymphocytic infiltrate around blood vessels in the papillary dermis (other features include increased fibroblasts and collagen in the papillary dermis) *(Low power view)*

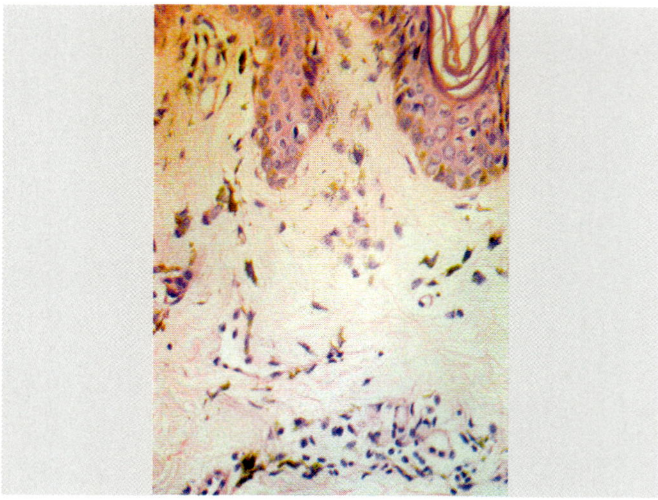

FIGURE 9.8.3

DIFFERENTIAL DIAGNOSIS

1. Hypopigmentation disorders
   a. Marked reduction in melanin with only marginally reduced melanocytes:
      i. Albinism
      ii. Pityriasis alba
      iii. Tinea versicolor
      iv. Hypomelanosis of Ito
   b. Significant reduction in number of melanocytes along with reduced melanin:
      i. Piebaldism
      ii. Halo nevus
      iii. Idiopathic guttate hypomelanosis (IGH)
2. Hyperpigmentation disorders
   a. Predominant increase in epidermal melanin
      i. Cafe-au-lait macules (CALM)
   b. Predominant increase in dermal melanin
      i. Prurigo pigmentosa
   c. Mixed dermal and epidermal melanin
      i. Postinflammatory
      ii. Melasma

DIAGNOSTIC PEARLS

1. Presence of some basilar melanocytes and melanin may be seen in repigmenting or trichrome vitiligo.
2. Nevus depigmentosus and hypomelanosis of Ito show poorly developed melanocytic dendrites.
3. Evidence of fibrosis may be a pointer to physical or chemical depigmentation.
4. IGH lesions may show atrophic epidermis.
5. Diffuse pigmentation due to endocrine causes shows heavily melanized cells in basal layer and stratum spinosum with pigment incontinence.
6. Patterned hypermelanosis may be associated with presence of collection of nevus cells at the base of rete ridges.

Panniculitis

10

Chapter Outline

10.1: Erythema Nodosum
10.2: Erythema Induratum (Nodular Vasculitis)
10.3: Subcutaneous Fat Necrosis of Newborn
10.4: Membranous Lipodystrophy
(Pseudomembranous Fat Necrosis)
10.5: Lipodermatosclerosis
10.6: Pancreatic Panniculitis

Pradeep Mahajan, Uday Khopkar,
Chirag Desai, KC Nischal

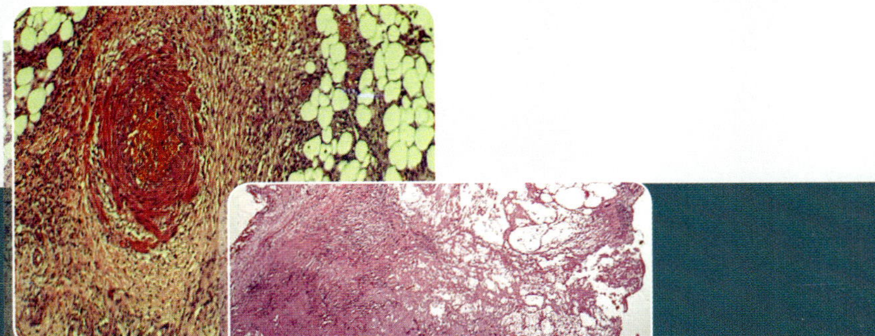

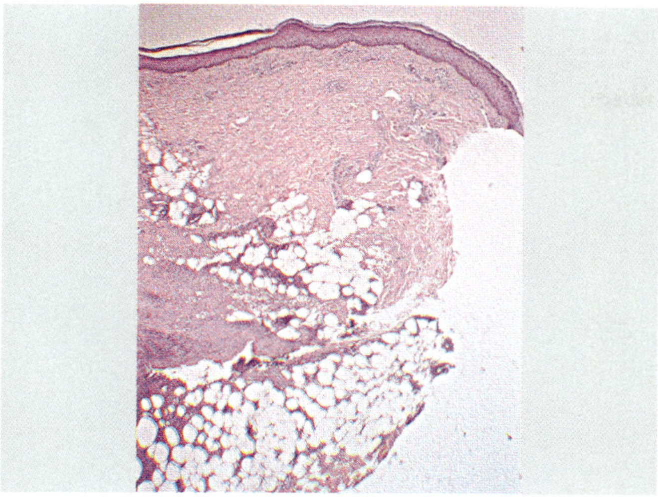

FIGURE 10.1.1

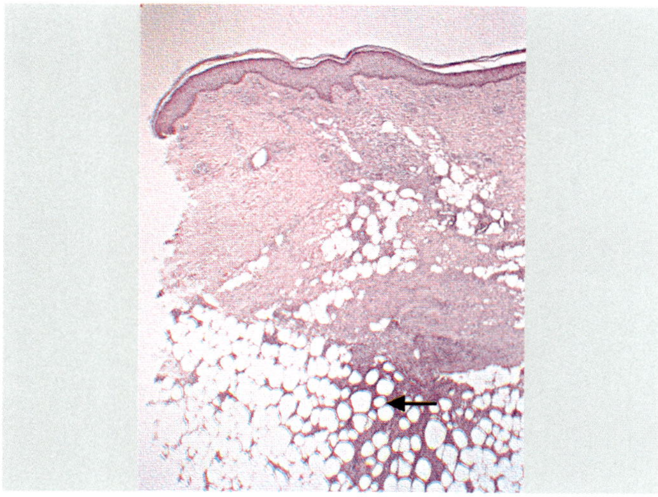

FIGURE 10.1.2

10.1: ERYTHEMA NODOSUM

10.1.1: Septal panniculitis—inflammatory infiltrate involving subcutaneous septa with septal thickening, dermis comparatively uninvolved *(Scanner view)*

10.1.2: Wedge like inflammatory infiltrate extending from subcutaneous septa *(Scanner view)*

10.1.3: Inflammation extends to lobule to some extent but there is sparing of center of the lobule *(Low power view)*

10.1.4: Thickening of septa with infiltrate *(Low power view)*

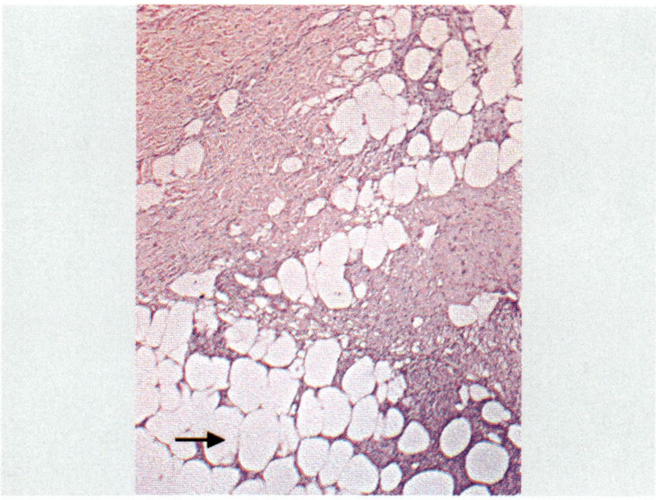

FIGURE 10.1.3

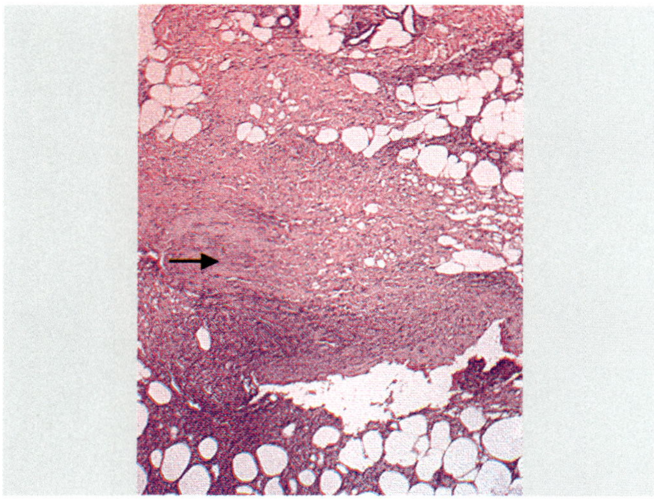

FIGURE 10.1.4

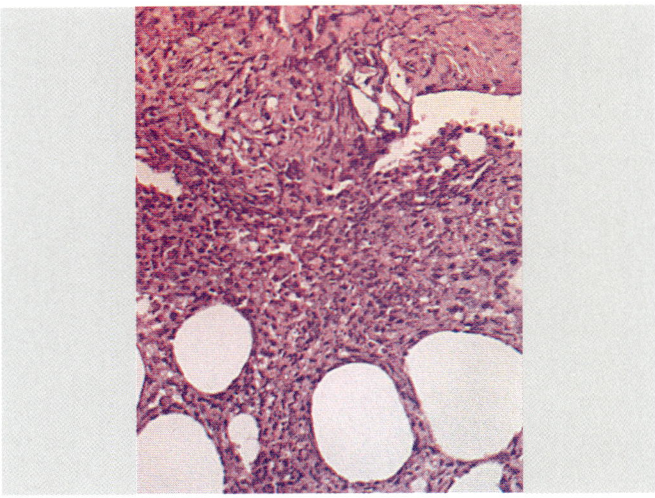

FIGURE 10.1.5

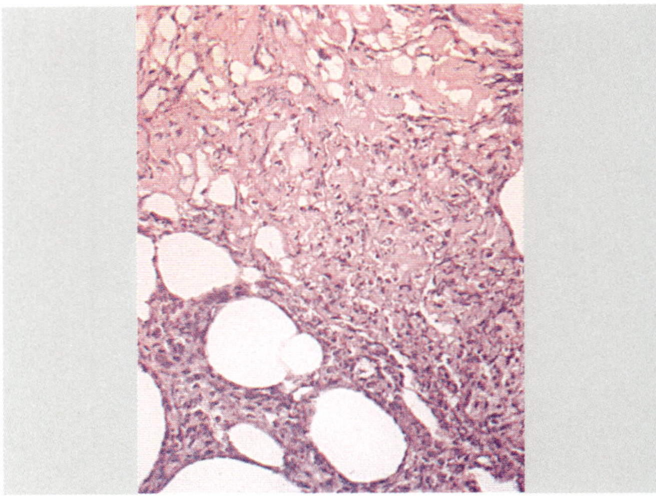

FIGURE 10.1.6

10.1.5: Neutrophilic infiltrate in early stages *(High power view)*

10.1.6: Another view of neutrophils and an occasional eosinophil *(High power view)*

10.1.7: Blood vessel shows endothelial thickening but no frank vasculitis *(High power view)*

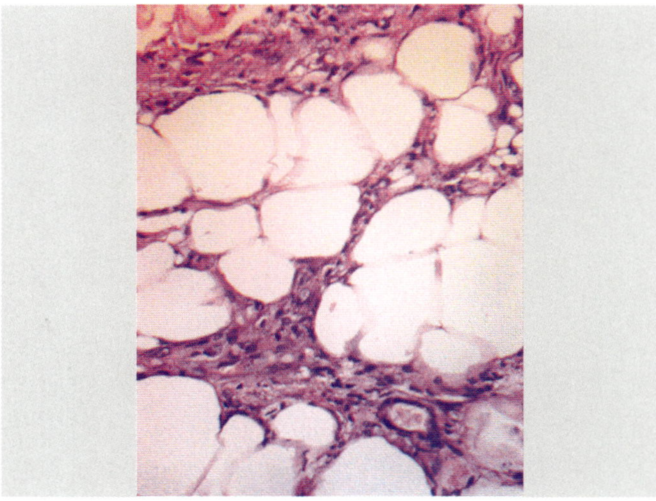

FIGURE 10.1.7

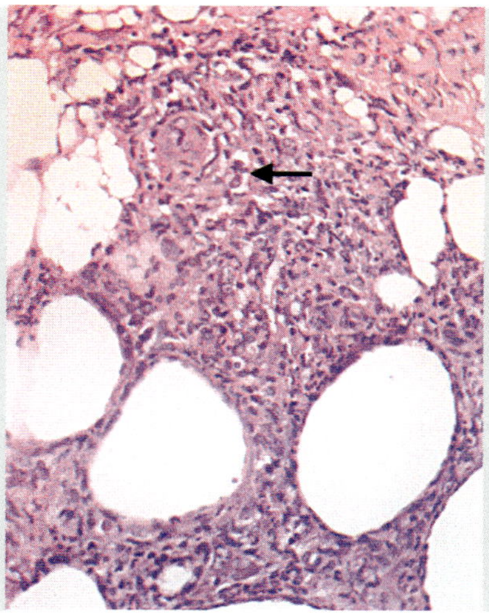

FIGURE 10.1.8

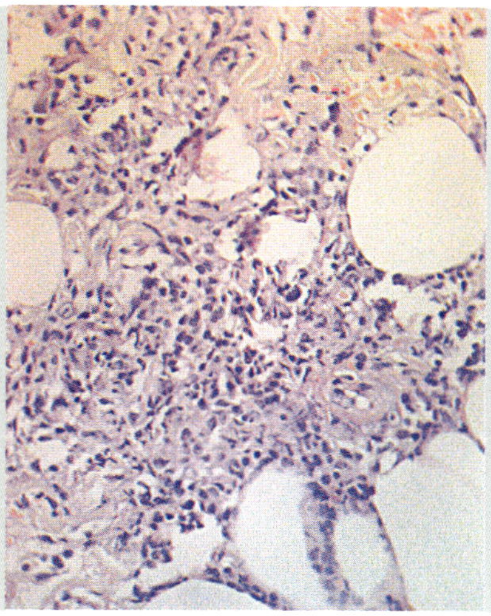

FIGURE 10.1.9

10.1.8: Shows structures like Miescher's granulomas which are histiocytes radiating around minute slits in the septa *(High power view)*

10.1.9: Another case with lymphocytic infiltrate and histiocytes (other histologic features include infiltrate composed of a few giant cells, usually of foreign body type however, true tuberculoid granuloma formation is very rare) *(High power view)*

10.1.10: Lymphocytes with a few eosinophils *(High power view)*

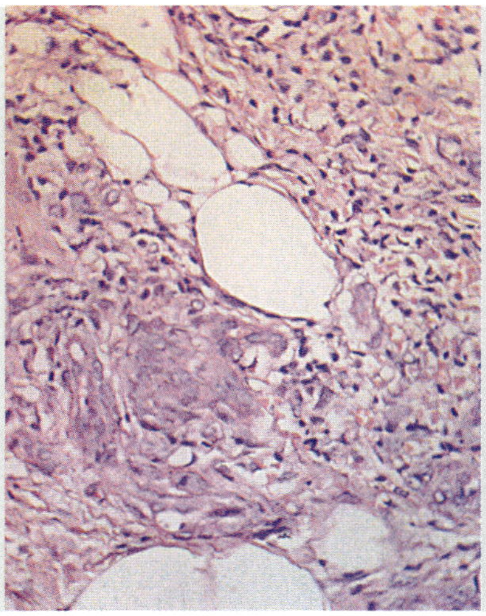

FIGURE 10.1.10

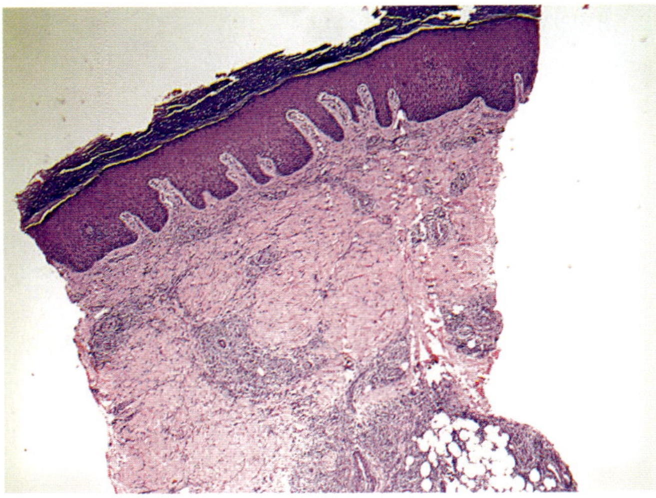

FIGURE 10.2.1

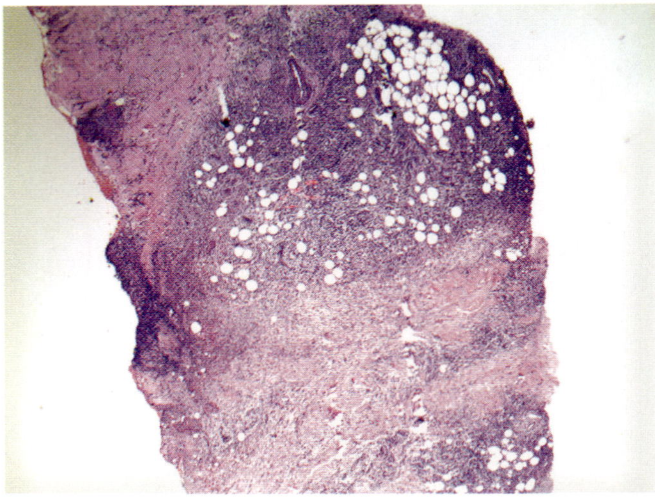

FIGURE 10.2.2

10.2: ERYTHEMA INDURATUM (NODULAR VASCULITIS)

10.2.1: Dermal infiltrate with lobular panniculitis *(Scanner view)*

10.2.2: Dense infiltrate around subcutaneous lobules and septal fibrosis *(Scanner view)*

10.2.3: Central lobule surrounded by infiltrate *(Low power view)*

10.2.4: Vascular changes *(Low power view)*

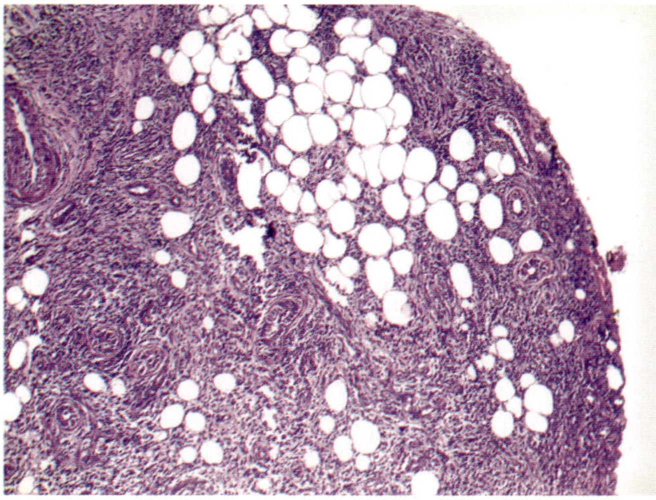

FIGURE 10.2.3

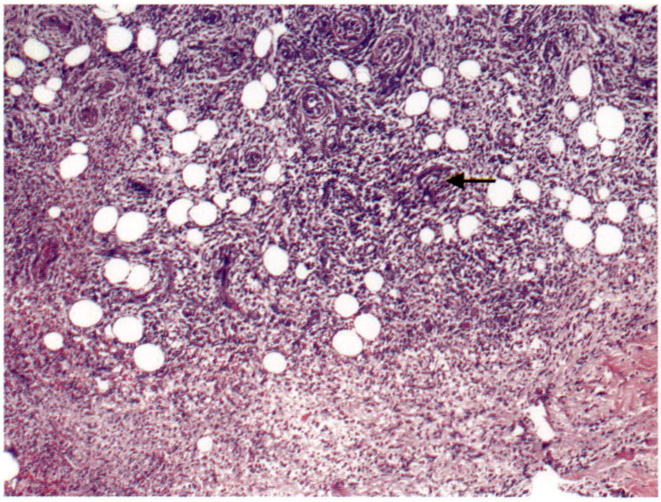

FIGURE 10.2.4

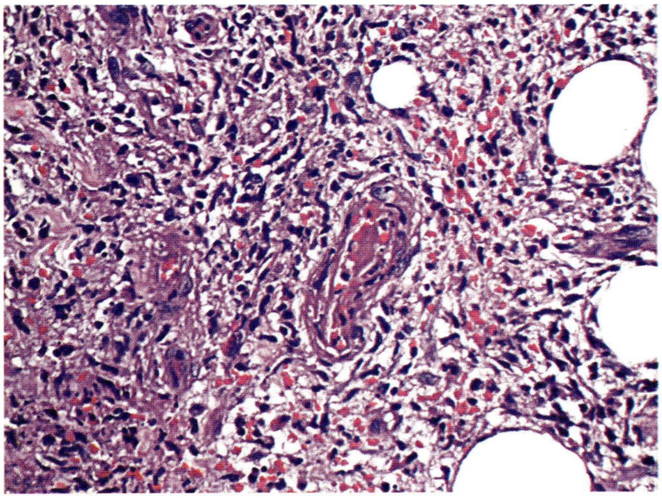

FIGURE 10.2.5

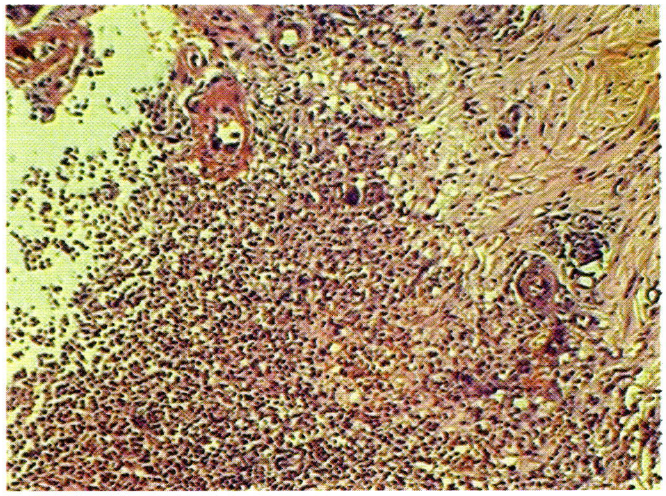

FIGURE 10.2.6

10.2.5: Closer view showing endothelial swelling and a mixed inflammatory cell infiltrate *(High power view)*

10.2.6: Another case with vasculitis (fibrinoid degeneration, neutrophilic infiltrate) *(Low power view)*

10.2.7: Vasculitis-endothelial cell thickening, fibrinoid degeneration, fibrin thrombus (nodular vasculitis) *(High power view)*

10.2.8: Another case with lobular panniculitis, clearly shows inflammatory infiltrate around the central lobule *(Scanner view)*

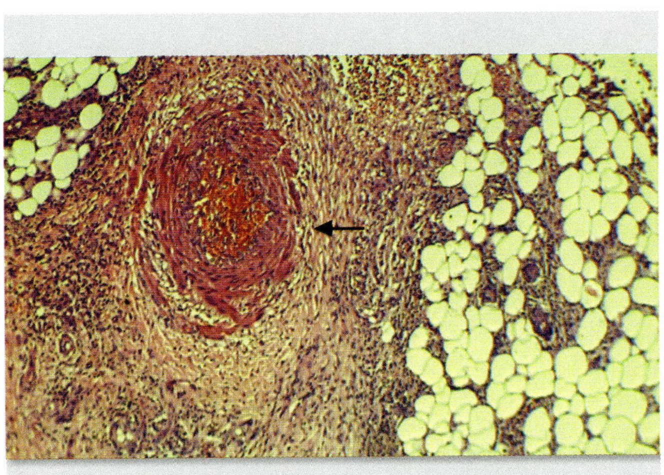

FIGURE 10.2.7

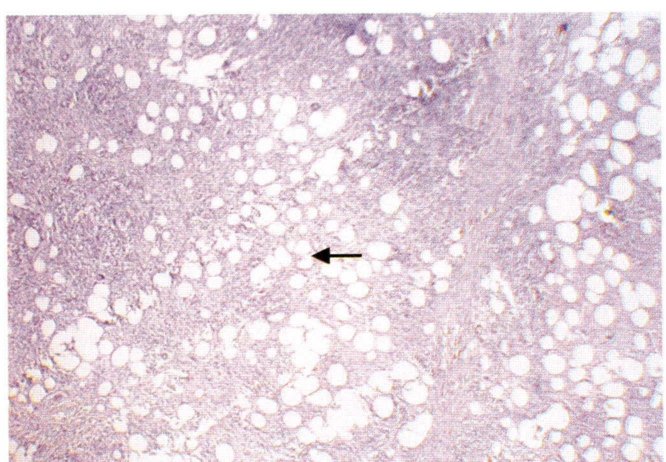

FIGURE 10.2.8

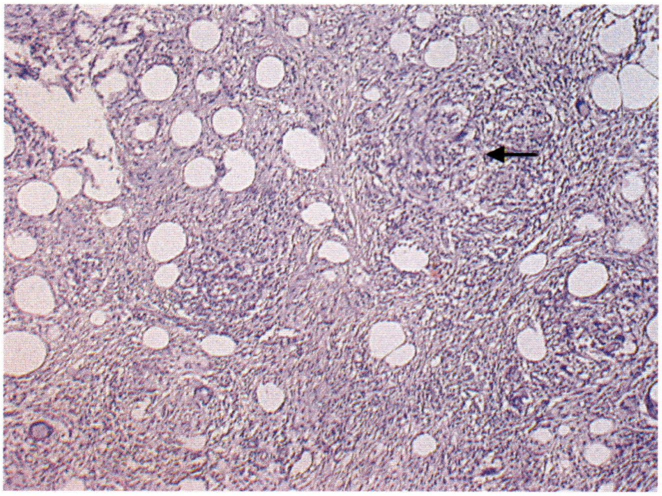

FIGURE 10.2.9

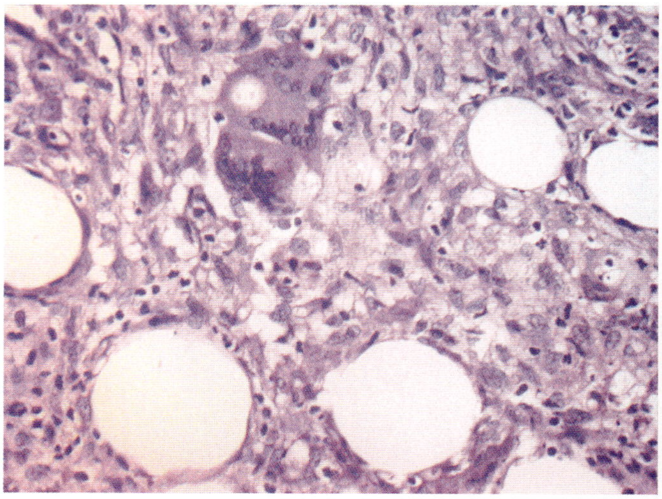

FIGURE 10.2.10

10.2.9: With granulomatous inflammation *(Low power view)*

10.2.10: Multinucleated giant cells *(High power view)*

10.2.11: Areas of caseation necrosis *(Low power view)*

10.2.12: Closer view of the same with caseation necrosis (may indicate tuberculoid etiology) *(High power view)*

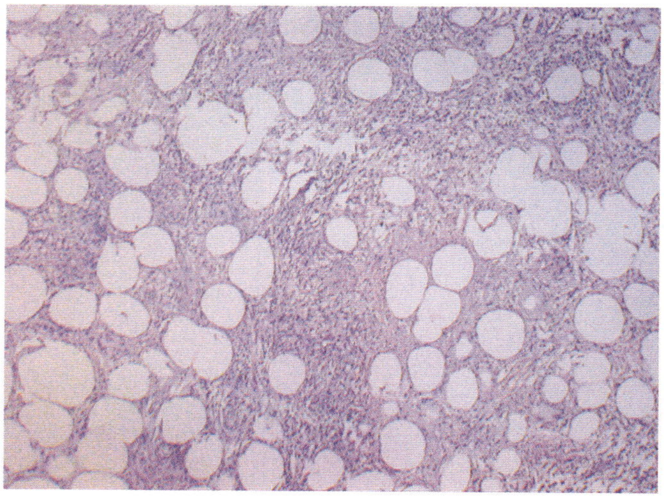

FIGURE 10.2.11

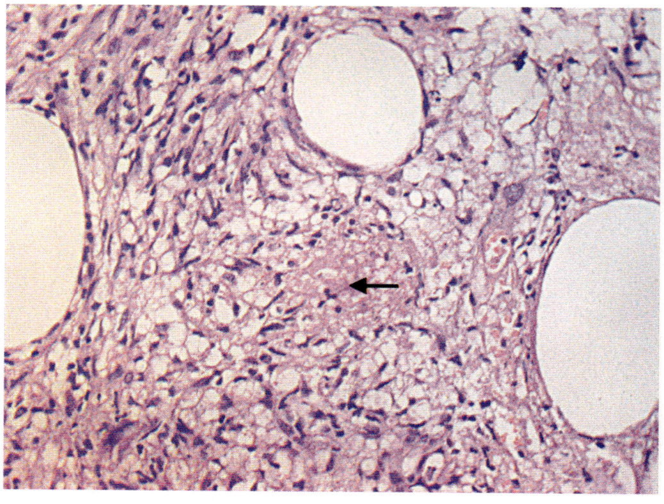

FIGURE 10.2.12

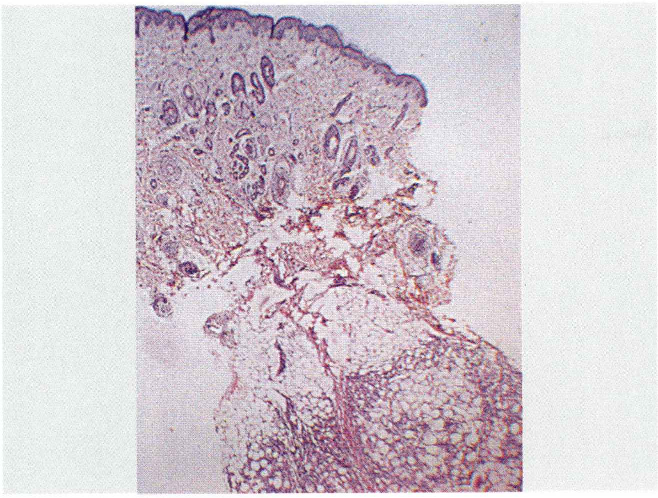

FIGURE 10.3.1

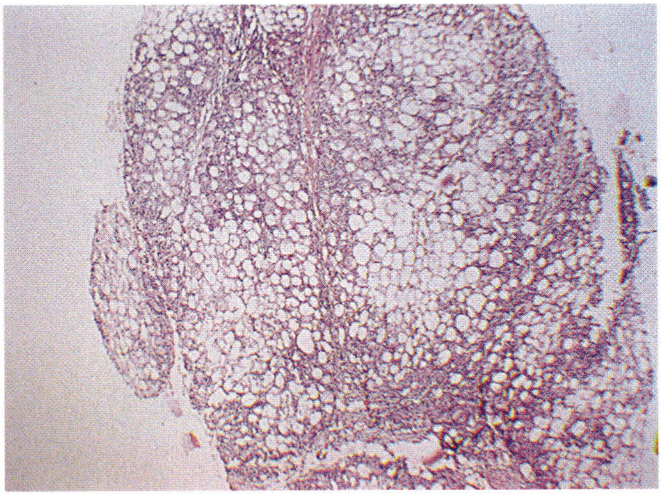

FIGURE 10.3.2

10.3: SUBCUTANEOUS FAT NECROSIS OF NEWBORN

10.3.1: Normal epidermis and dermis with an underlying lobular panniculitis *(Scanner view)*

10.3.2: Lobular panniculitis *(Scanner view)*

10.3.3: Focal fat cell necrosis leading to small cyst formation *(Low power view)*

10.3.4: Another view *(Low power view)*

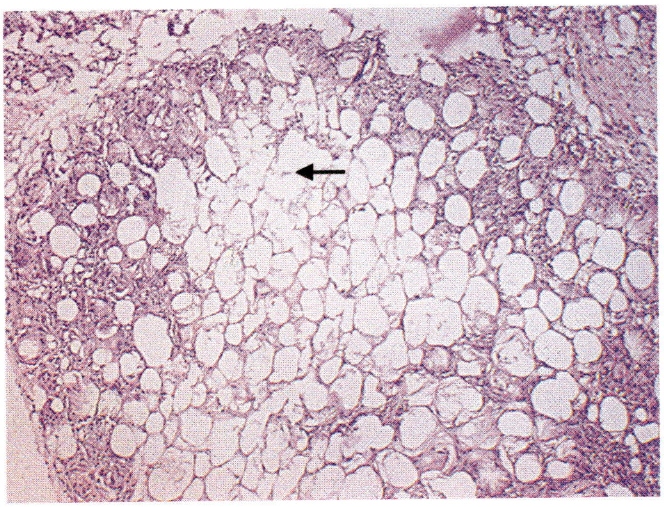

FIGURE 10.3.3

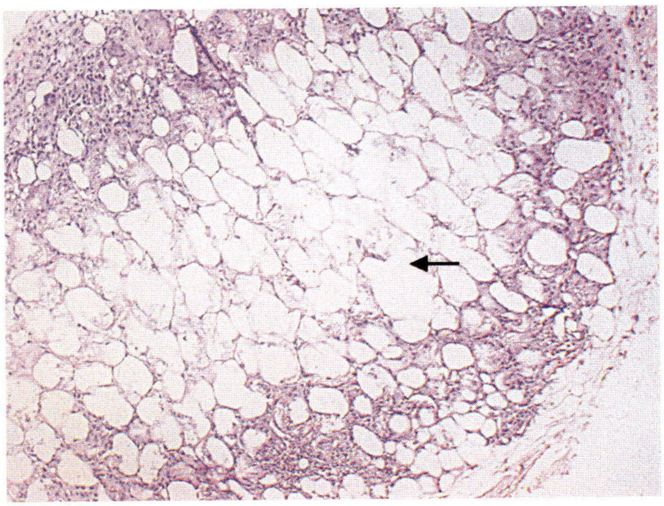

FIGURE 10.3.4

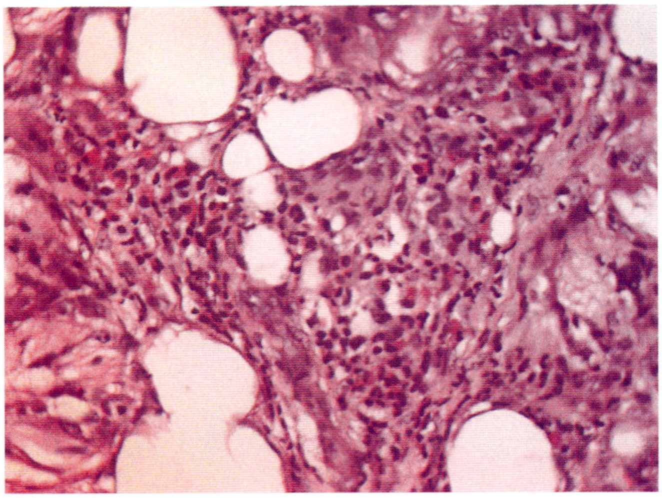

FIGURE 10.3.5

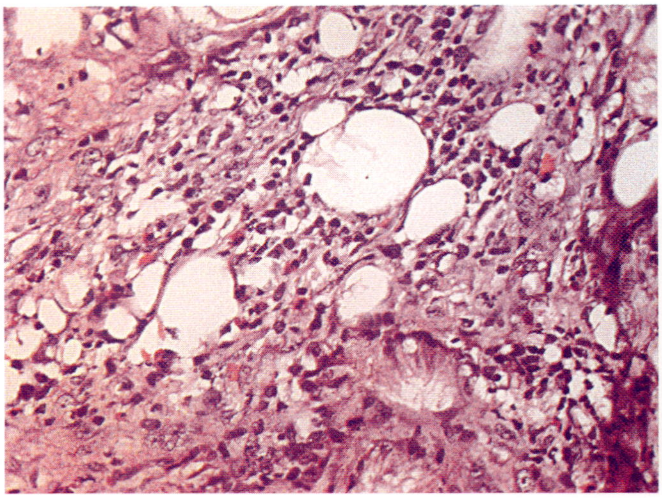

FIGURE 10.3.6

10.3.5: Inflammatory infiltrate of lymphocytes and eosinophils wedged between the fat cells *(High power view)*

10.3.6: Histiocytes and plasma cells *(High power view)*

10.3.7: Multinucleated giant cells *(High power view)*

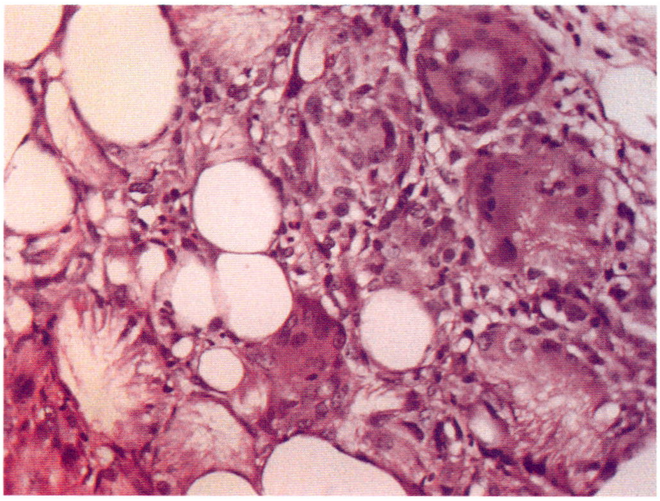

FIGURE 10.3.7

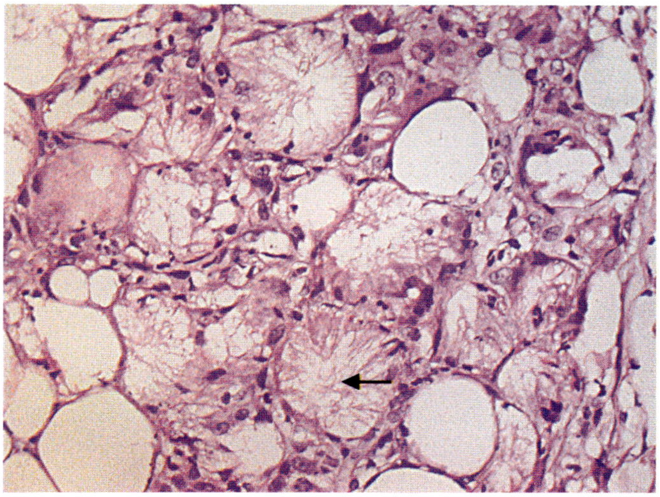

FIGURE 10.3.8

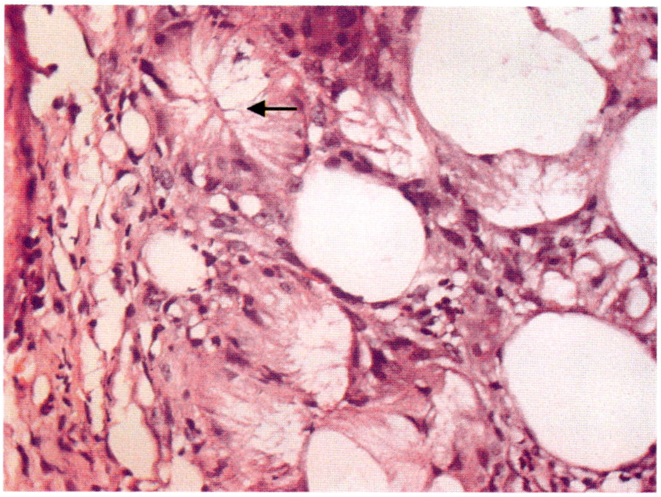

FIGURE 10.3.9

10.3.8: Another distinct feature is the presence of eosinophilic strands with clefts in between, strands are attached to the periphery of fat cells *(High power view)*

10.3.9: A closer view of the strands *(High power view)*

10.3.10: Strands with foreign body giant cells *(High power view)*

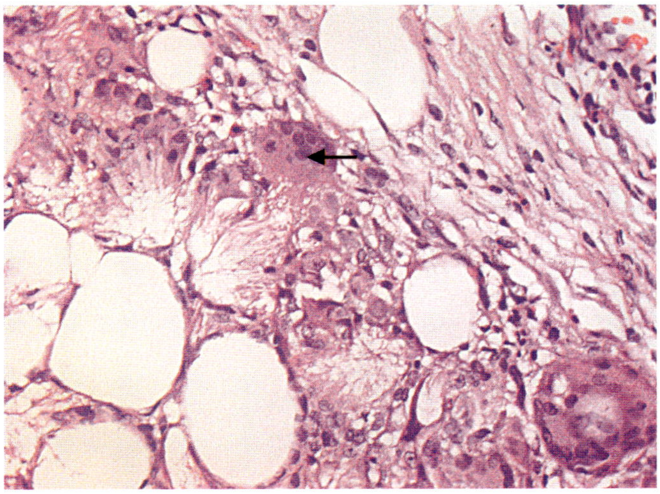

FIGURE 10.3.10

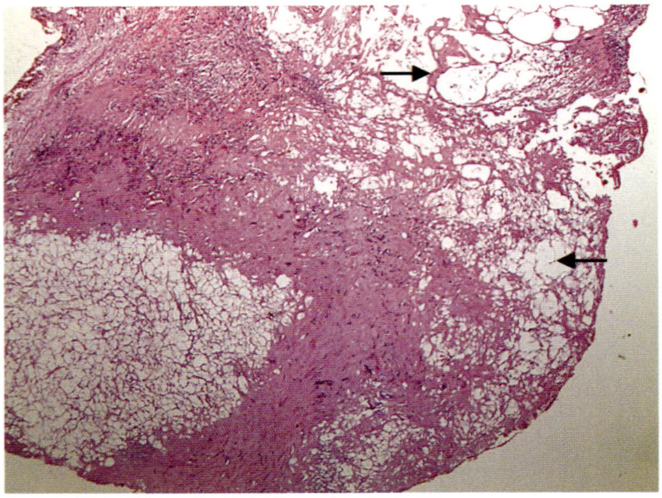

FIGURE 10.4.1

10.4: MEMBRANOUS LIPODYSTROPHY (PSEUDOMEMBRANOUS FAT NECROSIS)

10.4.1: Lipomembranous (membranocystic) change—H and E stain shows microcyst formation which are lined by eosinophilic material. (PAS and Sudan black stains highlight the material). Fibrous septa are present between these cysts. There is no evidence of inflammation *(Low power view)*

10.4.2: The membranes show small pseudopapillae (In secondary membranous lipodystrophy, changes of the underlying process are present) *(High power view)*

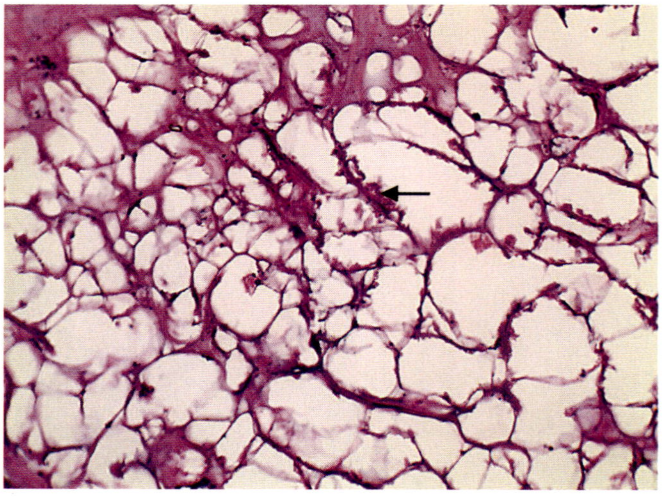

FIGURE 10.4.2

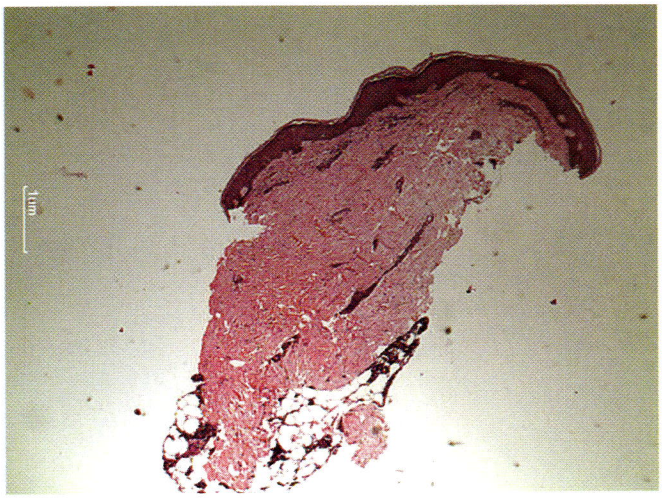

FIGURE 10.5.1

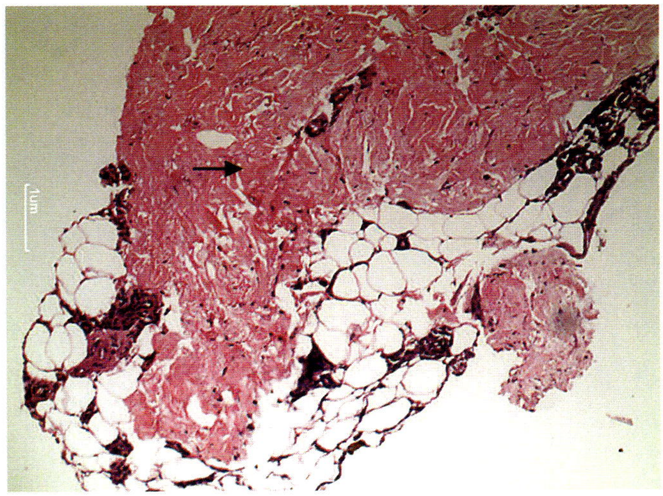

FIGURE 10.5.2

10.5: LIPODERMATOSCLEROSIS

10.5.1: Fibrosis of the dermis *(Scanner view)*

10.5.2: Dermal fibrosis and sclerosis extending to the subcutaneous tissue and microcyst formation in fat cells *(Low power view)*

10.5.3: Eosinophilic material, lining microcysts along with mild septal and lobular panniculitis (infiltrate composed mainly of lymphocytes) *(Low power view)*

10.5.4: Another case with dermal and septal fibrosis *(Scanner view)*

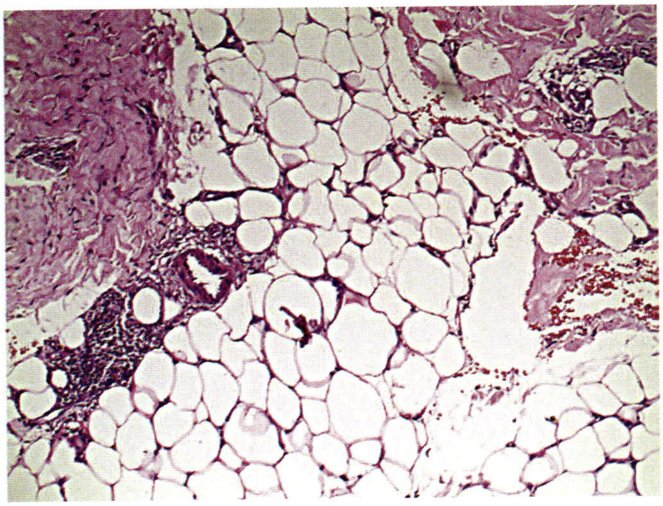

FIGURE 10.5.3

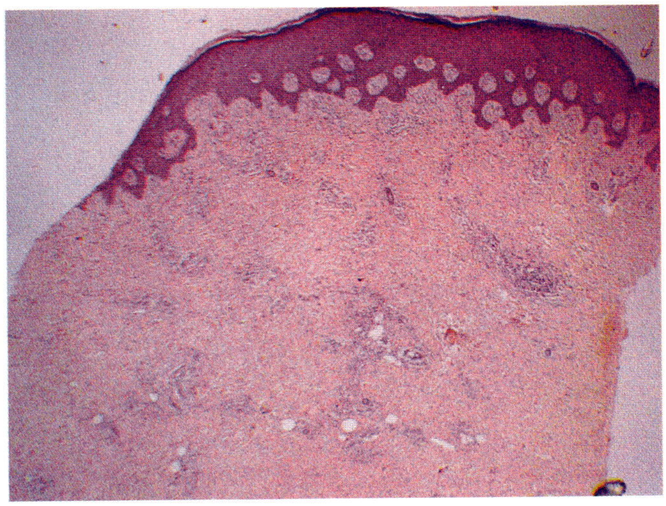

FIGURE 10.5.4

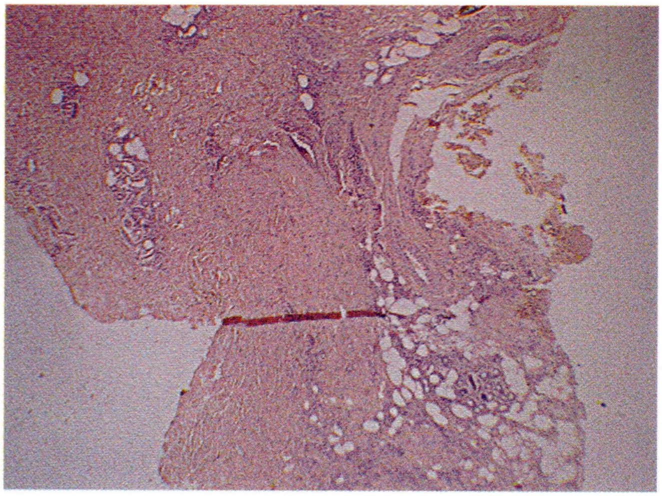

FIGURE 10.5.5

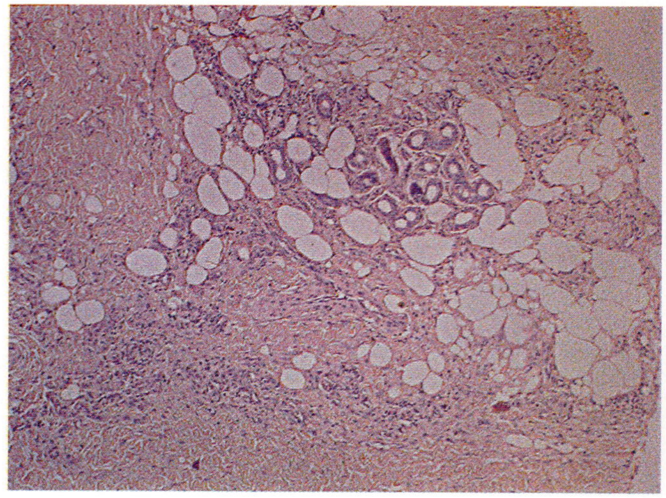

FIGURE 10.5.6

10.5.5: Septal fibrosis *(Scanner view)*

10.5.6: Mild septal and lobular panniculitis with lymphocytes *(Low power view)*

10.5.7: Microcysts with eosinophilic lining *(High power view)*

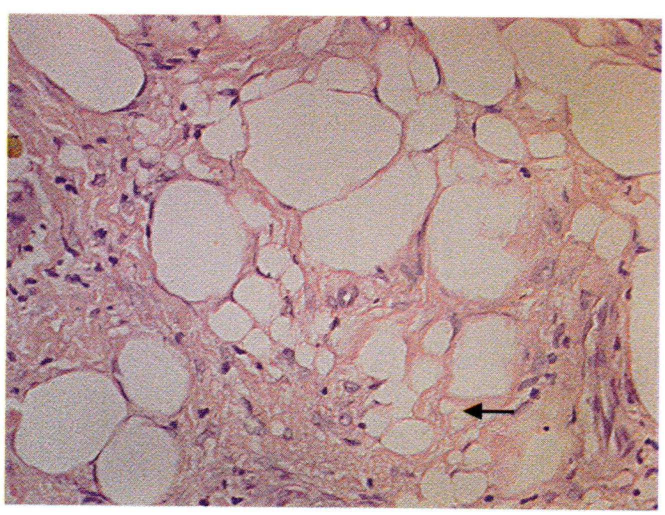

FIGURE 10.5.7

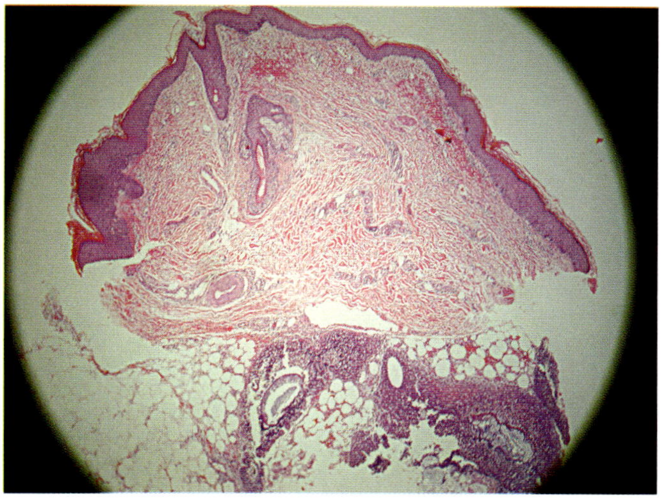

FIGURE 10.6.1

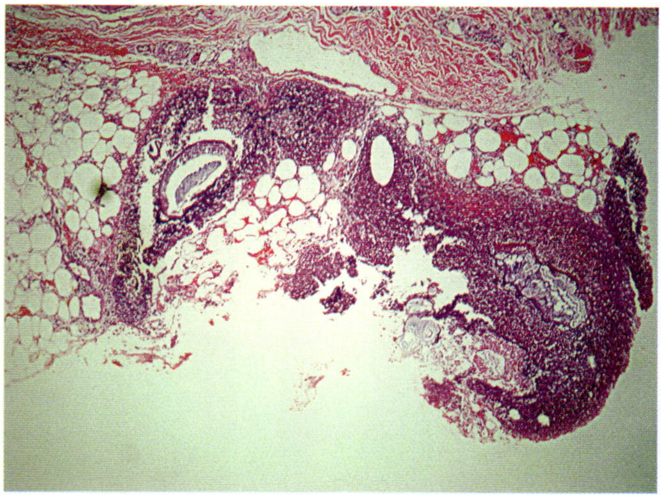

FIGURE 10.6.2

10.6: PANCREATIC PANNICULITIS

10.6.1: Mainly lobular panniculitis *(Scanner view)*

10.6.2: Fat cell necrosis *(Low power view)*

10.6.3: Inflammatory cell infiltrate and fat necrosis resulting in ghost-like contour *(Low power view)*

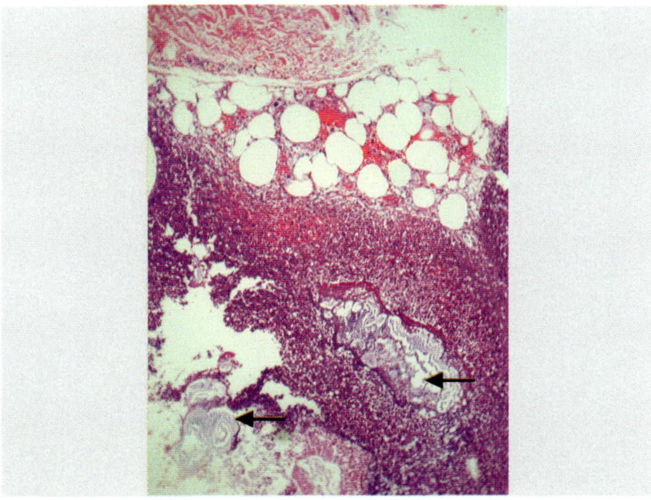

FIGURE 10.6.3

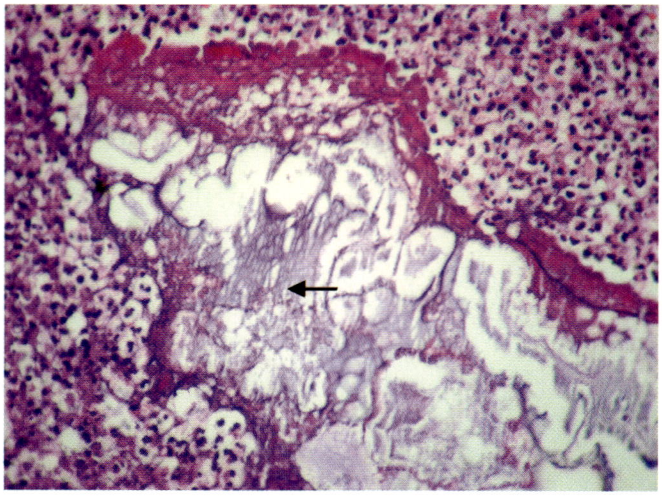

FIGURE 10.6.4

10.6.4: Calcium deposits give basophilic appearance to degenerated fat cells *(High power view)*

10.6.5: Neutrophils and RBC's around necrotic fat cells *(High power view)*

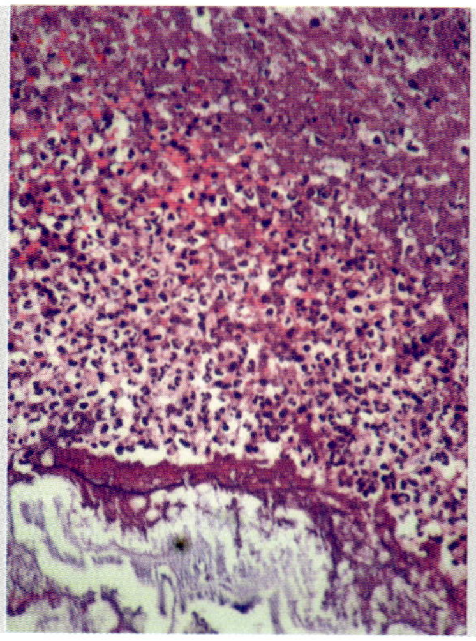

FIGURE 10.6.5

DIFFERENTIAL DIAGNOSIS

1. Septal Panniculitis
   a. Necrobiosis lipoidica (discussed elsewhere)
   b. Scleroderma (discussed elsewhere)
2. Lobular panniculitis
   a. Lupus panniculitis (discussed elsewhere)
   b. Panniculitis like T-cell lymphoma
   c. Sclerema neonatorum
   d. Alfa-1 antitrypsin deficiency
   e. Infective panniculitis

DIAGNOSTIC PEARLS

1. Well-formed tuberculoid granulomas are not a usual feature of erythema nodosum (EN).
2. Septal panniculitis with lymphocytic or leukocytoclastic type vasculitis is usually seen in EN like lesions of Behcet's disease.
3. Necrosis is more common in nodular vasculitis of tuberculoid etiology.
4. Polyarteritis nodosa shows panniculitis only around the involved blood vessels as against erythema induratum (nodular vasculitis) which involves multiple adjoining lobules.
5. Histiocytes showing phagocytosis of RBC's and leukocytes is a feature of cytophagic histiocytic panniculitis.
6. Alfa-1 antitrypsin deficiency panniculitis shows neutrophils between the collagen bundles of reticular dermis and presence of normal fat adjacent to foci of fat necrosis.

11

Diseases of Collagen, Elastin and Mucin

Chapter Outline

11.1: Collagen Disorders
11.2: Elastin Changes
11.3: Mucin Deposition

Asha Kubba, Atul Dongre, Uday Khopkar, Sara Edward, Nathan Lee, Jerad Gardner

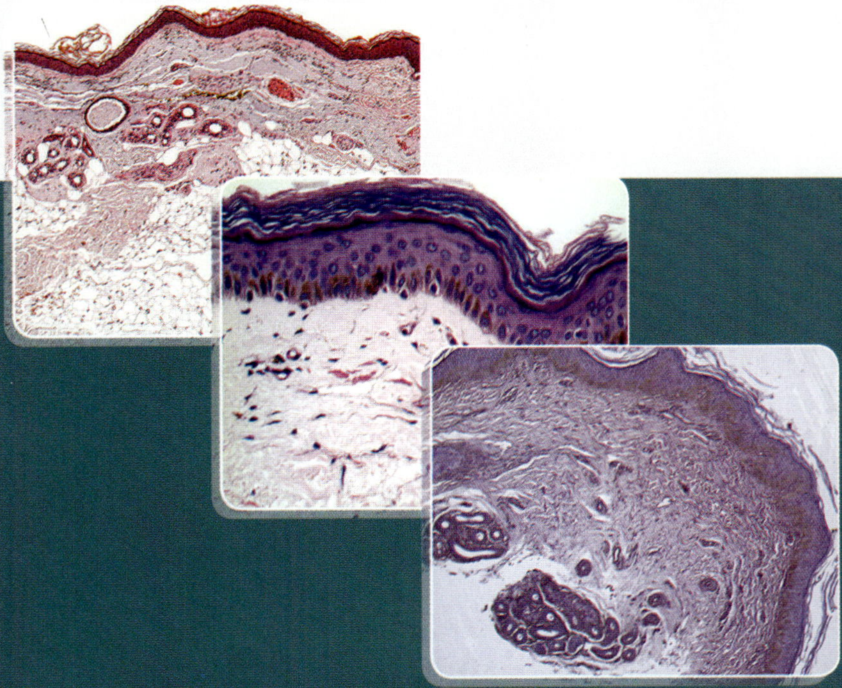

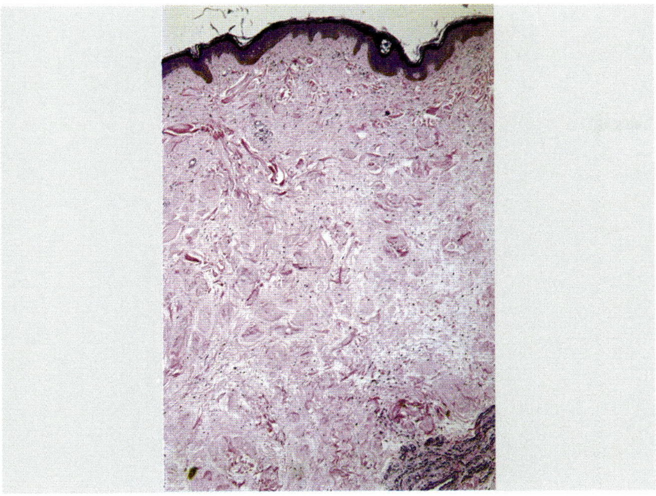

FIGURE 11.1.1.1

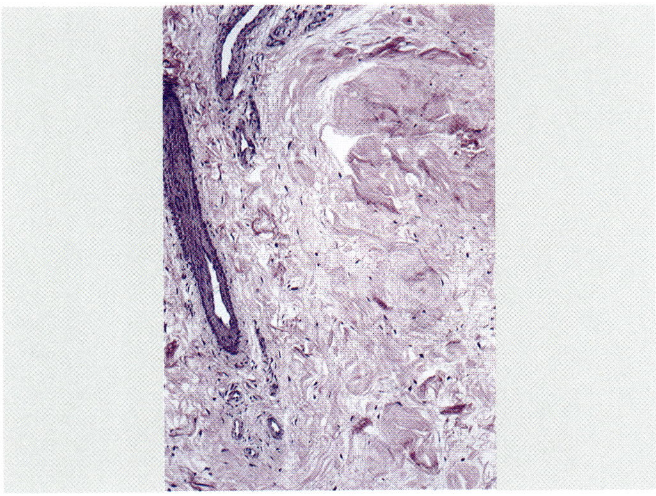

FIGURE 11.1.1.2

11.1: COLLAGEN DISORDERS

11.1.1: Collagen Tissue Nevi (Collagenoma)

11.1.1.1: Normal epidermis *(Scanner view)*

11.1.1.2: Densely packed broad collagen fibers in thickened dermis *(Low power view)*

11.1.1.3: Dermis is replaced by collagen fibers seen in blue (Masson trichrome) *(Scanner view)*

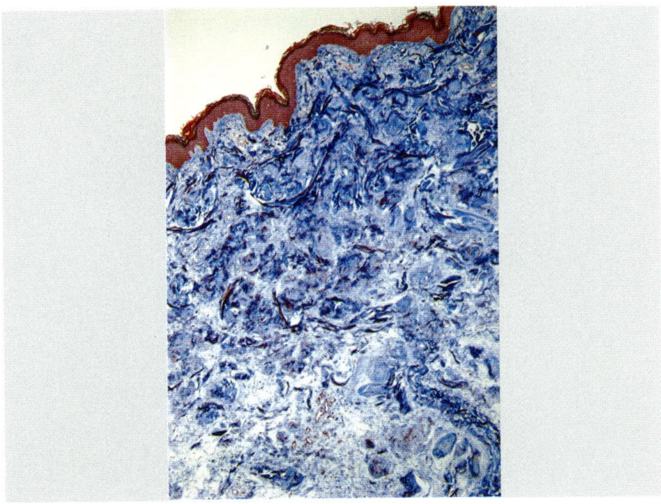

FIGURE 11.1.1.3

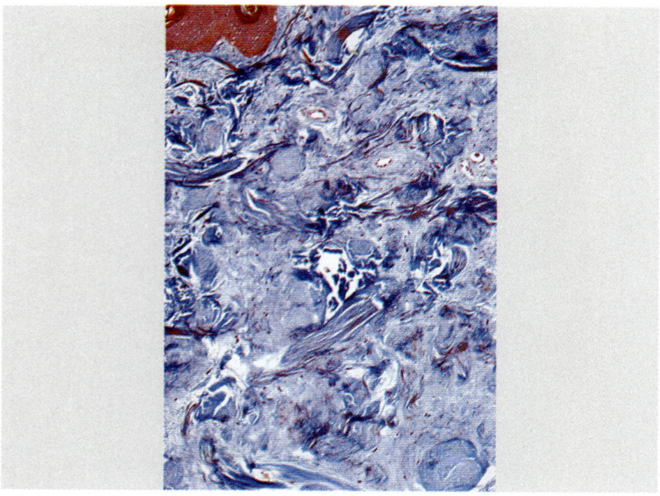

FIGURE 11.1.1.4

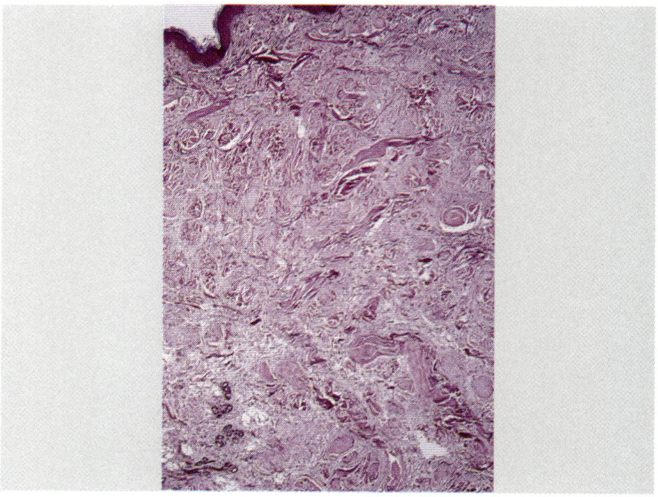

FIGURE 11.1.1.5

11.1.1.4: Low power view of the same
11.1.1.5: Elastic fibers diminished—elastin stain (orcein) *(Scanner view)*
11.1.1.6: Low power view of the same

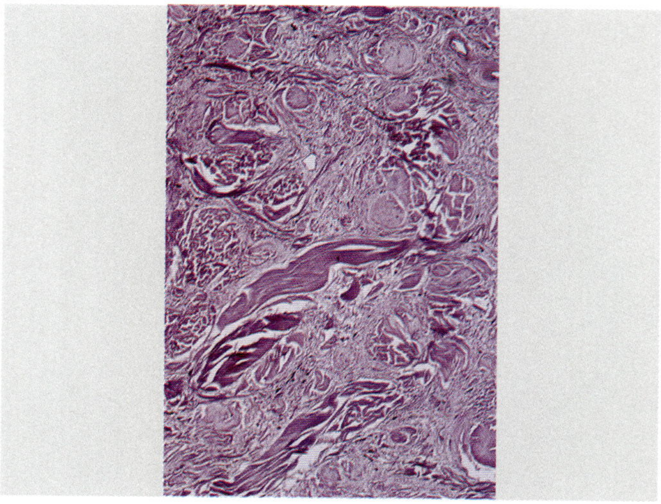

FIGURE 11.1.1.6

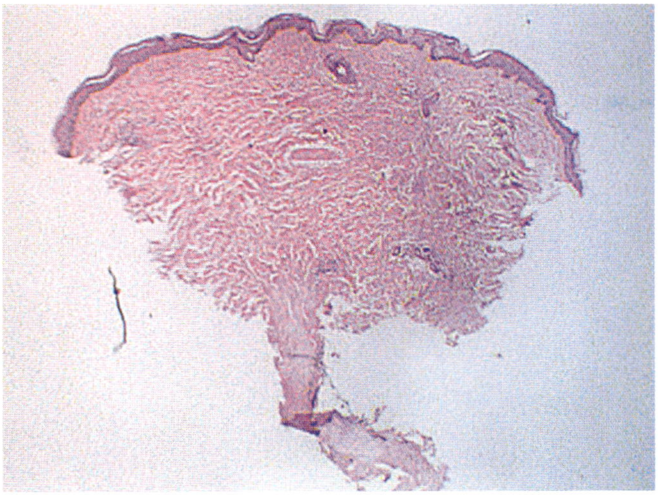

FIGURE 11.1.2.1

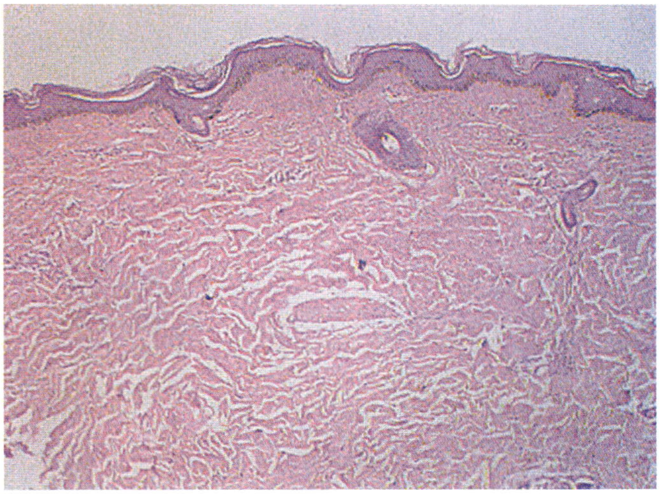

FIGURE 11.1.2.2

11.1.2: Morphea

11.1.2.1: The epidermis is atrophic, reticular dermis replaced by thick collagen extending to subcutaneous tissue *(Scanner view)*

11.1.2.2: Atrophic adnexal structures and thick dermis composed of hyalinized collagen bundles *(Low power view)*

11.1.2.3: Atrophic epidermis, increased pigmentation in basal cell layer, thick collagen *(High power view)*

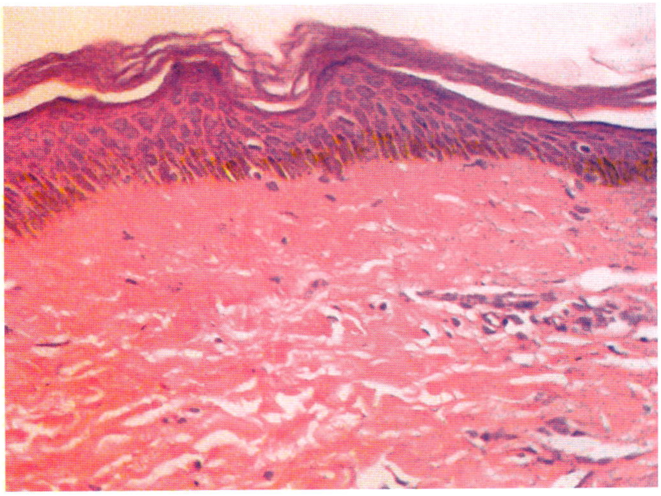

FIGURE 11.1.2.3

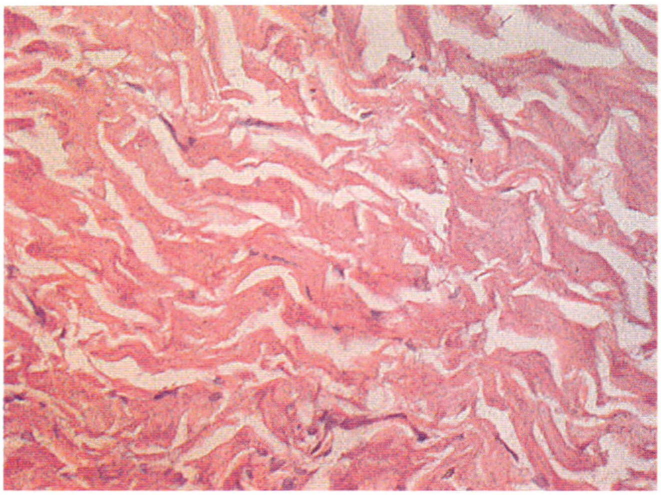

FIGURE 11.1.2.4

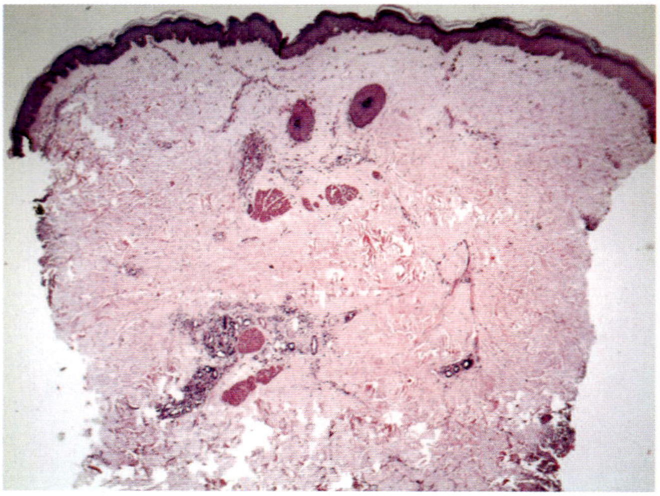

FIGURE 11.1.2.5

11.1.2.4: Late lesion with reduced fibroblast activity and sclerotic collagen *(High power view)*

11.1.2.5: Scleroderma—atrophic epidermis, thick collagen, adnexal atrophy *(Scanner view)*

11.1.2.6: Perivascular inflammatory cell infiltrate composed of lymphocytes and plasma cells *(Low power view)*

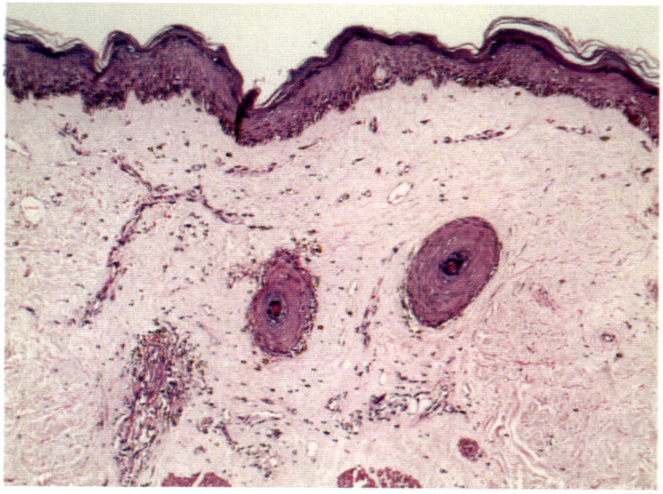

FIGURE 11.1.2.6

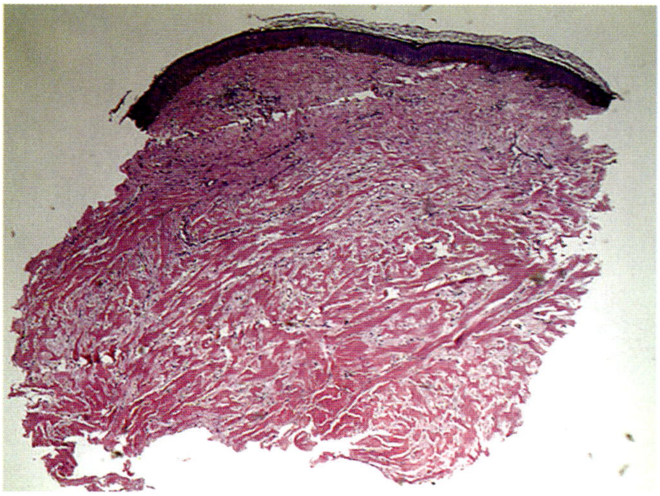

FIGURE 11.1.3.1

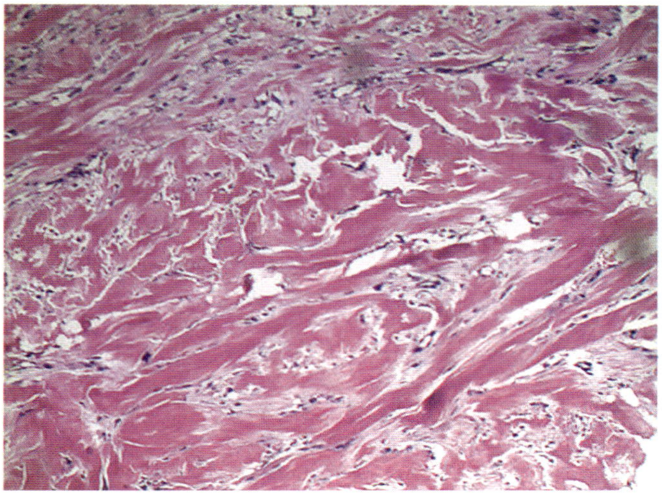

FIGURE 11.1.3.2

11.1.3: Keloid

11.1.3.1: Atrophic epidermis with broad collagen bundles *(Scanner view)*

11.1.3.2: Homogeneous, brightly eosinophilic collagen arranged in haphazard way *(Low power view)*

11.1.3.3: Increased fibroblasts located alongside the collagen bundles *(High power view)*

11.1.3.4: Hypertrophic scar—a circumscribed lesion composed of cells with scanty cytoplasm and elongated spindle-shaped nuclei (fibroblasts) with thickened bundles of collagen, perivascular inflammatory cell infiltrate *(Scanner view)*

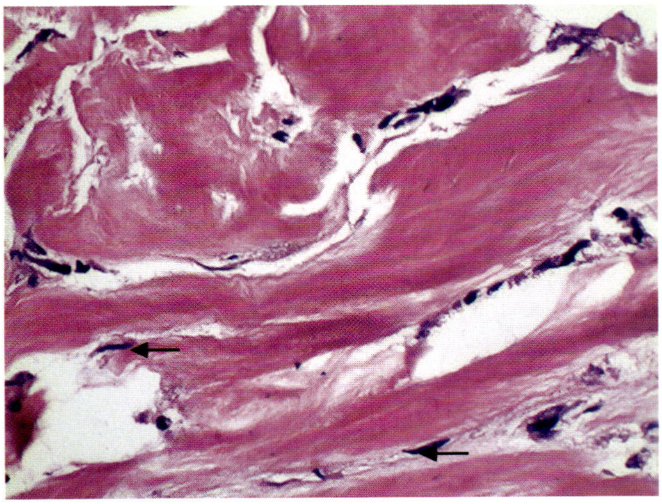

FIGURE 11.1.3.3

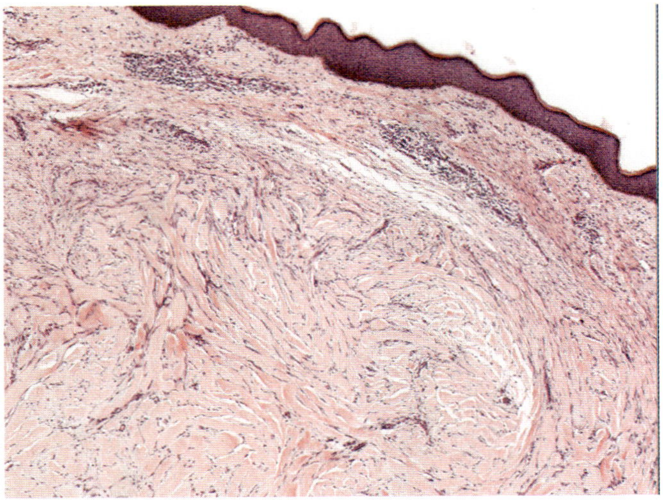

FIGURE 11.1.3.4

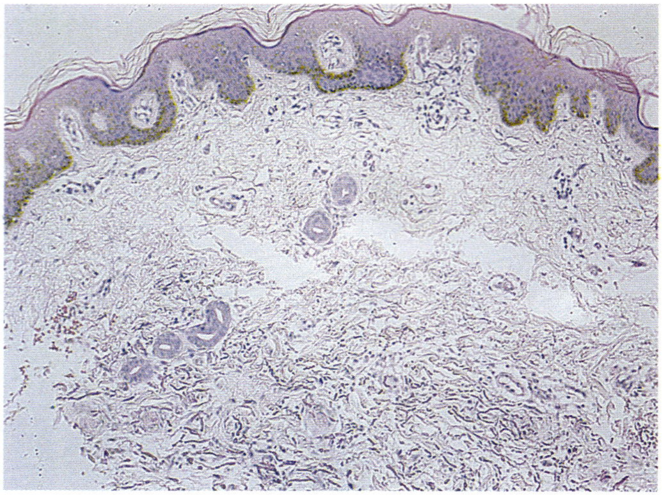

FIGURE 11.1.4.1

11.1.4: Ehler Danlos Syndrome

11.1.4.1: H & E stain shows essentially normal dermis (*Low power view*)

11.1.4.2: Orcein stain shows presence of elastic fibers (*Scanner view*)

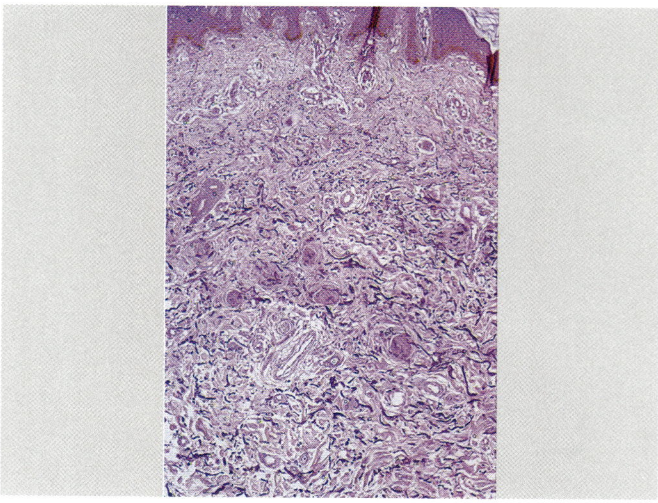

FIGURE 11.1.4.2

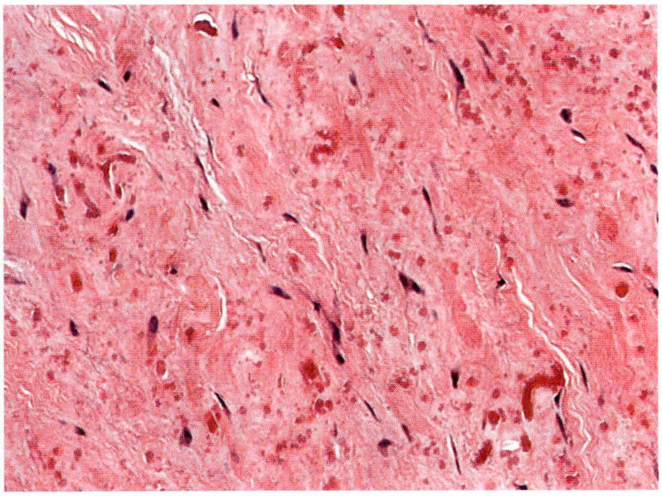

FIGURE 11.2.1.1

11.2: ELASTIN CHANGES

11.2.1: Elastofibroma

11.2.1.1: The dermal collagen is thickened and curled *(High power view)*

11.2.1.2: Dermal elastin highlighted by Verhoeff-van Gieson stain *(High power view)*

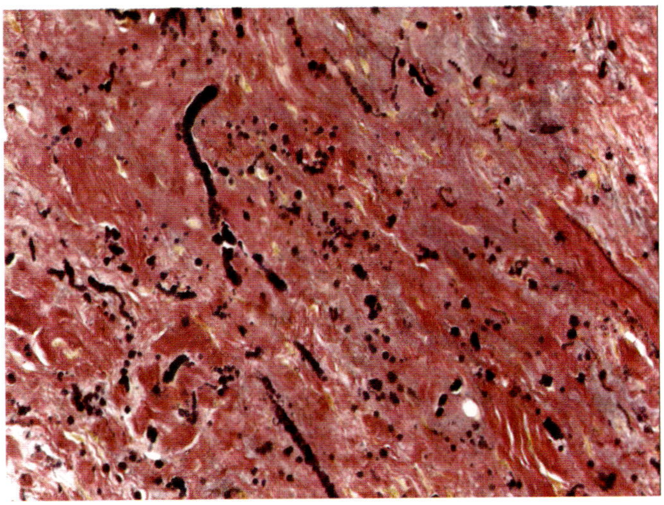

FIGURE 11.2.1.2

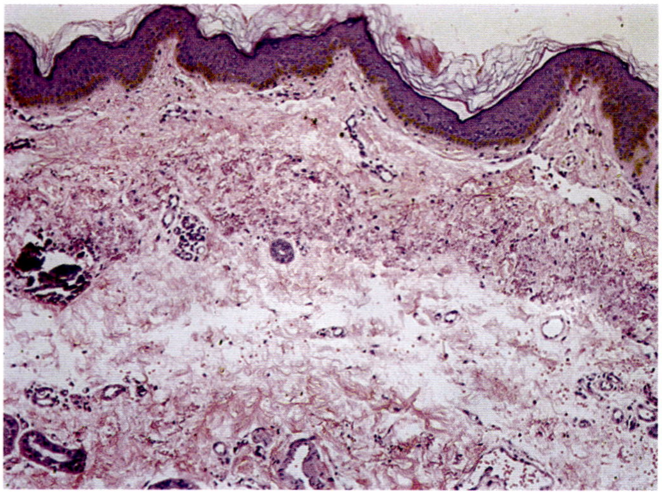

FIGURE 11.2.2.1

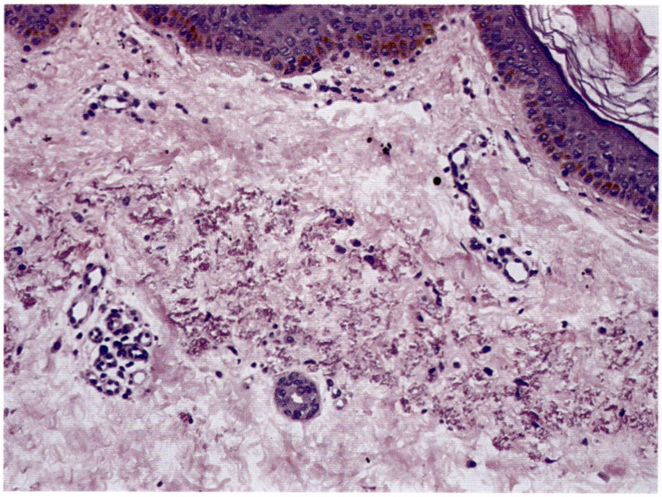

FIGURE 11.2.2.2

11.2.2: Pseudoxanthoma Elasticum

11.2.2.1: Broad band of eosinophilic degenerated elastic fibers below papillary dermis *(Scanner view)*

11.2.2.2: Closer view of the same *(Low power view)*

11.2.2.3: Orcein stain shows fragmented, thickened elastic fibers (dark brown) *(Scanner view)*

11.2.2.4: Closer view of the same *(Low power view)*

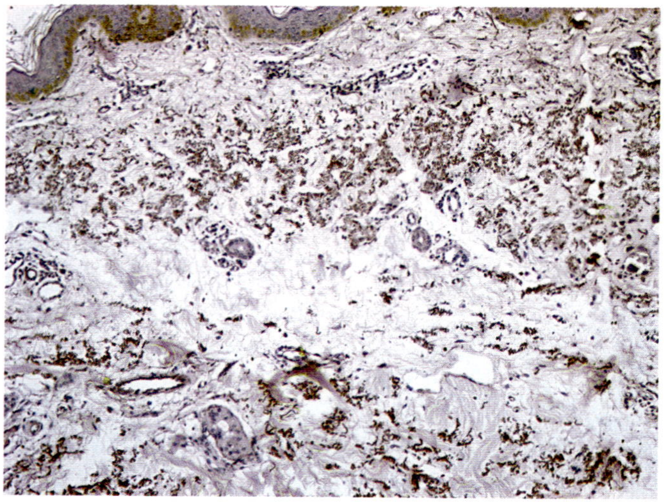

FIGURE 11.2.2.3

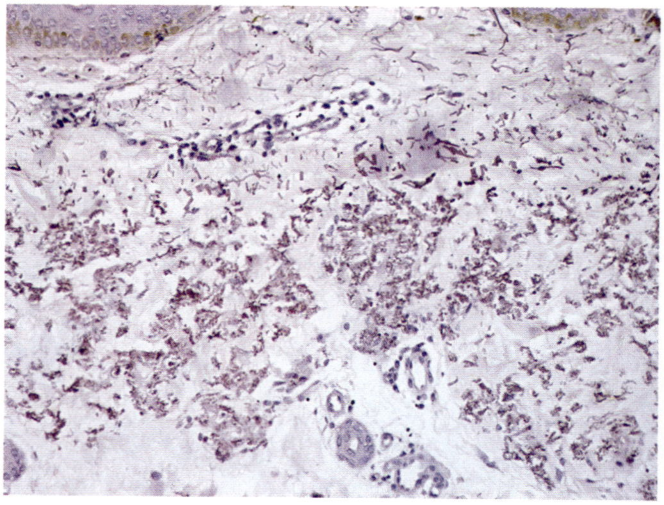

FIGURE 11.2.2.4

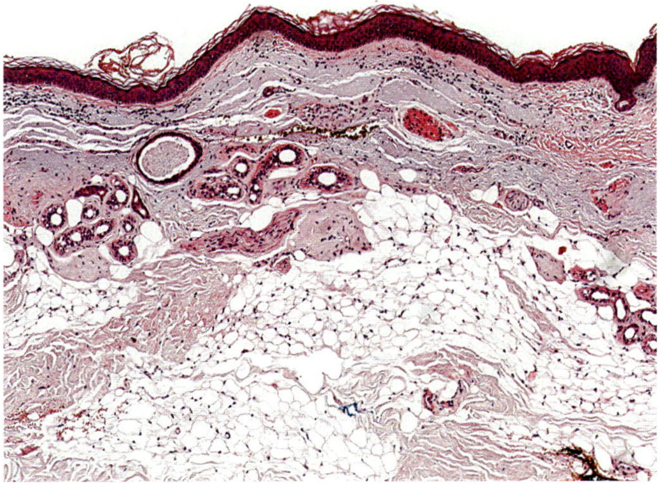

FIGURE 11.2.3.1

11.2.3: Solar Elastosis

11.2.3.1: The epidermis is flattened. The dermal collagen appears basophilic due to marked solar elastosis (with elastic tissue stain this basophilic degeneration stains like elastic tissue so referred as elastotic material)*(Scanner view)*

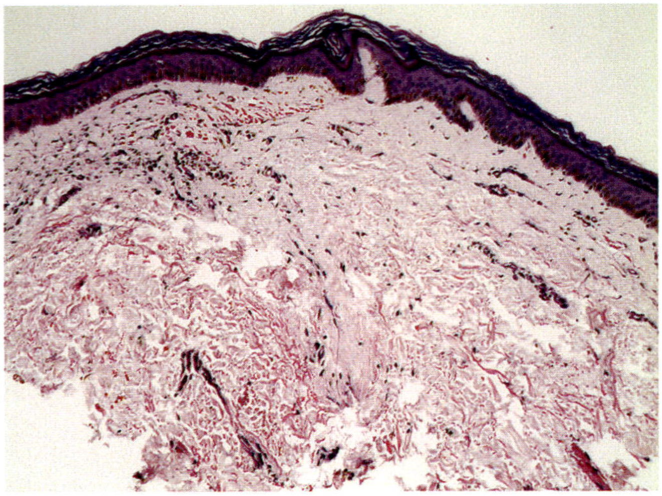

FIGURE 11.2.4.1

11.2.4: Anetoderma

11.2.4.1: Perivascular lymphocytic infiltrate *(Scanner view)*

11.2.4.2: Atrophic epidermis, elastic fibers reduced or absent (should be confirmed by elastic tissue stains) *(Low power view)*

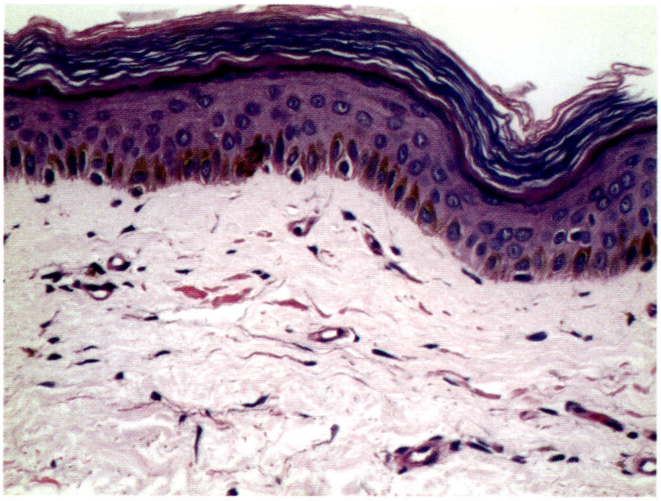

FIGURE 11.2.4.2

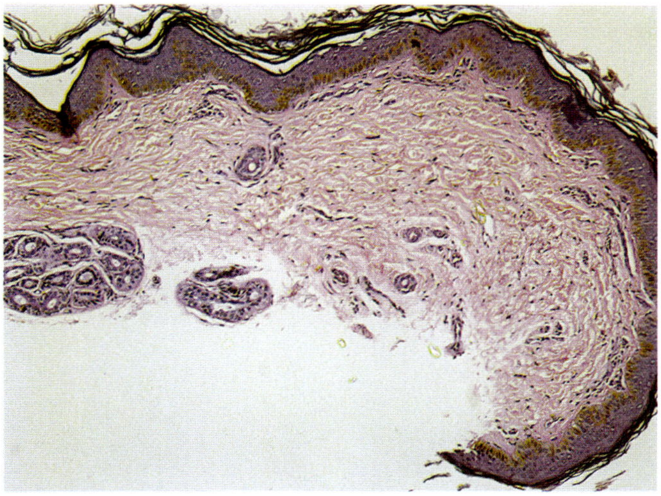

FIGURE 11.2.5.1

11.2.5: Cutis Laxa

11.2.5.1: Essentially normal skin on H & E *(Low power view)*

11.2.5.2: Elastic stain (orcein) showing absence of elastic fibers in dermis *(Low power view)*

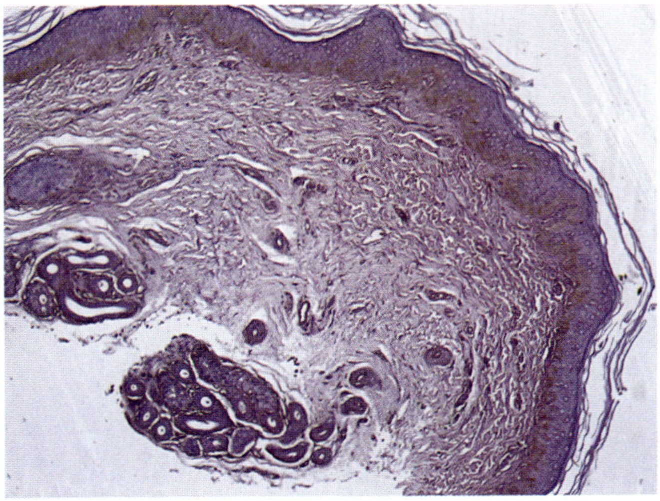

FIGURE 11.2.5.2

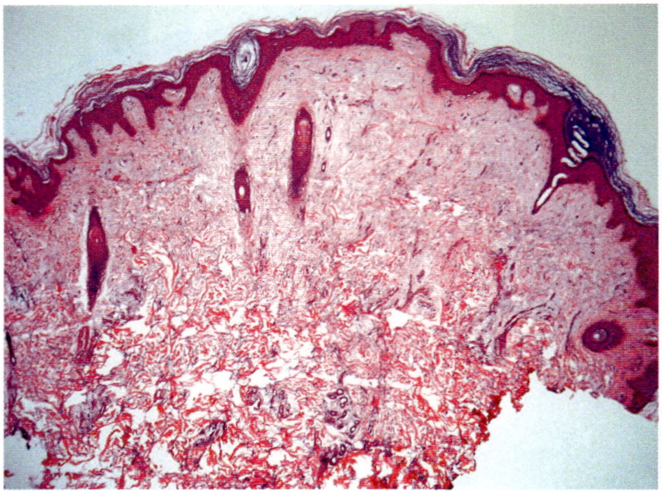

FIGURE 11.3.1.1

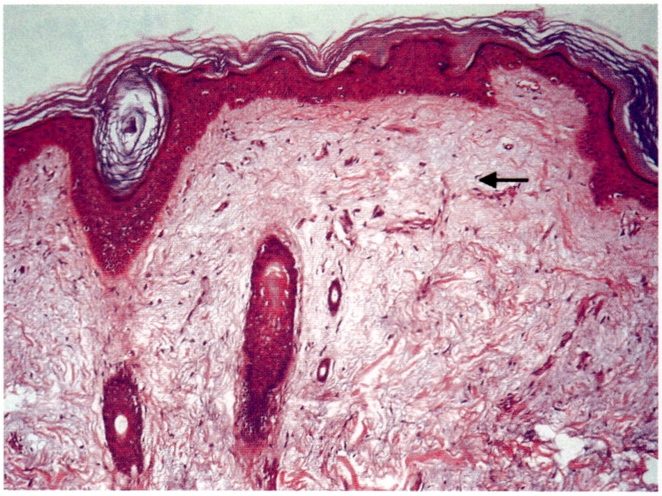

FIGURE 11.3.1.2

11.3: MUCIN DEPOSITION

11.3.1: Papular Mucinosis and Scleromyxoedema

11.3.1.1: Diffusely thick dermis, collagen bundles irregularly arranged, mucin deposits (bluish material) mainly in the upper dermis *(Scanner view)*

11.3.1.2: Closer view of mucin deposits, increased fibroblasts *(Low power view)*

11.3.1.3: Another case with thick dermis and mucin deposits in upper dermis *(Scanner view)*

11.3.1.4: Another case with unremarkable epidermis, shrinkage of mucin on routine H & E stain results in the gaps in between the collagen bundles *(Scanner view)*

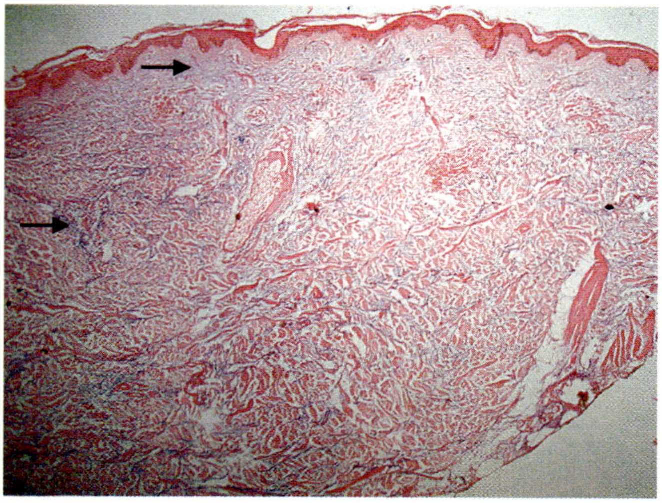

FIGURE 11.3.1.3

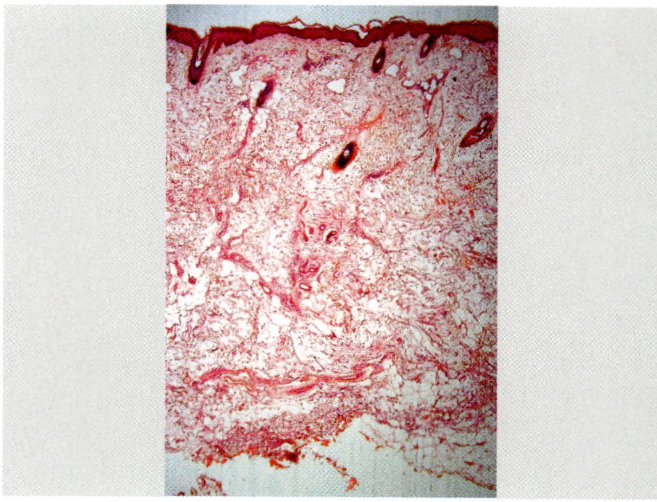

FIGURE 11.3.1.4

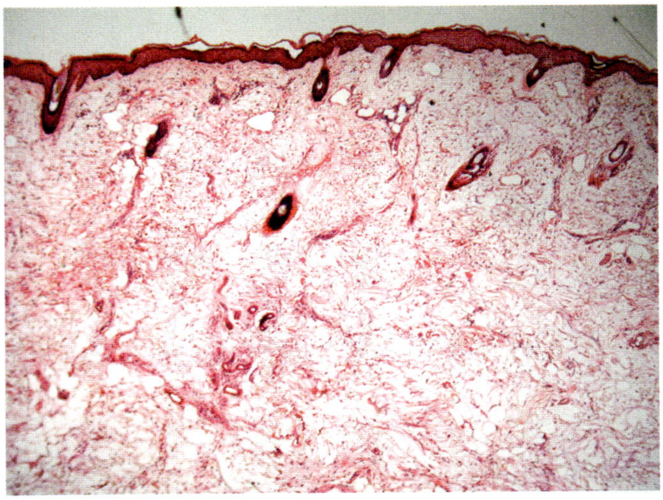

FIGURE 11.3.1.5

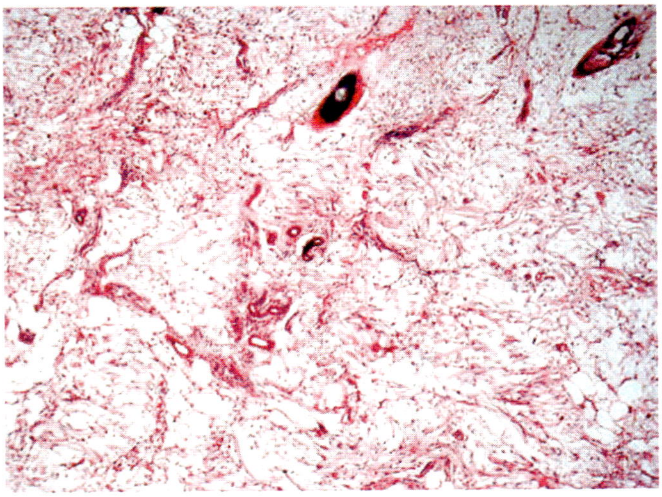

FIGURE 11.3.1.6

11.3.1.5: Thick dermis, irregular collagen bundles *(Low power view)*

11.3.1.6: Closer view showing splaying of collagen bundles due to mucin deposits *(High power view)*

11.3.1.7: Case of lichen myxedematosus with epidermal hyperplasia and thick dermis *(Scanner view)*

11.3.1.8: Mucin deposits, increased fibroblasts and irregular collagen fibers *(Low power view)*

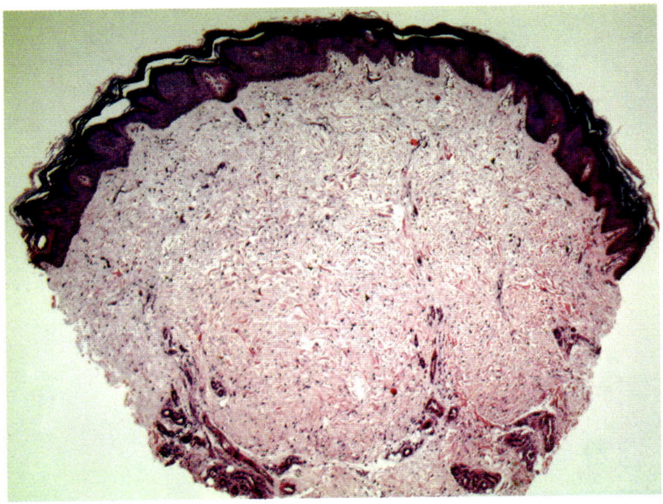

FIGURE 11.3.1.7

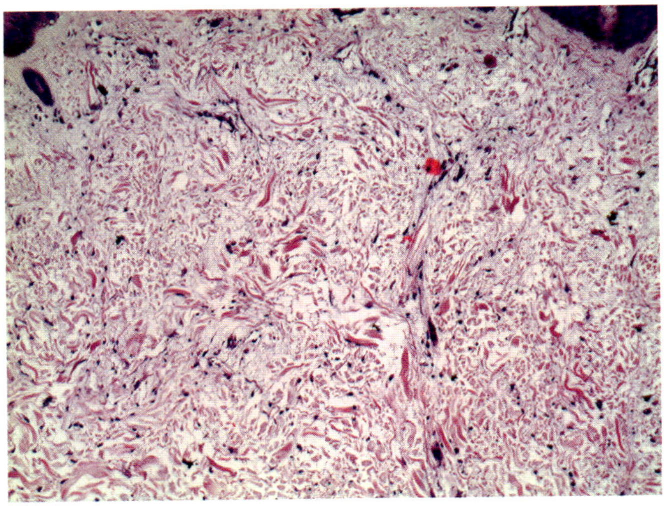

FIGURE 11.3.1.8

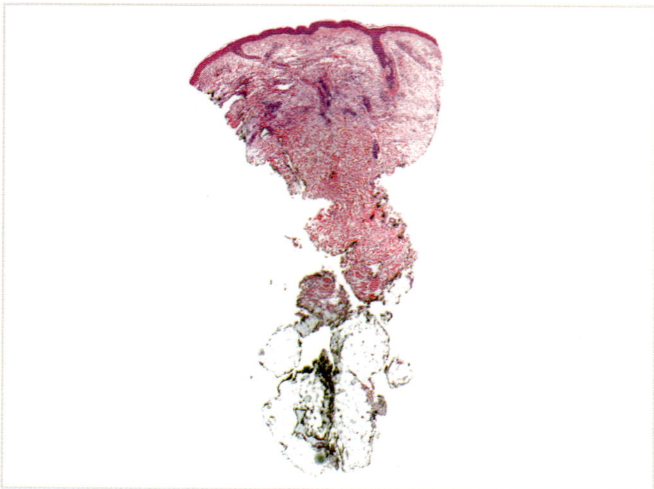

FIGURE 11.3.2.1

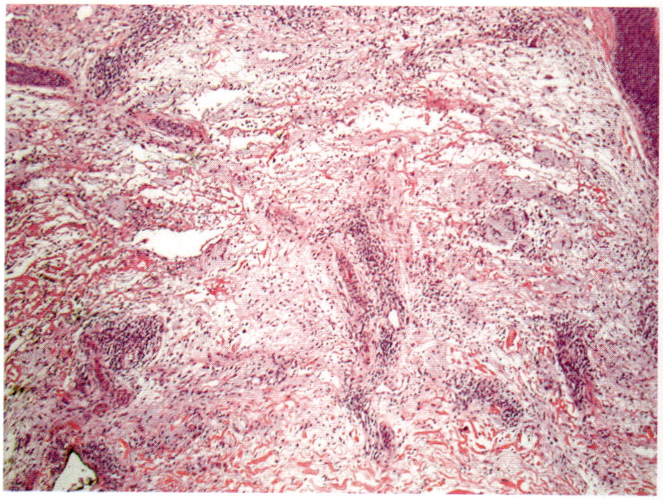

FIGURE 11.3.2.2

11.3.2: Reticulate Erythematous Mucinosis

11.3.2.1: Reticulate erythematous mucinosis shows superficial and deep perivascular lymphocytic infiltrate, epidermis unremarkable *(Scanner view)*

11.3.2.2: There is abundant dermal mucin between reticular dermal collagen fibers *(Low power view)*

11.3.2.3: Closer view of dermal infiltrate and mucin (histologic features closely mimic to those of tumid lupus erythematosus) *(High power view)*

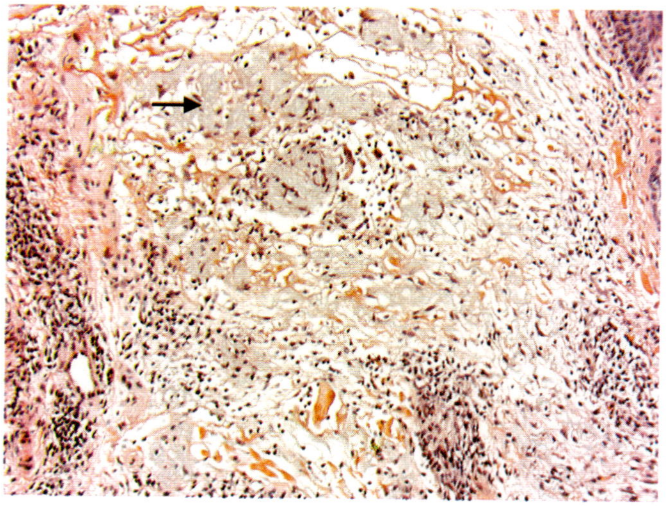

FIGURE 11.3.2.3

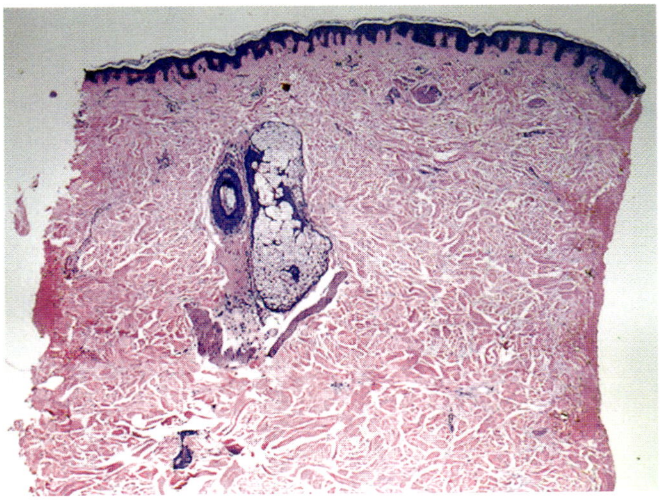

FIGURE 11.3.3.1

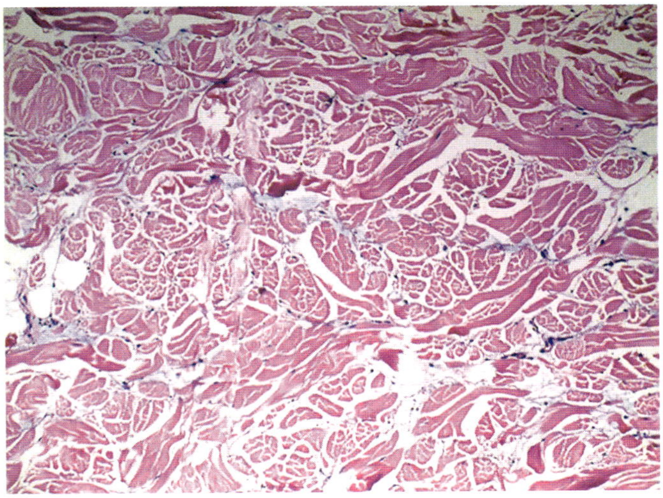

FIGURE 11.3.3.2

11.3.3: Scleredema

11.3.3.1: Unremarkable epidermis, dermis thick *(Scanner view)*

11.3.3.2: Thick collagen bundles with splaying (gaps in between) *(Low power view)*

11.3.3.3: Bluish mucin in between collagen bundles (H & E stain) *(High power view)*

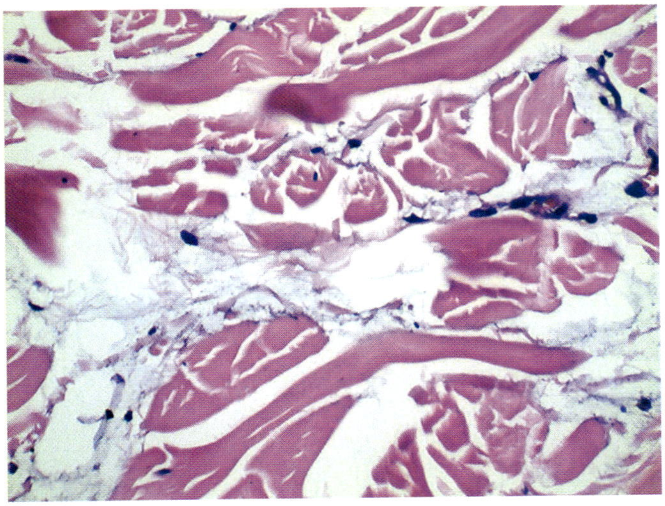

FIGURE 11.3.3.3

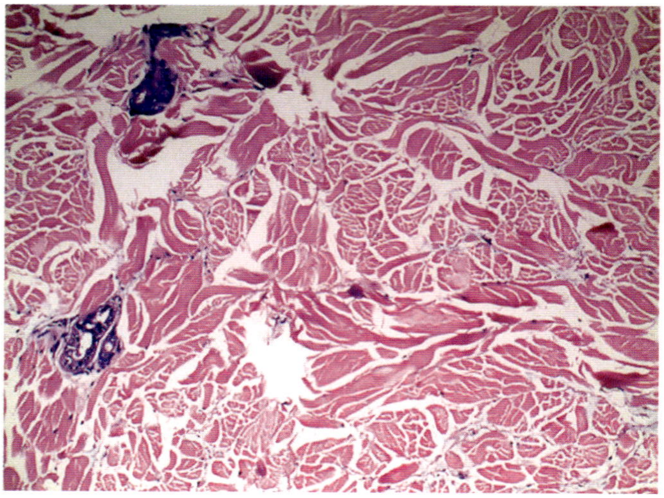

FIGURE 11.3.3.4

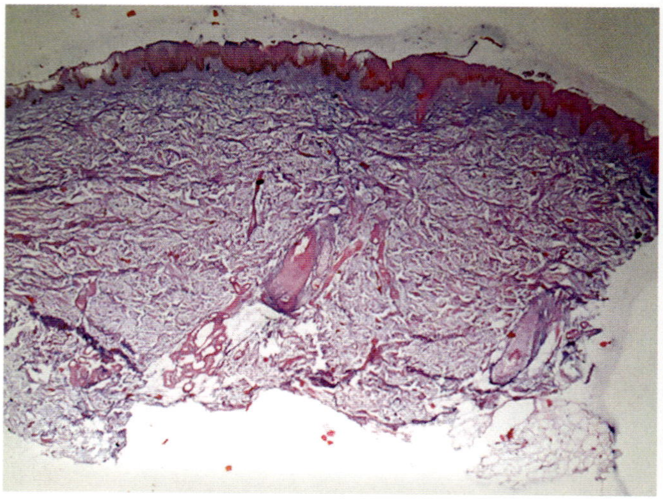

FIGURE 11.3.3.5

11.3.3.4: Adnexal structures normal, no infiltrate *(Low power view)*
11.3.3.5: Alcian blue stain highlighting mucin *(Scanner view)*
11.3.3.6: Closer view of the same *(Low power view)*

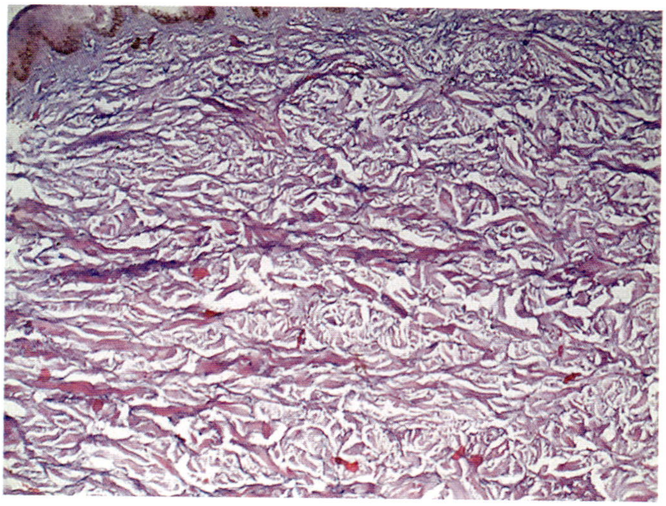

FIGURE 11.3.3.6

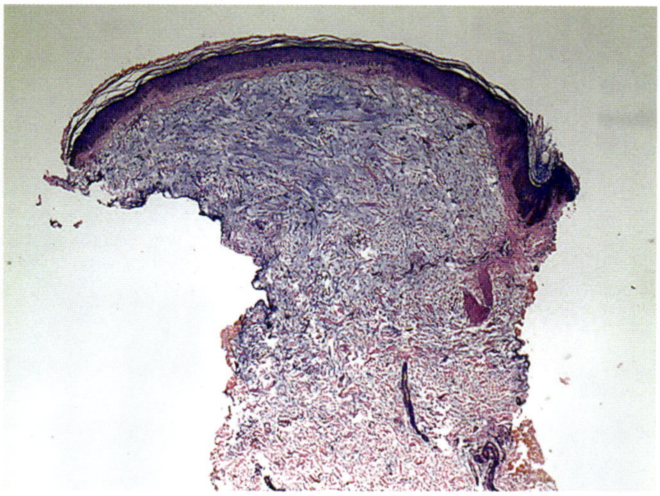

FIGURE 11.3.4.1

11.3.4: Focal Mucinosis

11.3.4.1: Dermal nodule, ill distinct margins *(Scanner view)*

11.3.4.2: Abundant mucin *(Low power view)*

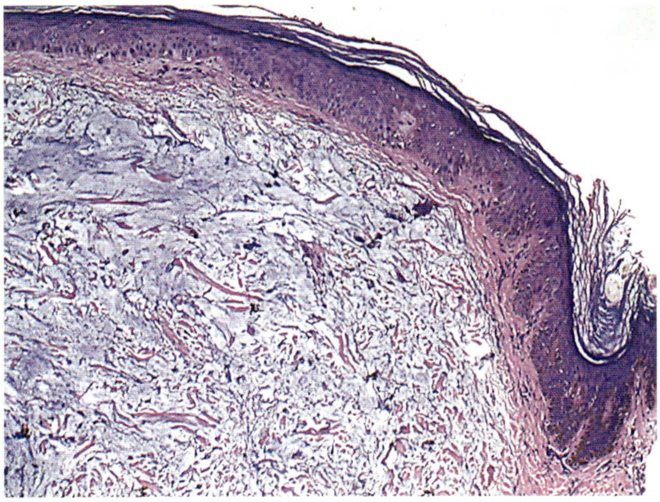

FIGURE 11.3.4.2

DIFFERENTIAL DIAGNOSIS

1. Eosinophilic fascitis
2. Atrophoderma
3. Aplasia cutis congenita
4. Lichen sclerosus
5. Sclerodermoid graft-versus-host reaction
6. Elastomas

DIAGNOSTIC PEARLS

1. Scleroderma does not exhibit sclerosis of the papillary dermis (morphea shows involvement of papillary dermis). Similarly elastic fibers are normal or increased in morphea as against scleroderma.
2. It is difficult to differentiate morphea and atrophoderma. It is preferred to include perilesional skin to compare with lesional skin.
3. Keloids are less vascular than hypertrophic scars and collagen is arranged haphazardly in keloid while in hypertrophic scar it is parallel to the epidermis.
4. Marked reduction in collagen seen in focal dermal hypoplasia is not a feature of nevus lipomatosus where collagen is normal.
5. Elastomas show thick branching elastic fibers.
6. Nephrogenic systemic fibrosis can be distinguished from scleromyxoedema by subcutaneous involvement and less mucin deposition.

Pilosebaceous Disorders and Cysts

12

Chapter Outline

12.1: Nonscarring Alopecia
12.2: Scarring Alopecias
12.3: Cysts
12.4: Acne Vulgaris

KC Nischal, Sujay Khandpur, Pradeep Mahajan, Venkataram Mysore, Nandakumar Gopinath

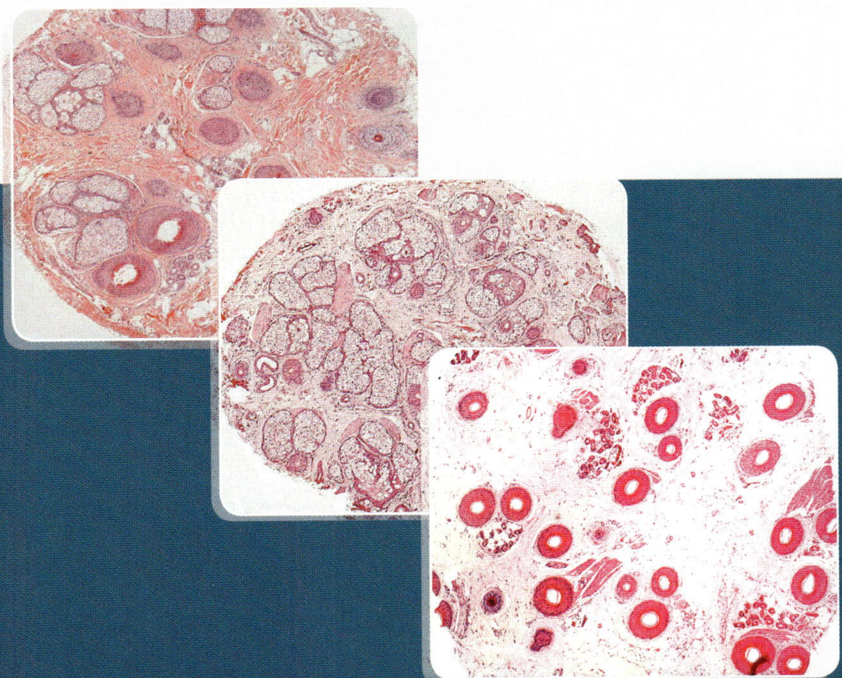

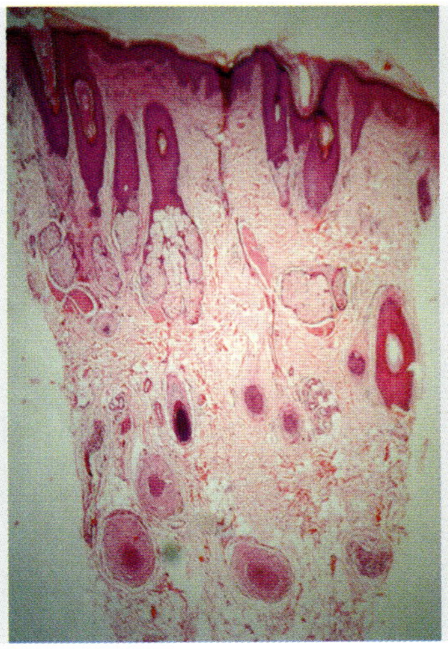

FIGURE 12.1.1.1

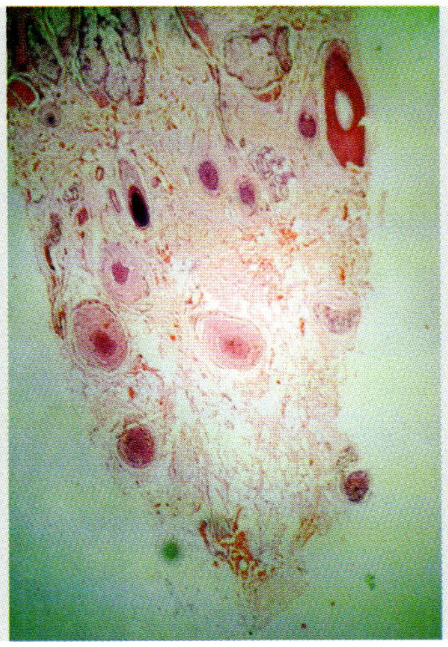

FIGURE 12.1.1.2

12.1: NONSCARRING ALOPECIA

12.1.1: Alopecia Areata

12.1.1.1: Hair follicles in late catagen and telogen (*Scanner view*)

12.1.1.2: Subcutaneous tissue shows a few anagen follicles (small miniaturized follicles in mid-dermis are seen) (*Scanner view*)

12.1.1.3: Another case showing larger anagen follicles with a peribulbar infiltrate of lymphocytes (a swarm of bees) (*Scanner view*)

12.1.1.4: *Low power view* of the same

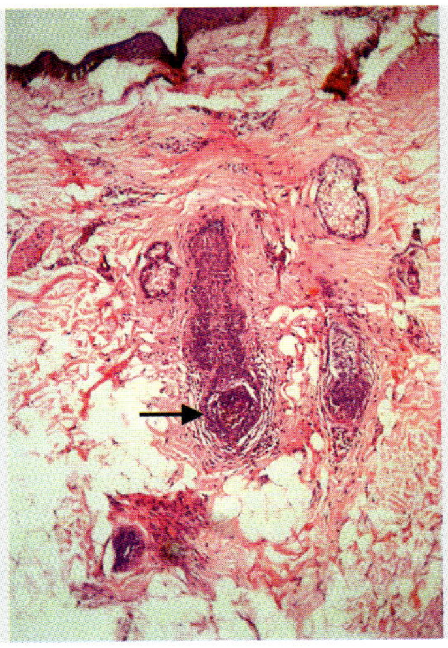

FIGURE 12.1.1.3

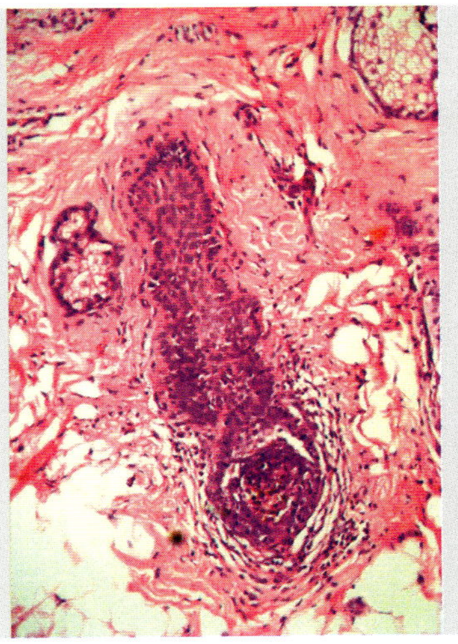

FIGURE 12.1.1.4

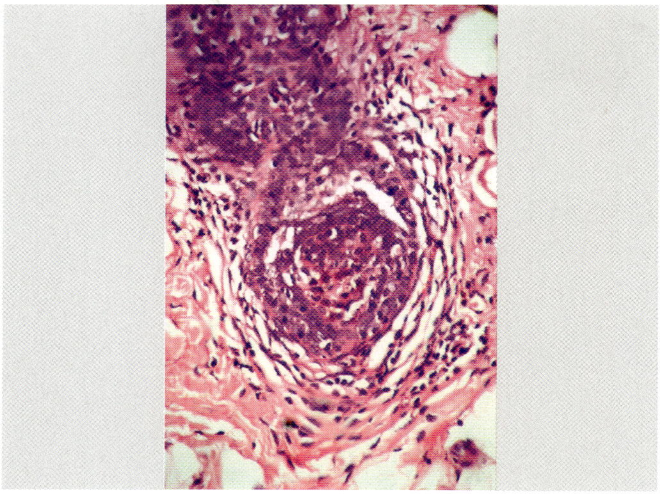

FIGURE 12.1.1.5

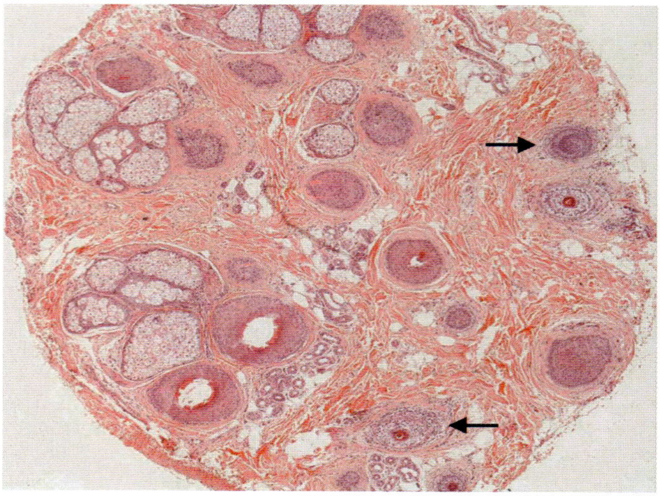

FIGURE 12.1.1.6

12.1.1.5: *High power view* of the same

12.1.1.6: Horizontal section showing peribulbar lymphocytes (*Low power view*)

12.1.1.7: Later on follicle is replaced by a collapsed fibrous root sheath and small deposits of melanin (*High power view*)

12.1.1.8: Old case showing damage to and fibrosis of follicular epithelium (*High power view*)

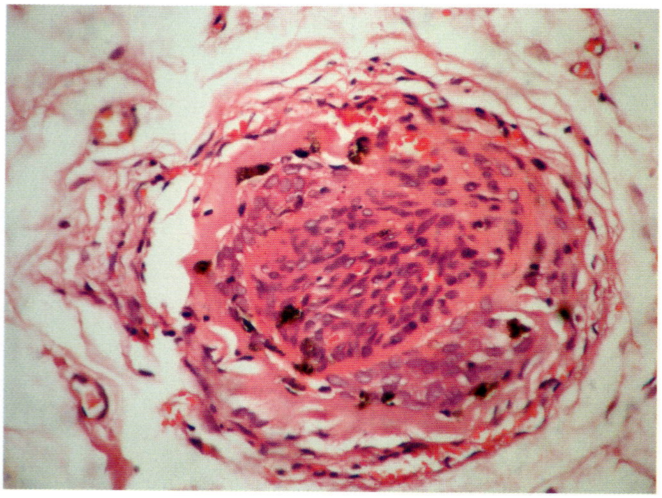

FIGURE 12.1.1.7

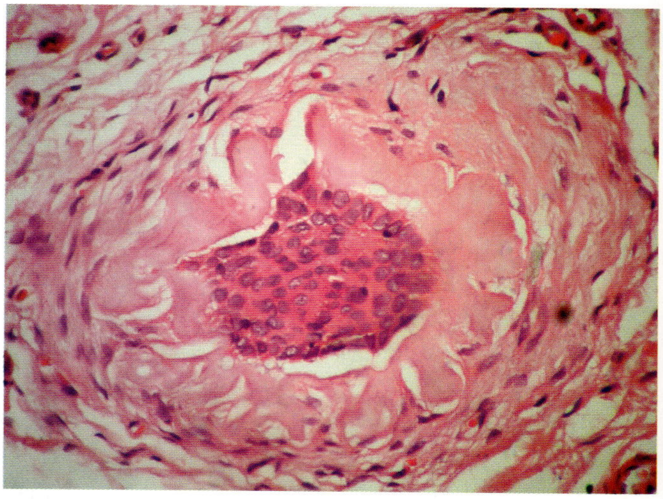

FIGURE 12.1.1.8

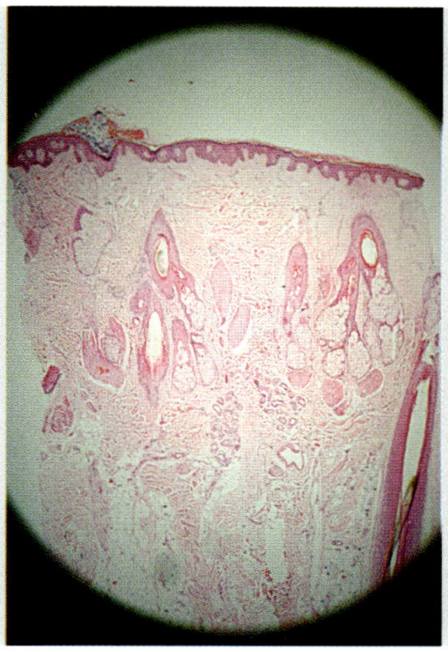

FIGURE 12.1.2.1

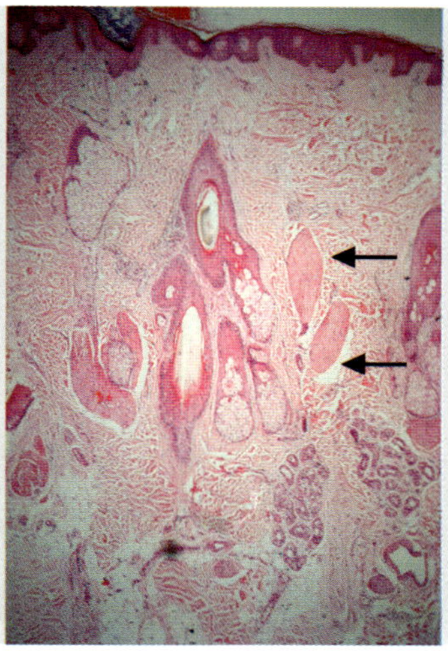

FIGURE 12.1.2.2

12.1.2: Androgenetic Alopecia

12.1.2.1: Degeneration of the connective tissue sheath of the lower one-third of anagen follicles and formation of miniaturized hair (terminal follicles become smaller and regress to vellus hair) (*Scanner view*)

12.1.2.2: Thick arrectores pilorum, increase in the number of telogen and catagen hairs relative to the number of anagen hairs (most of the follicles lie in the mid-dermis) (*Low power view*)

12.1.2.3: Thin fibrous strands replacing follicles and fibroplasia of the perifollicular sheath (*Scanner view*)

12.1.2.4: Horizontal section showing miniaturized hair, arrectores pilorum muscle, increased sebaceous gland structures and minimum inflammation (*Scanner view*)

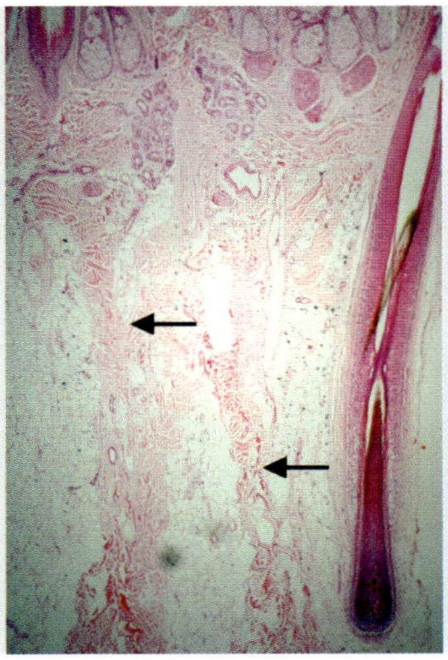

FIGURE 12.1.2.3

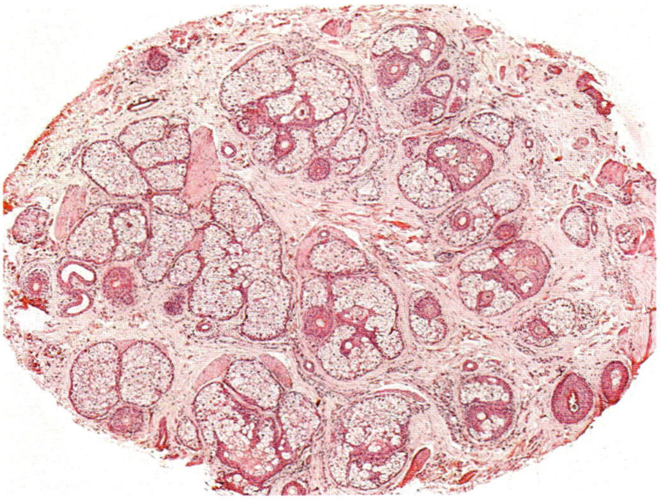

FIGURE 12.1.2.4

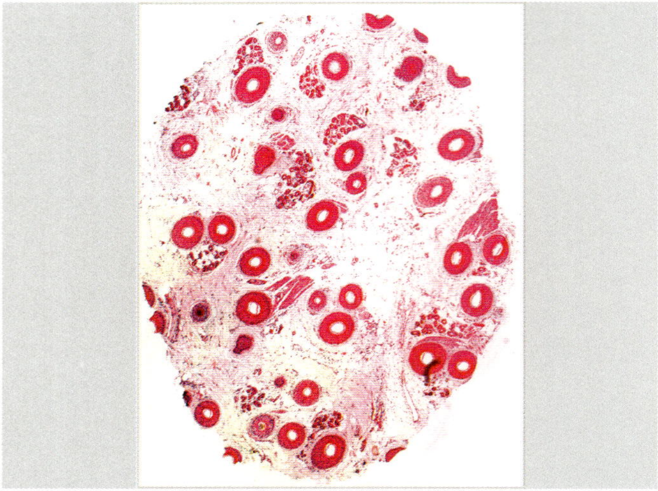

FIGURE 12.1.3.1

12.1.3: Telogen Effluvium

12.1.3.1: Horizontal sections of a scalp punch biopsy show a relatively normal number of follicles with an increase in the ratio of telogen to anagen follicles. There is no significant inflammation or fibrosis/scarring (*Scanner view*) (*Courtesy:* Nathan Lee and Jerad Gardner)

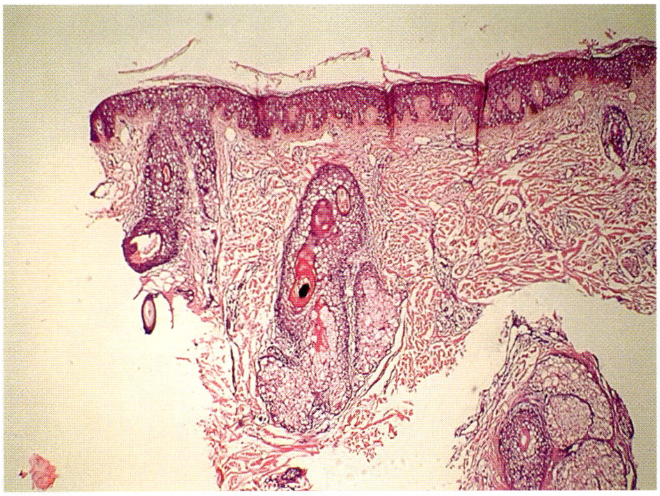

FIGURE 12.1.4.1

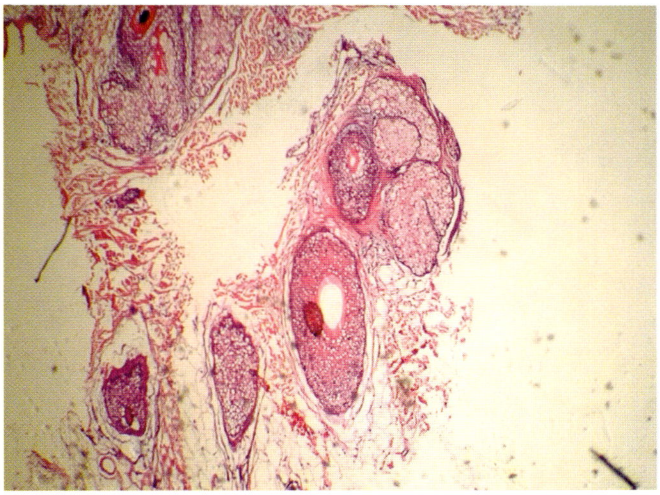

FIGURE 12.1.4.2

12.1.4: Trichotillomania

12.1.4.1: Damage to hair follicle, broken shaft, sparse inflammation (*Scanner view*)

12.1.4.2: Rupture of hair follicles, with clefts around hair follicles, hemorrhage and increased telogen hairs (*Low power view*)

12.1.4.3: Another case with distorted follicle (*scanner view*)—*Image contributed by Smita Ghate*

12.1.4.4: Melanin pigment casts referred as trichomalacia (*Low power view*)—*Image contributed by Smita Ghate*

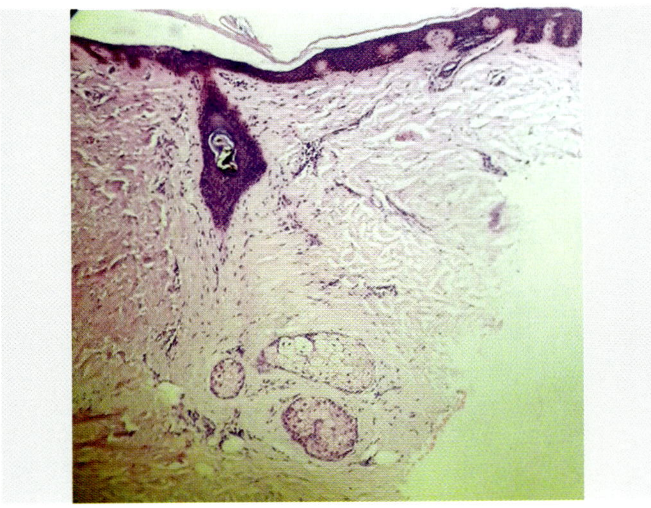

FIGURE 12.1.4.3

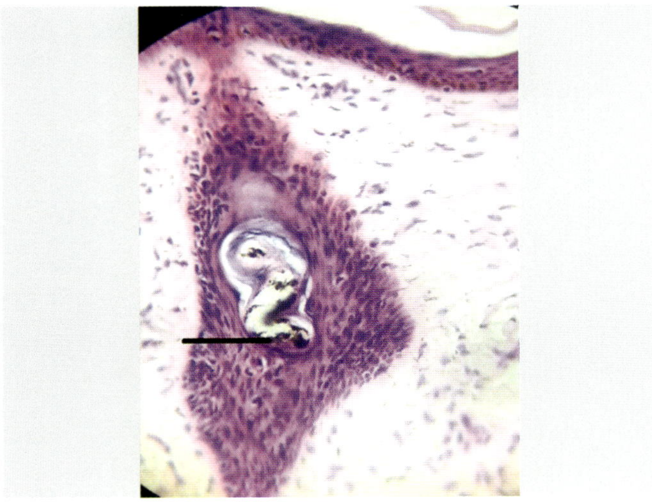

FIGURE 12.1.4.4

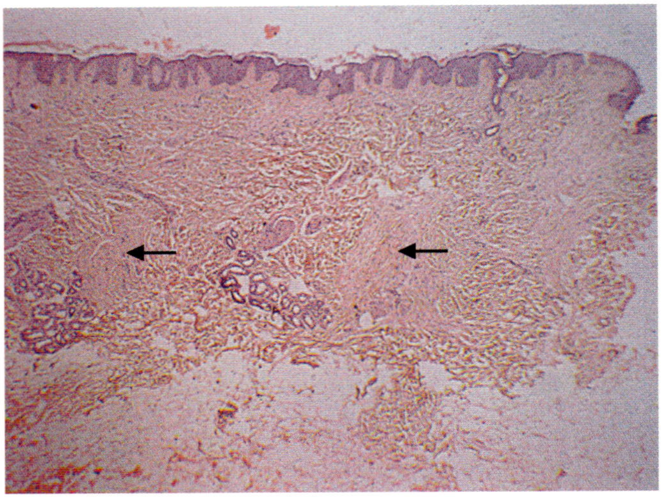

FIGURE 12.2.1.1

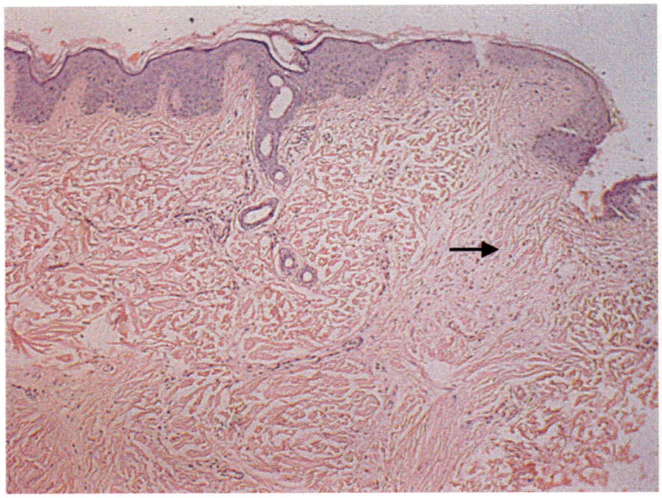

FIGURE 12.2.1.2

12.2: SCARRING ALOPECIAS

12.2.2: Pseudopelade

12.2.1.1: Late lesion showing absence of hair follicles with fibrous tracts replacing them. Note the absence of lymphocytic infiltrate at the dermoepidermal junction and basal cell degeneration (*Scanner view*)

12.2.1.2: Closer view showing fibrous tract replacing follicle (*Low power view*)

12.2.1.3: Infiltrate of lymphocytes around the upper part of damaged follicle still evident (*Low power view*)

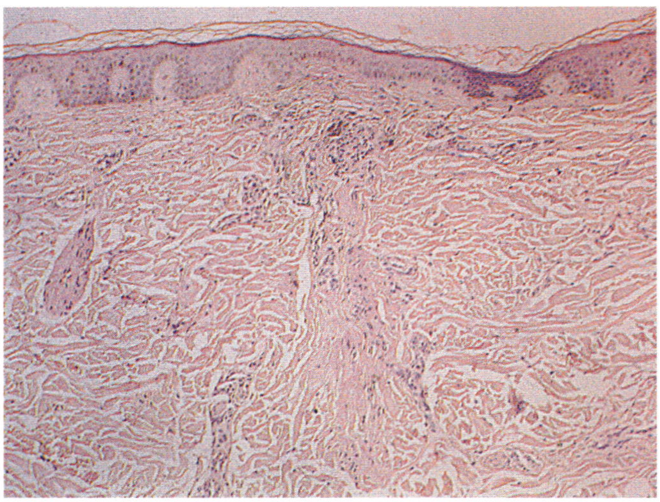

FIGURE 12.2.1.3

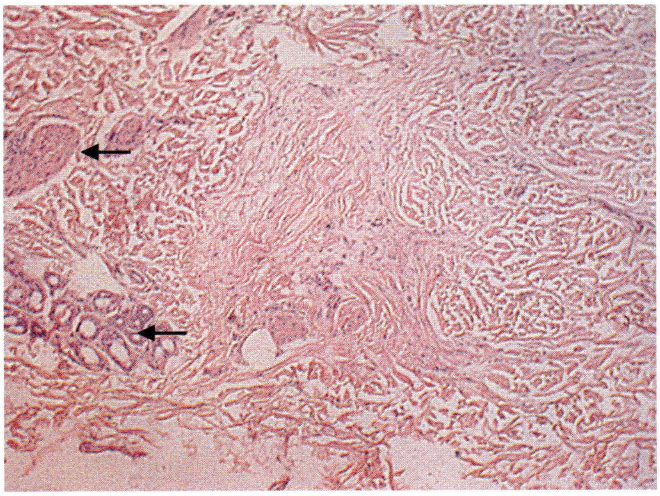

FIGURE 12.2.1.4

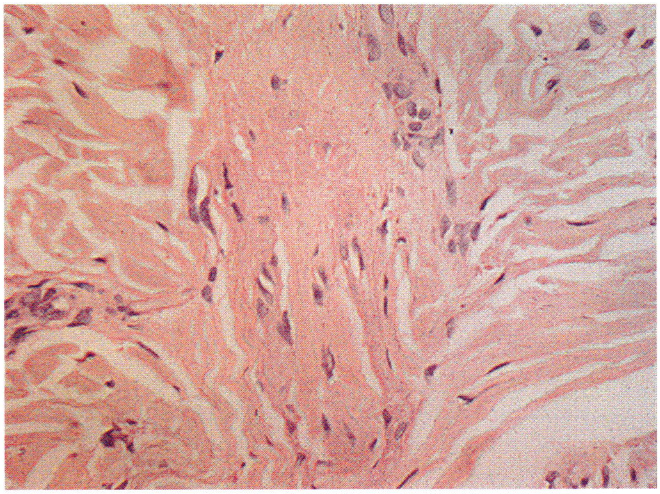

FIGURE 12.2.1.5

12.2.1.4: Loss of hair follicles and sebaceous glands, replaced by bands of fibrous tissue remnants of hair shaft, arrectores pilorum and sweat glands are seen even after destruction of hair, providing an important clue (*High power view*)

12.2.1.5: Closer view of vertical fibrous tract (*High power view*)

12.2.1.6: Horizontal section of scalp biopsy showing perifollicular fibrosis with lymphocytic infiltrate and pigment incontinence (suggests evolution from lichen planopilaris to pseudopelade). There is paucity of hair follicles—cicatricial alopecia (*Low power view*)

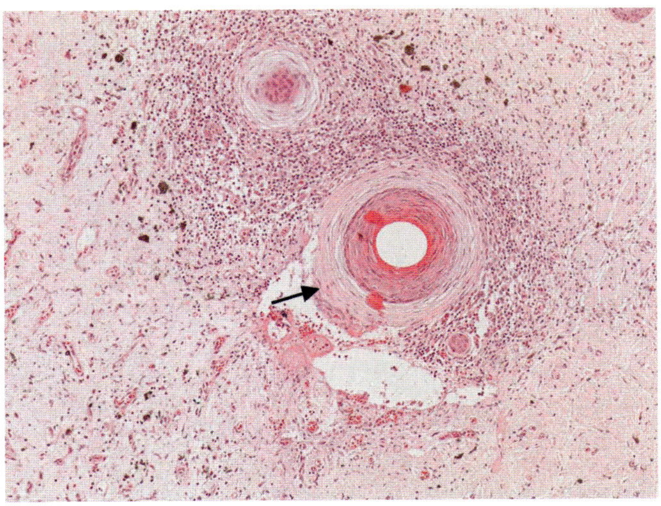

FIGURE 12.2.1.6

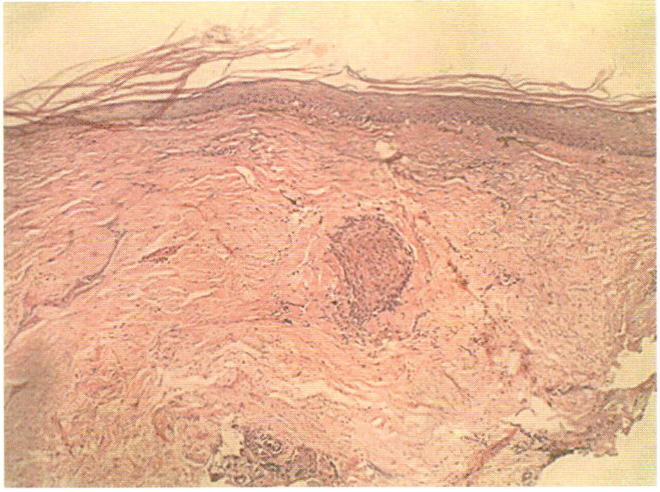

FIGURE 12.2.2.1

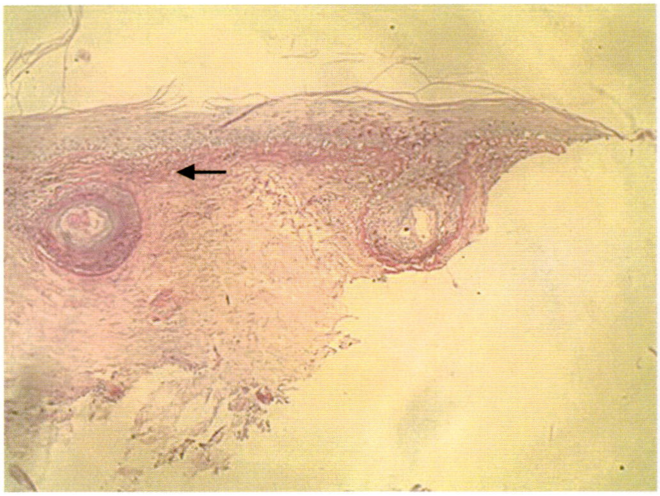

FIGURE 12.2.2.2

12.2.2: Scarring Alopecia Secondary to Discoid Lupus Erythematosus

12.2.2.1: Epidermal changes include hyperkeratosis and some atrophy of the malpighian layer and focal basal call vacuolation (*Scanner view*)

12.2.2.2: Keratotic follicular plugging and thickening of the basement membrane, seen with a periodic acid-Schiff (PAS) stain (*Scanner view*)

12.2.2.3: Closer view of thick basement membrane (PAS stain) (*High power view*)

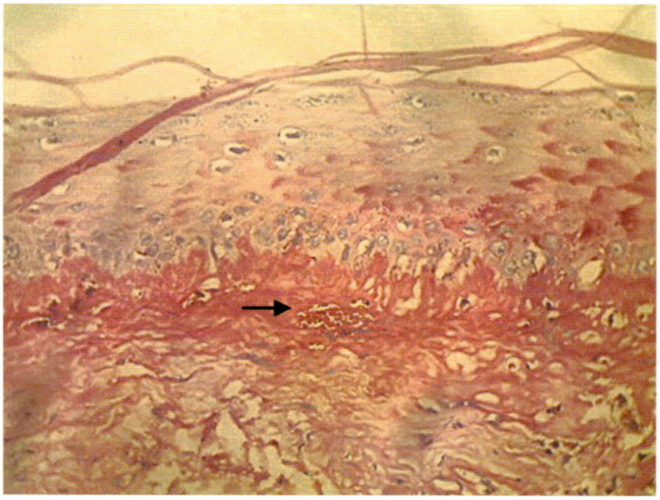

FIGURE 12.2.2.3

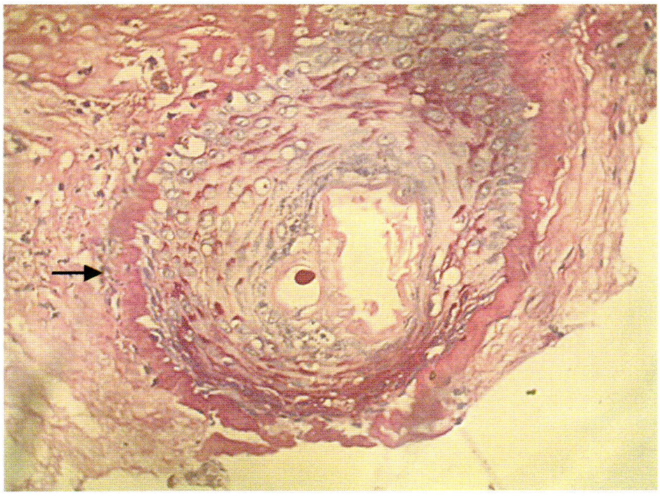

FIGURE 12.2.2.4

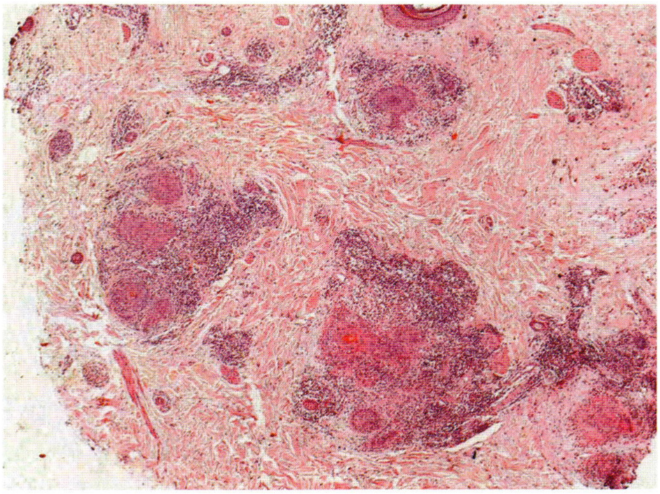

FIGURE 12.2.2.5

12.2.2.4: View of PAS positive thick basement membrane around the follicle (*High power view*)

12.2.2.5: Horizontal section showing infiltrate of inflammatory cells which have a tendency to accumulate around the pilosebaceous follicles. There is considerable reduction in the size of sebaceous glands (*Scanner view*)

12.2.2.6: Section shows significant follicular plugging, atrophic epidermis, vacuolar basal cell degeneration, inflammation and significant basement membrane thickening in discoid lupus erythematosus (*Low power view*)

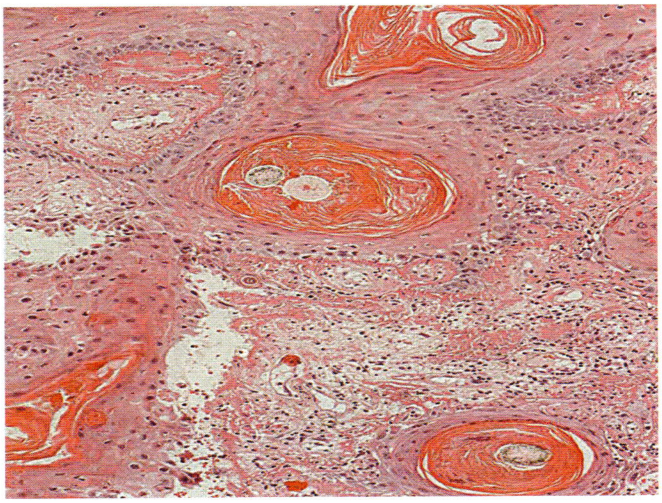

FIGURE 12.2.2.6

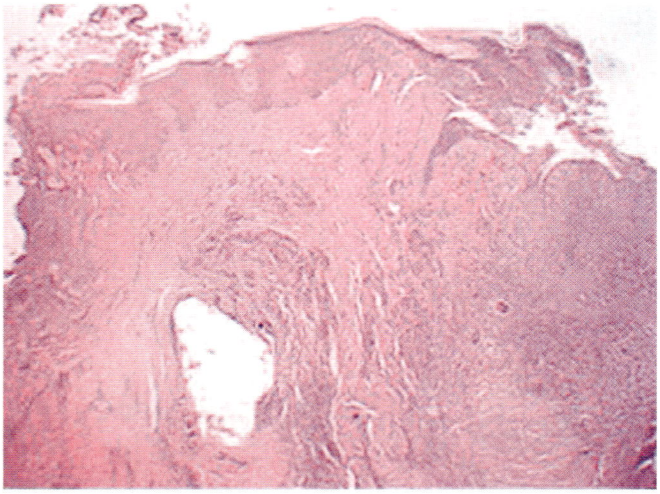

FIGURE 12.2.3.1

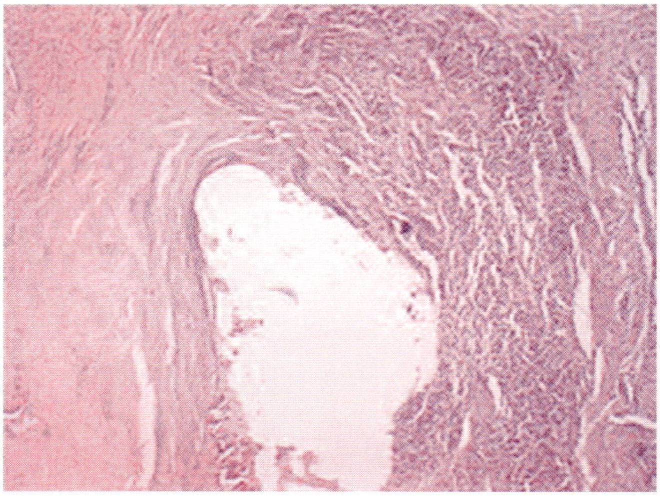

FIGURE 12.2.3.2

12.2.3: Folliculitis Decalvans

12.2.3.1: Perifollicular inflammation, disruption of the follicular wall (*Scanner view*)

12.2.3.2: Closer view of disrupted follicle and inflammation (*Low power view*)

12.2.3.3: Surrounding dermis has a mixed inflammatory cell infiltrate (*Low power view*)

12.2.3.4: Lymphocytes, plasma cells and giant cells with variable scarring (*High power view*)

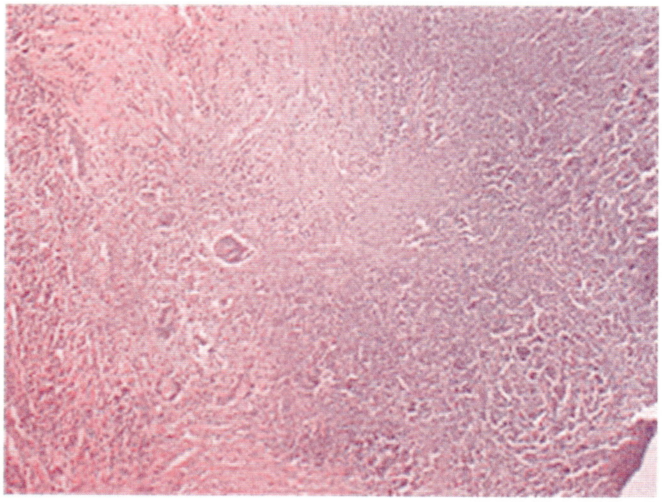

FIGURE 12.2.3.3

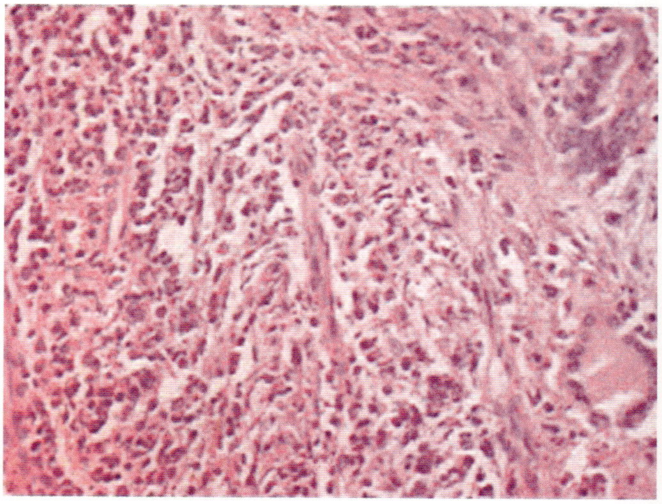

FIGURE 12.2.3.4

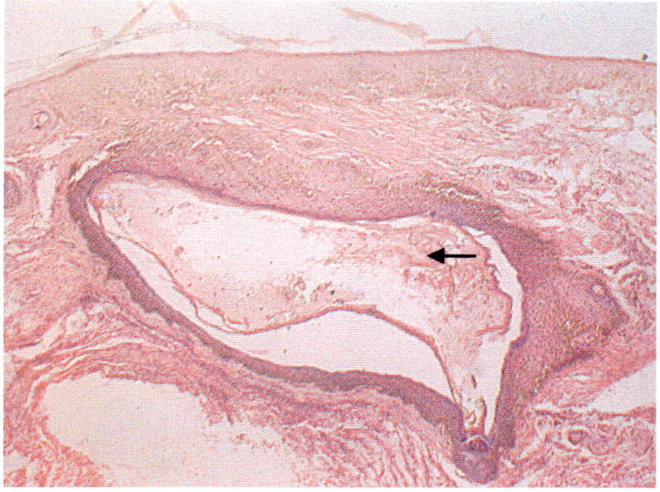

FIGURE 12.3.1.1

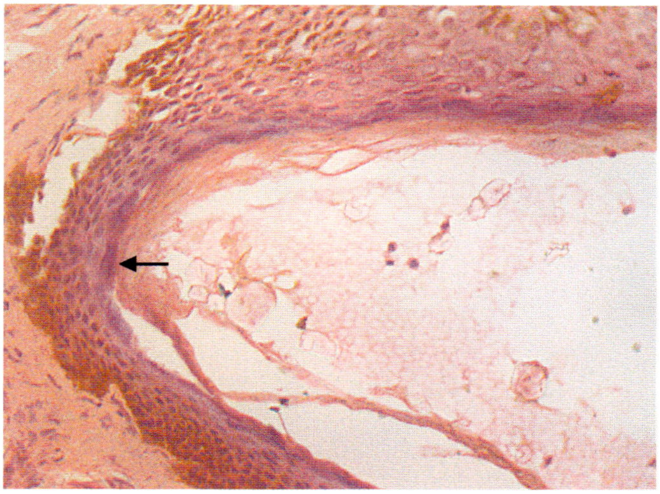

FIGURE 12.3.1.2

12.3: CYSTS

12.3.1: Epidermal Cyst (Infundibular Cyst)

12.3.1.1: Dermis shows a cyst lined by stratified squamous epithelium (*Scanner view*)

12.3.1.2: Cyst wall has all the layers of epidermis including granular cell layer (infundibular type of keratinization) (*Low power view*)

12.3.1.3: Another view of cyst wall with layers of epidermis including stratum granulosum and keratin in the cavity (*High power view*)

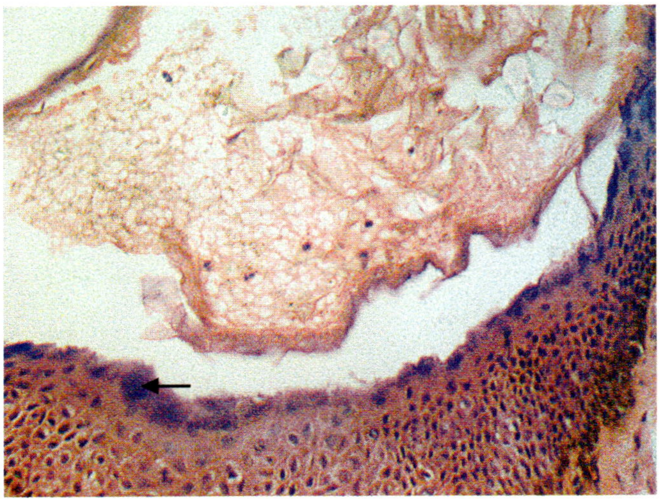

FIGURE 12.3.1.3

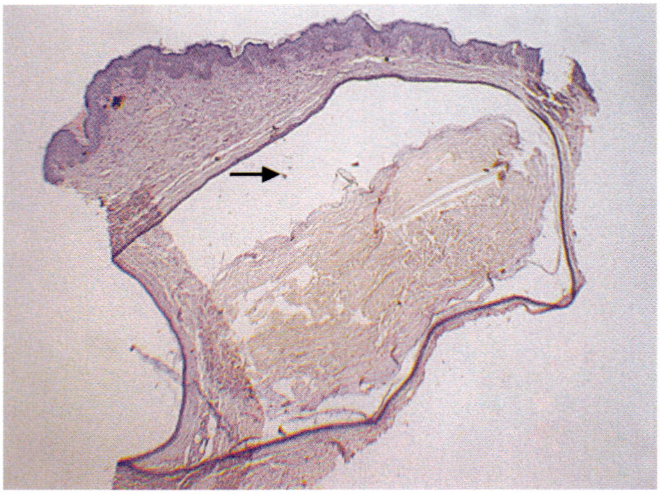

FIGURE 12.3.2.1

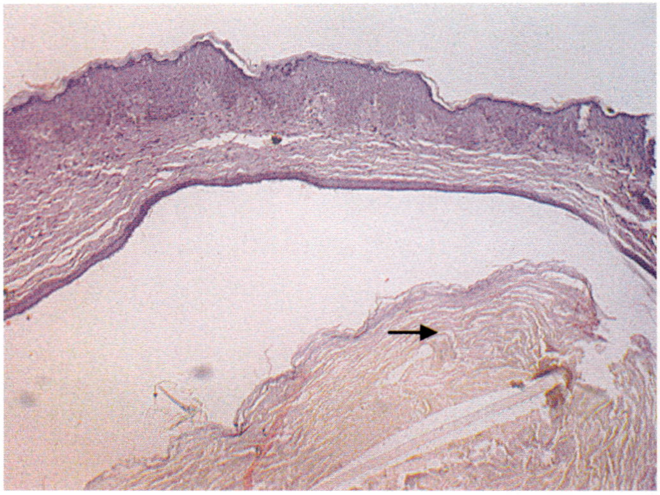

FIGURE 12.3.2.2

12.3.2: Trichilemmal (Sebaceous, Isthmus-Catagen, Pilar) Cyst

12.3.2.1: Dermis shows a cyst lined by stratified squamous epithelium (*Scanner view*)

12.3.2.2: Cavity contains keratin (*Low power view*)

12.3.2.3: Abrupt keratinization (lower part of section shows keratin) without the formation of keratohyaline granules (trichilemmal keratinization) (*High power view*)

12.3.2.4: Another view of cyst wall showing trichilemmal keratinization (lower part of section shows keratin) (Cholesterol clefts or calcification may be seen in the cavity) (*High power view*)

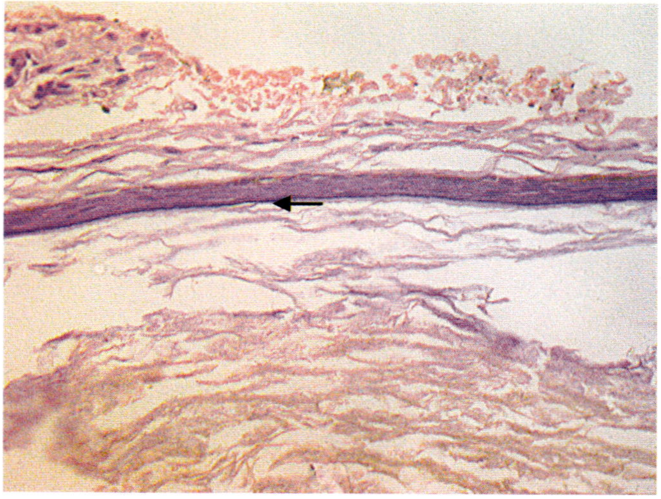

FIGURE 12.3.2.3

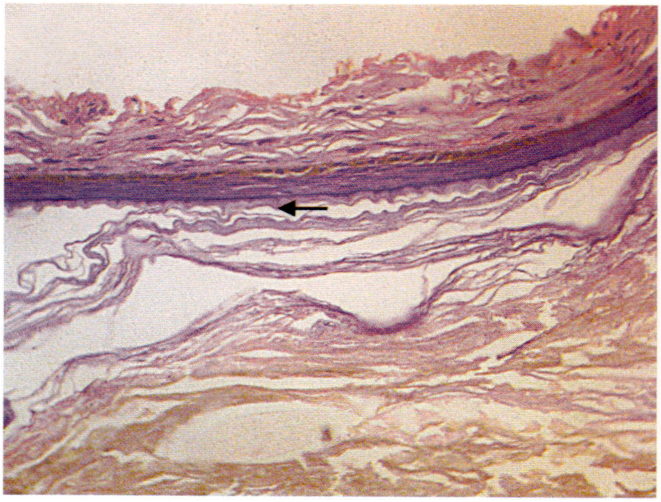

FIGURE 12.3.2.4

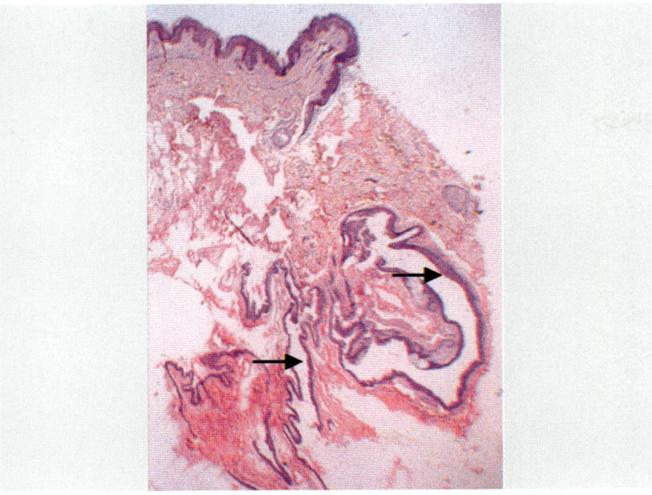

FIGURE 12.3.3.1

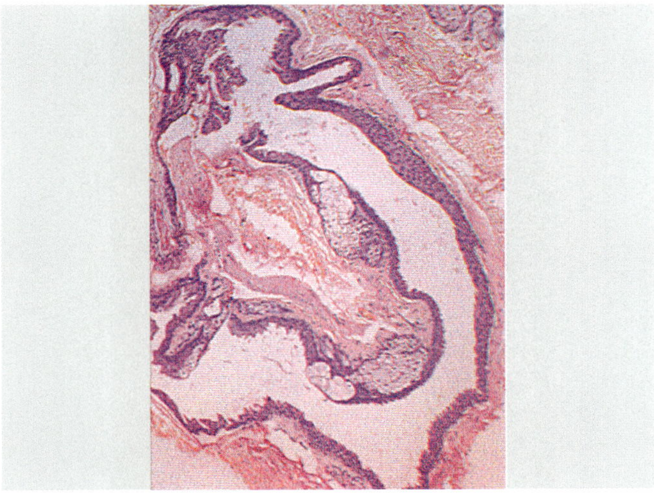

FIGURE 12.3.3.2

12.3.3: Steatocystoma Multiplex

12.3.3.1: Dermal cysts with wavy lining due to rupture of the cyst during processing (*Scanner view*)

12.3.3.2: Cyst wall composed of stratified squamous epithelium with 2–3 layers and without granular cell layer. Sometimes smooth muscle also seen in the wall (*Low power view*)

12.3.3.3: Sebaceous glands of varying size in the cyst wall, a typical feature (*High power view*)

12.3.3.4: Another view of sebaceous glands in the wall with red blood cells and keratin in the cyst cavity (*High power view*)

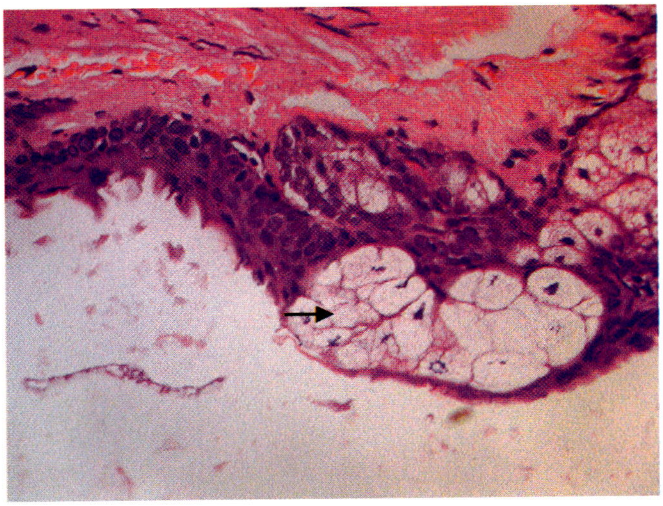

FIGURE 12.3.3.3

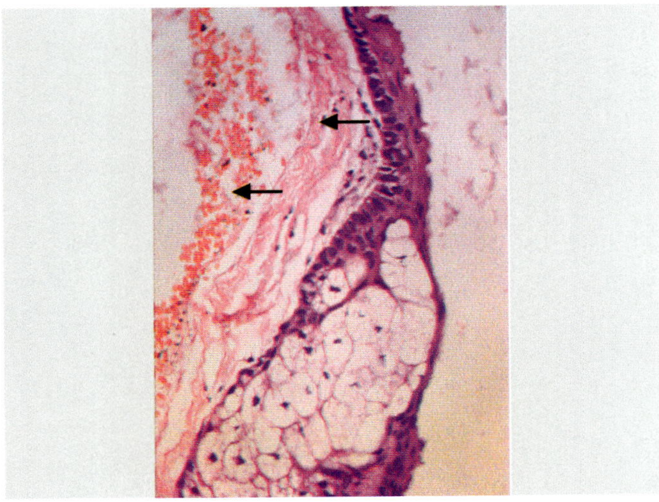

FIGURE 12.3.3.4

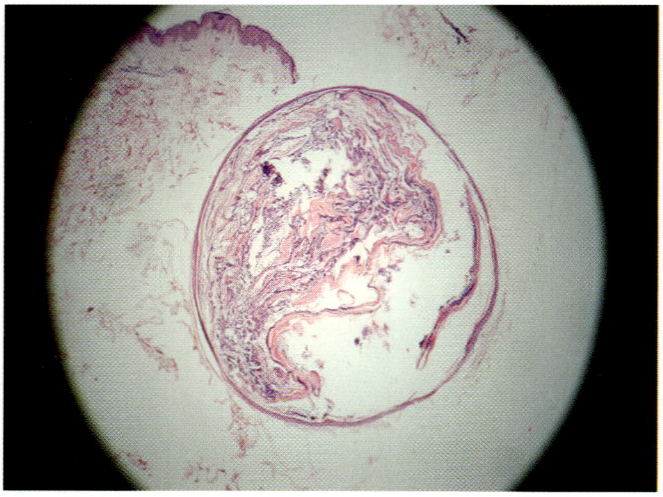

FIGURE 12.3.4.1

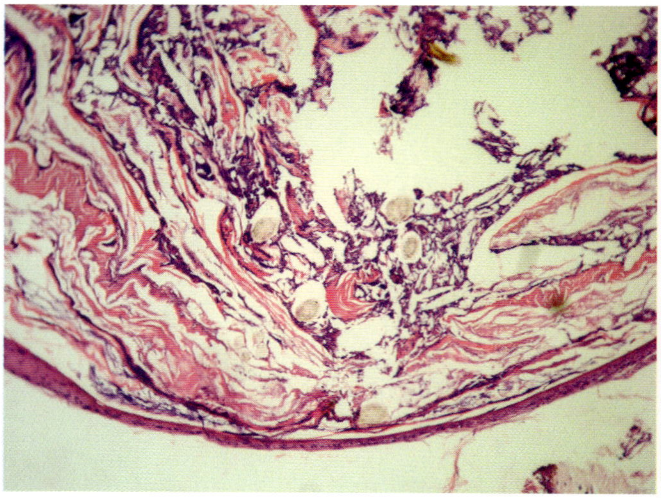

FIGURE 12.3.4.2

12.3.4: Vellus Hair Cyst

12.3.4.1: Dermal cyst lined by thin stratified squamous epithelium and containing keratin (*Scanner view*)

12.3.4.2: Cyst wall shows trichilemmal keratinization (*Low power view*)

12.3.4.3: The cavity contains keratin and many small vellus hair shafts seen with H & E stain (under polarized light shafts are doubly refractile) (*High power view*)

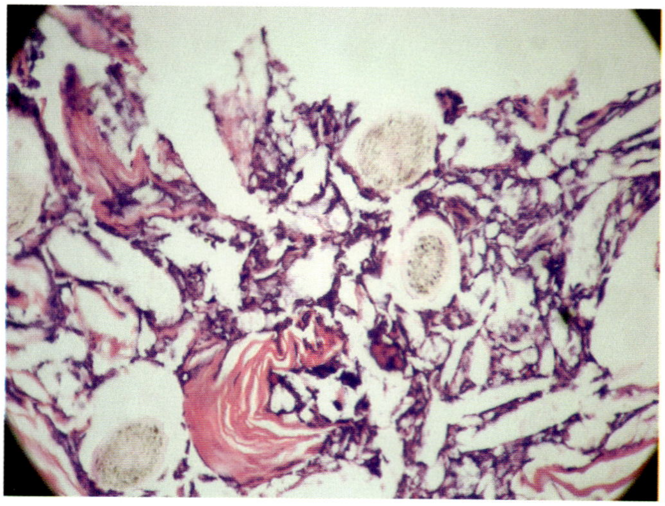

FIGURE 12.3.4.3

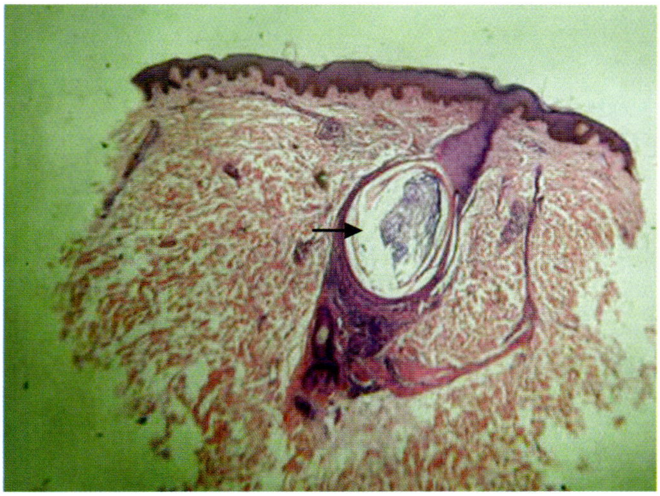

FIGURE 12.4.1

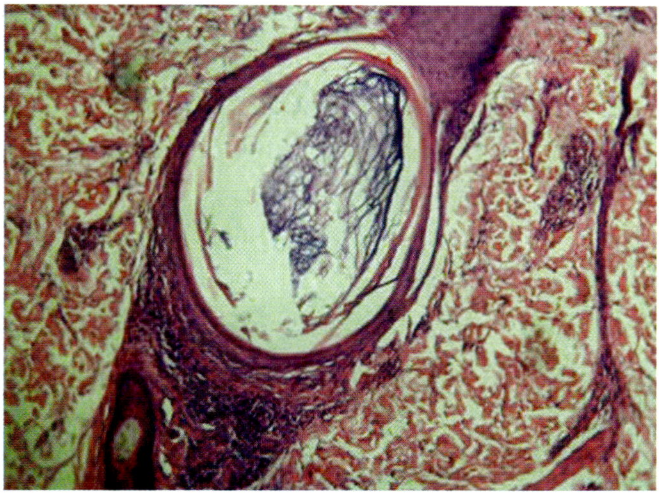

FIGURE 12.4.2

12.4: ACNE VULGARIS

12.4.1: Follicular plugging with perifollicular infiltrate—a comedone (*Scanner view*)

12.4.2: Close view of keratin plug (cyst formation) and focus of inflammatory infiltrate (*Low power view*)

12.4.3: Inflammatory lesions show accumulation of neutrophils and subsequent rupture of the follicle (*Scanner view*)

12.4.4: Another case with follicular plugging with perifollicular infiltrate (*Scanner view*)

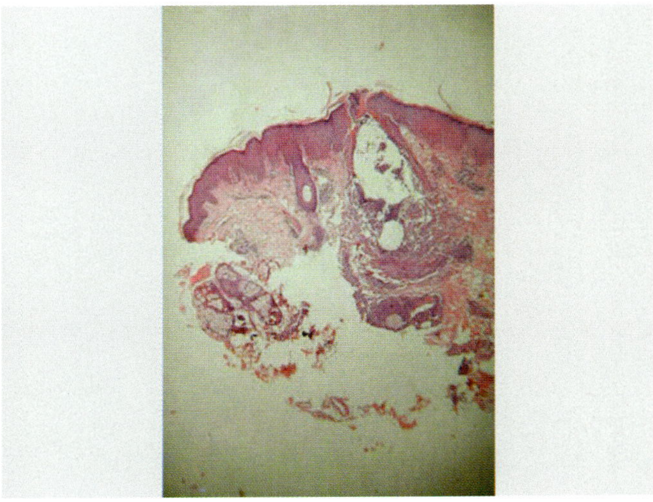

FIGURE 12.4.3

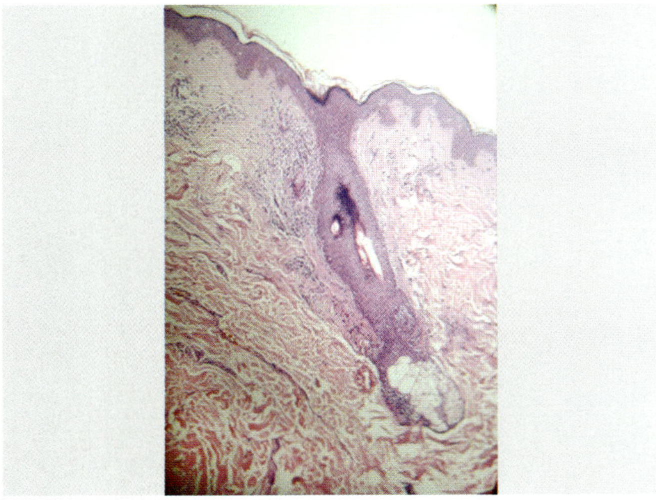

FIGURE 12.4.4

DIFFERENTIAL DIAGNOSIS

1. Frontal fibrosing alopecia
2. Keratosis pilaris atrophicans
3. Pseudofolliculitis
4. Folliculitis
5. Proliferating trichilemmal cyst
6. Milium

DIAGNOSTIC PEARLS

1. In telogen effluvium, examination of plucked hairs will reveal telogen counts greater than 25%.
2. An T : V of less than 4 : 1 is a feature of female pattern hair loss in horizontal scalp biopsy at the mid-isthmus level, whereas a ratio greater than 8 : 1 is seen in chronic telogen effluvium. Chronic telogen effluvium exhibits less inflammation as compared to androgenetic alopecia.
3. In lichen planopilaris lymphocytes extend up to the stem cells whereas in alopecia areata, lymphocytes infiltrate bulge region of the follicle.
4. Immunofluorescence in alopecia areata shows deposits of C3 and occasionally of IgG and IgM along the basement zone of the inferior segment of hair follicles.
5. In androgenetic alopecia, the connective tissue contains small elastin bodies (Arão-Perkins bodies) which indicate the sites of the papillae of each preceding generation of follicles. They stain with the acid orcein method, but not Verhoeff. Alopecia areata does not show these bodies.

13

Cutaneous Deposits

Chapter Outline

13.1: Calcinosis Cutis
13.2: Amyloidosis
13.3: Gouty Tophi
13.4: Lipoid Proteinosis
13.5: Colloid Milium
13.6: Ochronosis
13.7: Tattoo Pigment

Rajiv Joshi, Venkataram Mysore

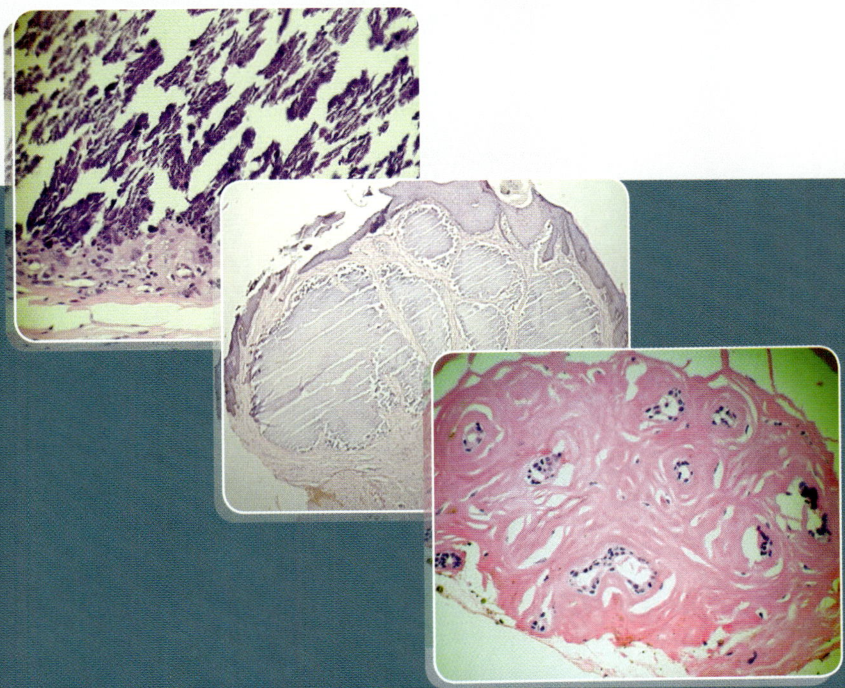

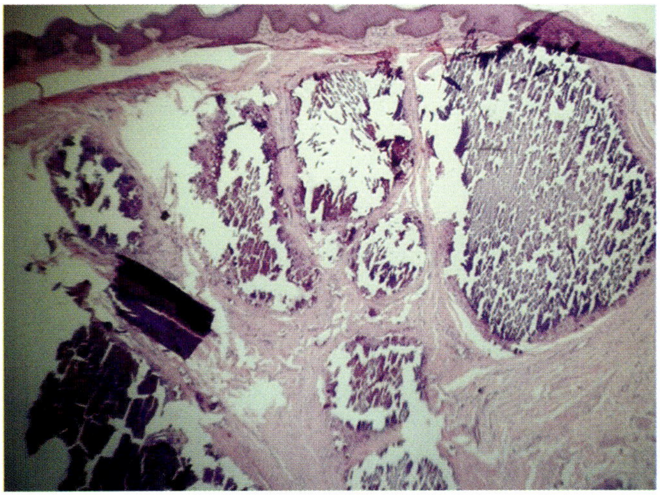

FIGURE 13.1.1

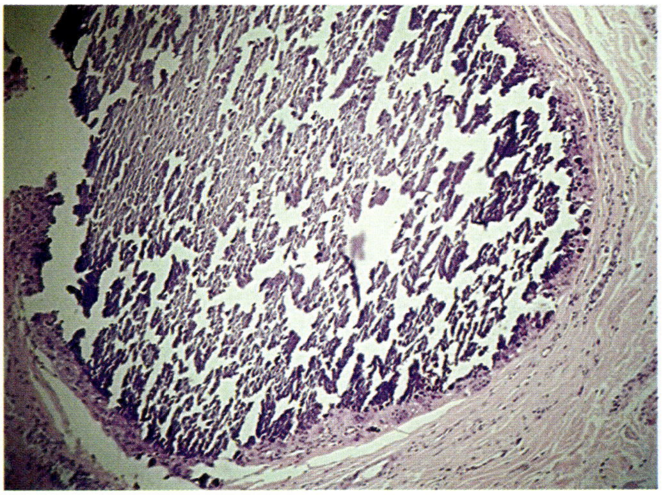

FIGURE 13.1.2

13.1: CALCINOSIS CUTIS

13.1.1: Calcinosis is seen as small and large deposits of basophilic material in the dermis (*Scanner view*)

13.1.2: A chronic inflammatory infiltrate surrounds the deposits (*Low power view*)

13.1.3: Closer view of deposits on H & E stain but deposits stain black with von Kossa stain (*High power view*)

13.1.4: Another case showing calcium deposits (but occasionally transepidermal elimination of calcium may be seen) (*Scanner view*)

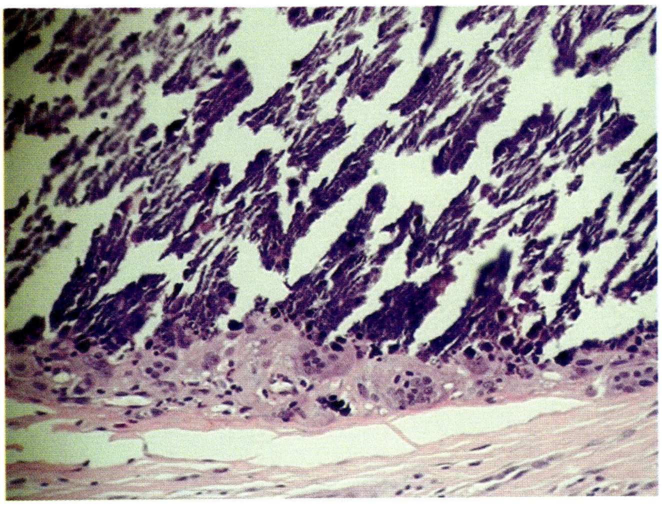

FIGURE 13.1.3

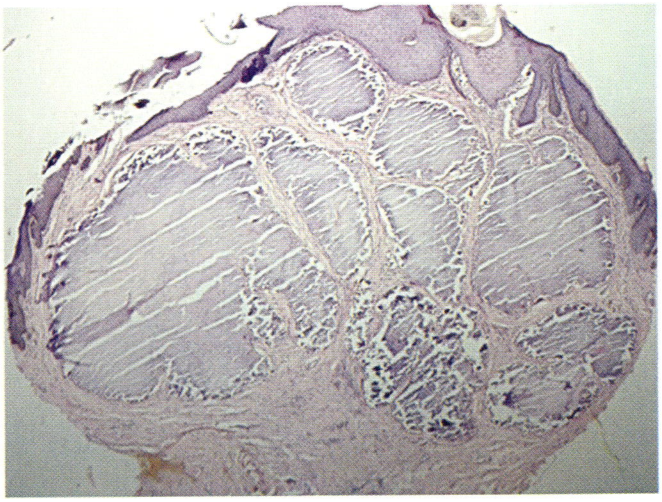

FIGURE 13.1.4

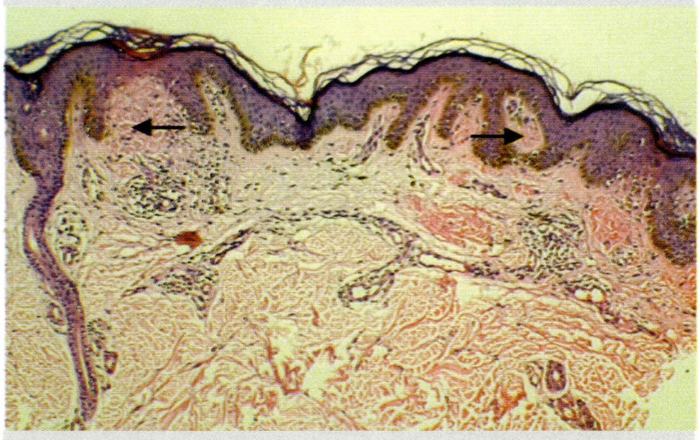

FIGURE 13.2.1.1

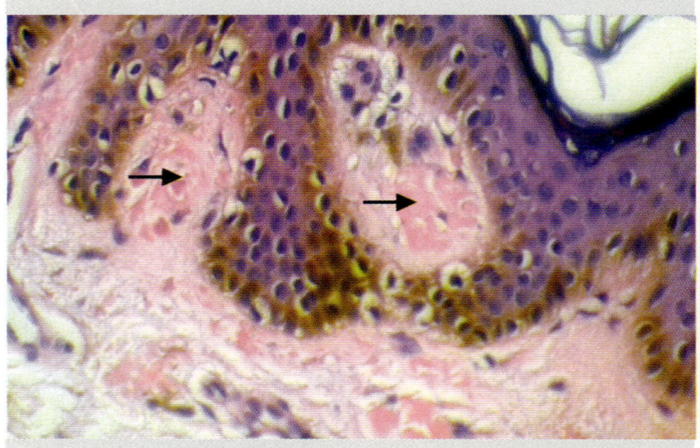

FIGURE 13.2.1.2

13.2: AMYLOIDOSIS

13.2.1: Lichen Amyloidosis

13.2.1.1: Dermal papillae contain globular deposits of amyloid and assume rounded contour, overlying epidermis shows hyperkeratosis and hyperplasia (lichenoid tissue reaction may be seen) (*Low power view*)

13.2.1.2: Closer view of hyaline deposits of amyloid (*High power view*)

13.2.1.3: Amyloid deposits stain positive with Congo red (*Low power view*)

13.2.1.4: Closer view of Congo red (*High power view*)

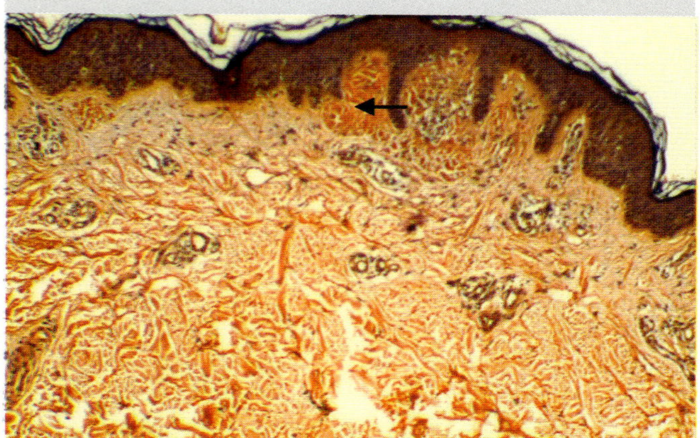

FIGURE 13.2.1.3

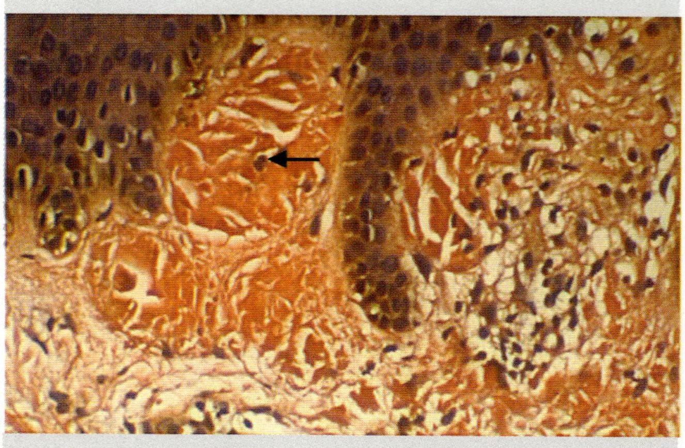

FIGURE 13.2.1.4

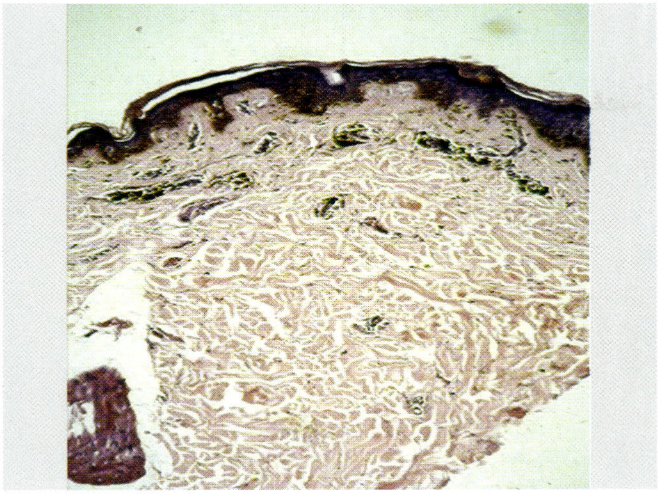

FIGURE 13.2.2.1

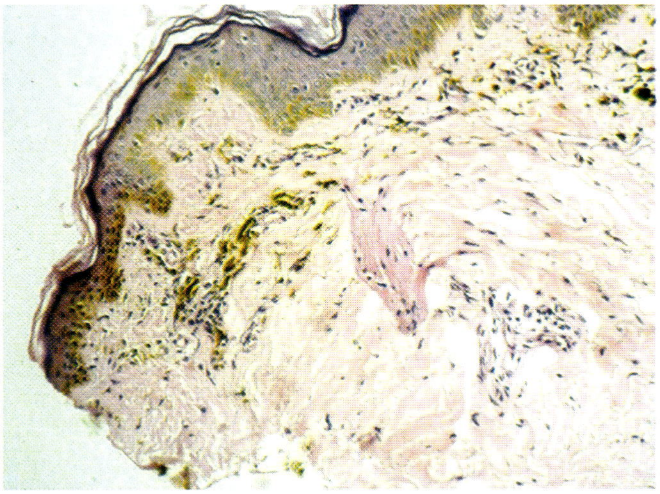

FIGURE 13.2.2.2

13.2.2: Macular Amyloidosis/Frictional Melanosis

13.2.2.1: Moderate epidermal hyperplasia, thinner basket weave stratum corneum (*Scanner view*)

13.2.2.2: Melanophages both in dermal papillae as well as deeper down in perivascular and interstitial locations (*Low power view*)

13.2.2.3: Sparse insignificant inflammatory infiltrate (*Low power view*)

13.2.2.4: Small clumps of amyloid in the dermal papillae (*High power view*)

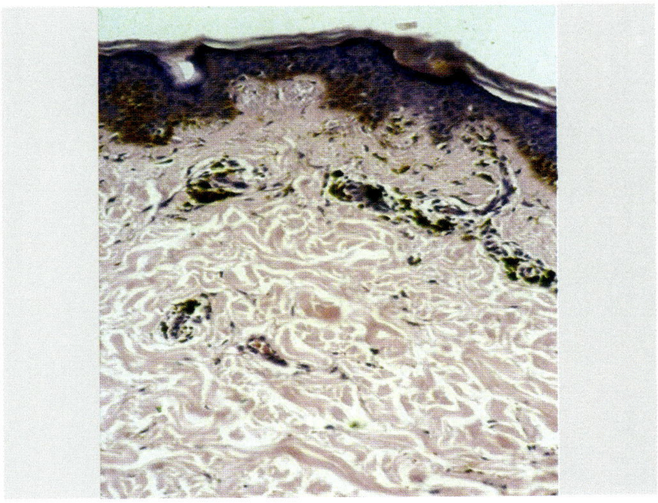

FIGURE 13.2.2.3

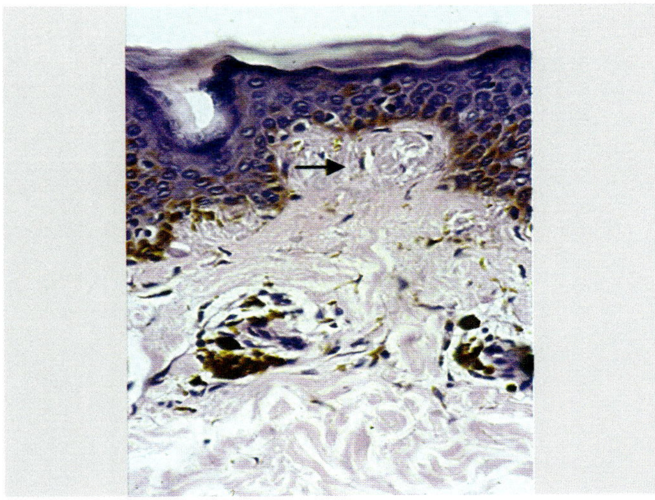

FIGURE 13.2.2.4

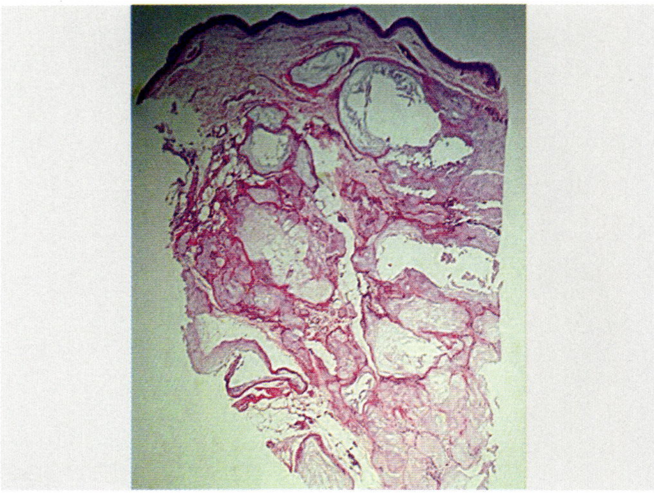

FIGURE 13.3.1

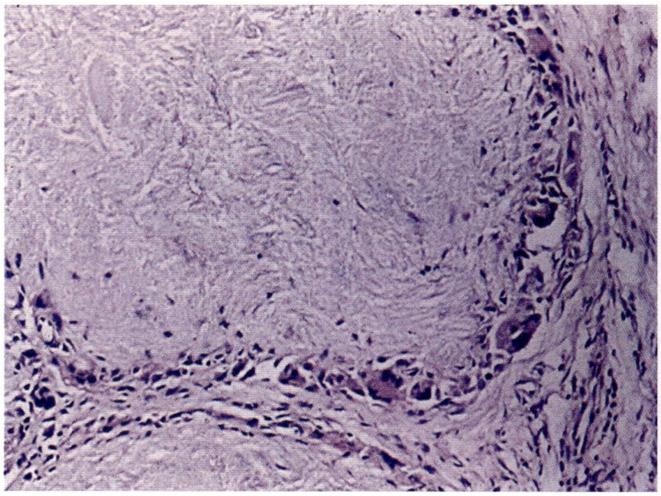

FIGURE 13.3.2

13.3: GOUTY TOPHI

13.3.1: Urates are seen as empty spaces on formalin fixed sections as they are dissolved during processing (*Scanner view*)

13.3.2: When present, seen as wispy, amorphous, bluish basophilic material, surrounded by palisades of histiocytes (*Low power view*)

13.3.3: Needle-shaped crystals are seen in alcohol fixed sections (*High power view*)

13.3.4: The crystals show birefringence under polarized light (*High power view*)

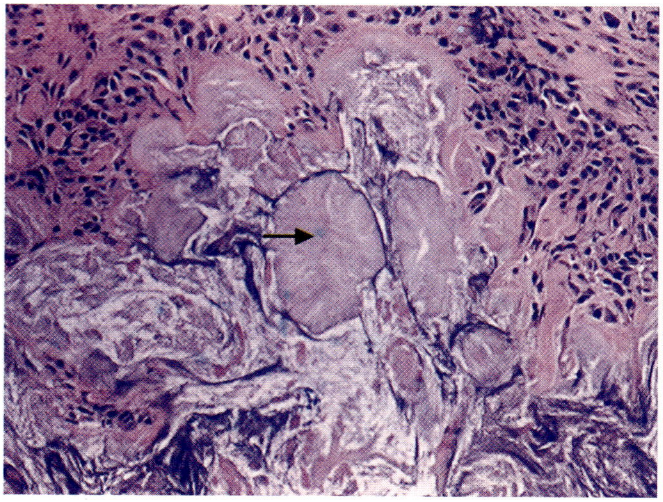

FIGURE 13.3.3

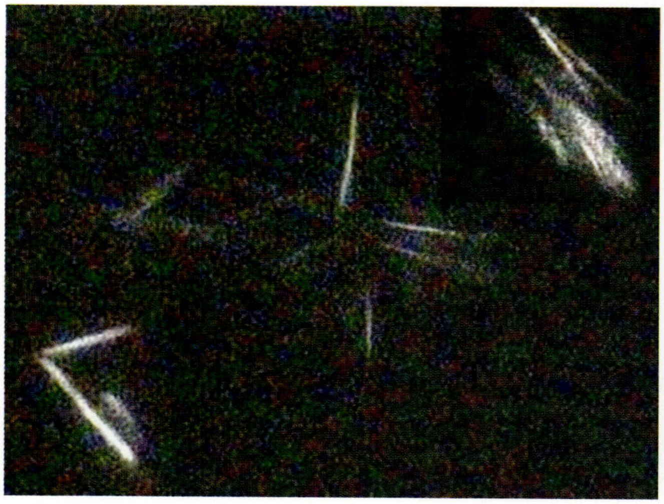

FIGURE 13.3.4

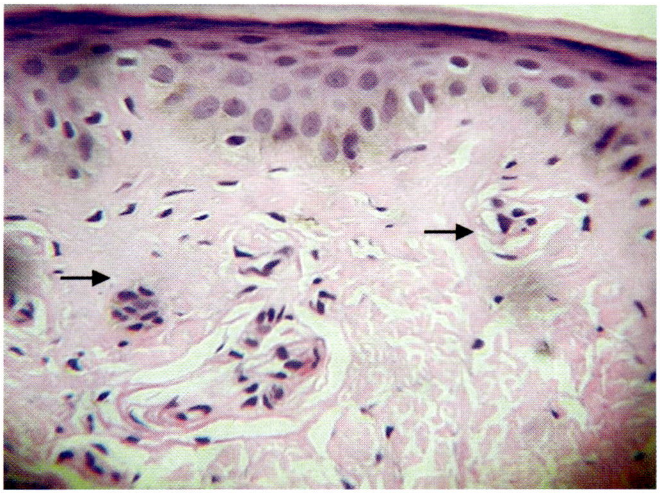

FIGURE 13.4.1

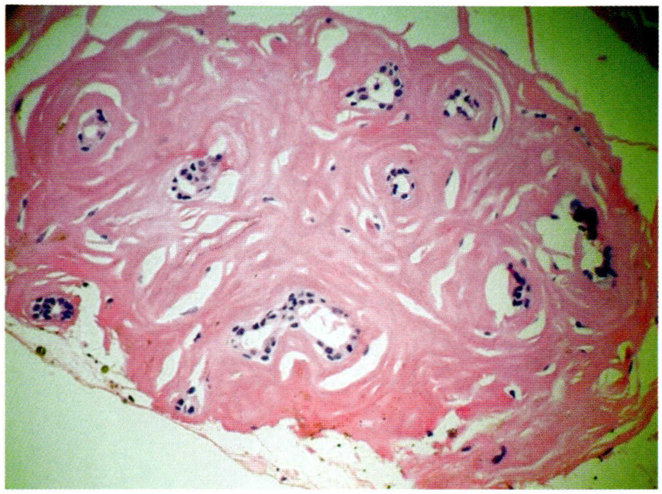

FIGURE 13.4.2

13.4: LIPOID PROTEINOSIS

13.4.1: Deposition of pale, eosinophilic material in the superficial dermis (*Low power view*)

13.4.2: Proliferation of capillaries with perivascular onion skin appearance of hyaline deposits in advanced cases (*High power view*)

13.4.3: Perivascular hyaline deposits are PAS positive (*High power view*)

13.4.4: PAS +ve deposit in superficial dermis and around the blood vessels. Deposit also seen around the hair follicles (*High power view*)

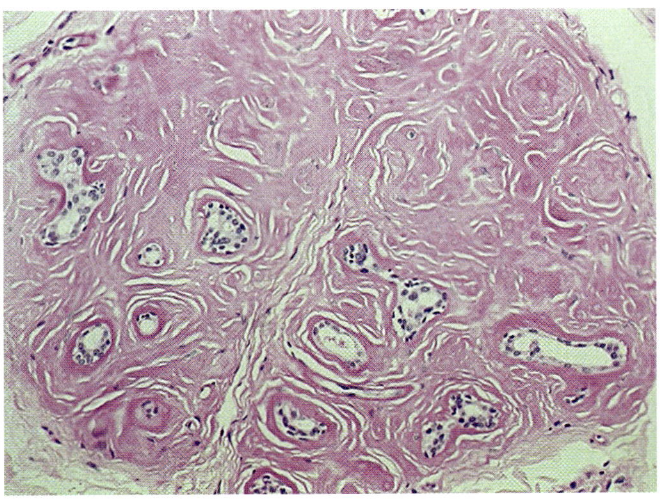

FIGURE 13.4.3

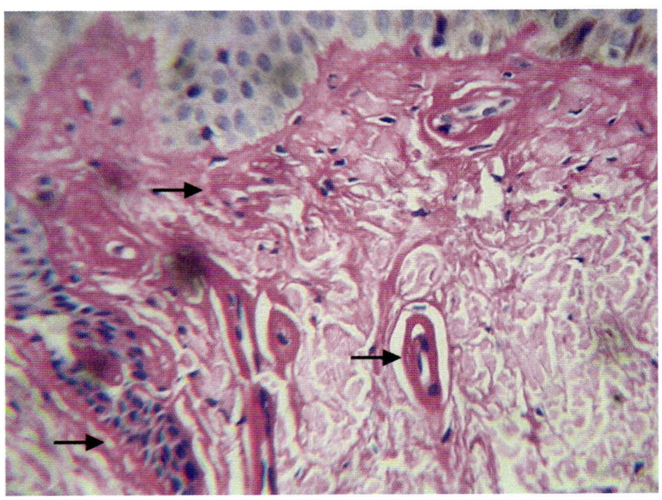

FIGURE 13.4.4

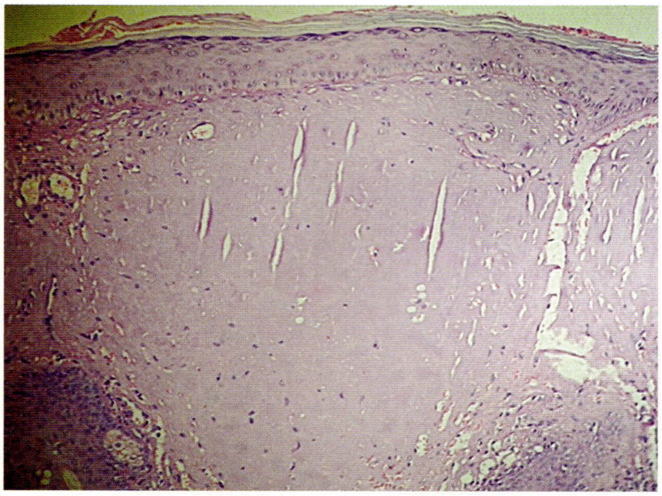

FIGURE 13.5.1

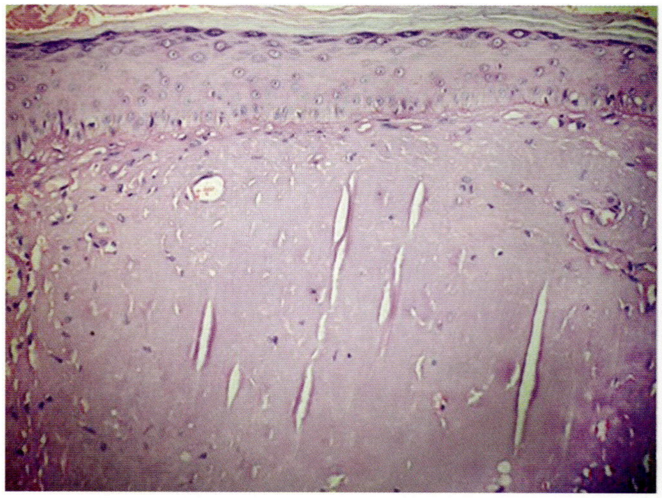

FIGURE 13.5.2

13.5: COLLOID MILIUM

13.5.1: Deposits of eosinophilic material are seen in superficial dermis (*Scanner view*)

13.5.2: The amorphous deposit appears faceted or clefted (*Low power view*)

13.5.3: Closer view of the same (*High power view*)

13.5.4: Another case with deposits along with adjacent solar elastosis seen in adult colloid milium (*Scanner view*)

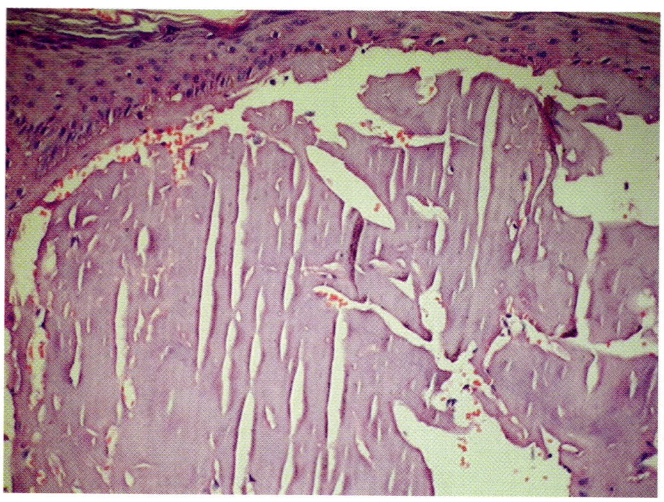

FIGURE 13.5.3

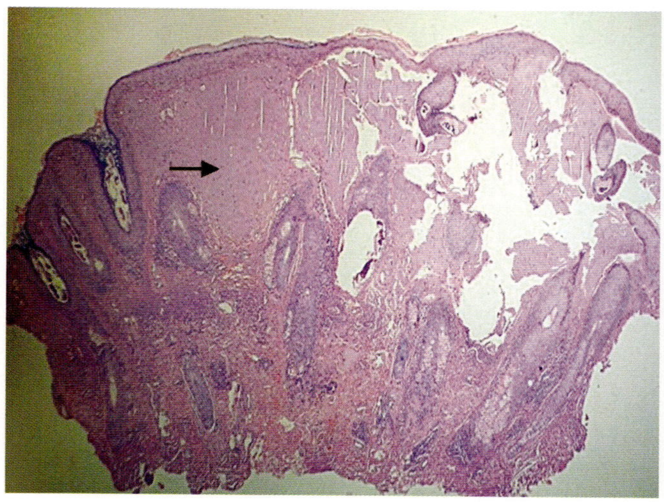

FIGURE 13.5.4

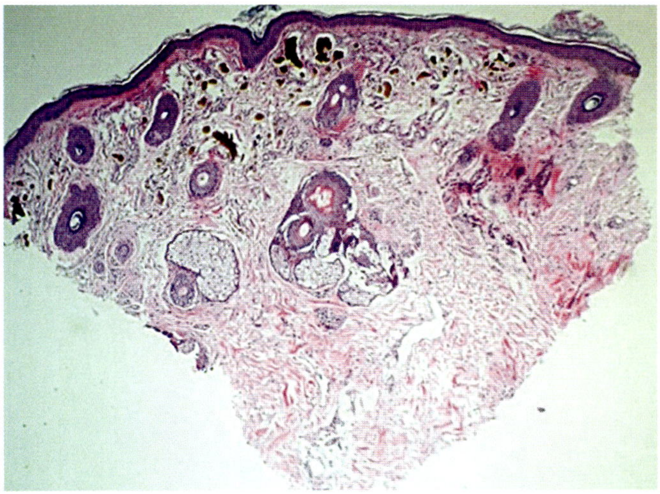

FIGURE 13.6.1

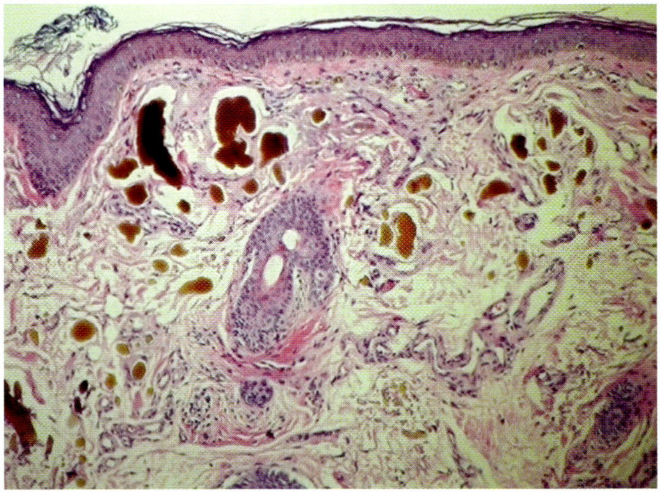

FIGURE 13.6.2

13.6: OCHRONOSIS

13.6.1: Initially collagen in the upper dermis appears swollen and basophilic (*Scanner view*)

13.6.2: Stout, sharply defined fibers of ochronosis in the dermis (*Low power view*)

13.6.3: Ochre-colored fibers of ochronosis, some of the fibers are fragmented (*High power view*)

13.6.4: Typical banana-shaped fiber (*High power view*)

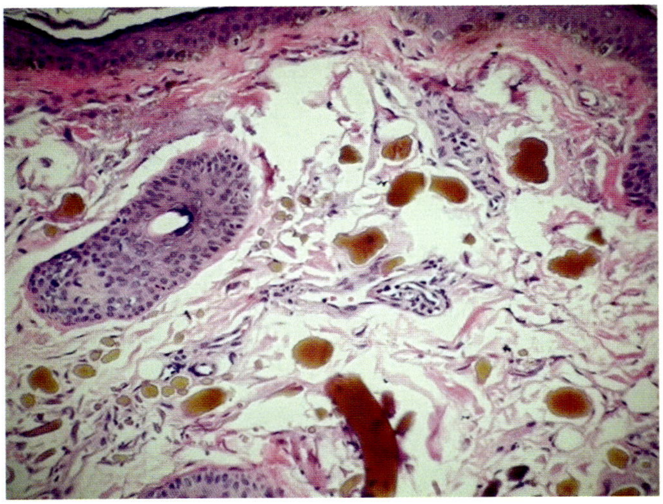

FIGURE 13.6.3

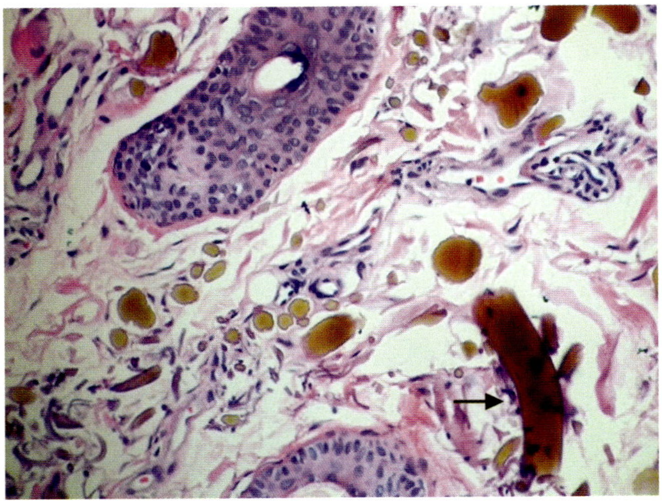

FIGURE 13.6.4

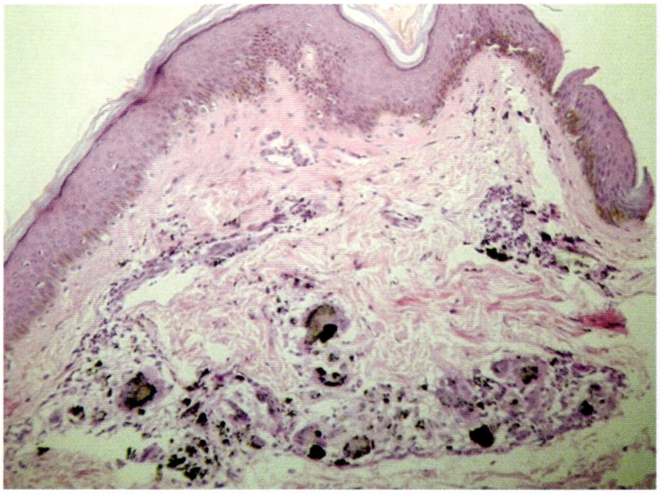

FIGURE 13.7.1

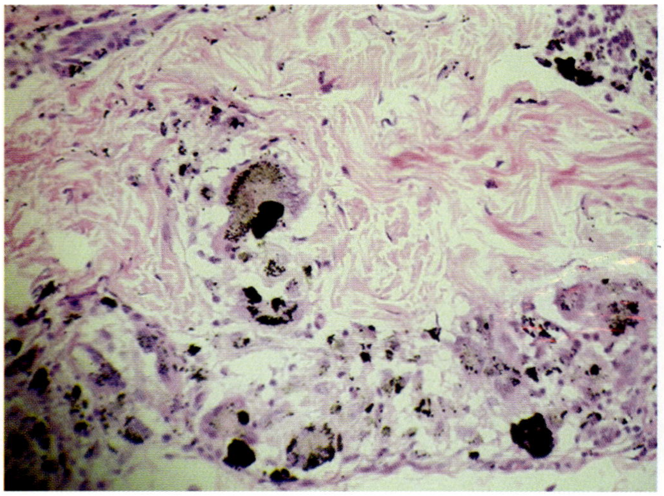

FIGURE 13.7.2

13.7: TATTOO PIGMENT

13.7.1: Histologically all pigments look black in color (*Scanner view*)

13.7.2: Pigment incites inflammatory response (can be granulomatous—foreign body or sarcoidal) (*Low power view*)

13.7.3: Granulomatous reaction with multinucleated giant cells (*Low power view*)

13.7.4: Closer view of granulomatous reaction (*High power view*)

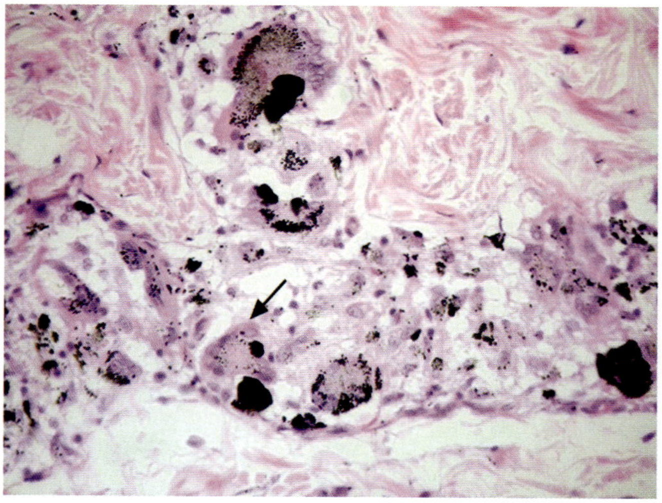

FIGURE 13.7.3

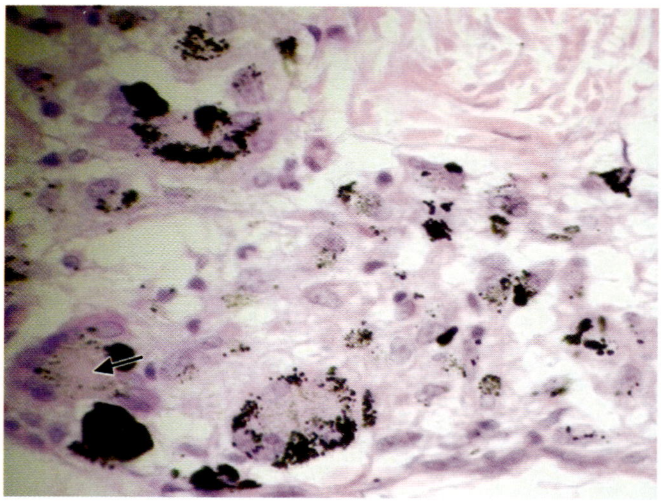

FIGURE 13.7.4

DIFFERENTIAL DIAGNOSIS

1. Osteomas
2. Chondromas
3. Argyria
4. Drug deposits
5. Cutaneous implants

DIAGNOSTIC PEARLS

1. In tumoral calcinosis, subcutaneous deposits of calcium are seen whereas deposits in metastatic and dystrophic calcification tend to be large and dense while those in subepidermal calcified nodule are multiple, small and globular in type.
2. Osteoma cutis shows Haversian systems and cement lines.
3. Primary cutaneous amyloidosis has pigmented cells within the dermal deposits.
4. Deposits in lipoid proteinosis extend to adjacent dermis from perivascular location as against porphyria. Also there is no involvement of the sweat glands in porphyria.
5. Colloid milium does not contain laminin or type IV collagen in contrast to lipoid proteinosis and primary cutaneous amyloidosis.
6. Exogenous ochronosis demonstrates variable number of macrophages, which are infrequent in alkaptonuria.

14

Perforating Disorders

Chapter Outline

14.1: Reactive Perforating Collagenosis

14.2: Kyrle's Disease (Hyperkeratosis Follicularis et Parafollicularis in Cutem Penetrans)

14.3: Perforating Folliculitis—Acquired Perforating Dermatoses

14.4: Elastosis Perforans Serpiginosa

Uday Khopkar, Chirag Desai, Atul Dongre, Nathan Lee, Jerad Gardner

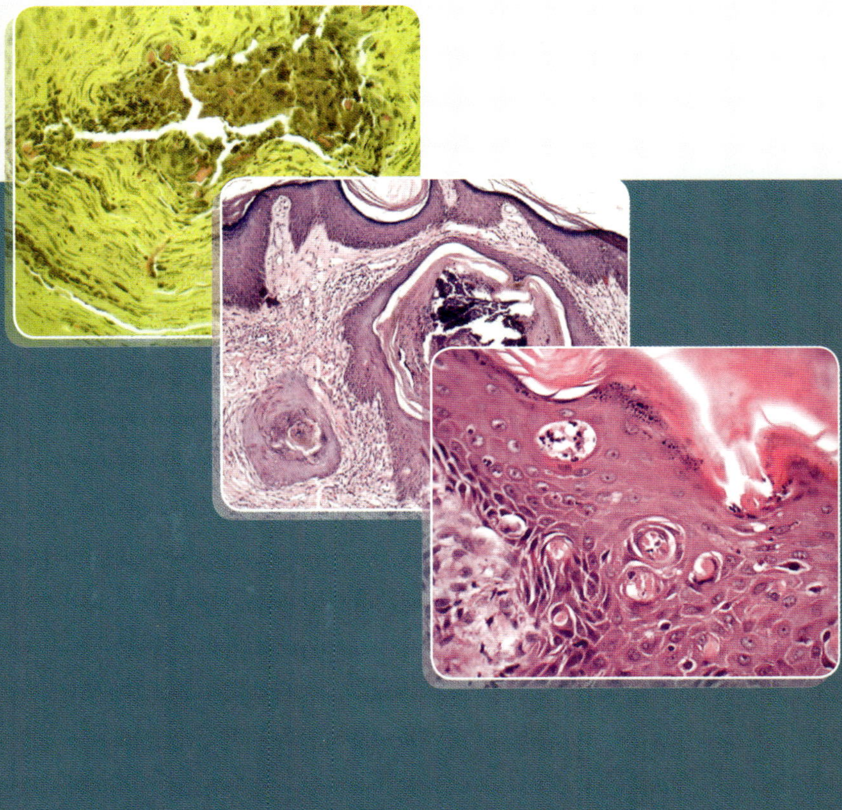

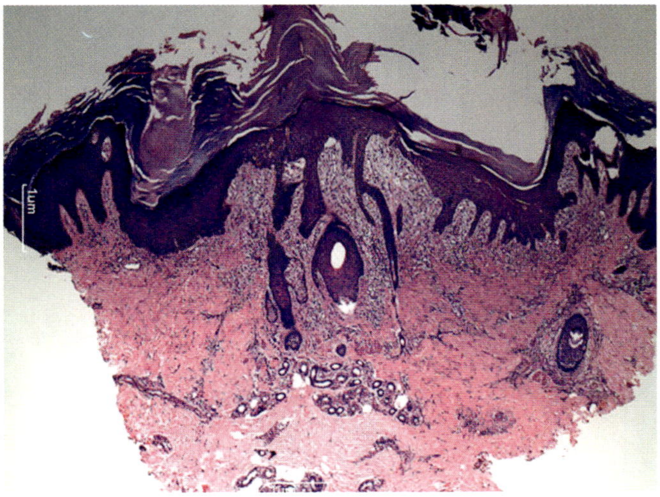

FIGURE 14.1.1

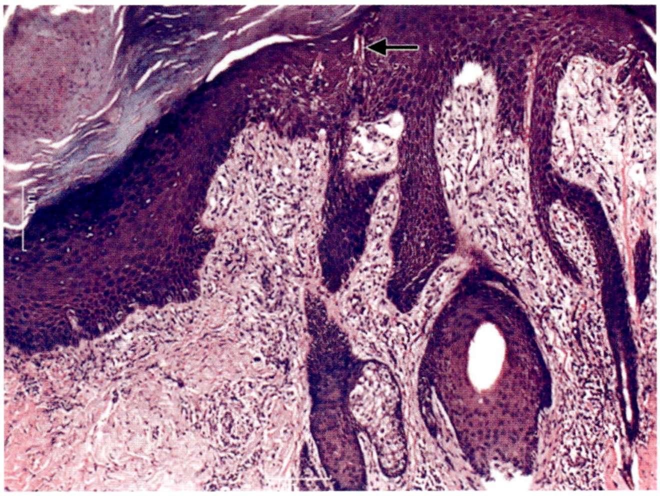

FIGURE 14.1.2

14.1: REACTIVE PERFORATING COLLAGENOSIS

14.1.1: Cup-shaped invagination of the epidermis usually filled with parakeratotic keratin, collagen and debris *(Scanner view)*

14.1.2: Underlying epidermis has fine slits through which basophilic collagen fibers are extruded in a vertical orientation *(Low power view)*

14.1.3: Closer view of the slit *(High power view)*

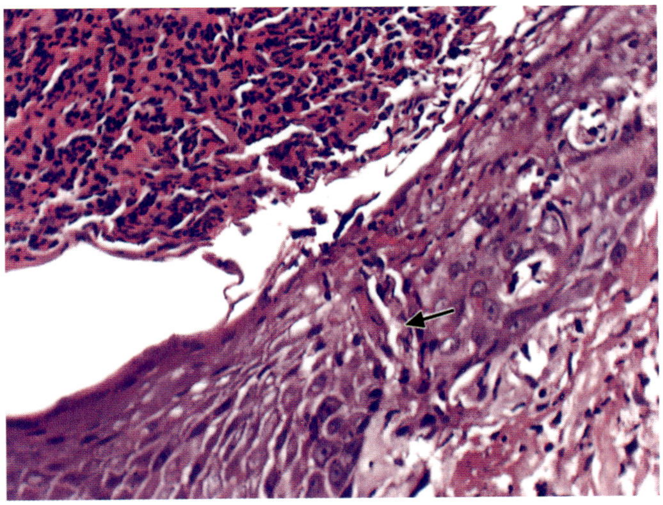

FIGURE 14.1.3

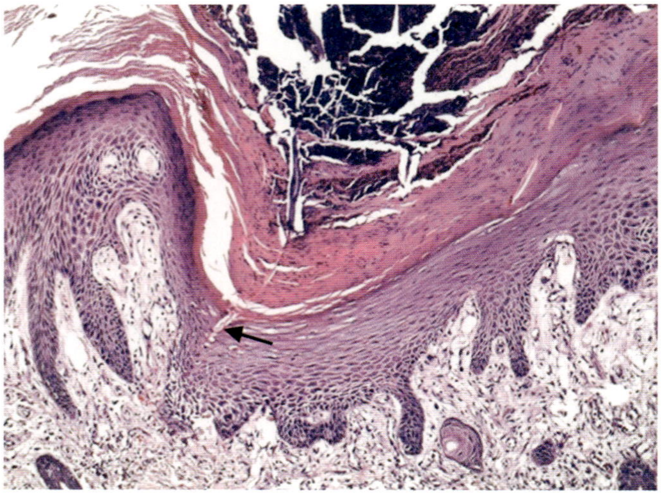

FIGURE 14.1.4

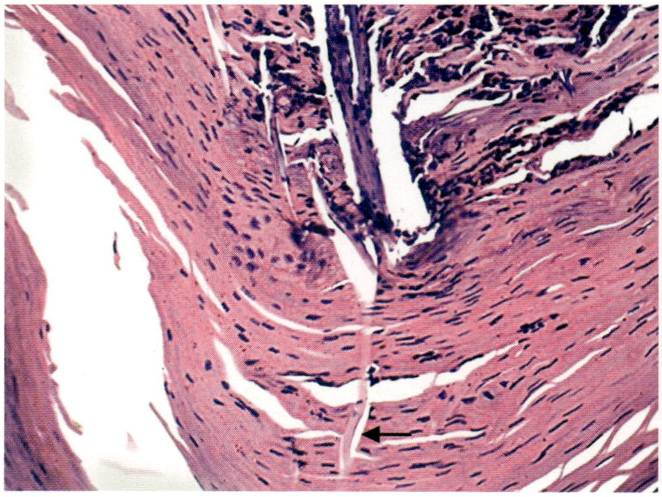

FIGURE 14.1.5

14.1.4: Case with depression and slit *(Low power view)*
14.1.5: Collagen in stratum corneum *(High power view)*
14.1.6: Verhoeff-van Gieson stain *(High power view)*

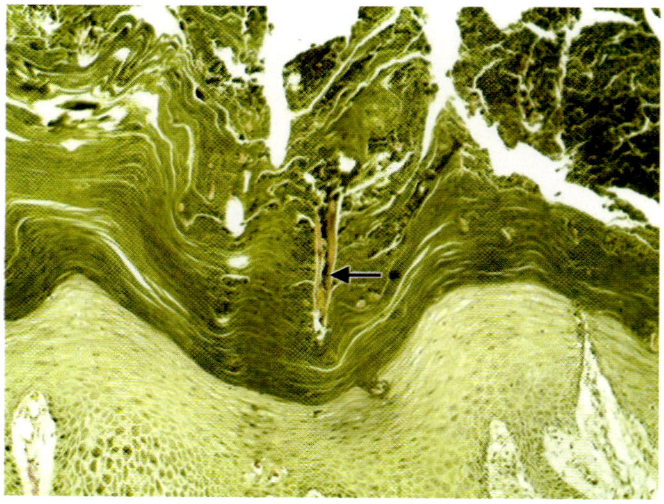

FIGURE 14.1.6

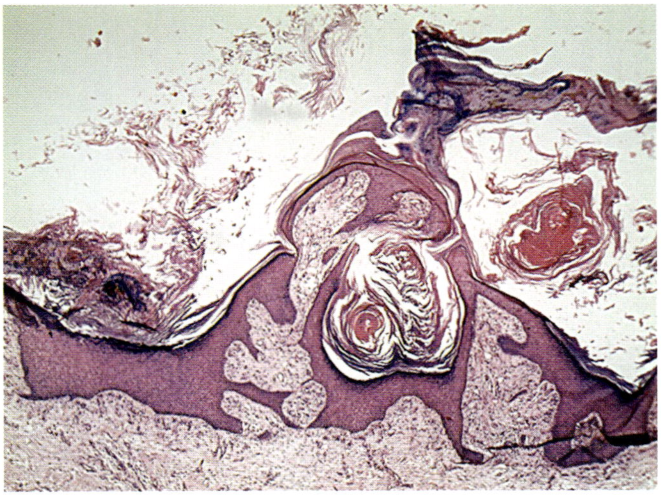

FIGURE 14.2.1

14.2: KYRLE'S DISEASE (HYPERKERATOSIS FOLLICULARIS ET PARAFOLLICULARIS IN CUTEM PENETRANS)

14.2.1: A follicular and extrafollicular cornified plug with focal parakeratosis embedded in an epidermal invagination, irregular epithelial hyperplasia *(Scanner view)*

14.2.2: Basophilic degenerated material identified in small collections throughout the plug with absence of demonstrable collagen and elastin, an inflammatory component may be granulomatous with small foci of suppuration *(Low power view)*

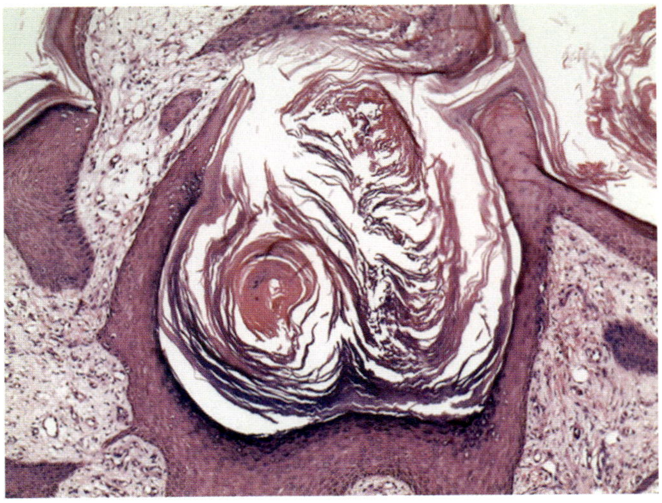

FIGURE 14.2.2

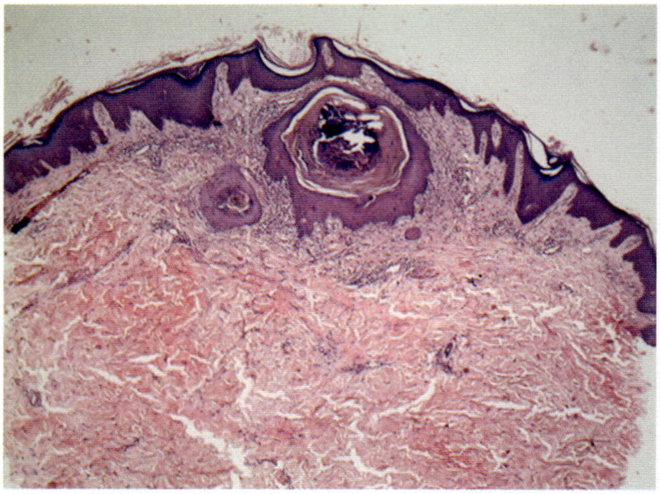

FIGURE 14.3.1

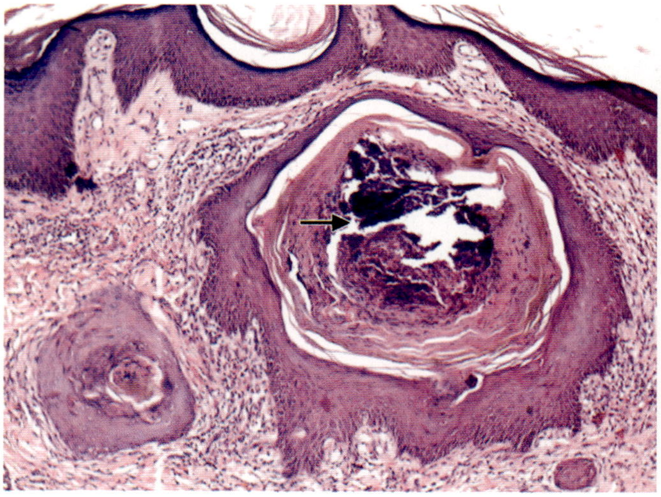

FIGURE 14.3.2

14.3: PERFORATING FOLLICULITIS—ACQUIRED PERFORATING DERMATOSES

14.3.1: Dermis shows enlarged follicle containing debris *(Scanner view)*

14.3.2: Basophilic debris composed of parakeratotic cells, inflammatory cells and degenerated collagen and elastin, perifollicular infiltrate of lymphocytes *(Low power view)*

14.3.3: Follicular epithelium showing perforations *(High power view)*

14.3.4: Verhoeff-Van Gieson (VVG) stain showing collagen/elastin *(High power view)*

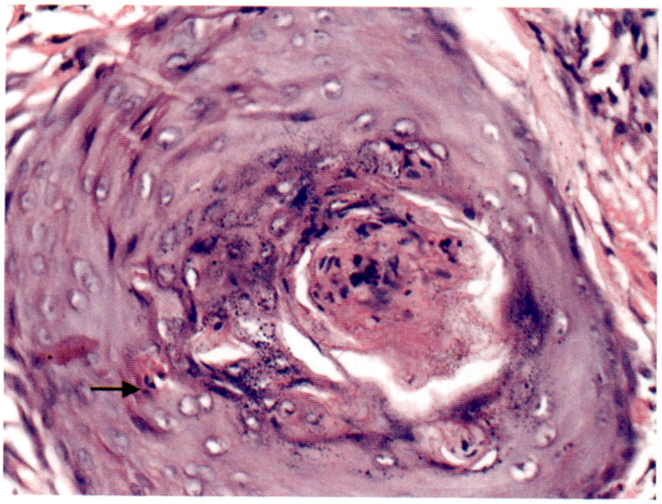

FIGURE 14.3.3

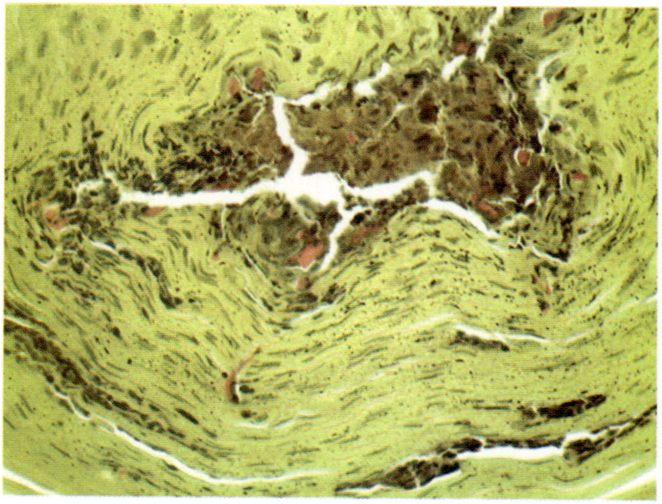

FIGURE 14.3.4

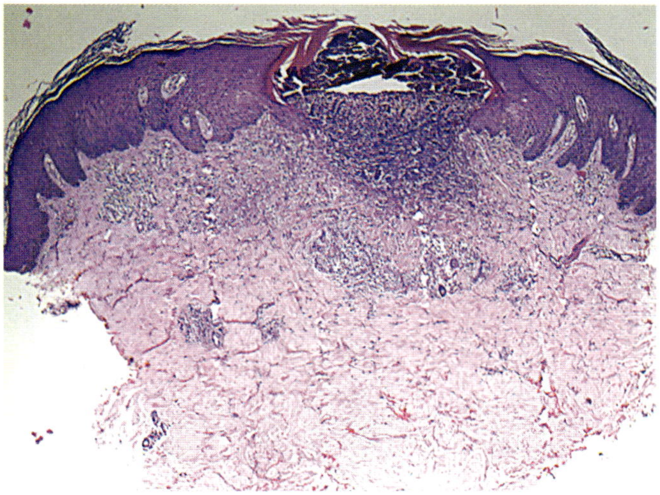

FIGURE 14.3.5

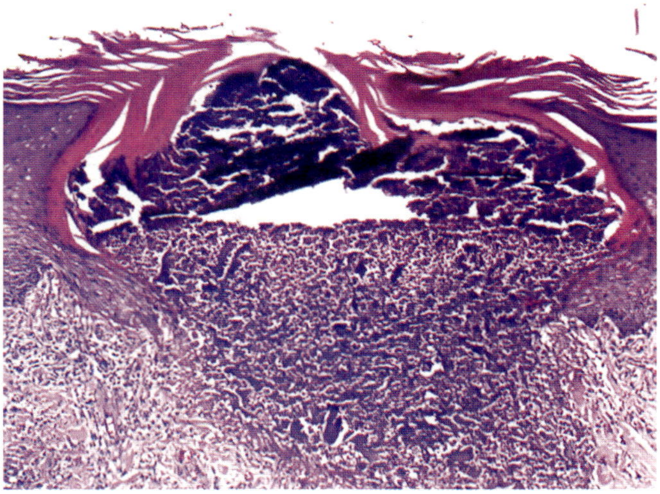

FIGURE 14.3.6

14.3.5: Acquired perforating dermatosis (APD) in diabetic and chronic renal failure—histologic features are overlapping with other perforating disorders *(Scanner view)*

14.3.6: Dilated follicle filled with debris and showing perforation (transepidermal elimination) *(Low power view)*

14.3.7: Transepidermal elimination of both collagen and elastin (special stain would confirm) *(High power view)*

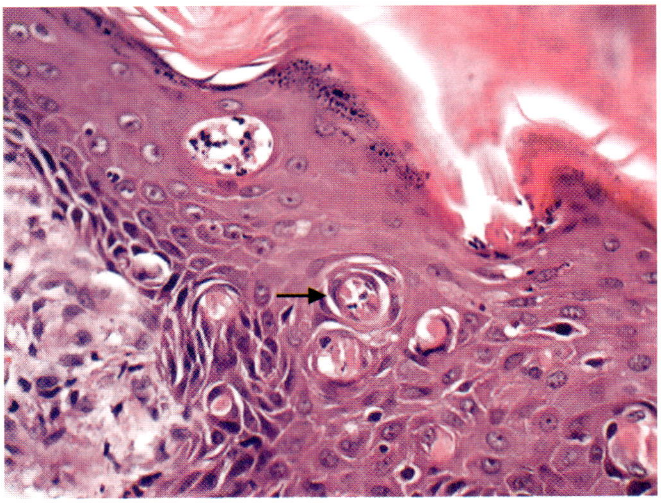

FIGURE 14.3.7

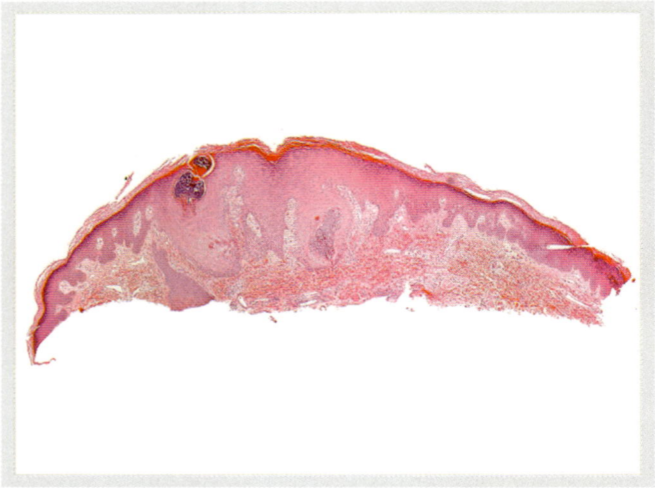

FIGURE 14.4.1

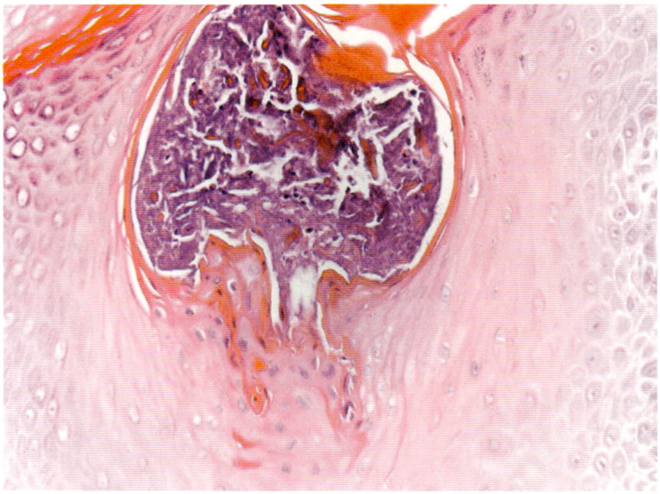

FIGURE 14.4.2

14.4: ELASTOSIS PERFORANS SERPIGINOSA

14.4.1: Transepidermal elimination is seen at two places *(Scanner view)*

14.4.2: Closer view shows an epidermal invagination with a central plug of necrotic debris. There is surrounding epidermal acanthosis *(Low power view)*

14.4.3: Degenerated fibers from the dermis are perforating into the epidermis. At the dermal/epidermal junction, these tangled degenerated fibers are clearly elastic fibers *(Low power view)*

14.4.4: Verhoeff-Van Gieson stain confirms elastic fibers, which stain black *(High power view)*

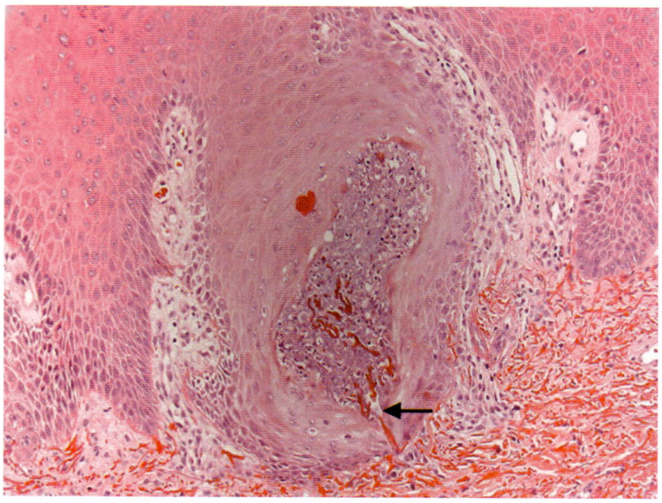

FIGURE 14.4.3

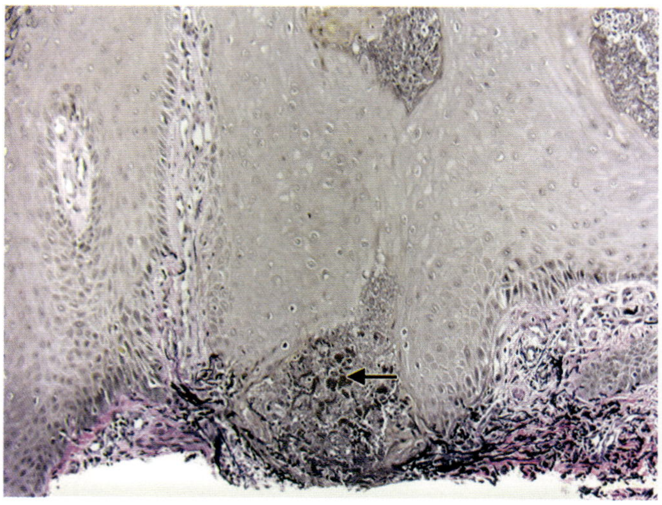

FIGURE 14.4.4

DIFFERENTIAL DIAGNOSIS

1. Chondrodermatitis nodularis helicis
2. Perforating granuloma annulare

DIAGNOSTIC PEARLS

1. If the follicular localization of perforating folliculitis is not appreciated, serial sections are advised.
2. In penicillamine induced EPS, there are thickened elastic fibers in the reticular dermis.
3. In the region of their transepidermal elimination, the elastic fibers may lose their staining properties and may become eosinophilic.
4. Pseudocarcinomatous lichenoid granulomatous diseases may result into transfollicular elimination, e.g. lupus vulgaris/tuberculosis verrucosa cutis/chromoblastomycosis.
5. In these diseases initiating event may be folliculitis and trauma, which may lead to dermal damage and subsequent dermal inflammation with epidermal and appendageal changes.
6. Such changes are not exclusive to only these perforating disorders but may also occur with prurigo nodularis/hypertrophic lichen planus/keratosis lichenoides chronica, etc.
7. In Kyrle's disease, keratotic plugs that develop in hair follicles and eccrine ducts, penetrate the epidermis and extend into the dermis.

15

Cutaneous Infections

Chapter Outline

15.1: Viral Infections
15.2: Fungal Infections
15.3: Bacterial Infections

Uma Nahar Saikia, Dipankar De,
KC Nischal, Pradeep Mahajan, Uday Khopkar

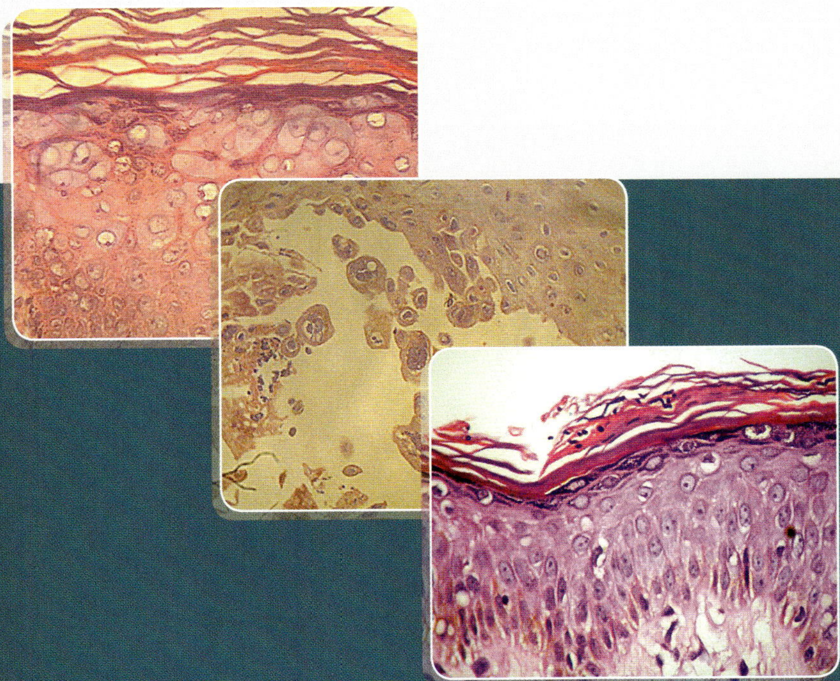

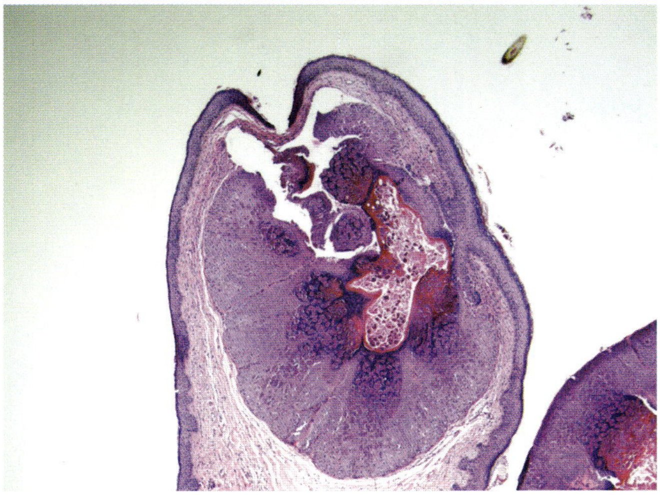

FIGURE 15.1.1.1

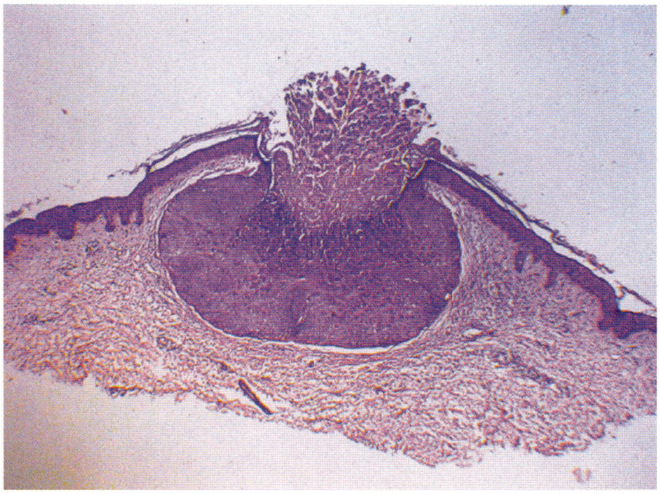

FIGURE 15.1.1.2

15.1: VIRAL INFECTIONS

15.1.1: Molluscum Contagiosum

15.1.1.1: Section shows lobule with epidermal hyperplasia extending into the dermis *(Scanner view)*

15.1.1.2: Another case with the lobules and extrusion of molluscum bodies over epidermal surface *(Scanner view)*

15.1.1.3: Closer view of the same showing eosinophilic inclusion bodies in the cytoplasm of cells in the stratum spinosum *(Low power view)*

15.1.1.4: The bodies become increasingly basophilic and enlarge as they approach the surface and are extruded *(Low power view)*

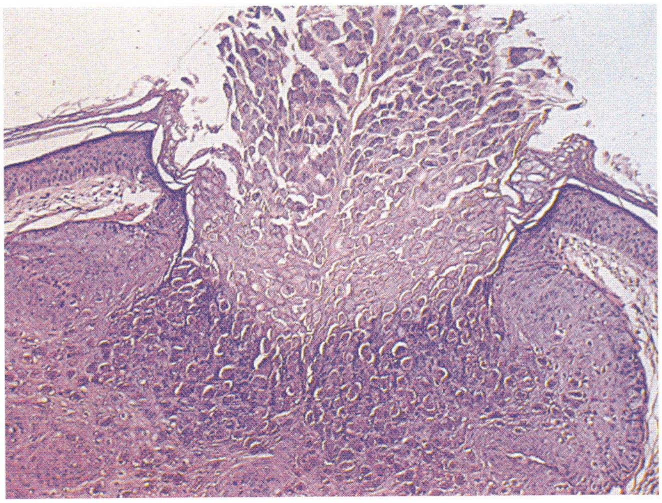

FIGURE 15.1.1.3

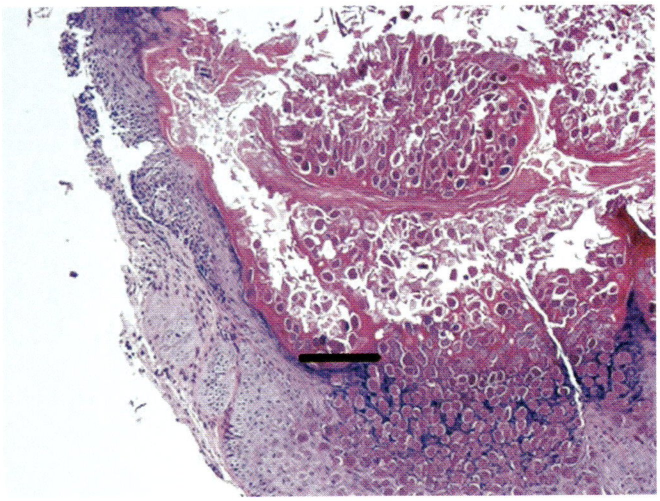

FIGURE 15.1.1.4

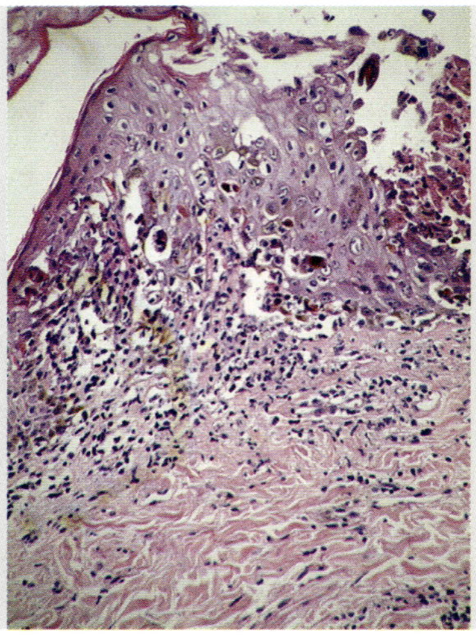

FIGURE 15.1.2.1

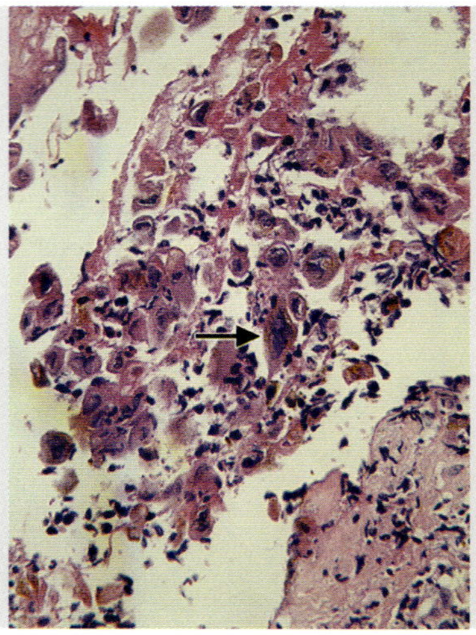

FIGURE 15.1.2.2

15.1.2: Herpesviridae Family

15.1.2.1: Herpes simplex, varicella, and herpes zoster show similar features histologically. Inflammation is more marked in simplex as compared to varicella or zoster as in this case which also shows ulcerated epidermis *(Low power view)*

15.1.2.2: Keratinocytes are swollen and have glassy cytoplasm (ballooning). They lose intercellular attachments and separate (secondary acantholysis). Progressive swelling also leads to rupture of the cells (reticular degeneration) (not seen in this section). All these changes lead to an intraepidermal vesicle formation *(Low power view)*

15.1.2.3: Another case with intraepidermal vesicle containing multinucleated keratinocytes admixed with inflammation *(Scanner view)*

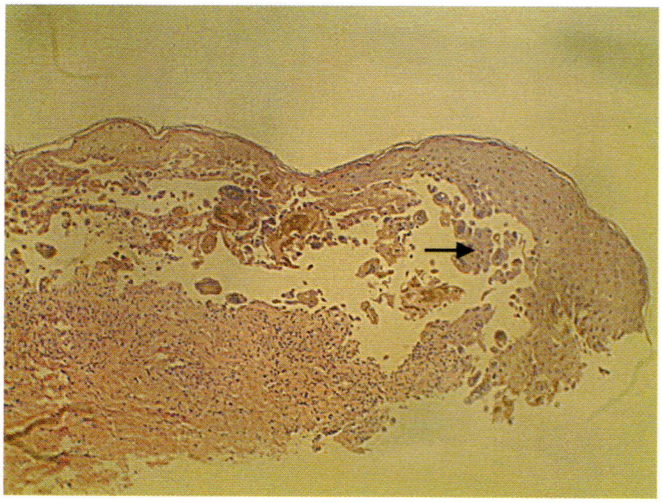

FIGURE 15.1.2.3

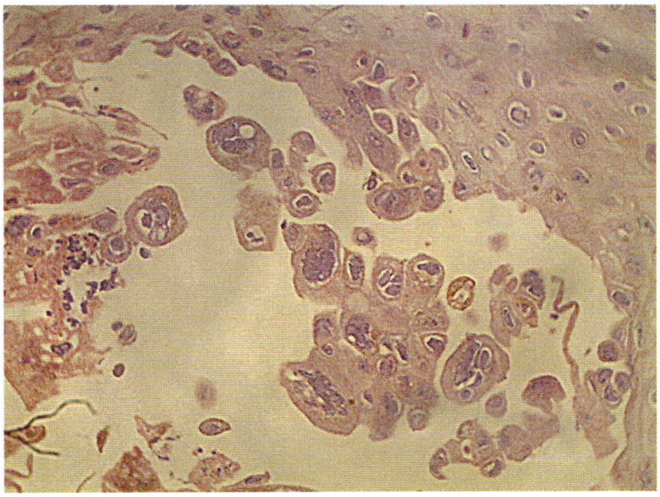

FIGURE 15.1.2.4

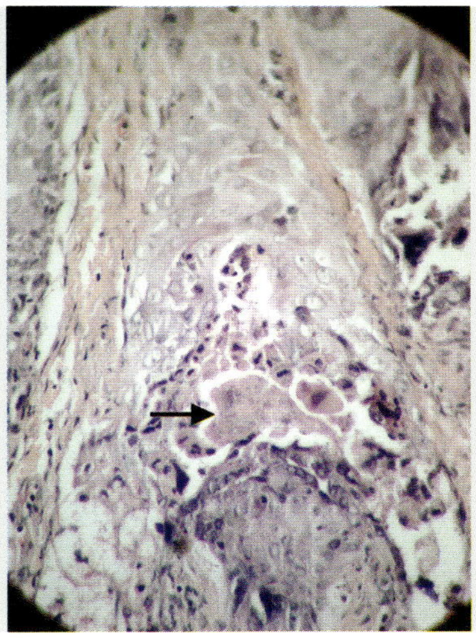

FIGURE 15.1.2.5

15.1.2.4: Closer view of multinucleated keratinocytes and intranuclear inclusions with margination of chromatin *(High power view)*

15.1.2.5: Case of herpes folliculitis with cells of the outer root sheath showing ballooning *(High power view)*

15.1.2.6: Extensive reticular degeneration leading to intraepidermal blister formation with minimal dermal inflammation in a case of varicella *(Scanner view)*

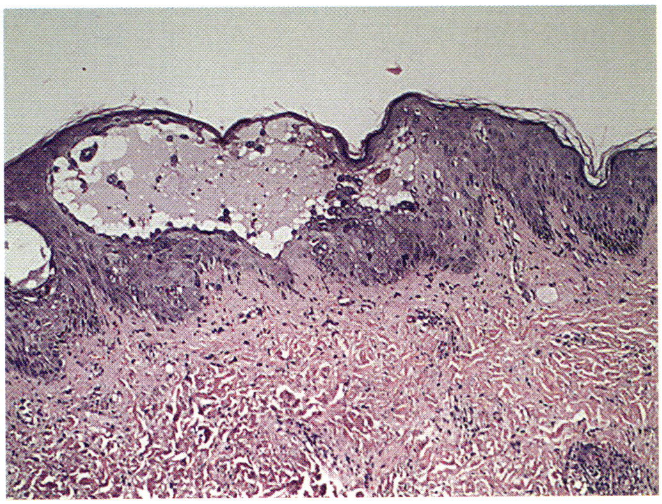

FIGURE 15.1.2.6

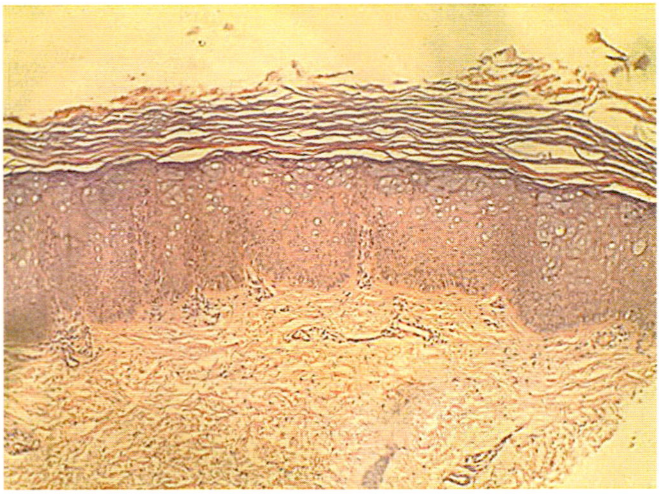

FIGURE 15.1.3.1

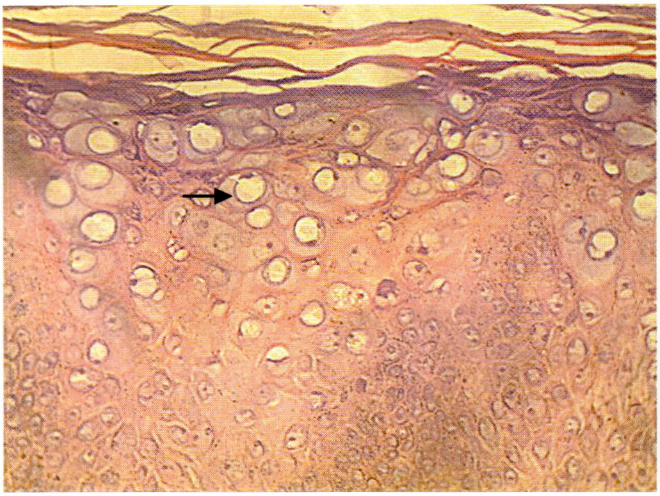

FIGURE 15.1.3.2

15.1.3: Verruca Plana

15.1.3.1: There is hyperkeratosis and acanthosis. The stratum corneum has a 'basket-weave' appearance. The dermis is usually normal *(Low power view)*

15.1.3.2: Vacuolation of the cells of the granular and upper malpighian layers with prominent keratohyaline granules *(High power view)*

15.1.3.3: Swollen cells in upper epidermis *(High power view)*

15.1.3.4: Cytoplasm has blue-gray pallor *(High power view)*

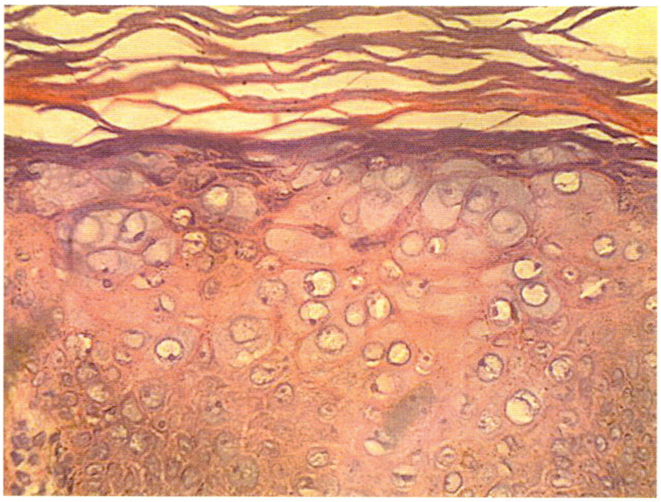

FIGURE 15.1.3.3

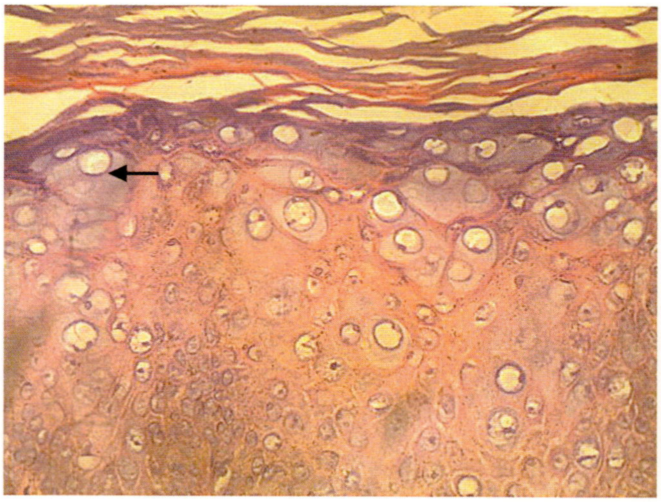

FIGURE 15.1.3.4

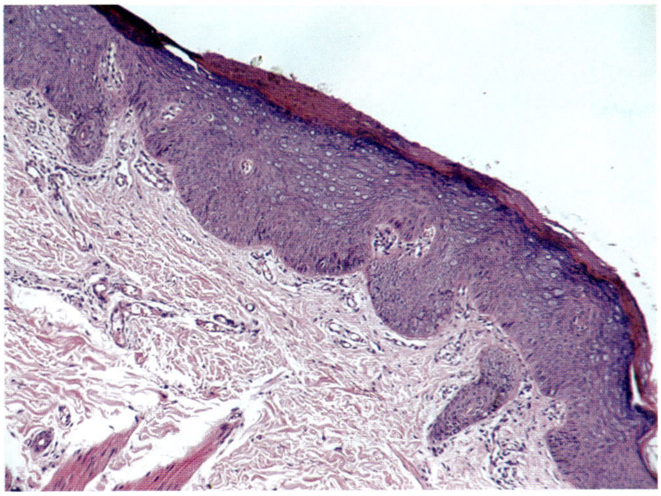

FIGURE 15.1.4.1

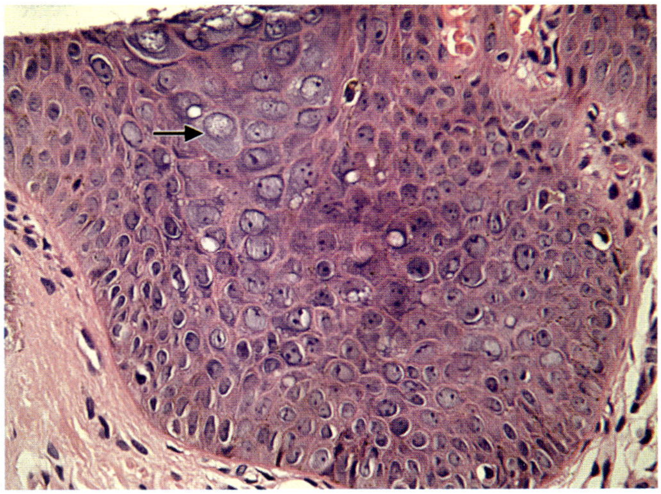

FIGURE 15.1.4.2

15.1.4: Epidermodysplasia Verruciformis

15.1.4.1: EDV shows acanthotic epidermis with compact hyperkeratosis. Histologic changes resemble plane warts *(Low power view)*

15.1.4.2: Groups of large cells in epidermis with blue cytoplasm and enlarged nuclei *(High power view)*

15.1.4.3: Swollen cells in the upper epidermal layers with pale blue cytoplasm and chromatin. Prominent keratohyaline granules also seen *(High power view)*

15.1.4.4: Another case showing a basket-weave appearance of *S. corneum* and swollen cells in *S. granulosum (High power view)*

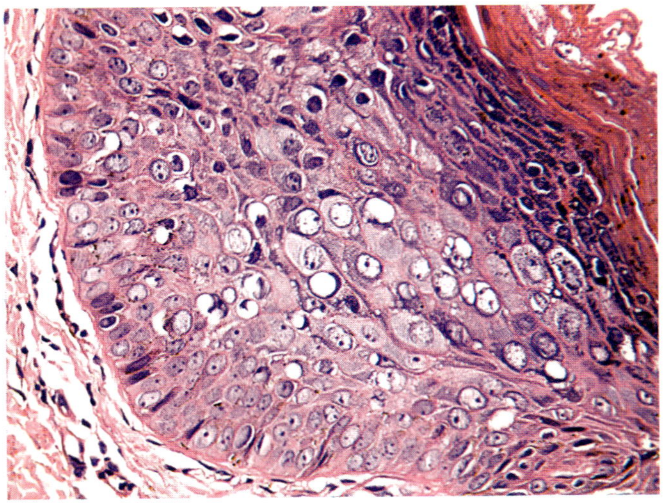

FIGURE 15.1.4.3

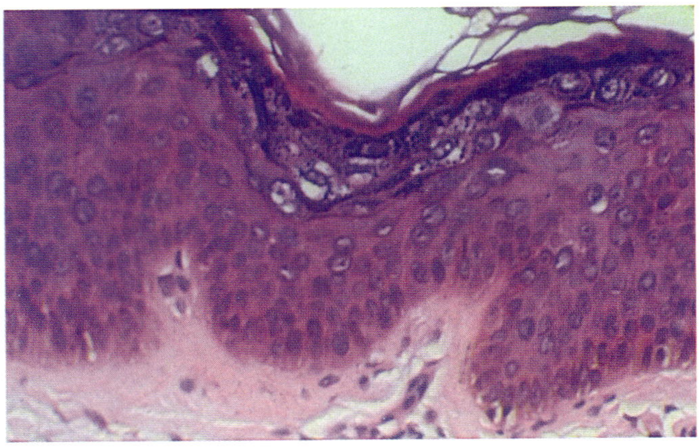

FIGURE 15.1.4.4

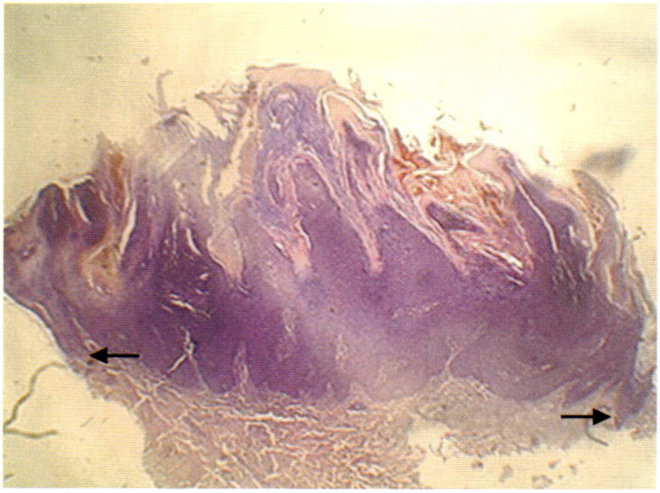

FIGURE 15.1.5.1

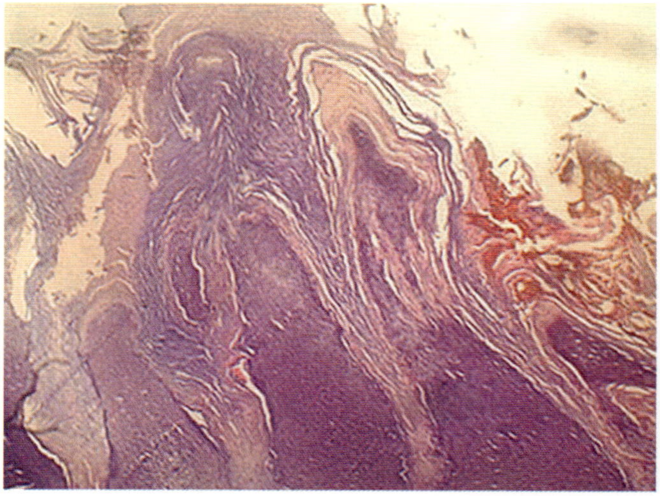

FIGURE 15.1.5.2

15.1.5: Verruca Vulgaris

15.1.5.1: Verruca vulgaris showing marked hyperkeratosis, acanthosis and papillomatosis with elongated rete ridges showing inward bending at the sides *(Scanner view)*

15.1.5.2: Stratum corneum above papillomatosis shows mounds of parakeratosis (filiform wart has distinct papillomatosis) *(Low power view)*

15.1.5.3: Large vacuolated cells in the granular cell layer with coarse keratohyaline granules *(High power view)*

15.1.5.4: Another case with hyperkeratosis, acanthosis and dermal infiltrate *(Scanner view)*

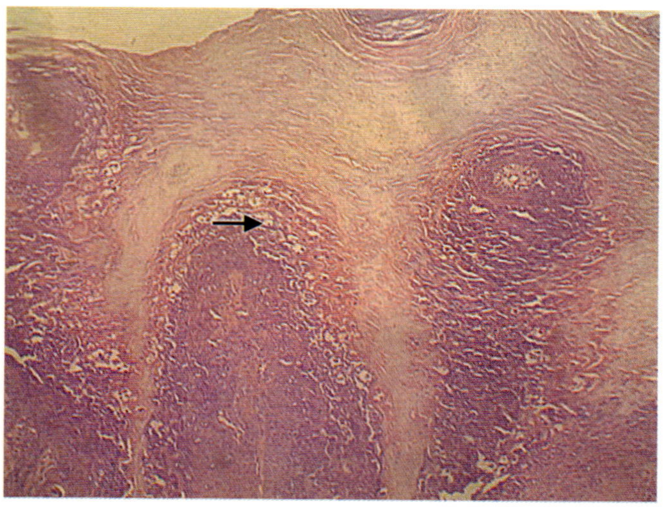

FIGURE 15.1.5.3

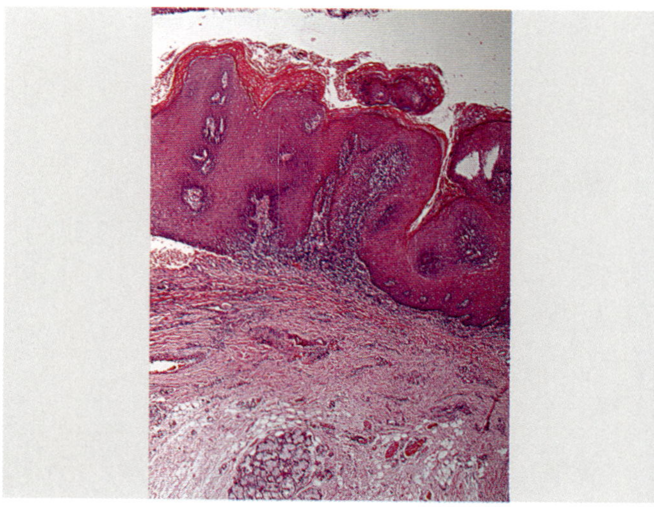

FIGURE 15.1.5.4

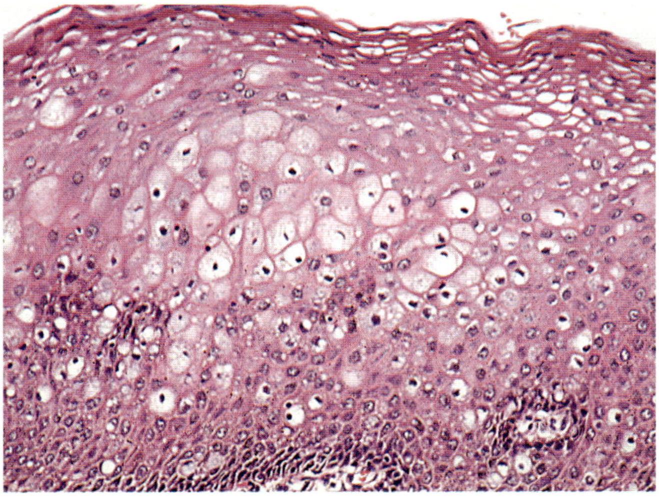

FIGURE 15.1.5.5

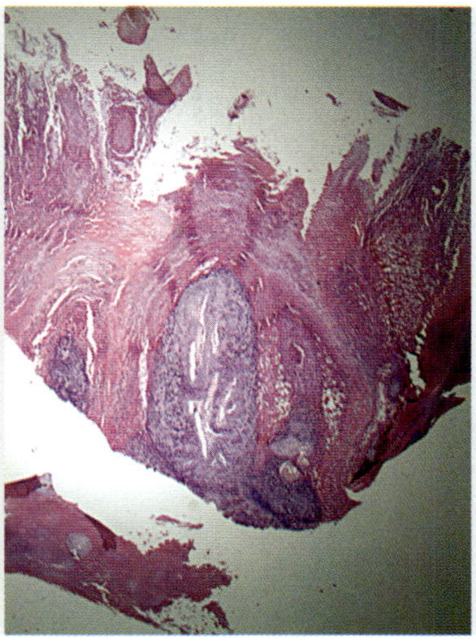

FIGURE 15.1.5.6

15.1.5.5: Koilocytic change with enlarged cell, pyknotic nucleus and clear cytoplasm (usually not seen in older lesions) *(High power view)*

15.1.5.6: Palmoplantar warts are situated deep enough to intrude in the dermis *(Scanner view)*

15.1.5.7: The cells containing coarse clumps of keratohyaline granules (hypergranulosis) *(Low power view)*

15.1.5.8: Prominent keratohyaline granules fuse to form eosinophilic inclusion bodies *(High power view)*

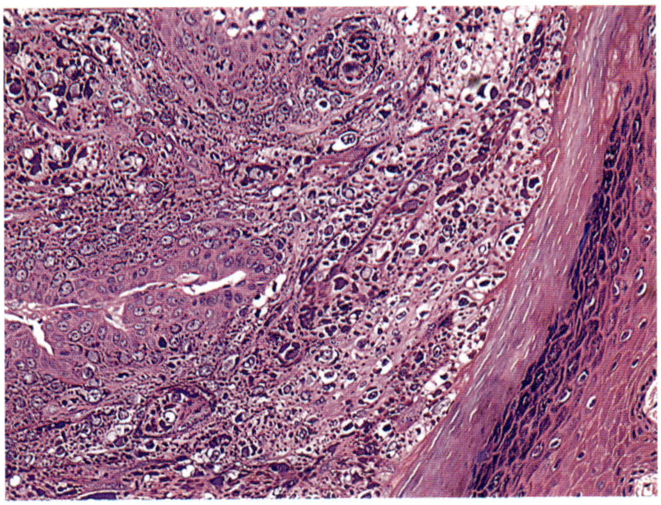

FIGURE 15.1.5.7

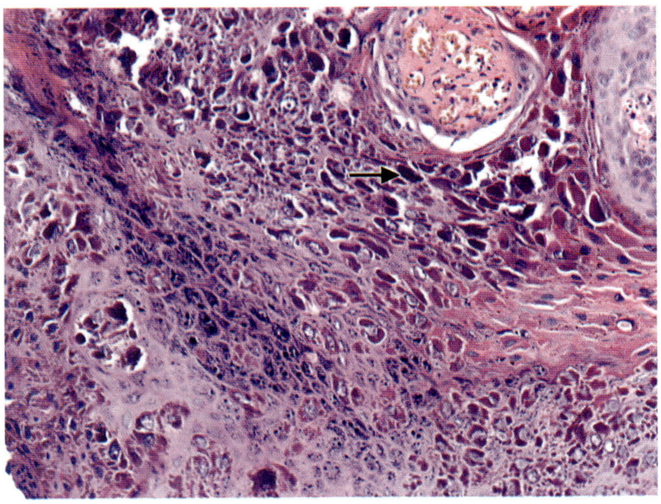

FIGURE 15.1.5.8

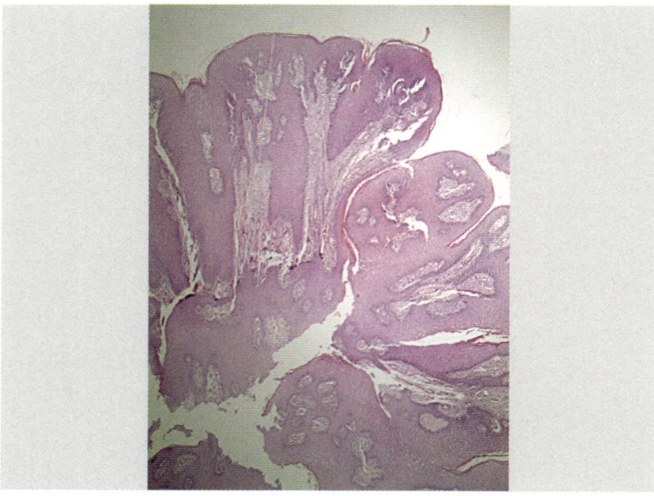

FIGURE 15.1.6.1

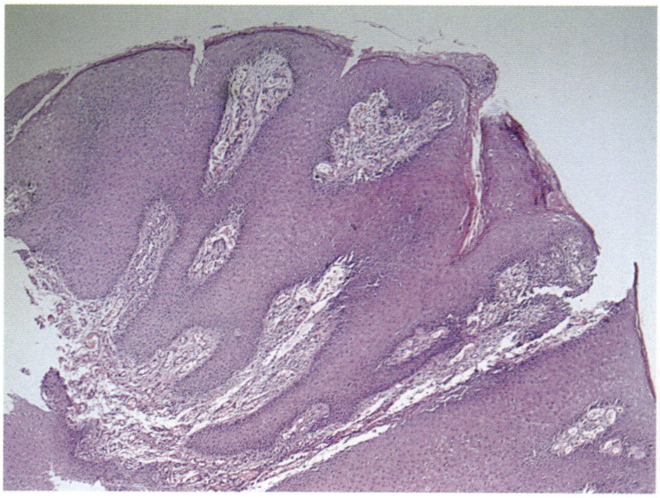

FIGURE 15.1.6.2

15.1.6: Condyloma Acuminatum

15.1.6.1: Marked papillomatous hyperplasia *(Scanner view)*

15.1.6.2: Closer view showing parakeratosis at the tips of papillae *(Low power view)*

15.1.6.3: Koilocytes seen as large keratinocytes with enlarged nucleus and perinuclear halo in the upper malpighian layer *(High power view)*

15.1.6.4: Dermis has dilated capillaries and chronic inflammation (podophyllin treated cases show epidermal pallor, degenerated keratinocytes and mitotic figures) *(High power view)*

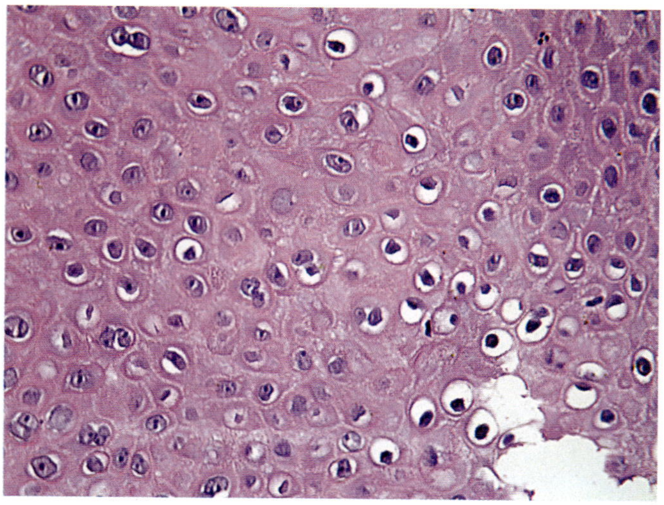

FIGURE 15.1.6.3

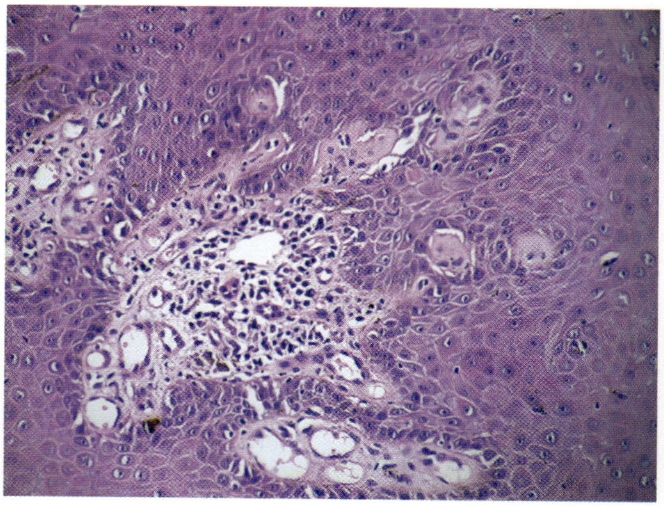

FIGURE 15.1.6.4

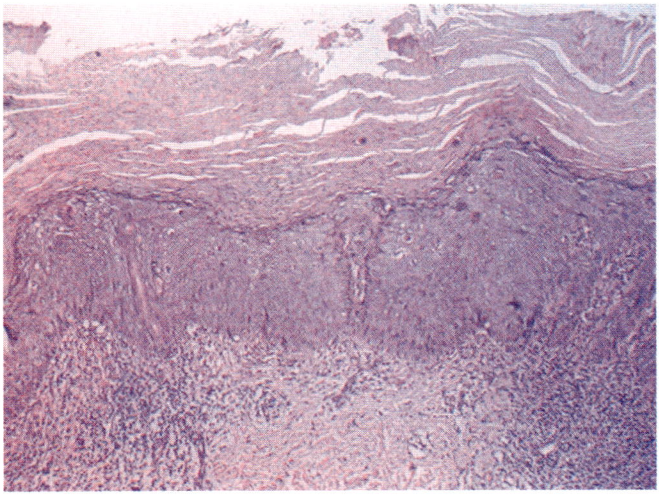

FIGURE 15.1.7.1

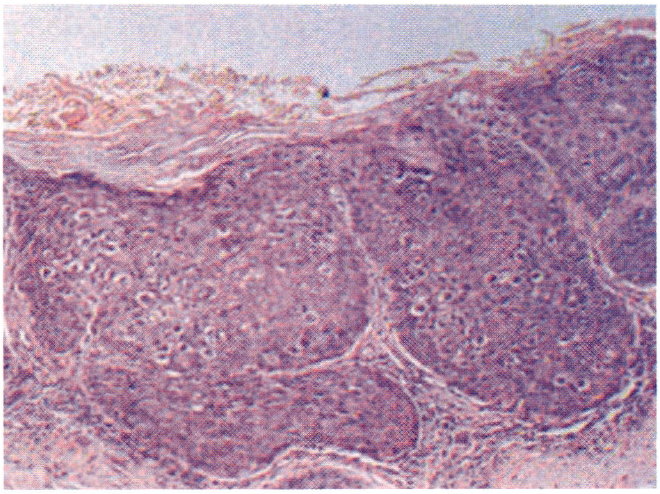

FIGURE 15.1.7.2

15.1.7: Bowenoid Papulosis

15.1.7.1: Parakeratosis, papillomatosis with acanthosis of epidermis, perivascular lymphocytes in the dermis *(Low power view)*

15.1.7.2: Full-thickness dysplastic changes with loss of polarity, however, the basement membrane is intact (difficult to differentiate from Bowen's) *(High power view)*

15.1.7.3: Frequent mitosis sometimes even atypical with many dyskeratotic cells *(High power view)*

15.1.7.4: Koilocytes like vacuolated cells and prominent keratohyaline granules *(High power view)*

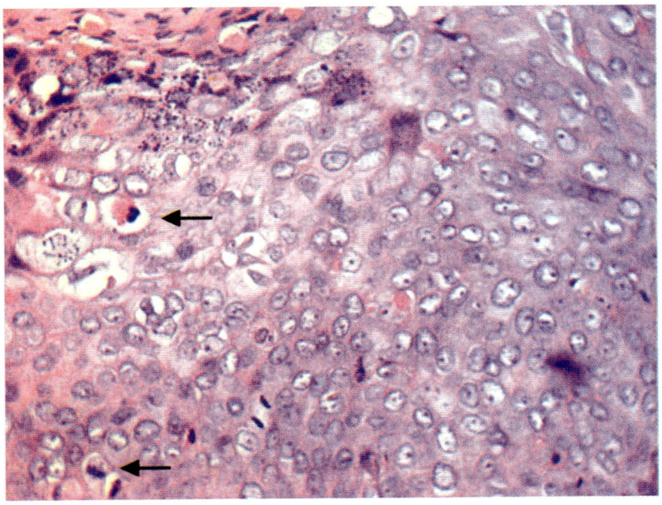

FIGURE 15.1.7.3

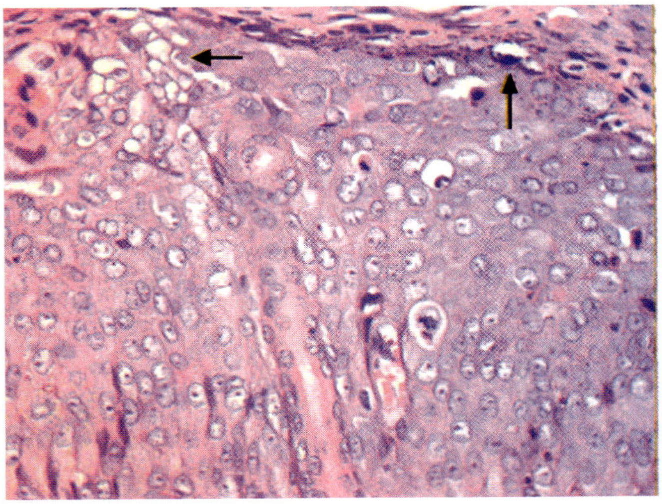

FIGURE 15.1.7.4

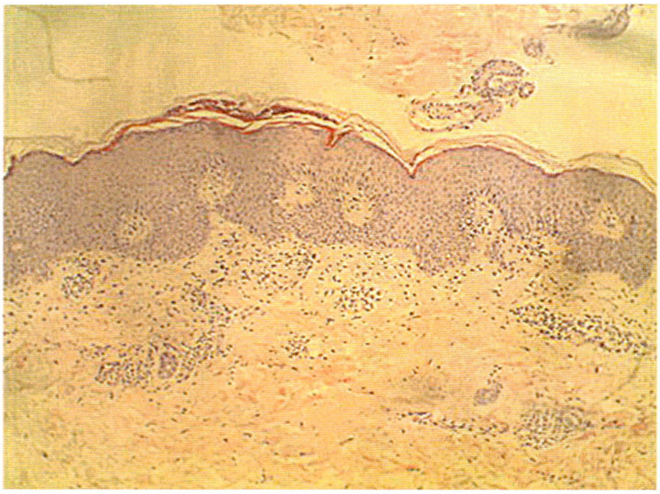

FIGURE 15.2.1.1

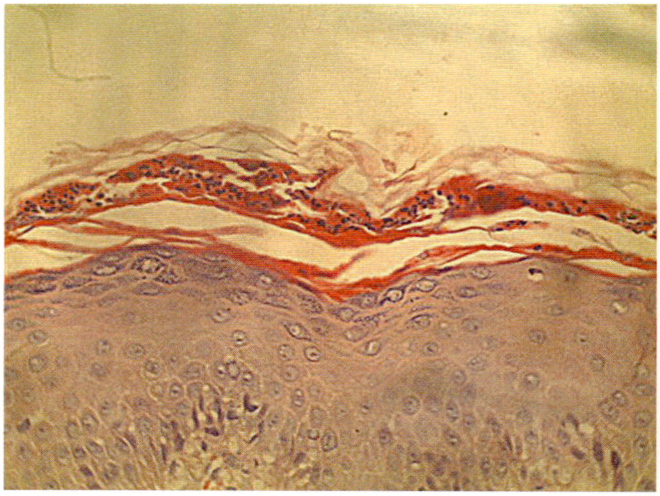

FIGURE 15.2.1.2

15.2: FUNGAL INFECTIONS

15.2.1: Dermatophytoses

15.2.1.1: Mild acanthosis and dermal inflammation (histologic features of dermatophytosis vary from psoriasiform to spongiotic tissue reaction pattern *(Low power view)*

15.2.1.2: The stratum corneum shows neutrophils and parakeratosis. 'Sandwich sign' refers to the presence of hyphae between upper basket-weave stratum corneum and lower compact orthokeratotic or parakeratotic stratum corneum *(High power view)*

15.2.1.3: PAS stain positive dermatophytes seen within crust as bright pink hyphal forms *(High power view)*

15.2.1.4: Another case with positive PAS stain. Neutrophils within stratum corneum with fungal hyphae [Gomori methenamine silver (GMS) stain is another stain for demonstrating the organisms] *(High power view)*

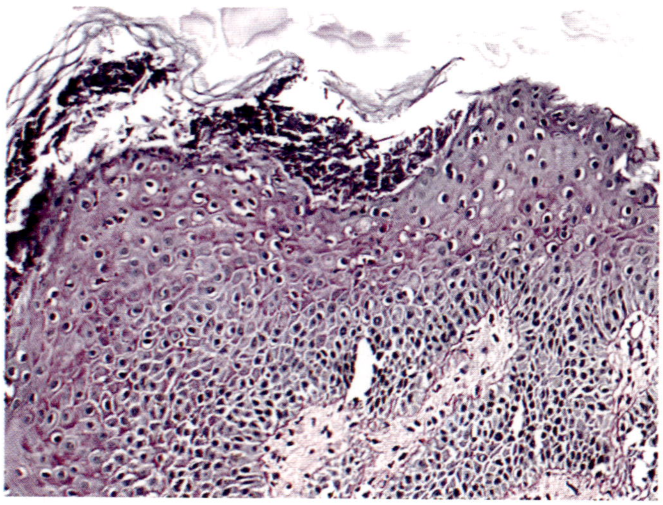

FIGURE 15.2.1.3

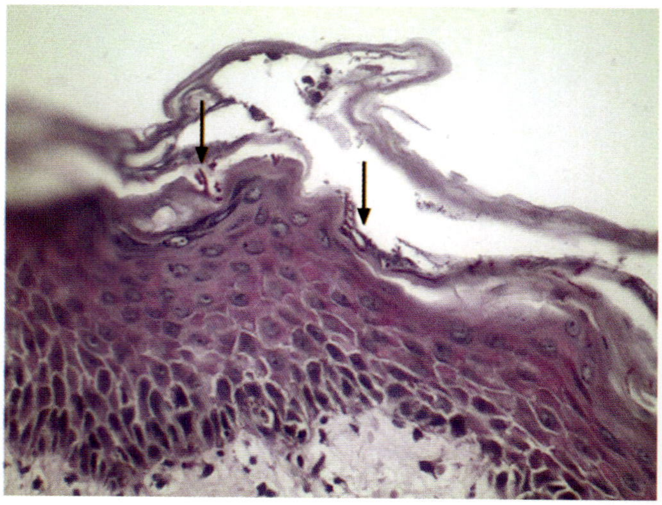

FIGURE 15.2.1.4

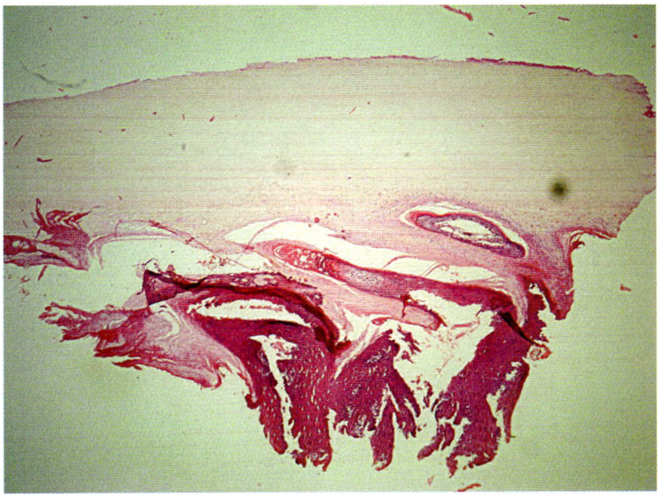

FIGURE 15.2.1.5

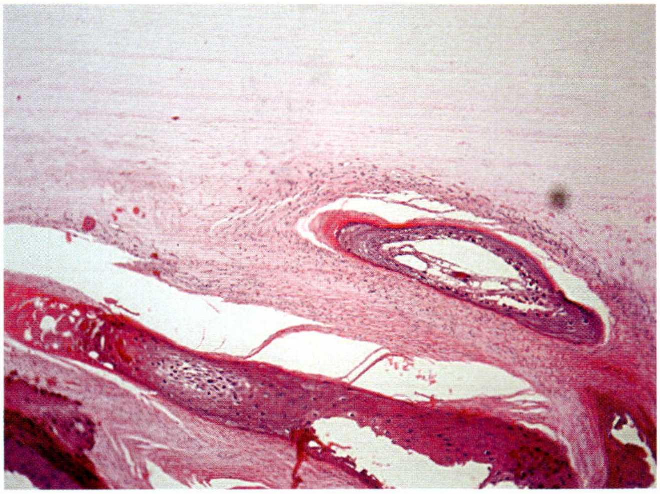

FIGURE 15.2.1.6

15.2.1.5: Nail biopsy showing keratinized epithelium *(Scanner view)*

15.2.1.6: Stratum corneum has parakeratosis and a few neutrophils *(Low power view)*

15.2.1.7: Shows hyphae and spores *(High power view)*

15.2.1.8: PAS stain positive for fungus *(High power view)*

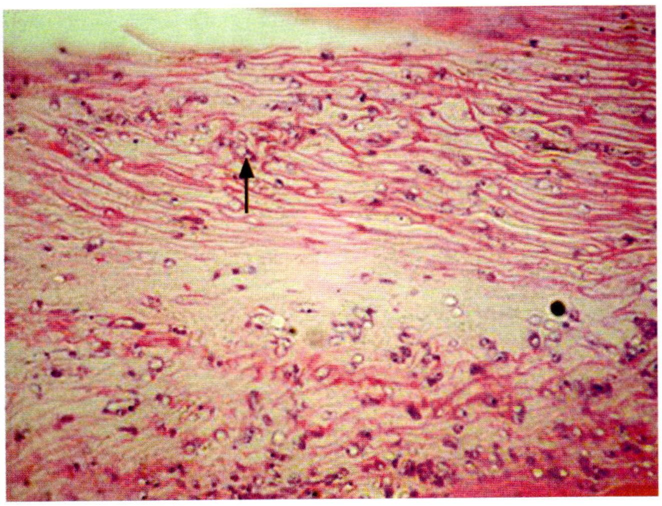

FIGURE 15.2.1.7

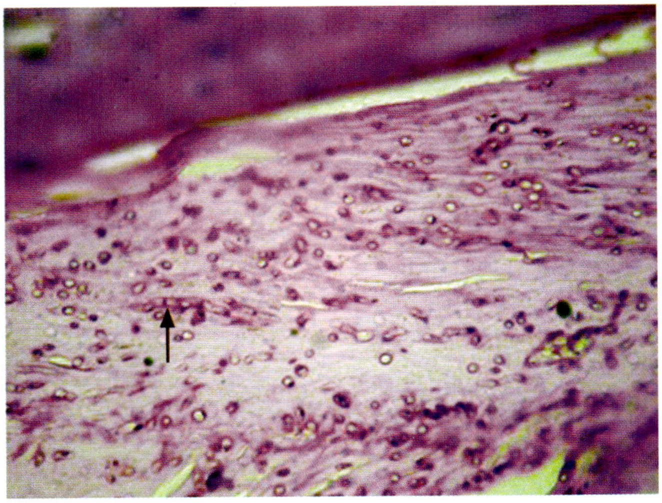

FIGURE 15.2.1.8

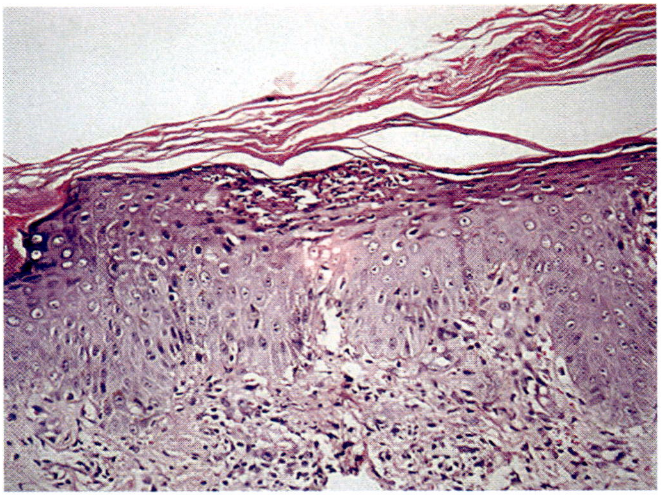

FIGURE 15.2.2.1.1

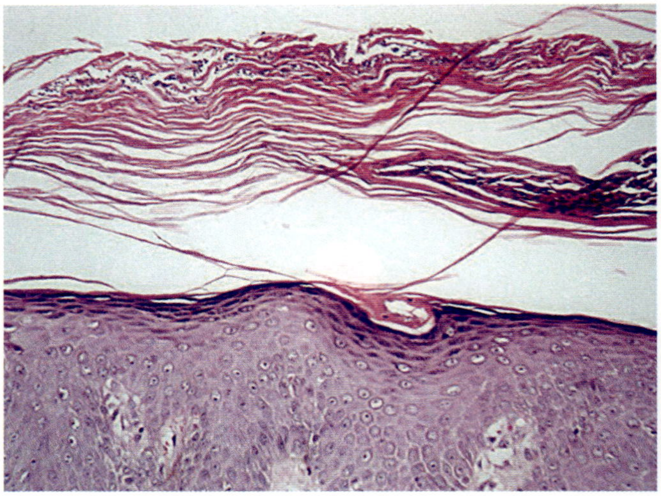

FIGURE 15.2.2.1.2

15.2.2: Candidosis (Candidiasis)

15.2.2.1: Acute Superficial Candidosis

15.2.2.1.1: Neutrophils below the stratum corneum in the form of subcorneal pustule with spongiosis *(Low power view)*

15.2.2.1.2: Fungal elements seen in the stratum corneum *(Low power view)*

15.2.2.1.3: Mycelia as well as spores *(High power view)*

15.2.2.1.4: Oil immersion microscopy shows spores

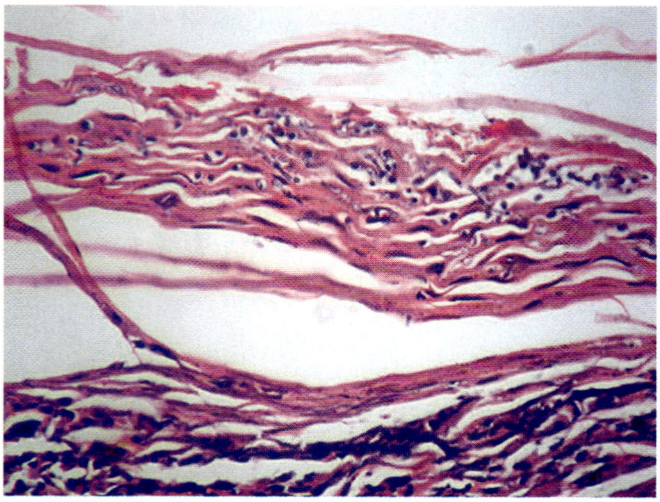

FIGURE 15.2.2.1.3

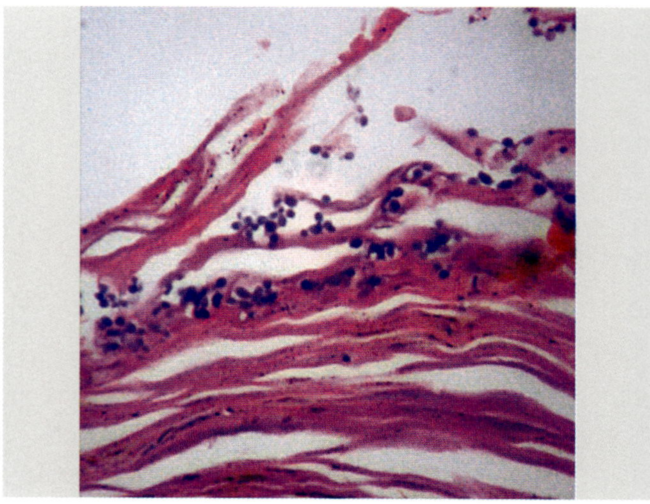

FIGURE 15.2.2.1.4

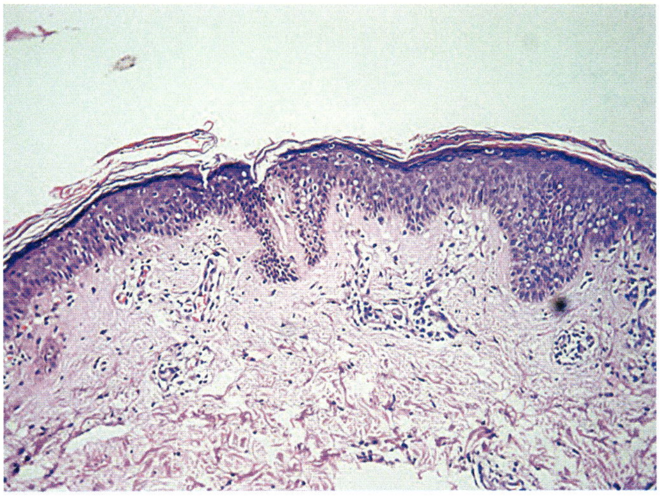

FIGURE 15.2.3.1

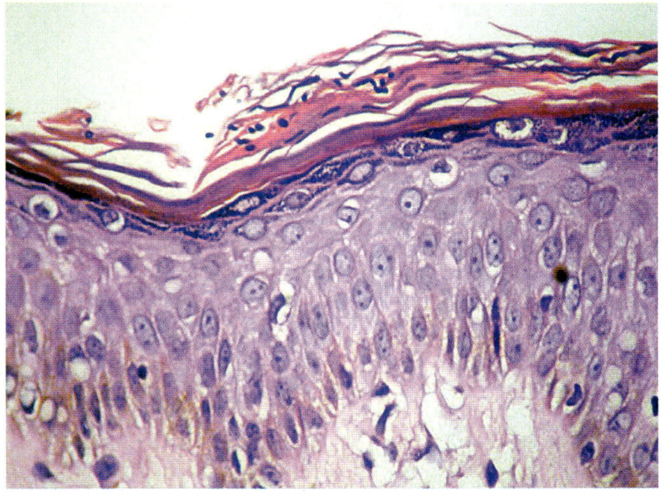

FIGURE 15.2.3.2

15.2.3: Pityriasis Versicolor

15.2.3.1: Epidermis shows hyperkeratosis and acanthosis. The dermis contains a mild, superficial perivascular lymphocytic infiltrate *(Low power view)*

15.2.3.2: Stratum corneum shows round budding yeasts (blastoconidia) and short-septate hyphae (pseudomycelium), giving a 'spaghetti and meatballs' appearance *(High power view)*

15.2.3.3: Another case with oil immersion microscopy showing hyphae and budding yeasts

15.2.3.4: PAS stain (pityrosporum are clearly seen in PAS preparations) (They also stain with Alcian blue, Congo red, and the Masson–Fontana stain. They are not acid fast) *(High power view)*

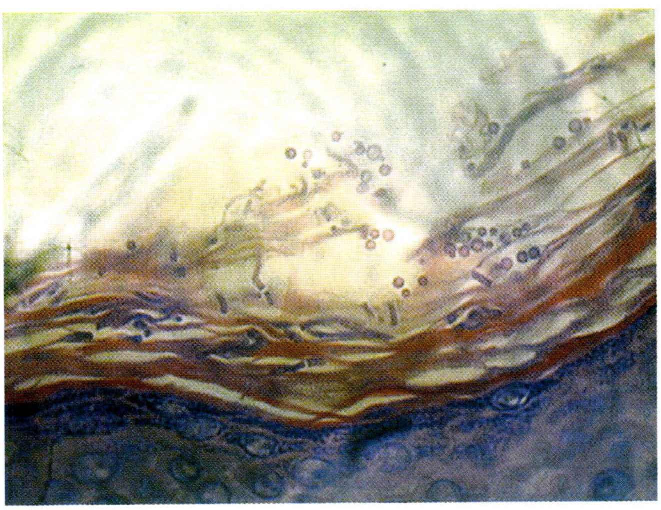

FIGURE 15.2.3.3

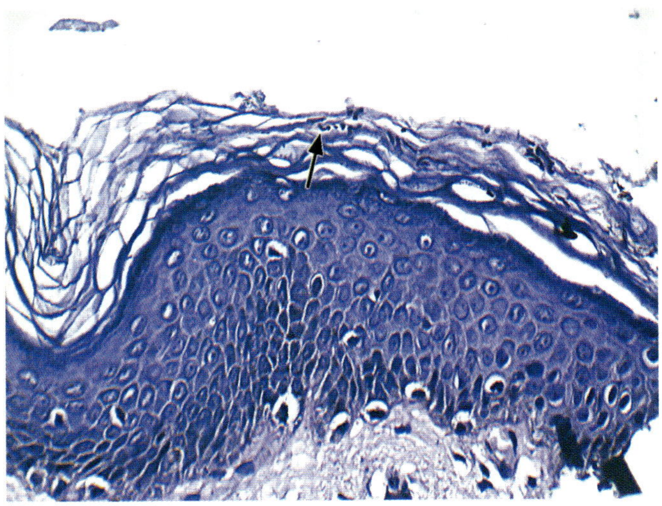

FIGURE 15.2.3.4

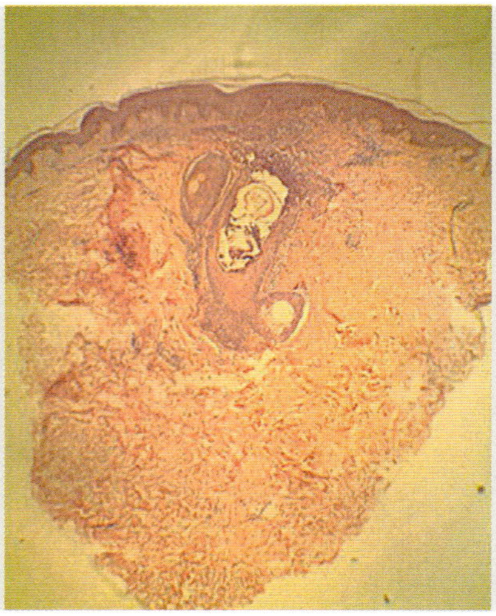

FIGURE 15.2.4.1

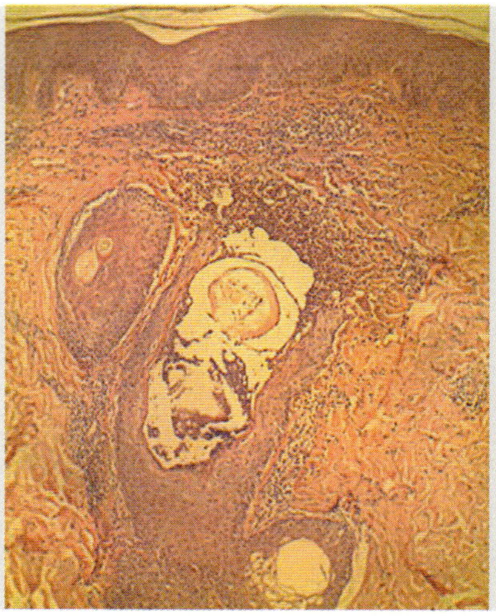

FIGURE 15.2.4.2

15.2.4: Fungal Folliculitis

15.2.4.1: Pityrosporum folliculitis—involved follicle is dilated and plugged with keratinous material and debris *(Scanner view)*

15.2.4.2: There is mild chronic inflammatory cell infiltrate around the infundibular portion of the follicle *(Low power view)*

15.2.4.3: Disruption of the follicular epithelium is sometimes found with keratinous material, neutrophils, and other inflammatory cells in the perifollicular dermis *(High power view)*

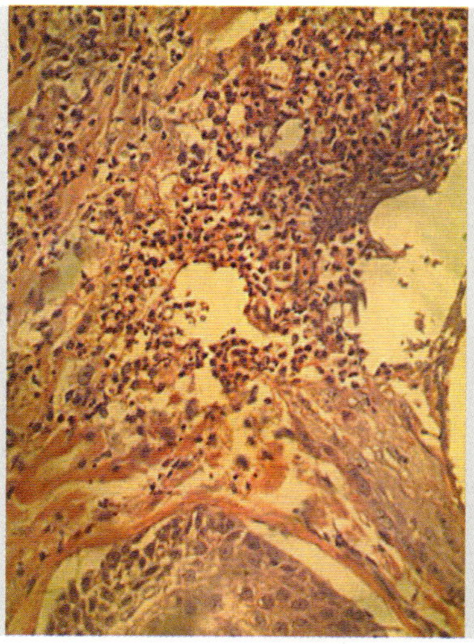

FIGURE 15.2.4.3

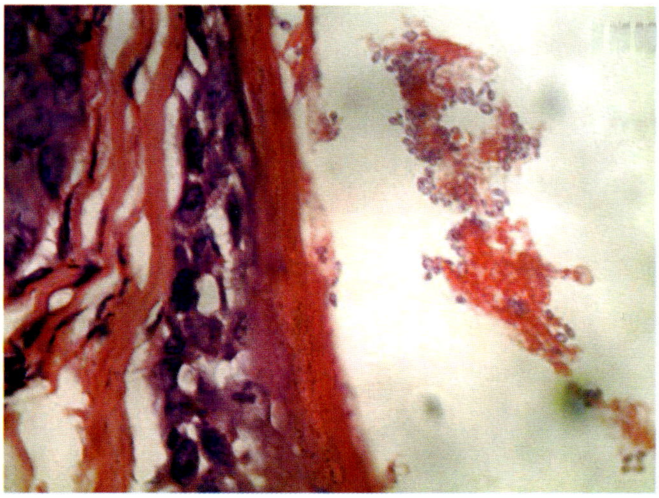

FIGURE 15.2.4.4

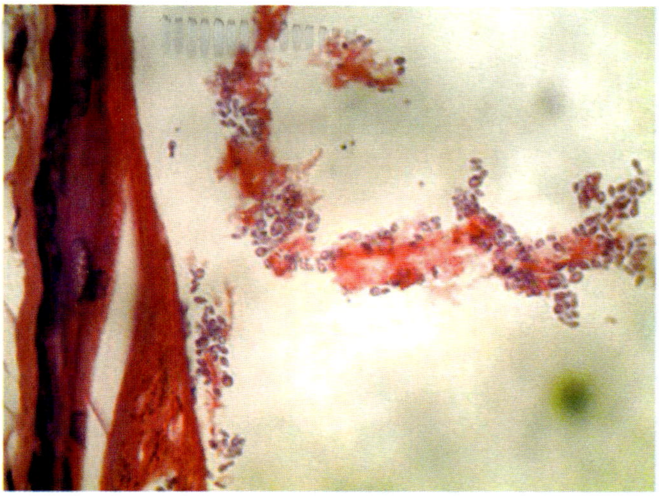

FIGURE 15.2.4.5

15.2.4.4: Section reveals spherical to oval yeast-like organisms, 2–4 µm in diameter found inside the follicle *(High power view)*

15.2.4.5: Another view showing spherical yeast like organisms *(High power view)*

15.2.4.6: This section shows endothrix infection with organisms and inflammatory infiltrate *(High power view)*

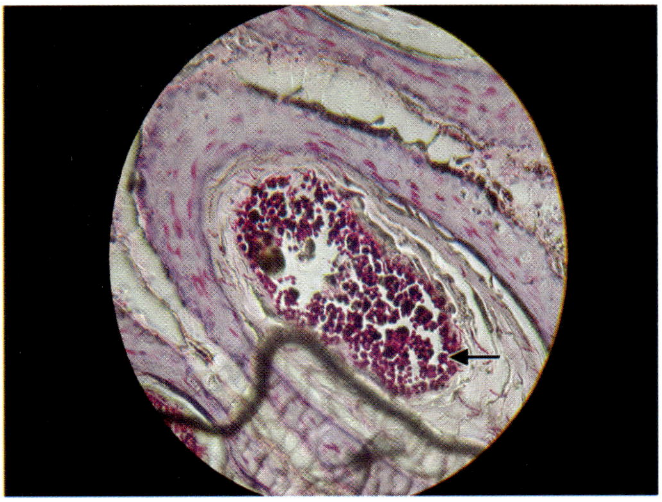

FIGURE 15.2.4.6

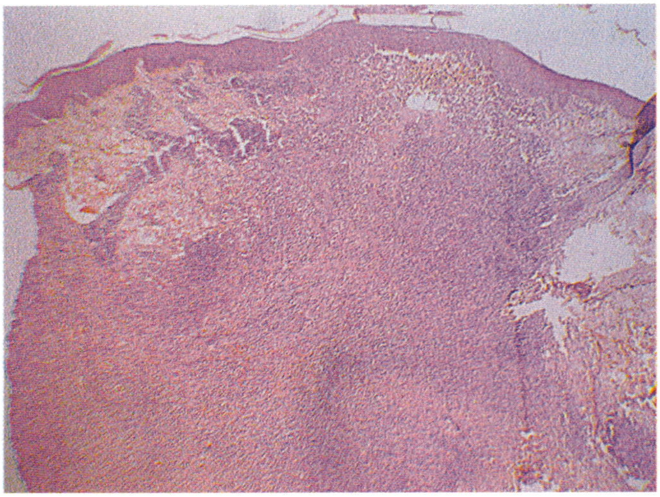

FIGURE 15.3.1.1

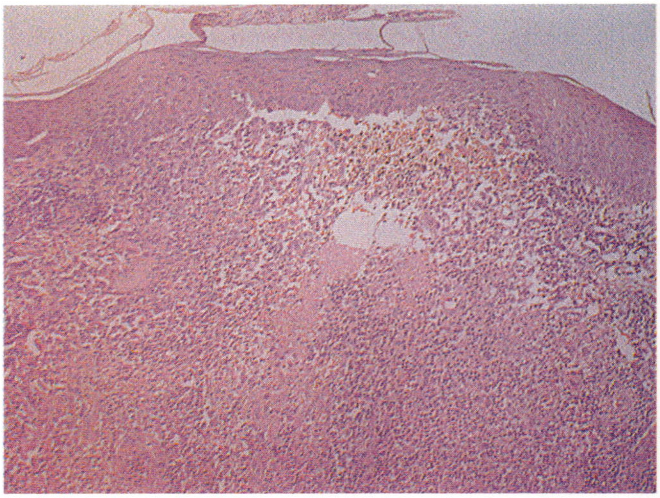

FIGURE 15.3.1.2

15.3: BACTERIAL INFECTIONS

15.3.1: Cellulitis

15.3.1.1: The cellulitides are characterized histopathologically by an infiltrate of neutrophils throughout the dermis and/or the subcutaneous tissue *(Scanner view)*

15.3.1.2: Sections show subepidermal edema and vascular ectasia *(Low power view)*

15.3.1.3: Low power view of dense and diffuse neutrophilic infiltrate *(Low power view)*

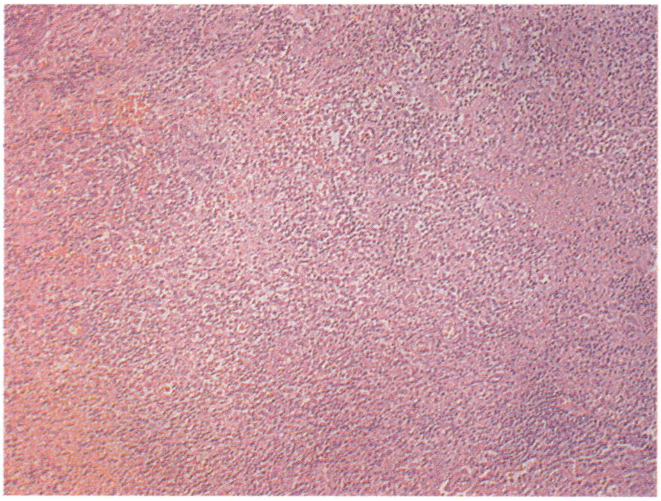

FIGURE 15.3.1.3

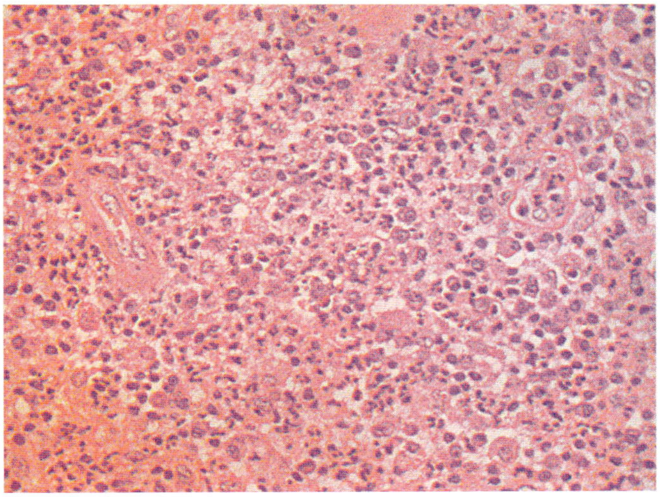

FIGURE 15.3.1.4

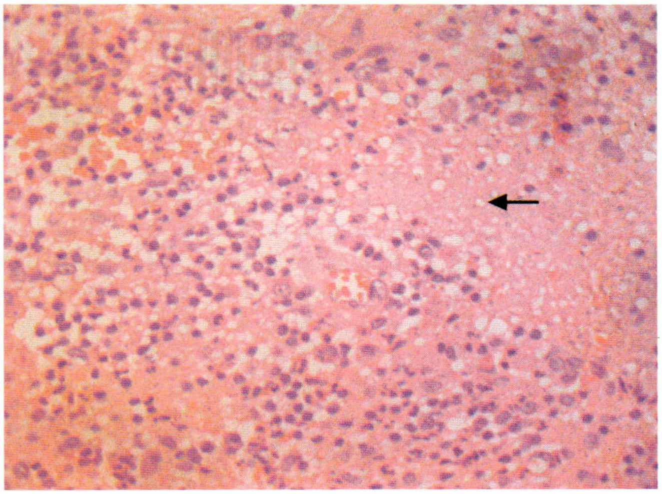

FIGURE 15.3.1.5

15.3.1.4: Closer view of neutrophilic abscesses *(High power view)*

15.3.1.5: There may be foci of necrosis *(High power view)*

15.3.1.6: Involvement of the subcutis may lead to a predominantly septal panniculitis *(Low power view)*

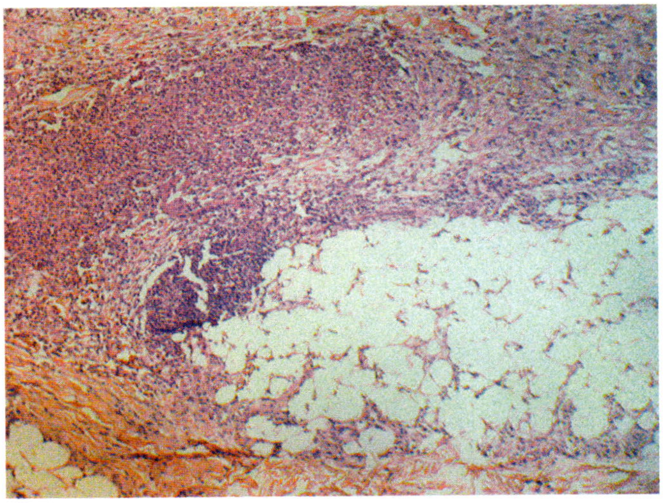

FIGURE 15.3.1.6

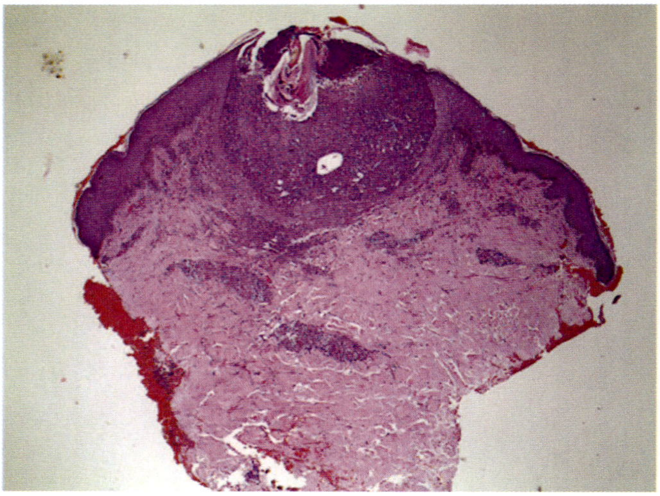

FIGURE 15.3.2.1

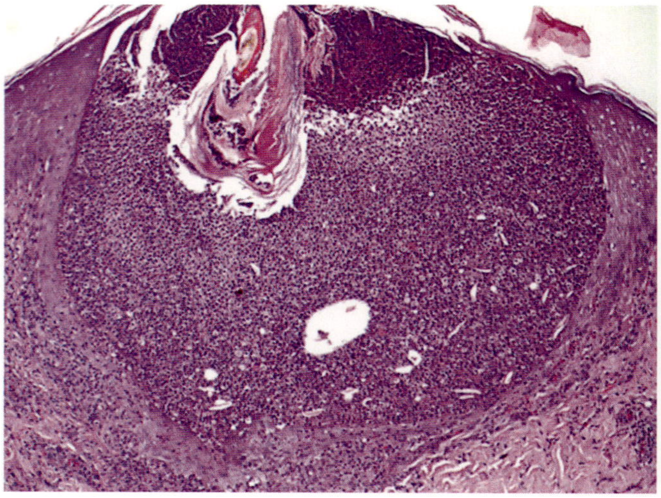

FIGURE 15.3.2.2

15.3.2: Folliculitis

15.3.2.1: Dermal abscess centered on a hair follicle. Extension to deep dermis *(Scanner view)*

15.3.2.2: Hair follicle usually destroyed, although a residual hair shaft is sometimes present in the center of the abscess. The overlying epidermis is eventually destroyed and the surface is covered by an inflammatory crust *(Low power view)*

15.3.2.3: Closer view of neutrophilic abscess *(High power view)*

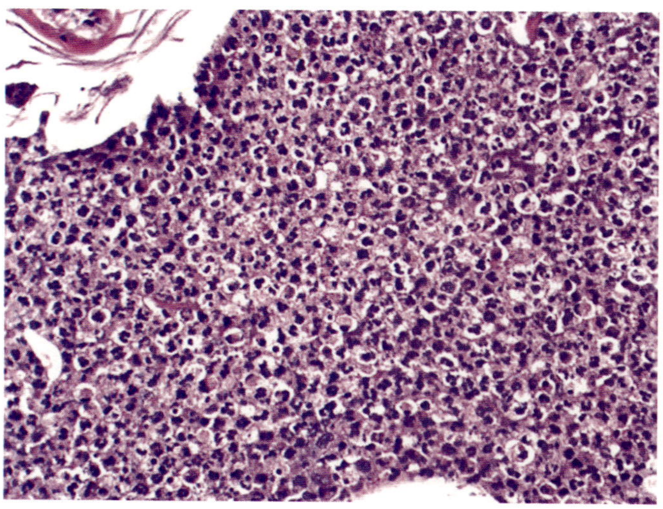

FIGURE 15.3.2.3

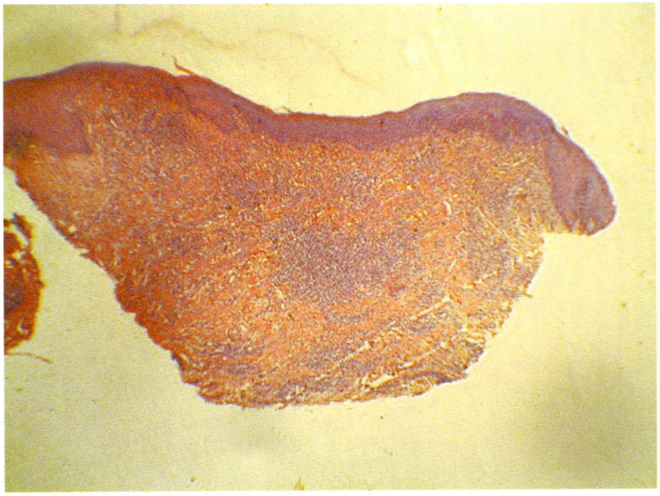

FIGURE 15.3.3.1

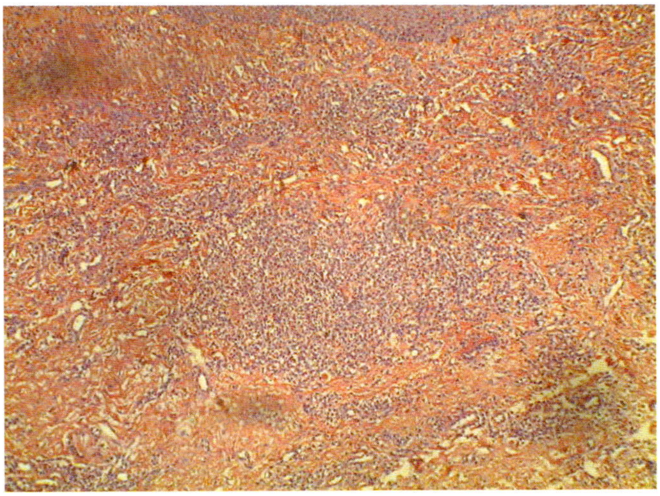

FIGURE 15.3.3.2

15.3.3: Rhinoscleroma

15.3.3.1: Dense inflammatory infiltrate in the dermis *(Scanner view)*

15.3.3.2: Low power view of polymorphous infiltrate *(Low power view)*

15.3.3.3: Many plasma cells with Russell bodies *(High power view)*

15.3.3.4: High power view of plasma cells

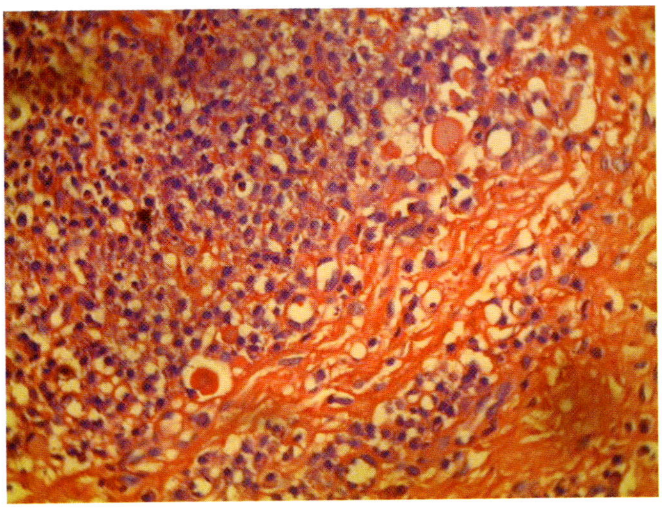

FIGURE 15.3.3.3

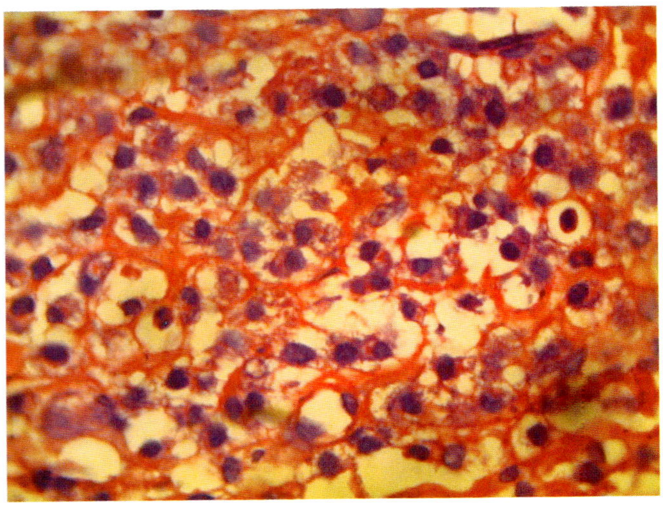

FIGURE 15.3.3.4

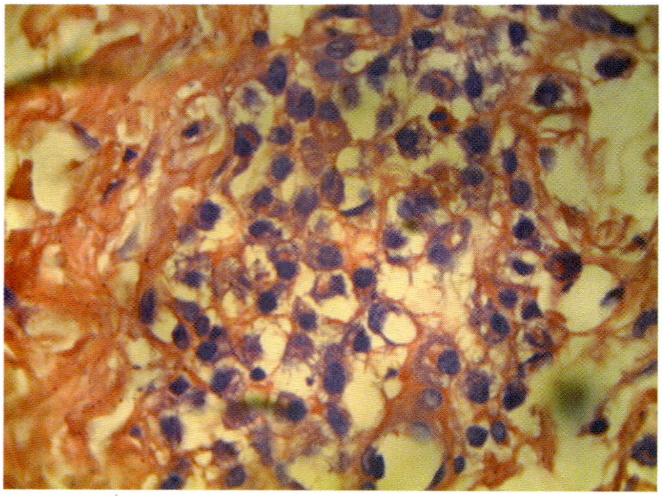

FIGURE 15.3.3.5

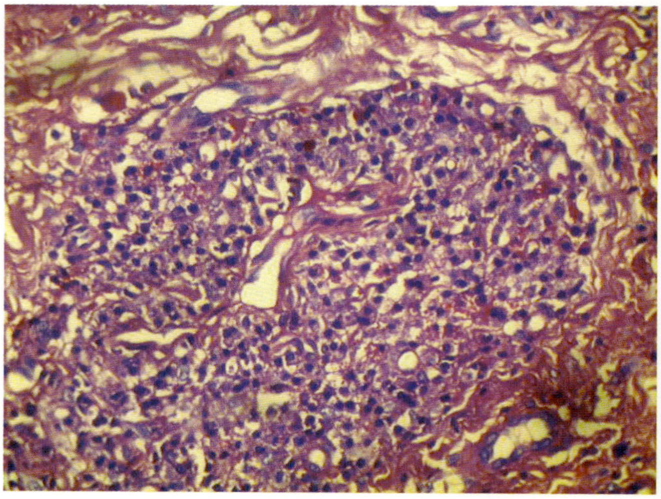

FIGURE 15.3.3.6

15.3.3.5: Large macrophages with vacuolated cytoplasm (Mikulicz cells) *(High power view)*

15.3.3.6: PAS positive organisms in the cytoplasm of these cells *(High power view)*

15.3.3.7: High-power view of PAS positive organisms

15.3.3.8: Gram stain showing organisms (orgtanisms are best visualized with silver impregnation methods, Warthin–Starry stain) *(High power view)*

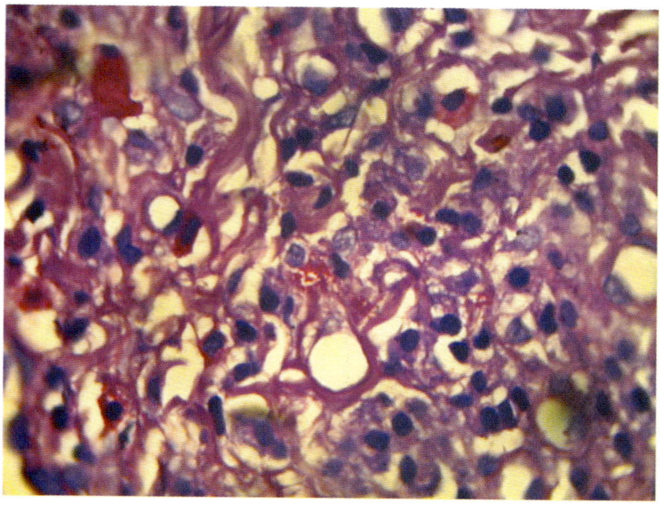

FIGURE 15.3.3.7

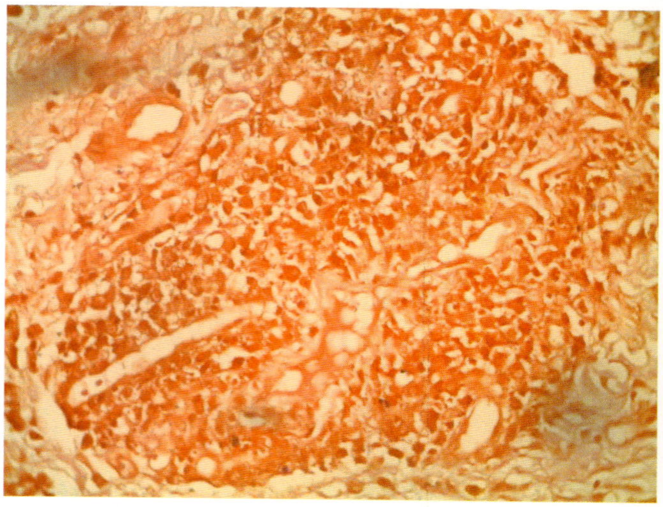

FIGURE 15.3.3.8

DIFFERENTIAL DIAGNOSIS

1. Infections without remarkable epidermal or dermal changes
   a. Superficial dermatophytes
   b. Tinea versicolor
   c. Erythrasma
2. Infections with predominant plasma cells
   a. Chancroid
   b. Lymphogranuloma venereum
   c. Granuloma inguinale
   d. Syphilis
   e. Yaws
3. Infections with predominant neutrophils
   a. Anthrax
   b. Ecthyma
   c. Type 2 lepra reaction
   d. Deep fungal infections

DIAGNOSTIC PEARLS

1. Impetigo: Acantholysis is not prominent and Gram-positive cocci seen.
2. Chancroid: Tissue necrosis, fibrin, red cells, and neutrophils in the upper part. Middle zone of vascular proliferation and inflammatory infiltrate. Plasma cells and lymphocytes in the deep.
3. Malakoplakia: Macrophages containing PAS-positive inclusions called von Hansemann cells. A few cells contain calcospherites with a homogeneous appearance—the Michaelis-Gutmann bodies.
4. In rhinosporidiosis, there are large spherical sporangia containing hundreds to thousands of endospores.
5. Milkers nodule: Demonstrates vacuolization and ballooning of the cells in the upper epidermis, leading to multilocular vesicles. Later on it shows papillary edema, acanthosis and chronic inflammation.
6. Inclusion bodies are present in the cytoplasm of the keratinocytes in the upper epidermis in orf.
7. There is follicular dilatation, perifollicular chronic inflammation and eosinophilic material surrounding the mites in demodicidosis.

16

Epidermal Premalignant and Malignant Conditions

Chapter Outline

16.1: Seborrheic Keratosis
16.2: Actinic Keratosis
16.3: Bowen's Disease
16.4: Erythroplasia
16.5: Basal Cell Carcinoma
16.6: Squamous Cell Carcinoma
16.7: Verrucous Carcinoma
16.8: Keratoacanthoma

*Pradeep Mahajan, Nandakumar Gopinath,
Nathan Lee, Jerad Gardner, Rathnam Attilee*

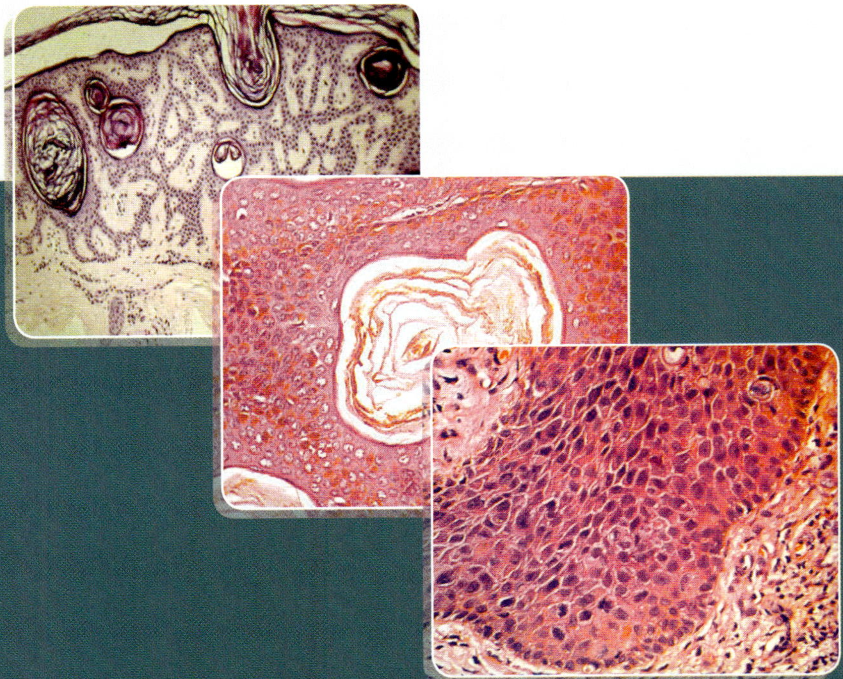

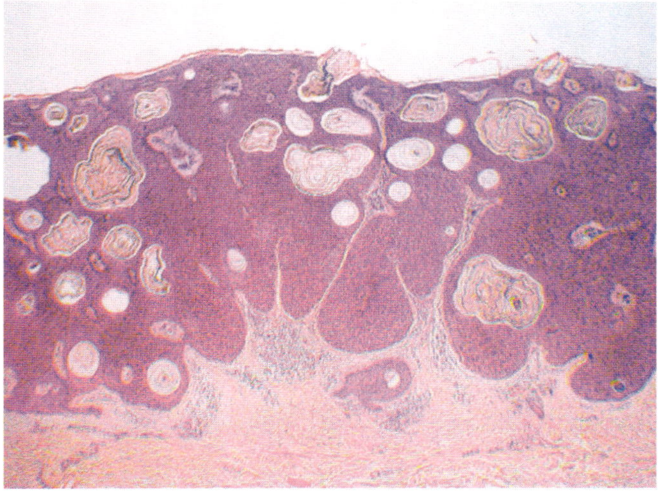

FIGURE 16.1.1

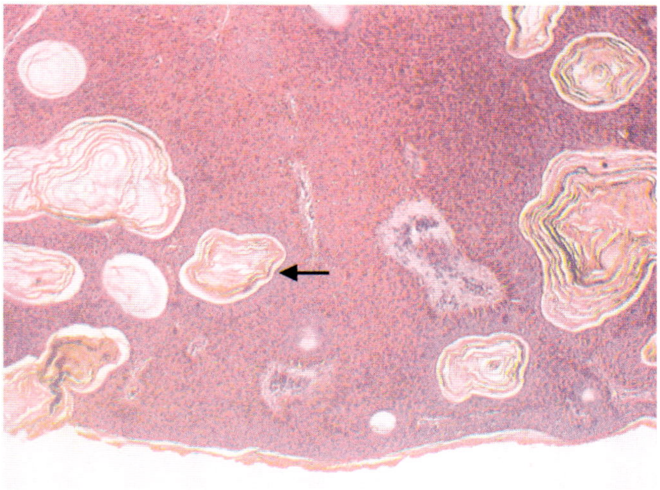

FIGURE 16.1.2

16.1: SEBORRHEIC KERATOSIS*

16.1.1: Composed of broad columns of basaloid cells, horny invaginations which appear as pseudo horn cysts on cross section and true horn cysts (both demonstrate thin granular cell layer with sudden and complete keratinization)—acanthotic type *(Scanner view)*

16.1.2: Basaloid cells and horn cysts *(Low power view)*

16.1.3: Pigmented basaloid cells *(High power view)*

16.1.4: Horn cyst *(High power view)*

*Seborrheic keratosis is a benign tumor of the epidermis but is included in this chapter for convenience.

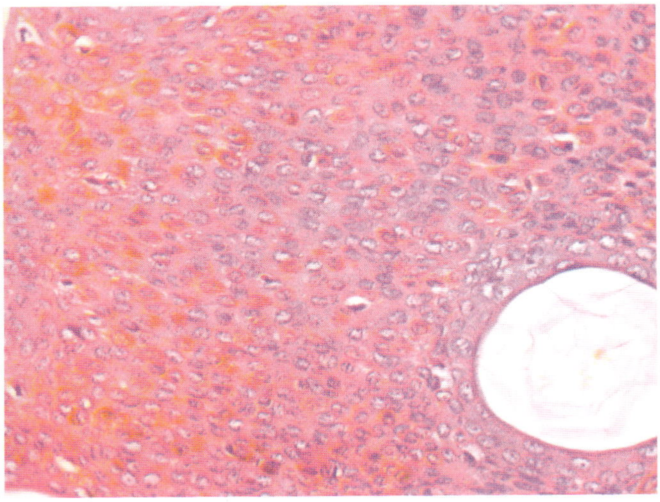

FIGURE 16.1.3

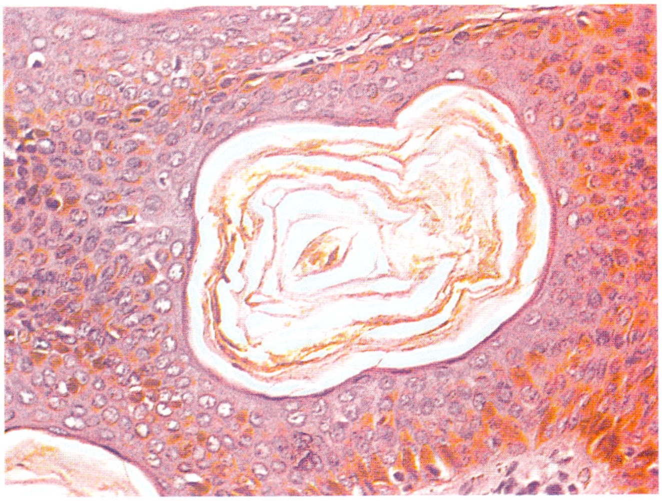

FIGURE 16.1.4

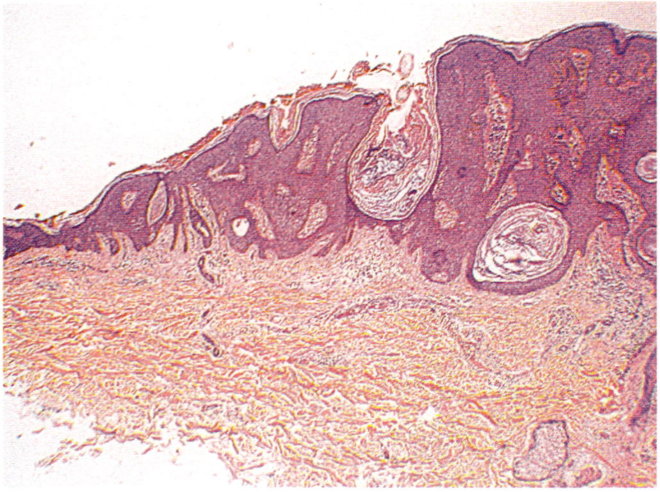

FIGURE 16.1.5

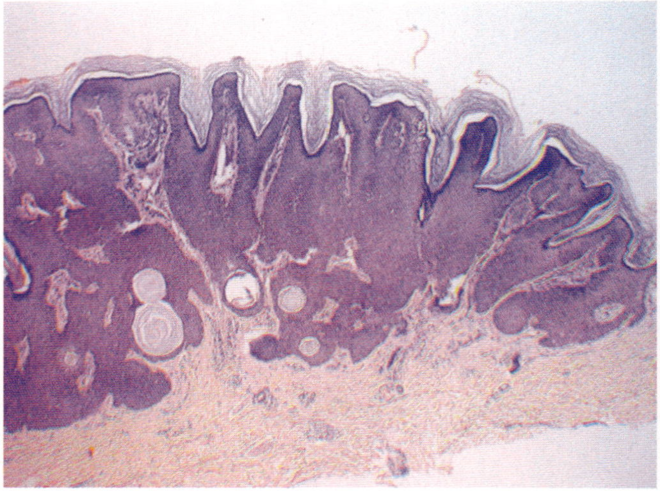

FIGURE 16.1.6

16.1.5: Exophytic growth with lower margin of the lesion and surrounding normal epidermis are in line *(Scanner view)*

16.1.6: Hyperkeratotic type with varying degrees of hyperkeratosis, papillomatosis, and acanthosis *(Scanner view)*

16.1.7: Hyperkeratosis and papillomatosis *(Low power view)*

16.1.8: Irritated type with areas of squamous differentiation (there is also a heavy inflammatory cell infiltrate, with lichenoid features, in the upper dermis) *(Scanner view)*

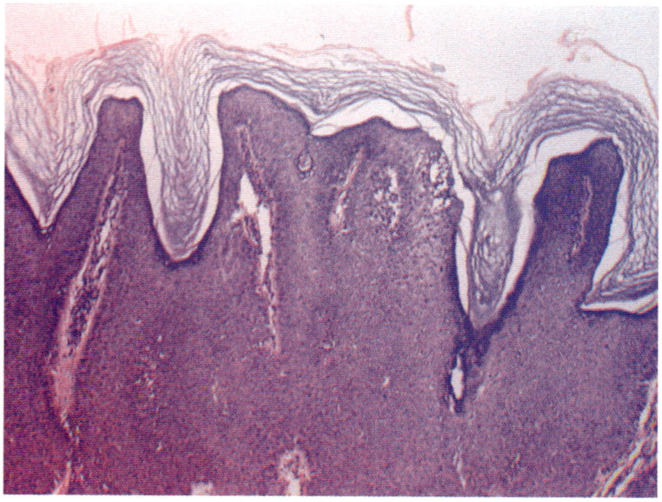

FIGURE 16.1.7

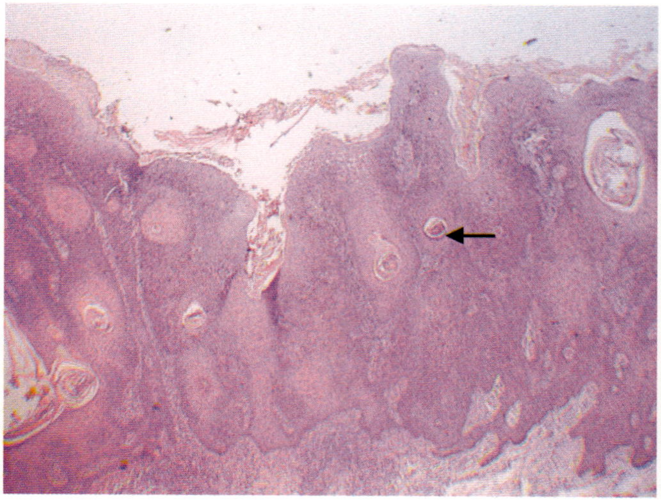

FIGURE 16.1.8

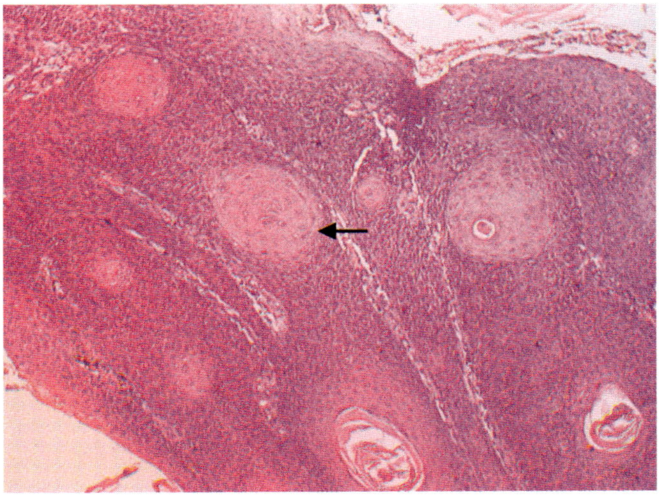

FIGURE 16.1.9

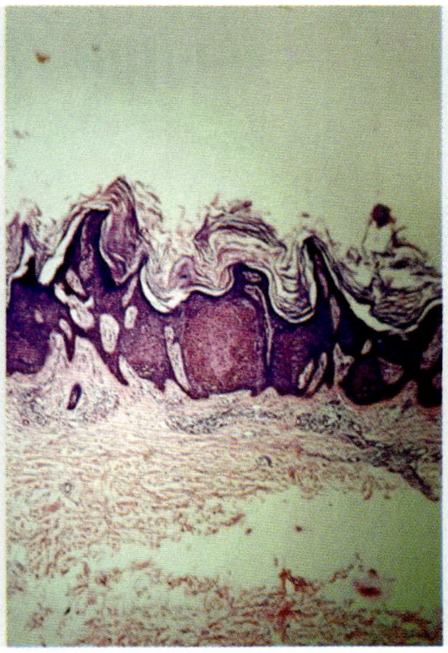

FIGURE 16.1.10

16.1.9: Closer view of squamous eddies *(Low power view)*

16.1.10: Clonal type—have intraepidermal nests of basaloid cells resembling the Borst-Jadassohn phenomenon *(Scanner view)*

16.1.11: Intraepidermal nests of basaloid cells *(Low power view)*

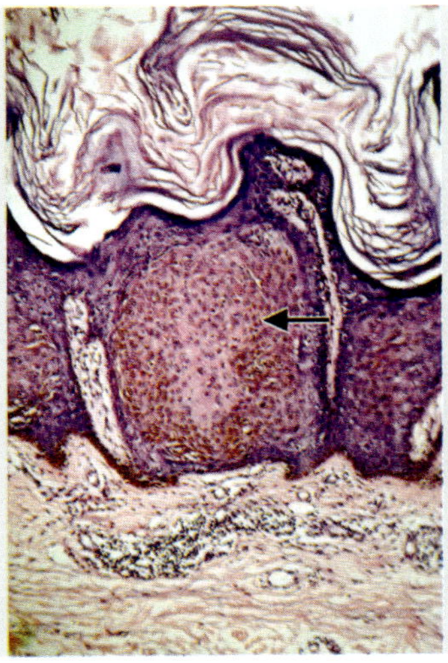

FIGURE 16.1.11

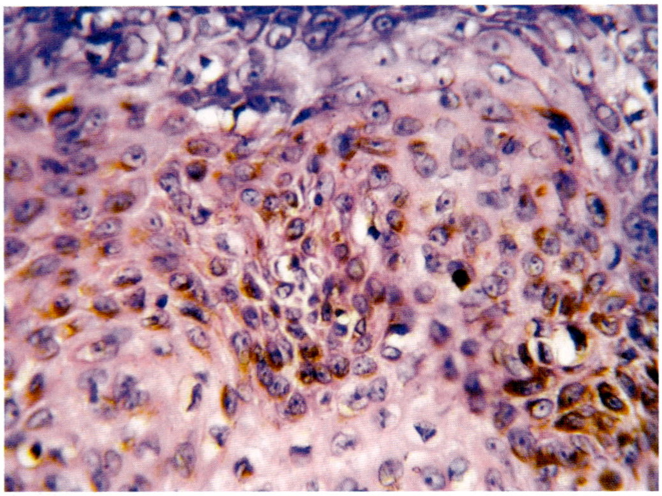

FIGURE 16.1.12

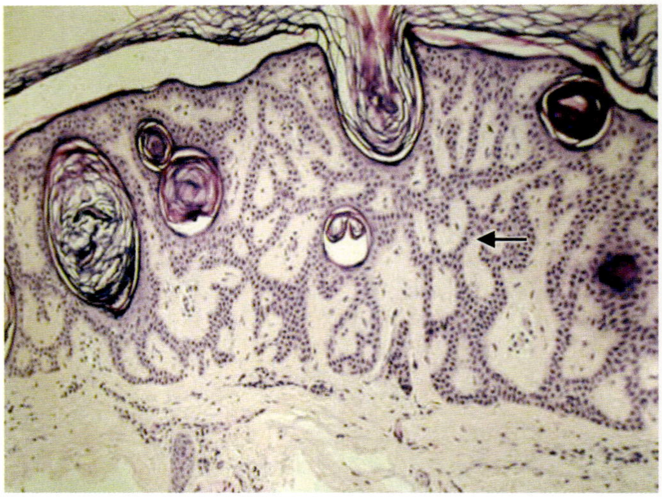

FIGURE 16.1.13

16.1.12: Variable amounts of melanin pigment are present within the cytoplasm of the basaloid cells. These are epithelial cells not melanocytes *(High power view)*

16.1.13: Adenoid variant—interlacing thin strands of basaloid cells, often pigmented, enclosing small horn cysts *(Low power view)*

16.1.14: Adenoid variant—interconnected strands of basaloid cells are punctuated by horn cysts. This variant often evolves from a solar lentigo *(High power view)*

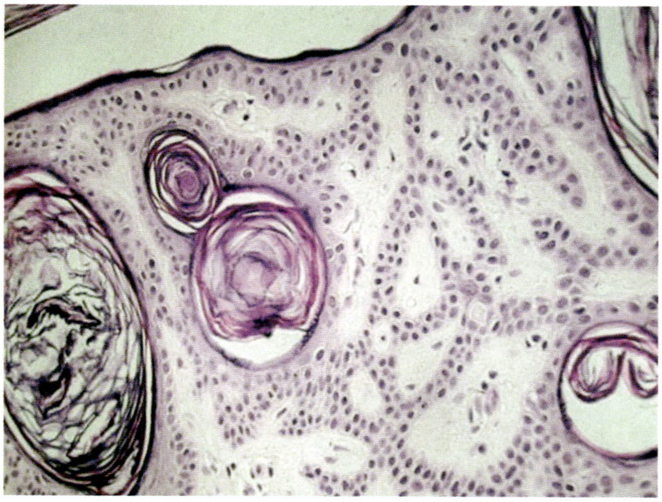

FIGURE 16.1.14

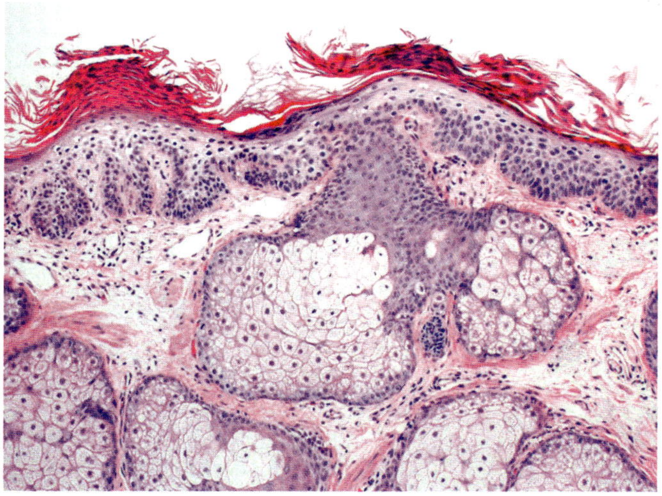

FIGURE 16.2.1

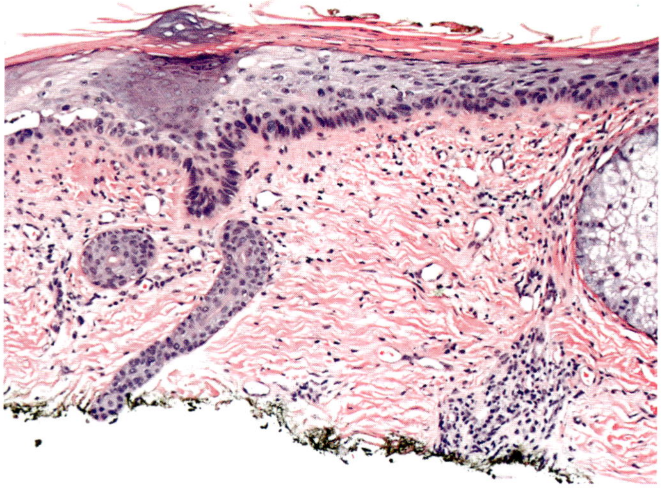

FIGURE 16.2.2

16.2: ACTINIC KERATOSIS

16.2.1: Actinin keratosis—disorganized keratinocytes with nuclear atypia seen mostly in lower epidermis, overlying parakeratosis and diminished granular cell layer *(Low power view)*

16.2.2: Actinic keratosis—atypical nuclei crowding along the basal layer, sparing of adnexal outlets such as follicular ostia and acrosyringium (shown here) *(High power view)*

16.2.3: Crowding of nuclei at basal cell layer, intact basement membrane, dilated capillaries and lymphocytic infiltrate in the dermis. Types—hypertrophic, proliferative, atrophic *(High power view)*

16.2.4: Acantholytic type—case showing hyperkeratosis, papillomatosis, atypia *(Low power view)*

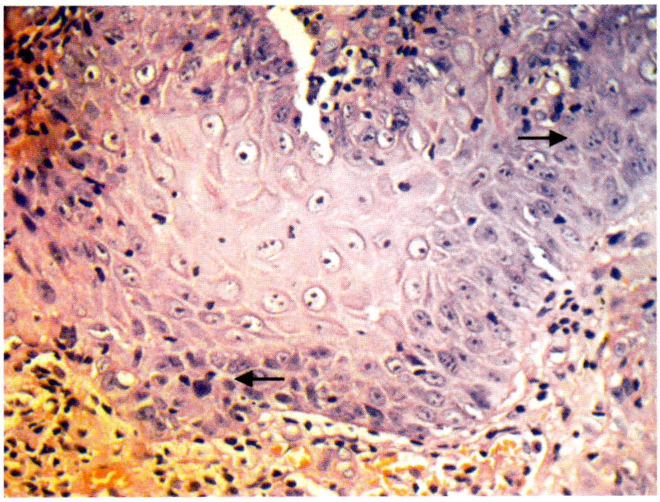

FIGURE 16.2.3

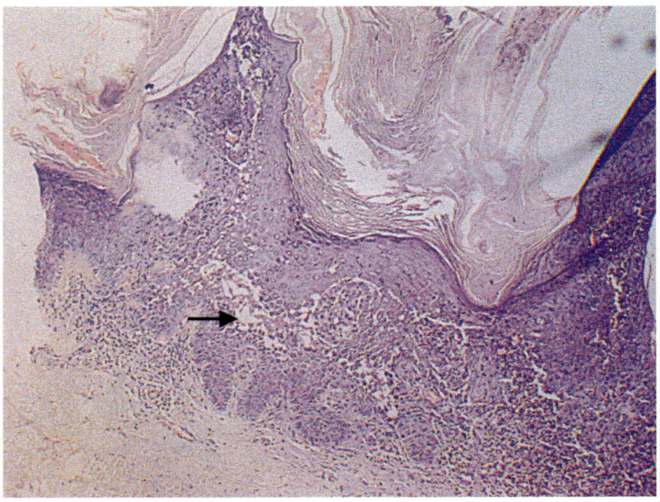

FIGURE 16.2.4

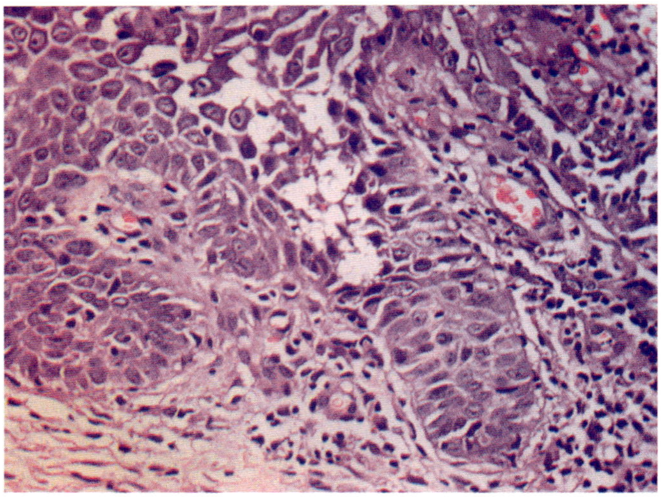

FIGURE 16.2.5

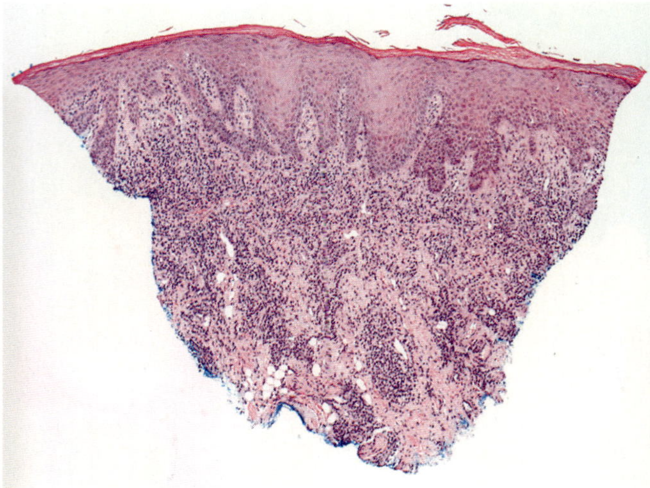

FIGURE 16.2.6

16.2.5: Closer view of acantholytic type—in addition to cytologic atypia, there are suprabasal clefts with acantholytic cells, may involve upper layers of the epidermis also *(High power view)*

16.2.6: Actinic cheilitis—histologic appearance that is nearly identical to that of an actinic keratosis with underlying dermal inflammation composed of lymphocytes and plasma cells *(Scanner view)*

16.2.7: Actinic cheilitis—disorganized atypical keratinocytes in the basilar portion of the epidermis along with spongiosis and dermal inflammation *(Low power view)*

16.2.8: Variable cytological atypia of keratinocytes, from slight to extreme *(Low power view)*

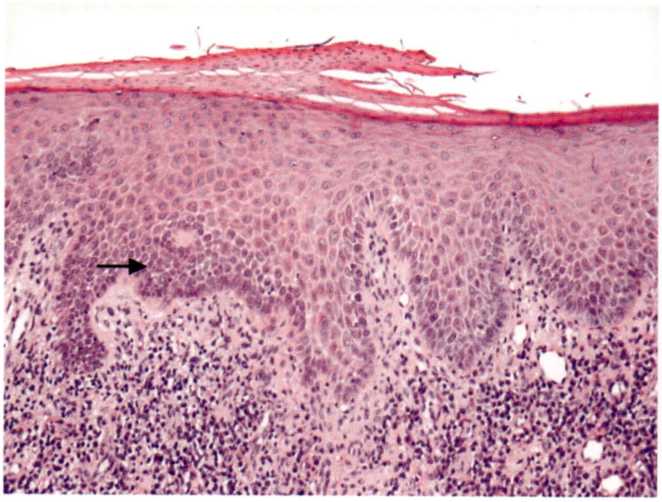

FIGURE 16.2.7

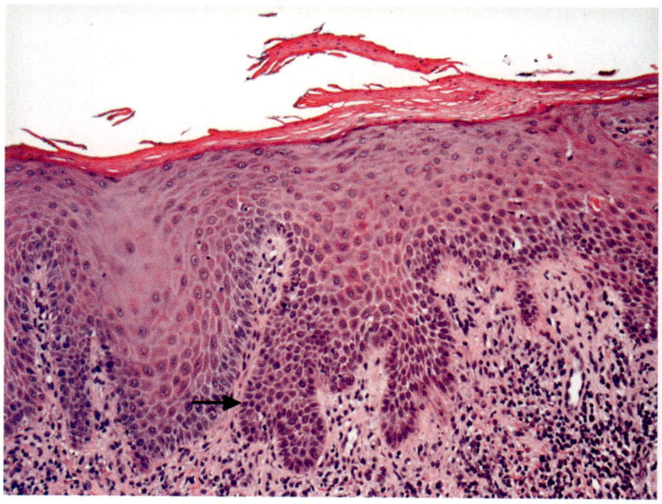

FIGURE 16.2.8

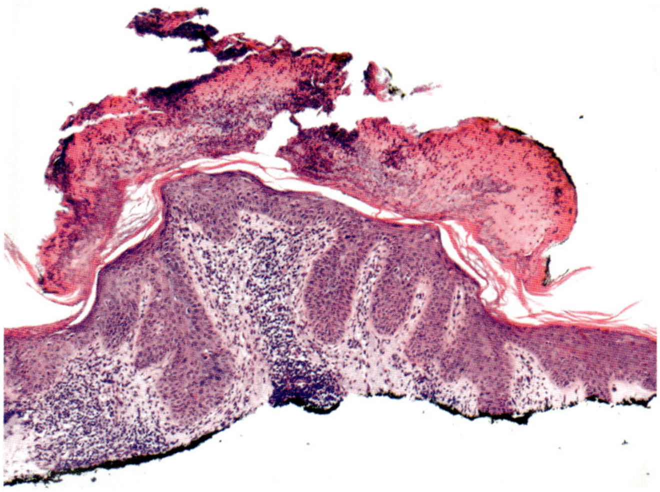

FIGURE 16.3.1

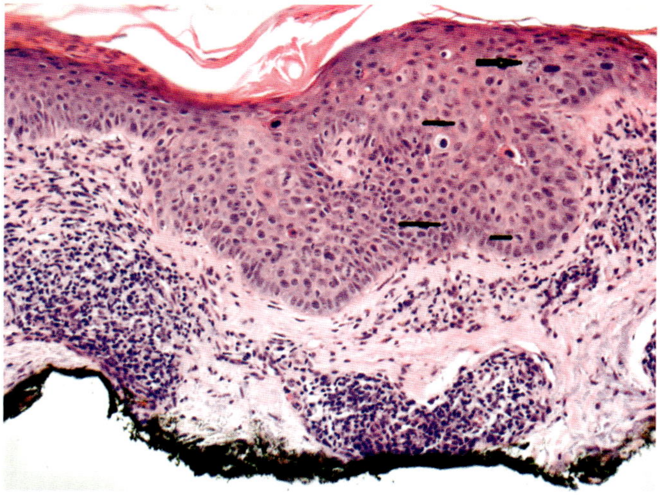

FIGURE 16.3.2

16.3: BOWEN'S DISEASE

16.3.1: Psoriasiform pattern with disorderly maturation of the epidermis *(Low power view)*

16.3.2: Mitoses at different levels *(High power view)*

16.3.3: Variant with irregular acanthosis, and extensive chronic inflammation in the dermis *(Low power view)*

16.3.4: Dyskeratotic cells *(High power view)*

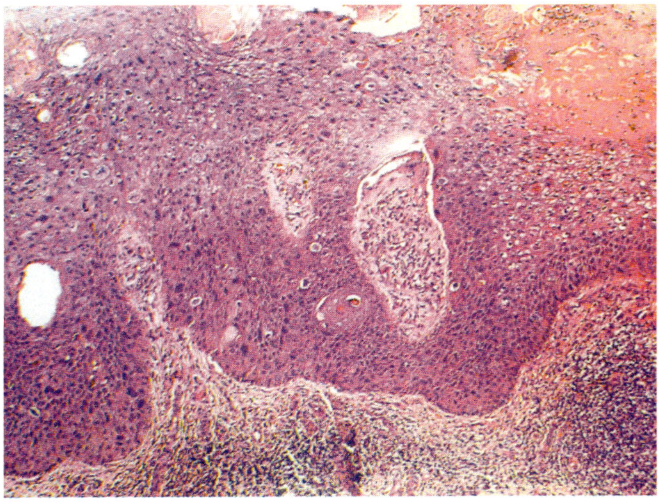

FIGURE 16.3.3

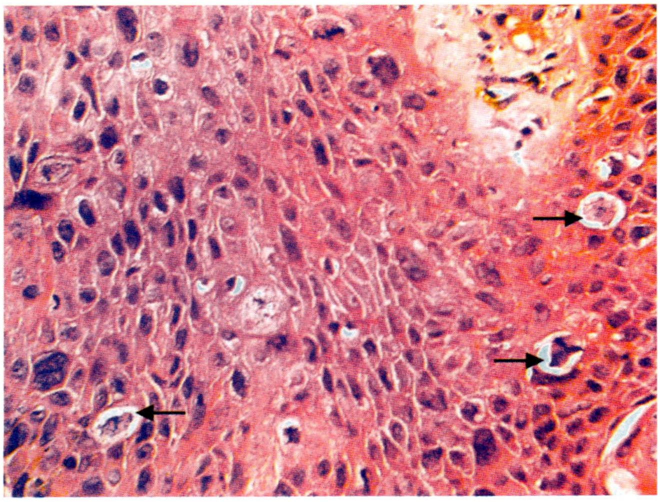

FIGURE 16.3.4

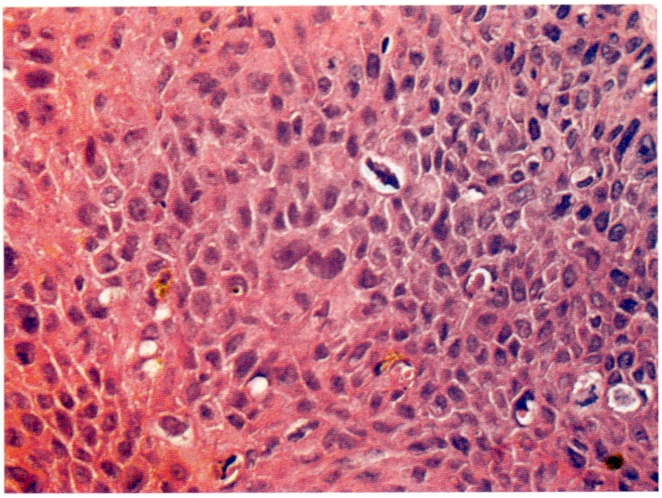

FIGURE 16.3.5

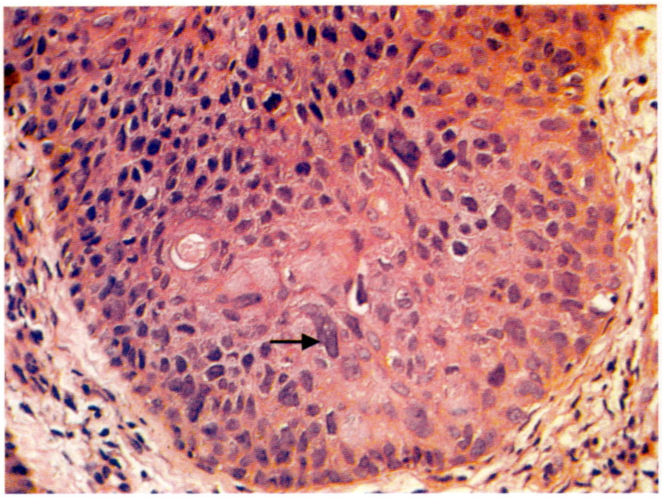

FIGURE 16.3.6

16.3.5: Full-thickness atypia and disorganization *(High power view)*

16.3.6: Multinucleated keratinocytes *(High power view)*

16.3.7: Relative sparing of basal cell layer—eye liner sign *(High power view)*

16.3.8: Usually, there is loss of the granular layer, with overlying parakeratosis and sometimes hyperkeratosis *(Low power view)*

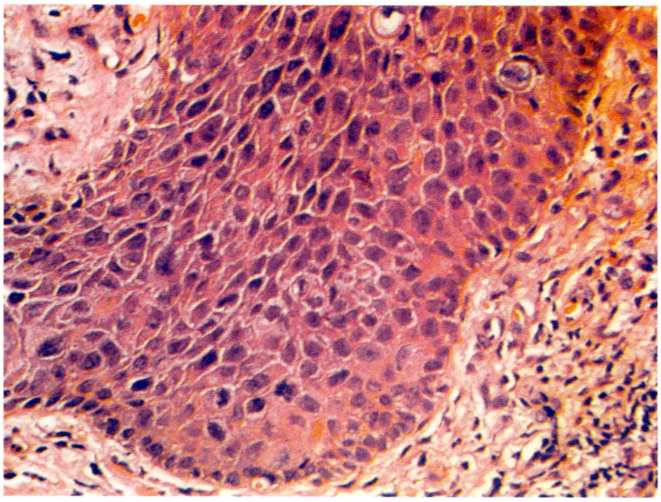

FIGURE 16.3.7

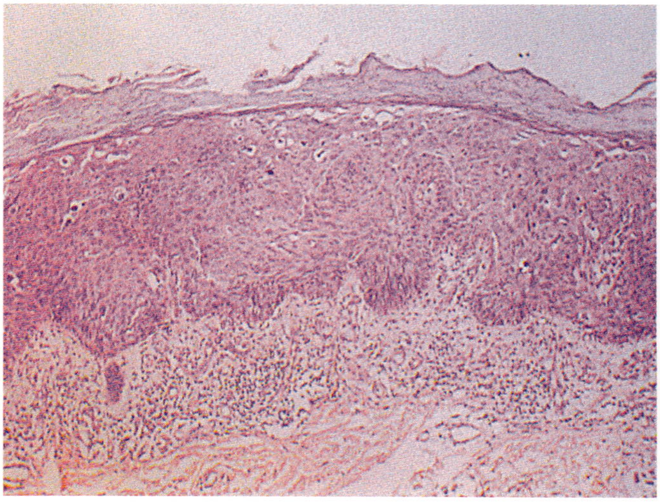

FIGURE 16.3.8

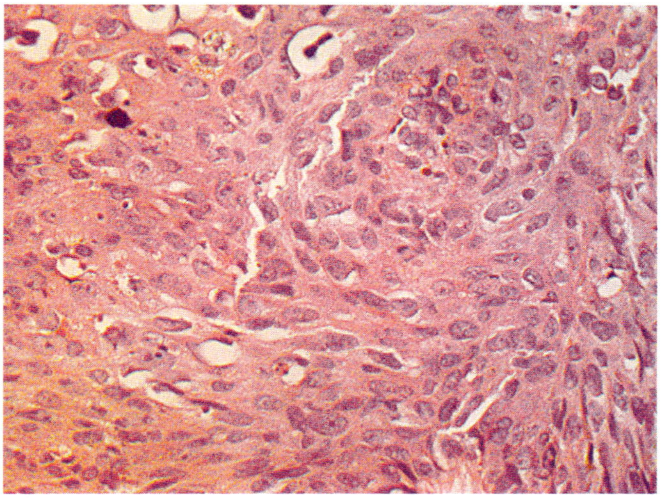

FIGURE 16.3.9

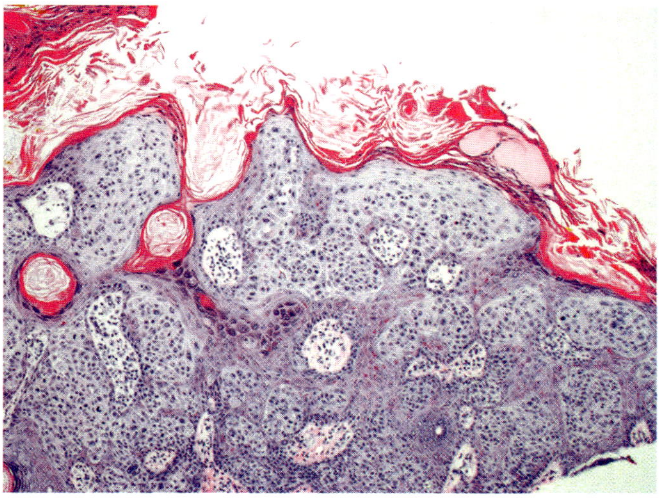

FIGURE 16.3.10

16.3.9: Windblown appearance *(High power view)*

16.3.10: Pagetoid variant has nests of cells with pale cytoplasm *(Low power view)*

16.3.11: Closer view of pale pagetoid nests of atypical keratinocytes. There is sparing of the basal layer (eyeliner sign) *(High power view)*

16.3.12: Pigmented variant—there may be melanin in individual tumor cells and melanophages in the underlying dermis *(High power view)* (*Source:* Image contributed by Venkataram Mysore)

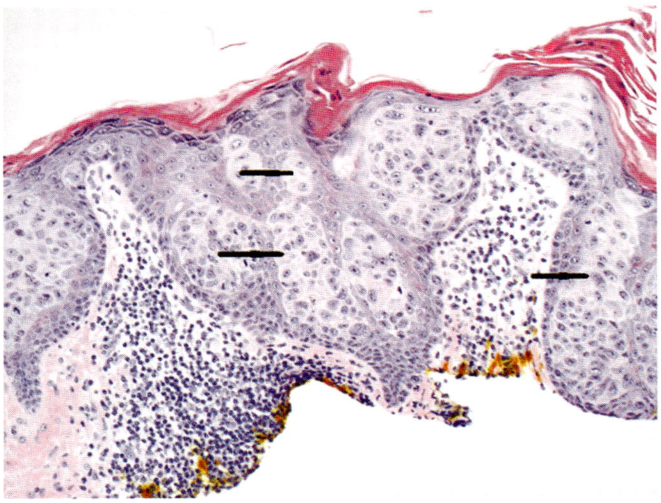

FIGURE 16.3.11

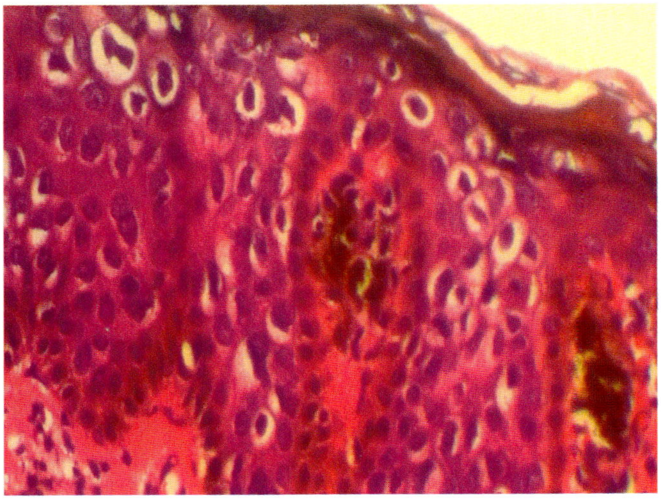

FIGURE 16.3.12

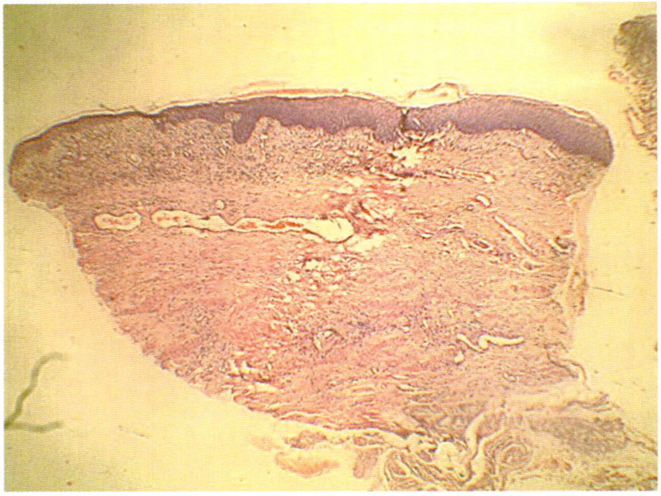

FIGURE 16.4.1

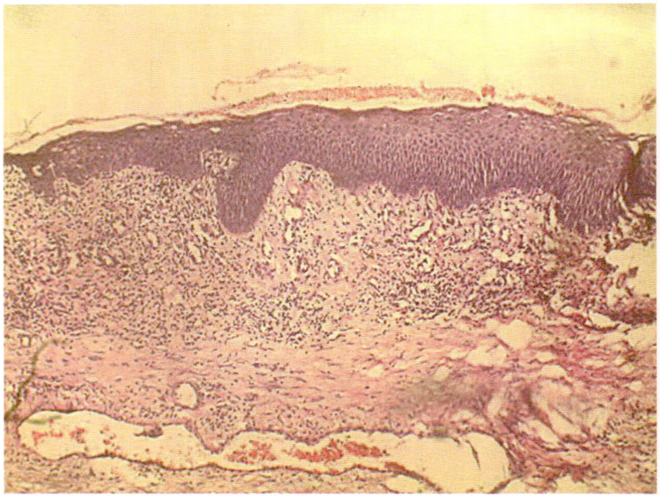

FIGURE 16.4.2

16.4: ERYTHROPLASIA

16.4.1: The changes are similar to Bowen's disease *(Scanner view)*

16.4.2: Inflammatory infiltrate is usually rich in plasma cells *(Low power view)*

16.4.3: There are fewer multinucleate and dyskeratotic cells than in Bowen's disease *(High power view)*

16.4.4: Full thickness dysplasia *(High power view)*

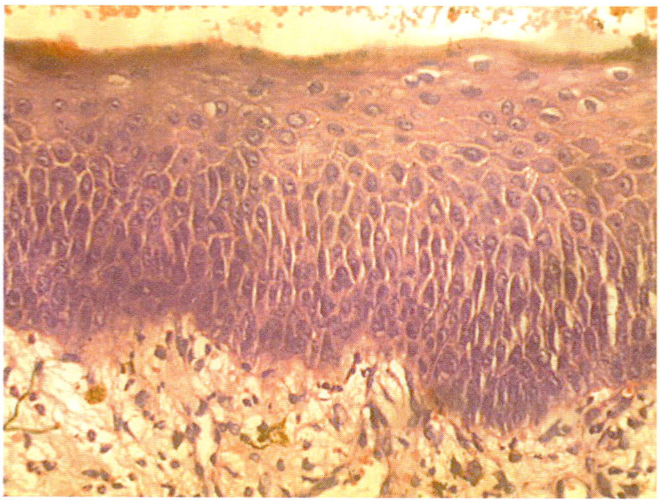

FIGURE 16.4.3

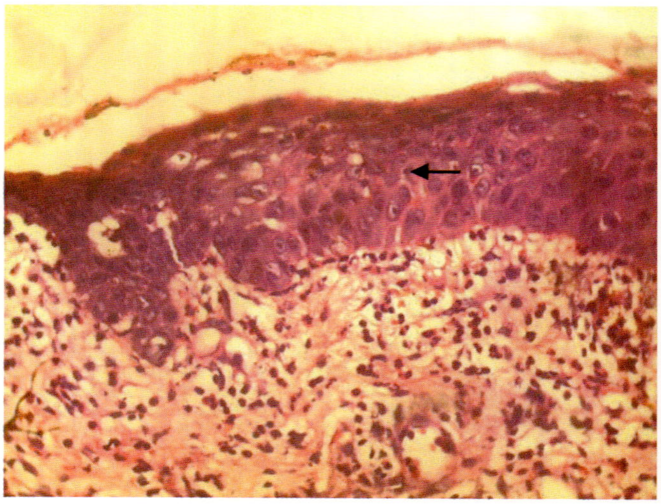

FIGURE 16.4.4

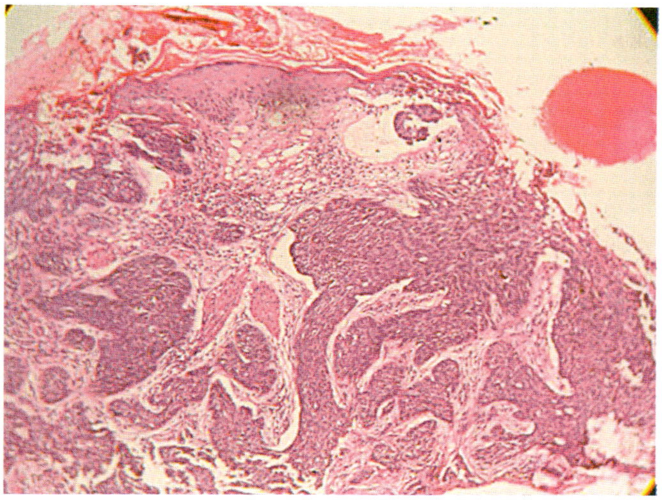

FIGURE 16.5.1

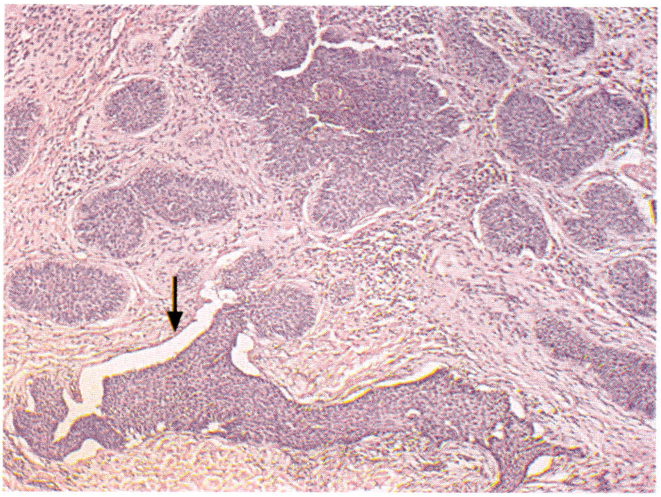

FIGURE 16.5.2

16.5: BASAL CELL CARCINOMA

16.5.1: Shows islands of basaloid cells arising from the undersurface of epidermis *(Scanner view)*

16.5.2: Retraction between the tumor islands and the surrounding stroma *(Low power view)*

16.5.3: Palisading of the cells at the periphery and haphazard arrangement towards the center of the islands. The tumor cells have hyperchromatic nuclei and scant cytoplasm *(High power view)*

16.5.4: Superficial (multifocal) type—small islands of basaloid cells attached to the undersurface of the epidermis *(Scanner view)*

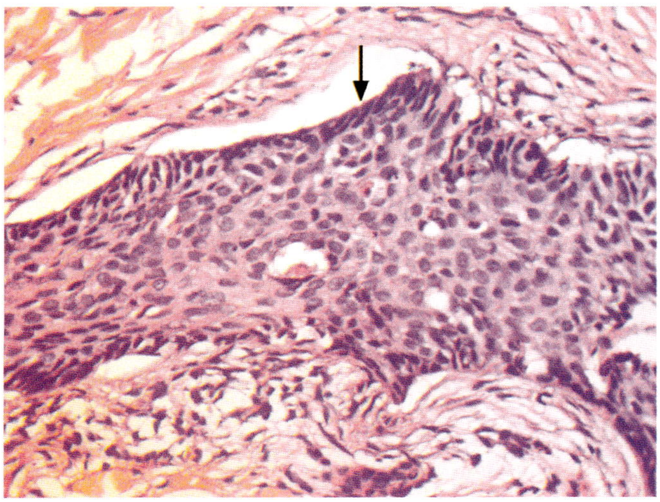

FIGURE 16.5.3

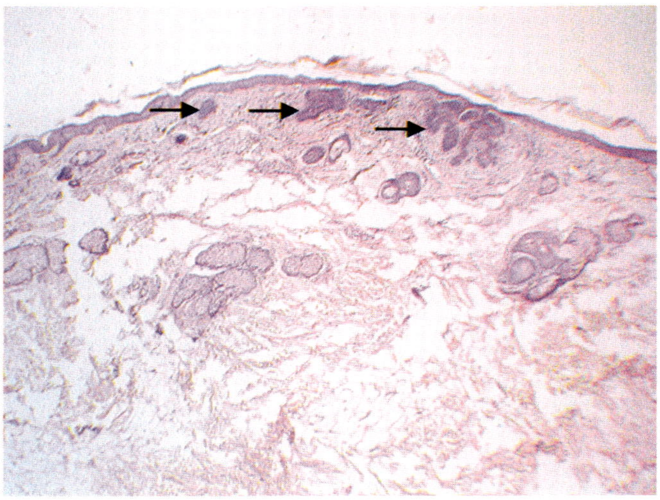

FIGURE 16.5.4

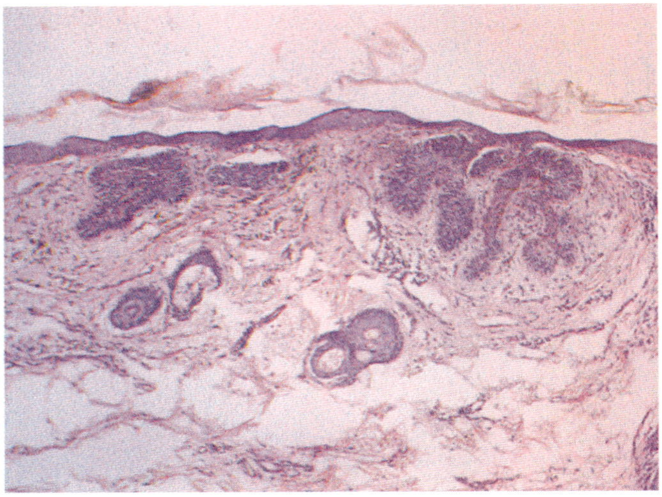

FIGURE 16.5.5

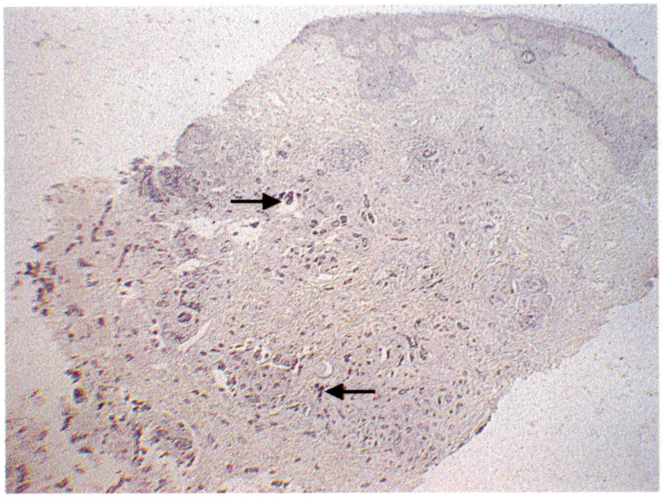

FIGURE 16.5.6

16.5.5: Multiple islands confined to the papillary dermis *(Low power view)*

16.5.6: Sclerosing type—islands of tumor cells embedded in a dense fibrous stroma *(Scanner view)*

16.5.7: Infiltrative angulated islands and strands of basaloid tumor cells infiltrate the dense sclerotic stroma *(Low power view)*

16.5.8: Narrow elongated strands of basaloid tumor cells with dense sclerctic stroma *(High power view)*

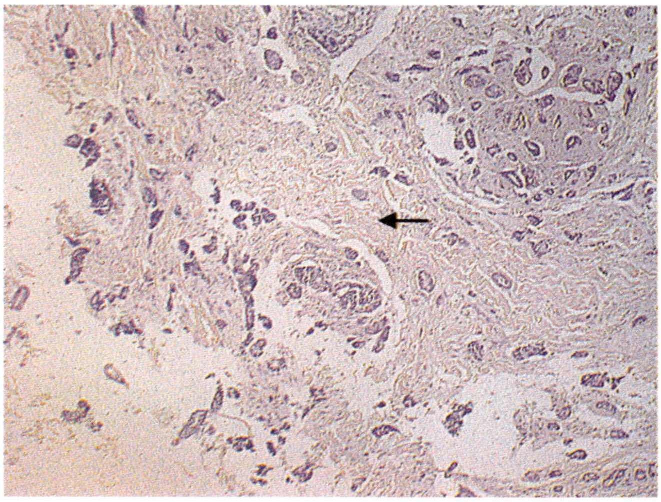

FIGURE 16.5.7

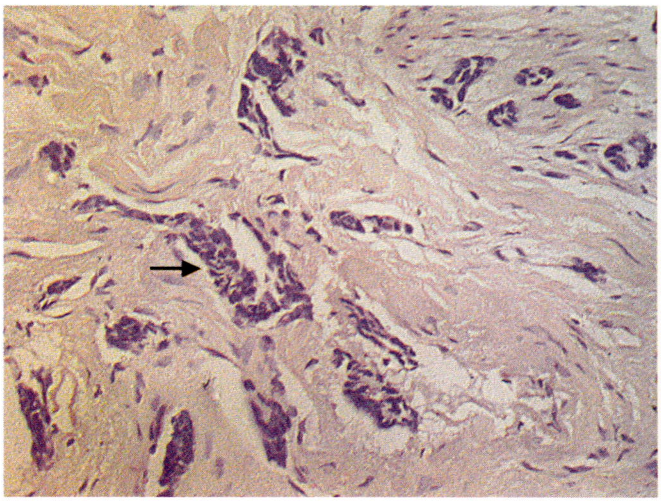

FIGURE 16.5.8

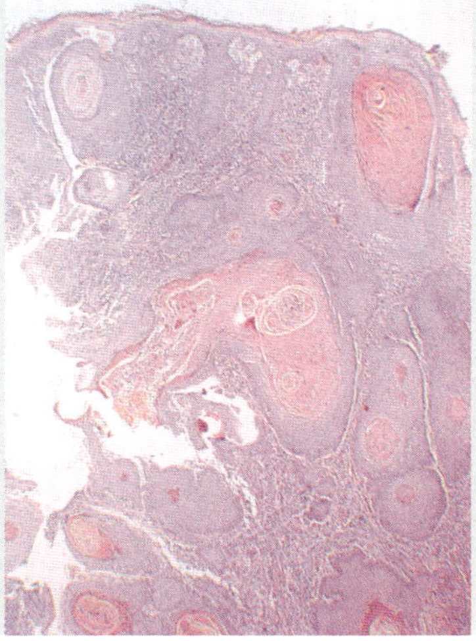

FIGURE 16.6.1

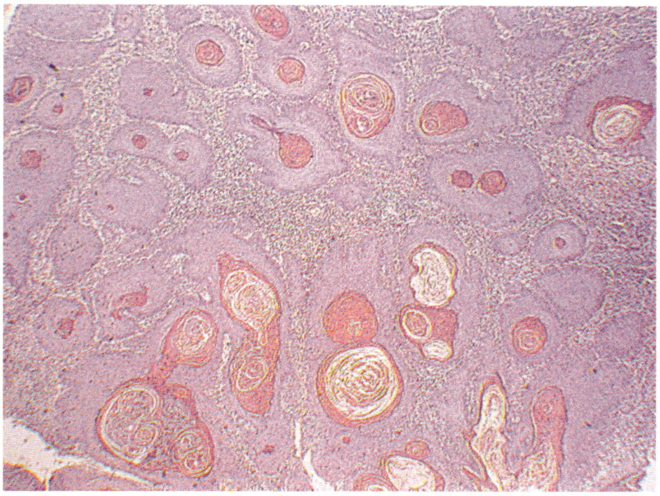

FIGURE 16.6.2

16.6: SQUAMOUS CELL CARCINOMA

16.6.1: Nests of squamous epithelial cells which arise from the epidermis *(Scanner view)*

16.6.2: Extend into the dermis for a variable distance *(Low power view)*

16.6.3: Tumor cells show marked nuclear atypia. The dense pink cytoplasm is evidence of squamous differentiation *(High power view)*

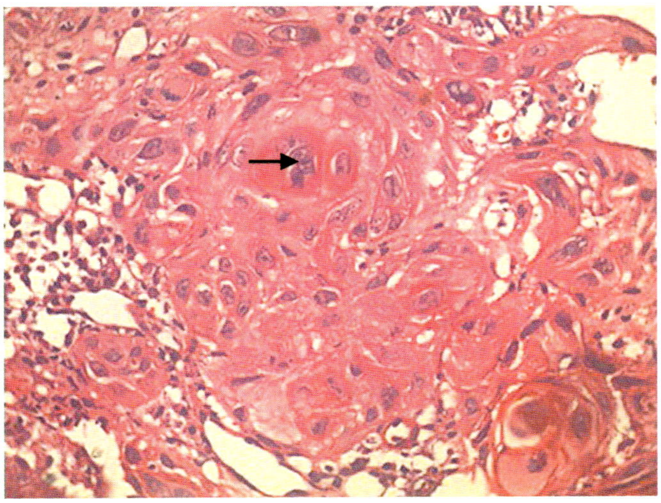

FIGURE 16.6.3

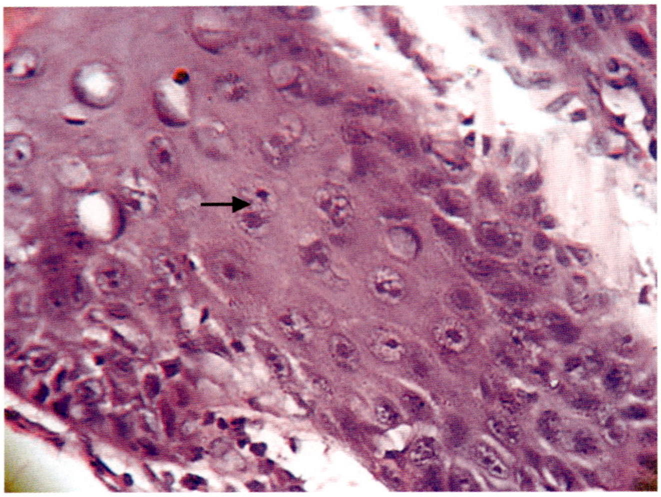

FIGURE 16.6.4

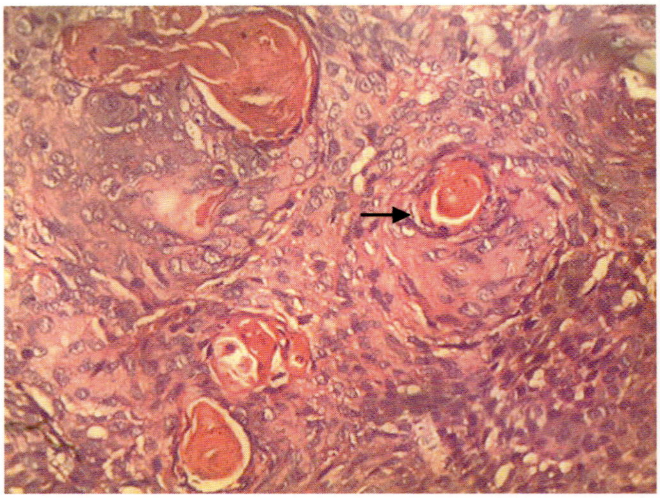

FIGURE 16.6.5

16.6.4: Marked nuclear atypia and large nucleoli *(High power view)*

16.6.5: Central keratinization and horn pearl (keratin pearl) formation *(High power view)*

16.6.6: Closer view of keratin pearl *(High power view)*

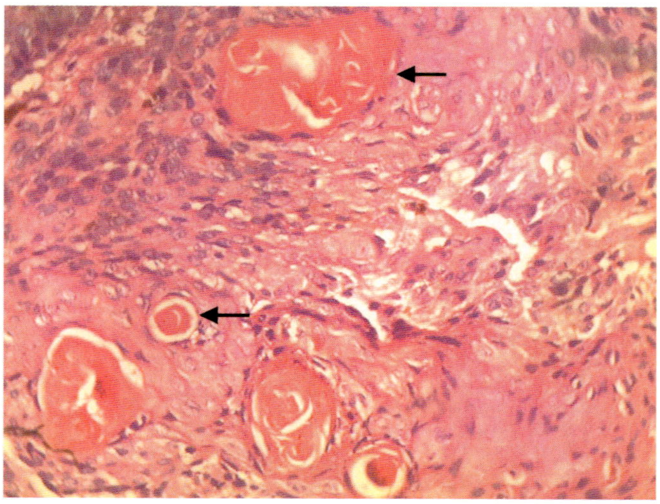

FIGURE 16.6.6

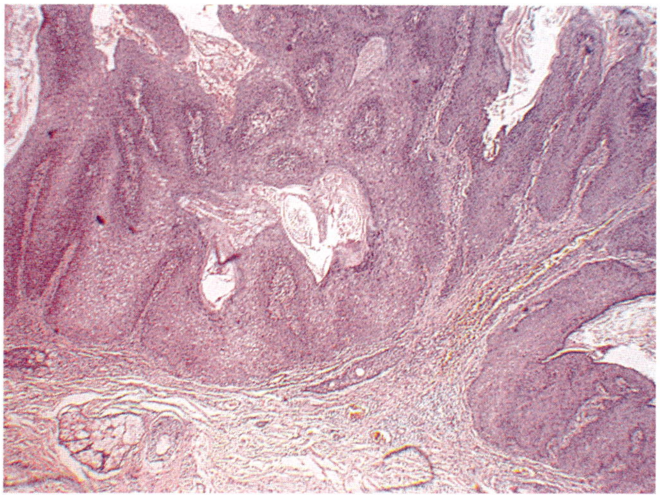

FIGURE 16.7.1

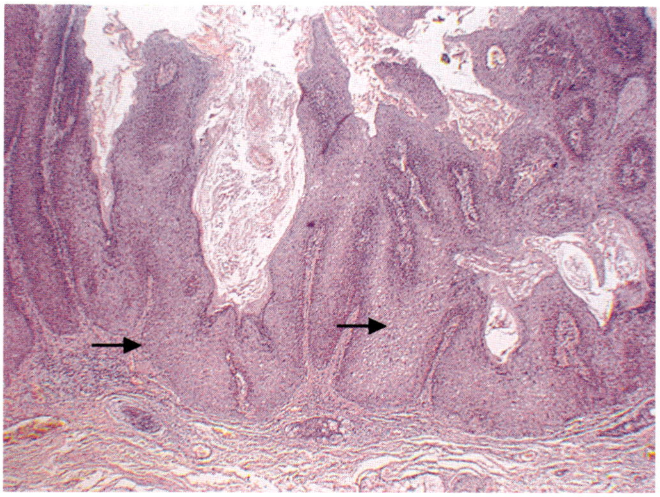

FIGURE 16.7.2

16.7: VERRUCOUS CARCINOMA

16.7.1: Exophytic growth showing hyperkeratosis and papillomatous hyperplasia (tumor has both exophytic and endophytic component) *(Scanner view)*

16.7.2: Acanthotic downgrowths *(Scanner view)*

16.7.3: Rete pegs have a bulbous appearance *(Low power view)*

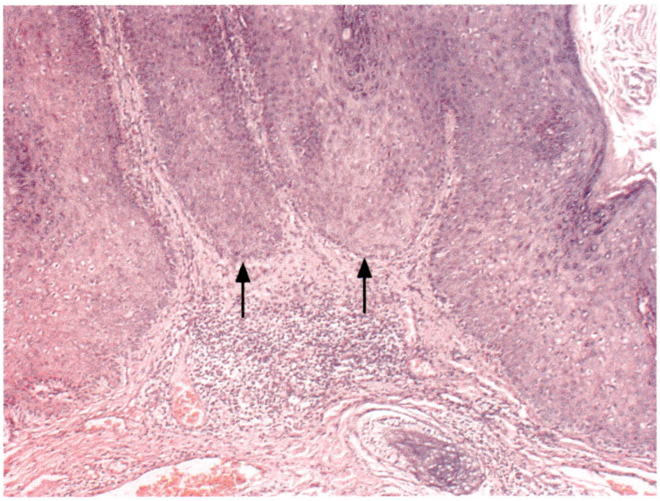

FIGURE 16.7.3

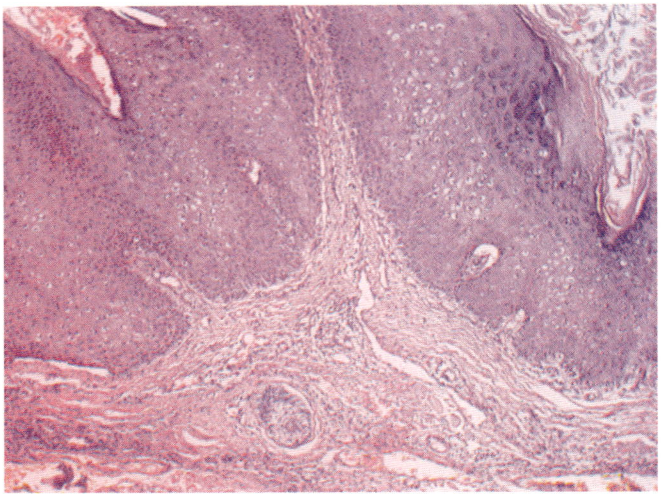

FIGURE 16.7.4

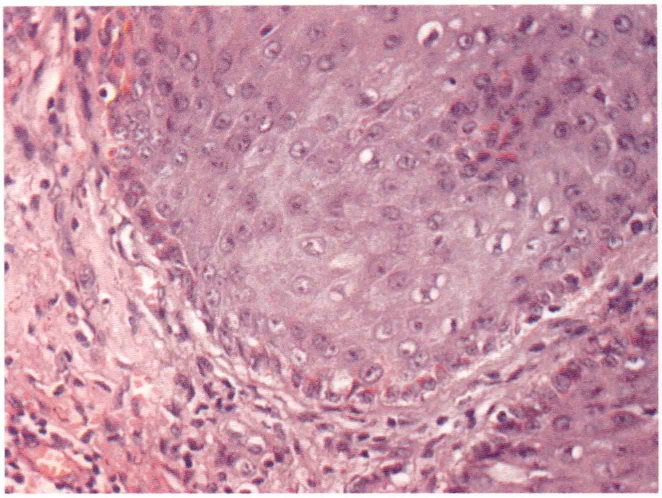

FIGURE 16.7.5

16.7.4: Blunted projections *(Low power view)*

16.7.5: Large well-differentiated squamous epithelial cells with very little nuclear atypia *(High power view)*

16.7.6: Low mitotic activity. The downgrowths are mostly contained by an intact basement membrane *(High power view)*

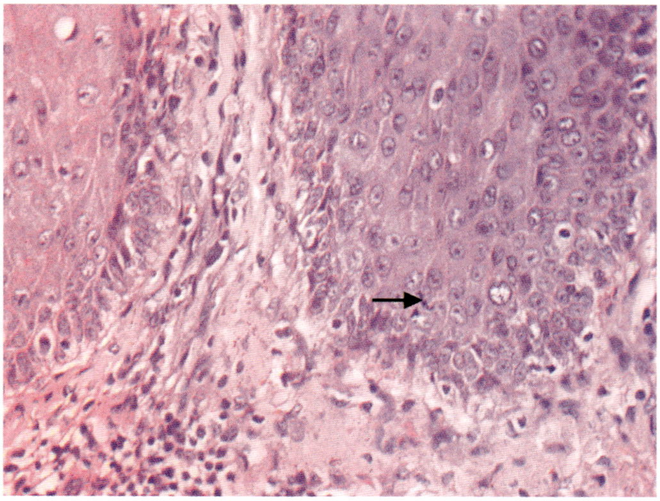

FIGURE 16.7.6

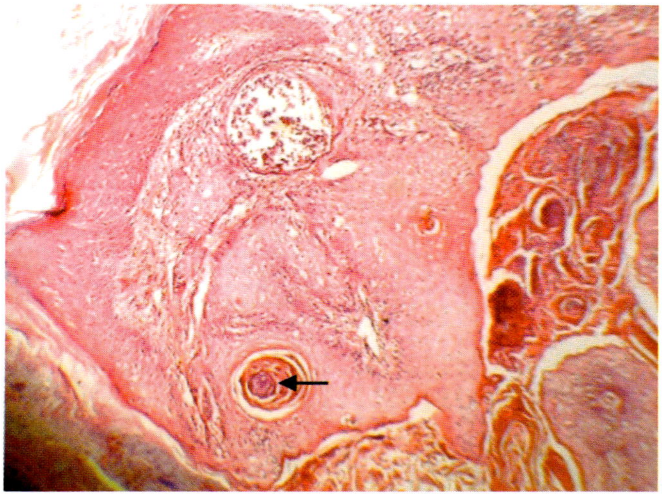

FIGURE 16.8.1

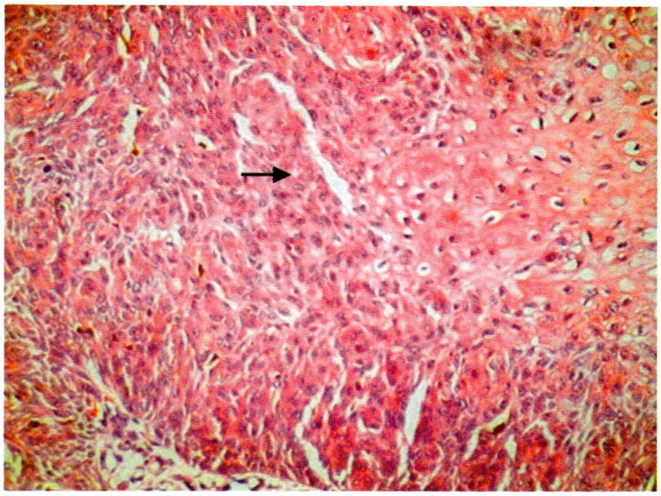

FIGURE 16.8.2

16.8: KERATOACANTHOMA

16.8.1: The lesion is mostly exophytic and partially endophytic. Cells are atypical, pale, pink and glassy *(Scanner view)*

16.8.2: Keratinocytes appear large, atypical and may have mitotic figures. Many polymorphonuclear cells may be seen within epidermis *(Low power view)*

16.8.3: Another case showing a central cup-shaped crater. It is also described as a 'volcano-shaped lesion' *(Scanner view)*

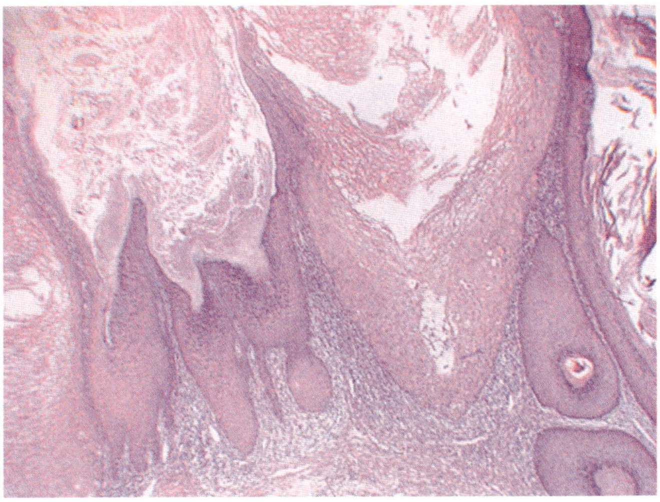

FIGURE 16.8.3

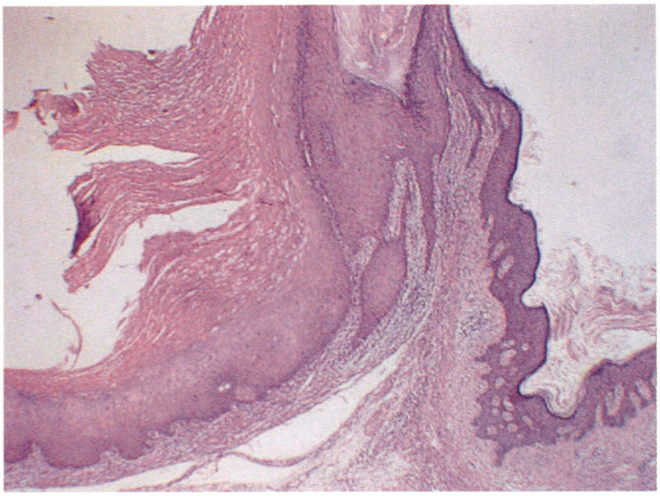

FIGURE 16.8.4

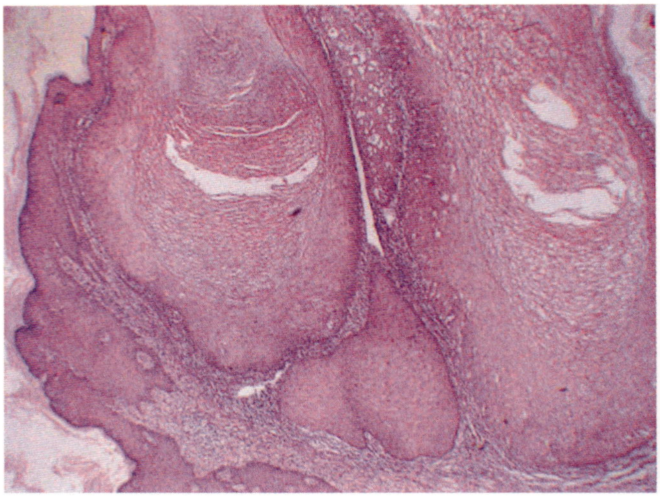

FIGURE 16.8.5

16.8.4: On both sides of the invagination is an epidermal lip, which rises above the lesion as a buttress *(Low power view)*

16.8.5: Other side of lipping *(Low power view)*

16.8.6: Epithelial atypia and mitoses at places only (Squamous eddies and keratin pearls may be present, causing confusion with well-differentiated squamous cell carcinoma) (There is debate over whether some or all keratoacanthomas are variants of squamous cell carcinoma) *(High power view)*

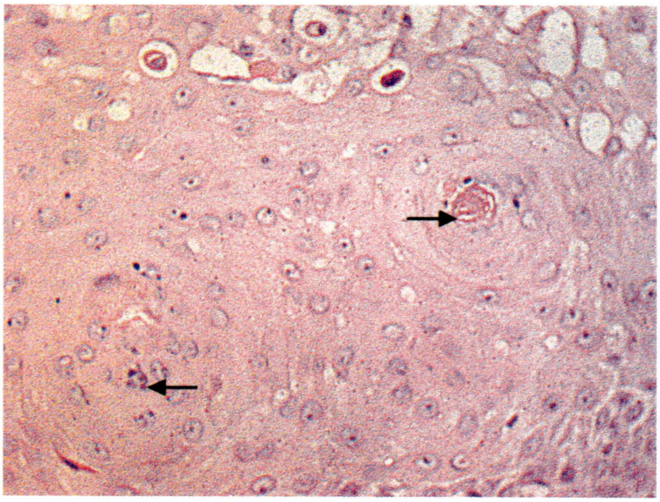

FIGURE 16.8.6

DIFFERENTIAL DIAGNOSIS

1. Seborrheic keratosis
   a. Large clear cell acanthoma
   b. Dermatosis papulosa nigra
   c. Stucco keratosis
   d. PUVA keratosis
   e. Verruca vulgaris
2. Actinic keratosis
   a. Paget's disease
   b. SCC
   c. Lentigo maligna (Pigmented actinic keratosis)
3. Bowen's disease
   a. Podophyllin treated condylomata acuminata
4. Erythroplasia of Queyrat
   a. Bowenoid papulosis
5. Squamous cell carcinoma (SCC)
   a. Eccrine porocarcinoma
   b. Inverted follicular keratosis
   c. Keratoacanthoma
   d. Pilar tumor
   e. Hidradenocarcinoma
6. Basal cell carcinoma (BCC)
   a. Trichoblastoma
   b. Trichoepithelioma
   c. Clear cell hidradenoma
   d. Trichilemmoma
   e. Sebaceoma
7. Verrucous carcinoma
   a. Viral warts
   b. SCC

DIAGNOSTIC PEARLS

1. Presence of buds at the base in proliferative actinic keratosis should not be confused with SCC.
2. Presence of mitotic figures differentiates lichenoid actinic keratosis from lichen planus.
3. Bowen's disease can be distinguished from podophyllin treated condylomata acuminata by the presence of metaphase figures.
4. Lymphovascular invasion in SCC is associated with poor prognosis.
5. Erythrophagocytosis of tumor cells may be seen in SCC.
6. SCC should be graded based on the least differentiated area of the section.
7. Marked intercellular edema in verrucous carcinoma gives the cytoplasm a glassy appearance.
8. Mitosis in keratoacanthoma are generally limited to basal layer.
9. Pagetoid Bowen's, Paget's disease and superficial spreading malignant melanoma are sometimes difficult to differentiate histologically. Immunohistochemistry can be very useful: Bowen's (CK 5/6+, p63+, CK7 negative or focal, CK66+, CK54 negative), Paget's (CK7+, CEA+, CK45+, CK66, CK5/6 and p63 negative), melanoma (S100 protein and MART-1 positive, negative for deratins and p63).

17 Appendageal Tumors

Chapter Outline

17.1: Follicular Differentiation
17.2: Sebaceous Differentiation
17.3: Apocrine Differentiation
17.4: Eccrine Differentiation

Deepa Gharpuray Pandit, Pradeep Mahajan,
Nandakumar Gopinath, Jag Bhawan,
Ying Guo, Asha Kubba

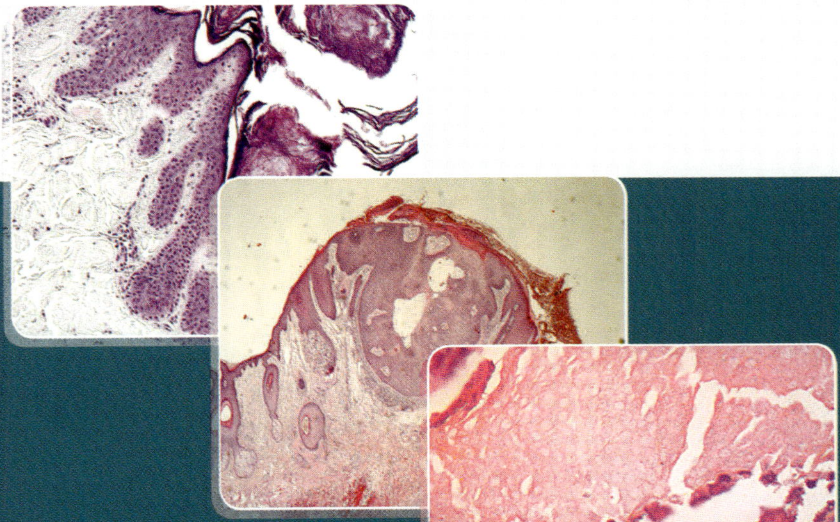

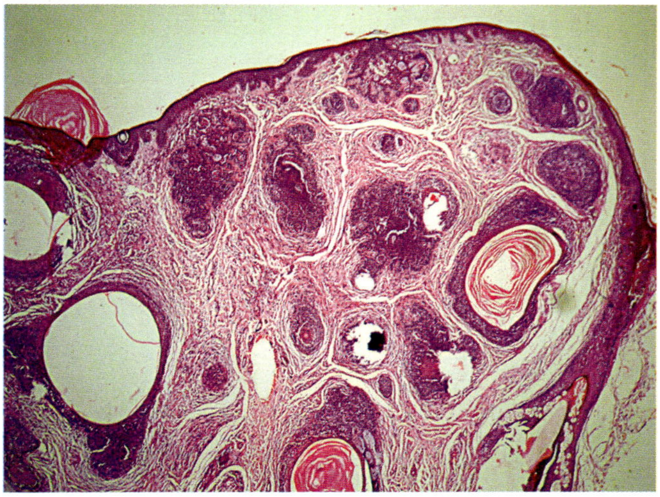

FIGURE 17.1.1.1

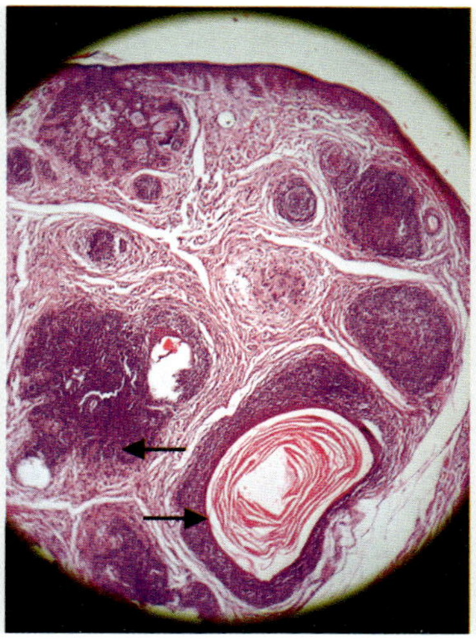

FIGURE 17.1.1.2

17.1: FOLLICULAR DIFFERENTIATION

17.1.1: Trichoepithelioma

17.1.1.1: Epithelial structures resembling different portions of hair follicle (*Scanner view*)

17.1.1.2: Horn cysts and basaloid islands (*Low power view*)

17.1.1.3: Branching nests of basaloid structures with germ and papilla (*High power view*)

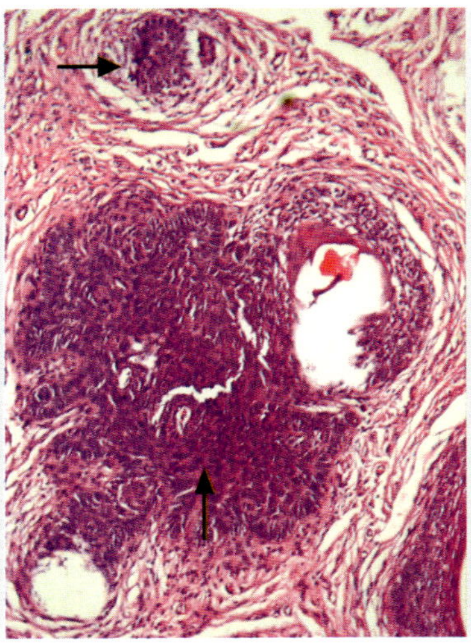

FIGURE 17.1.1.3

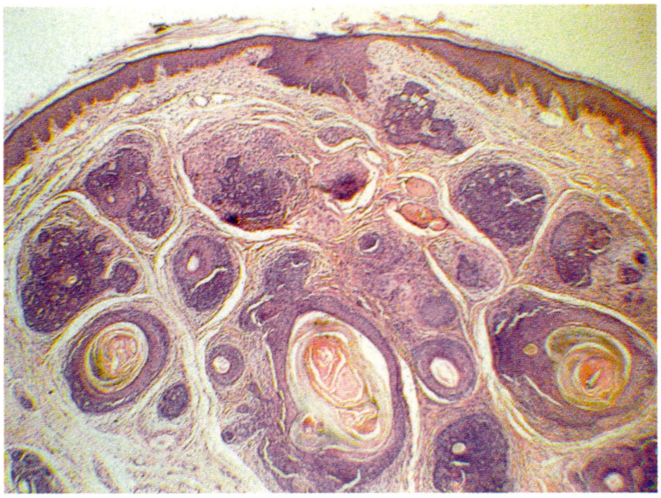

FIGURE 17.1.1.4

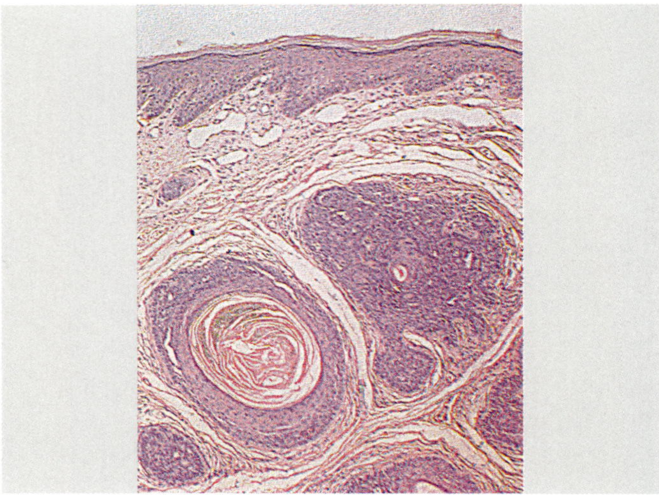

FIGURE 17.1.1.5

17.1.1.4: Another case showing almost symmetric arrangement of hair structures (*Scanner view*)

17.1.1.5: Horn cysts, basaloid structures (*Low power view*)

17.1.1.6: Fibrotic stroma in close proximity of the tumor, branching nests (*High power view*)

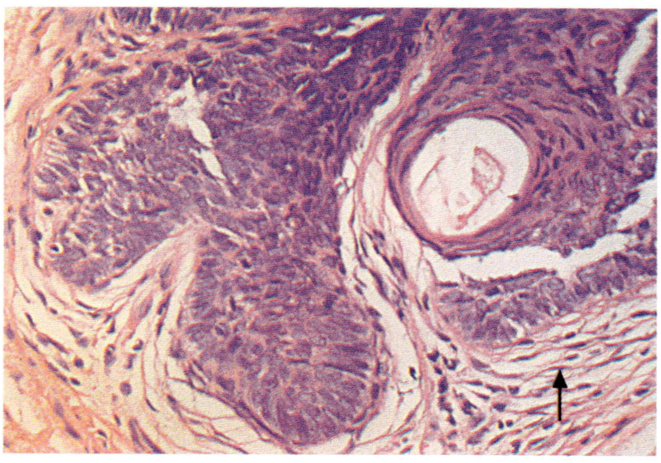

FIGURE 17.1.1.6

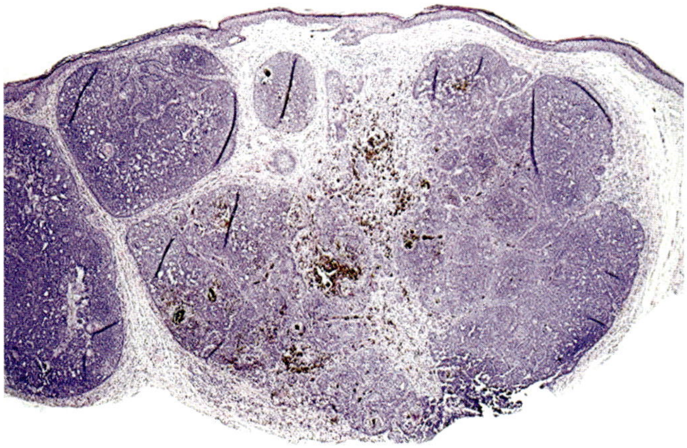

FIGURE 17.1.2.1

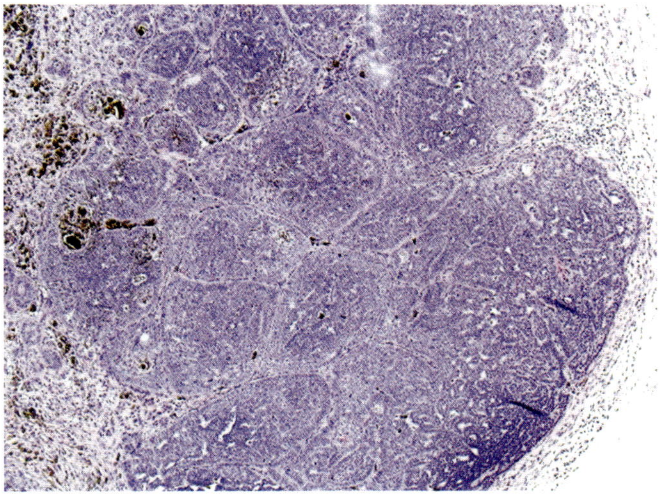

FIGURE 17.1.2.2

17.1.2: Trichoblastoma

17.1.2.1: Basaloid tumor in mid and lower dermis with extension to subcutis, no connection to the epidermis *(Scanner view)*

17.1.2.2: Nests of basaloid cells; no peripheral palisading; no clefting around the nests *(Low power view)*

17.1.2.3: Another case showing primitive hair papilla formation (papillary mesenchymal body) *(High power view)*

17.1.2.4: Nests of basaloid cells with pilar differentiation *(High power view)*

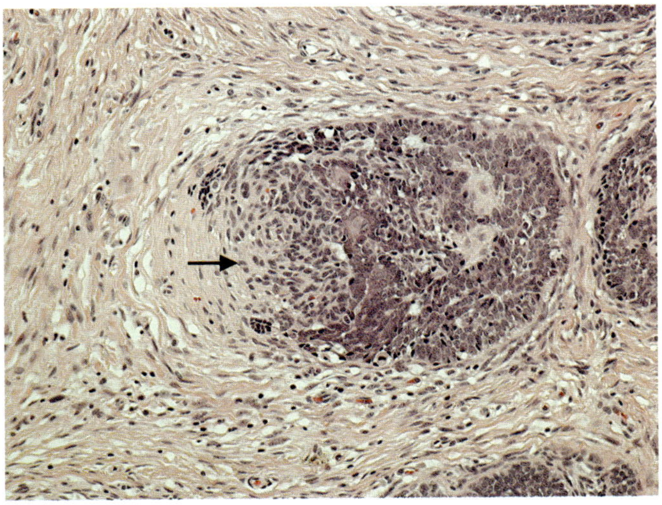

FIGURE 17.1.2.3

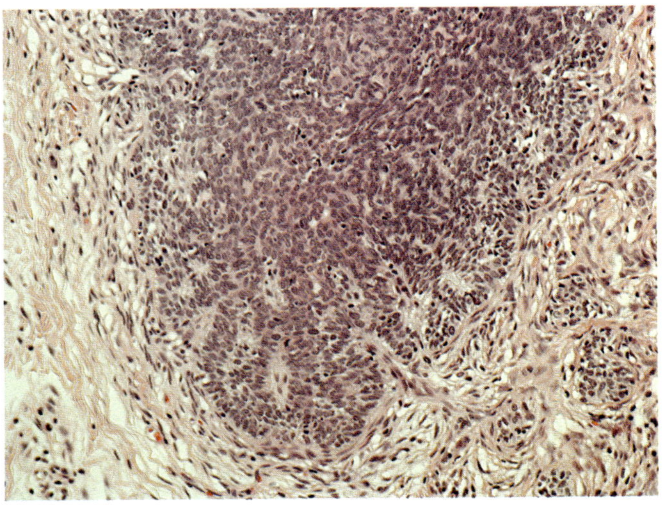

FIGURE 17.1.2.4

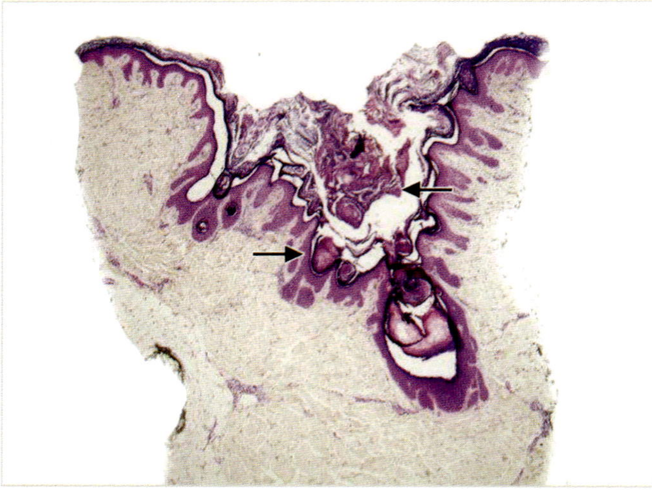

FIGURE 17.1.3.1

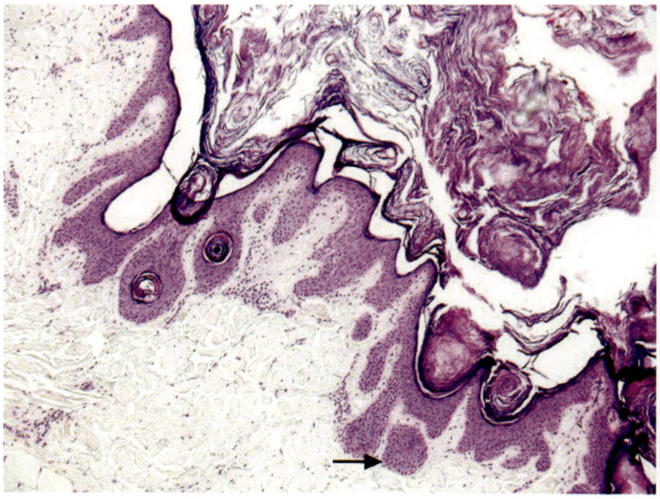

FIGURE 17.1.3.2

17.1.3: Dilated Pore of Winer

17.1.3.1: Dilated hair follicle with keratin plugging and radiating strands of epithelium at the base and sides of the pore *(Scanner view)*

17.1.3.2: Lining epithelium shows irregular budding *(Low power view)*

17.1.3.3: Hyperplastic epithelium and keratin plugs *(High power view)*

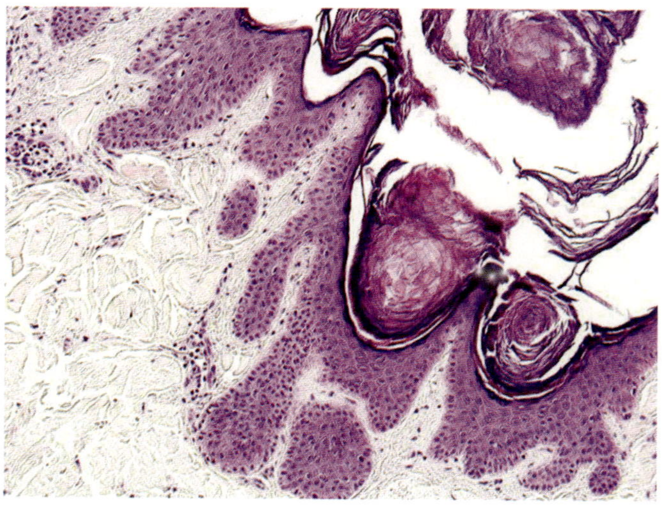

FIGURE 17.1.3.3

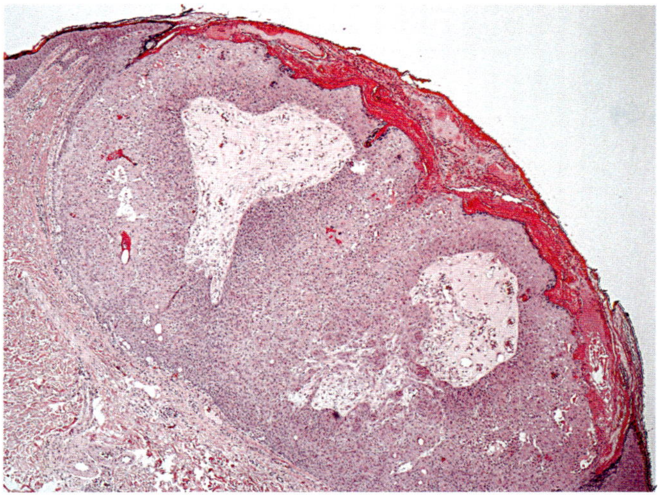

FIGURE 17.1.4.1

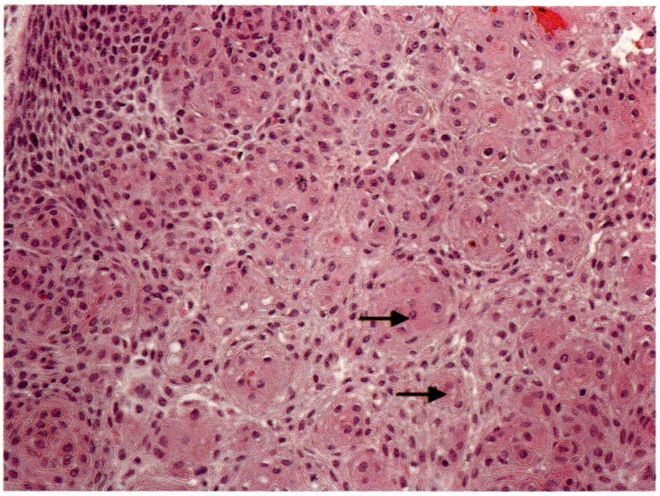

FIGURE 17.1.4.2

17.1.4: Inverted Follicular Keratosis

17.1.4.1: Endophytic lesion connected to epidermis *(Scanner view)*

17.1.4.2: Characteristic squamous eddies *(High power view)*

17.1.4.3: Another lesion with endophytic and exophytic appearance *(Scanner view)*

17.1.4.4: Squamous eddies and few horn cysts *(High power view)*

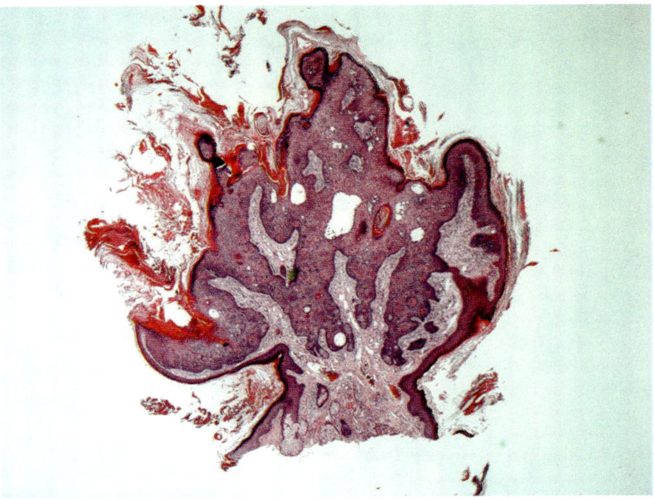

FIGURE 17.1.4.3

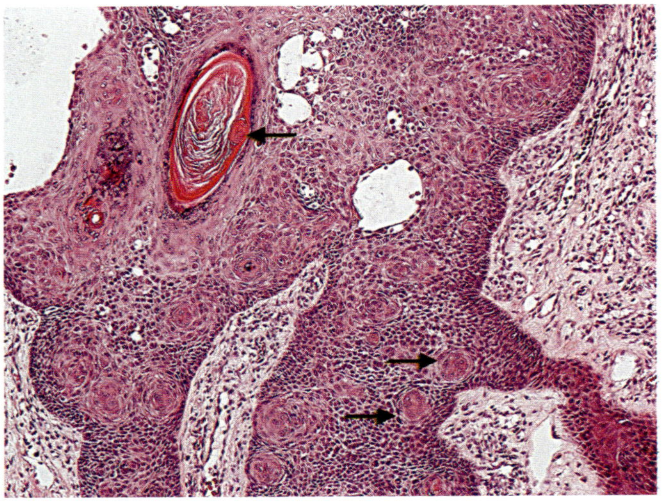

FIGURE 17.1.4.4

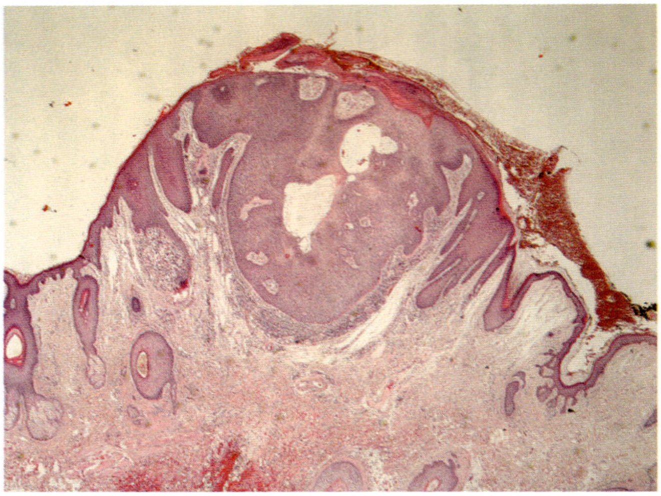

FIGURE 17.1.5.1

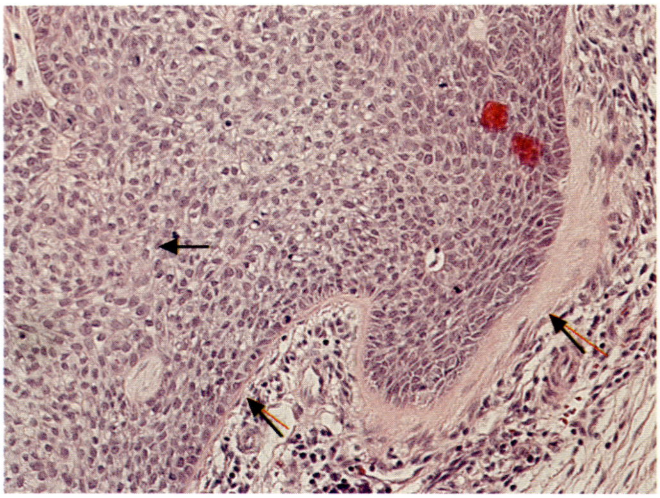

FIGURE 17.1.5.2

17.1.5: Trichilemmoma

17.1.5.1: Small circumscribed solid nodule connecting to the epidermis 'folliculocentric tumor' *(Scanner view)*

17.1.5.2: Uniform cells with clear/vacuolated cytoplasm. Hyaline eosinophilic basement membrane around the tumor (marked with arrow) *(High power view)*

17.1.5.3: Peripheral palisade of cells *(High power view)*

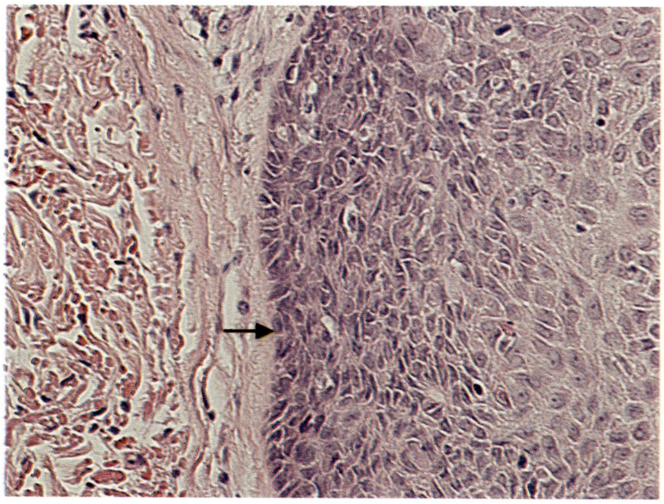

FIGURE 17.1.5.3

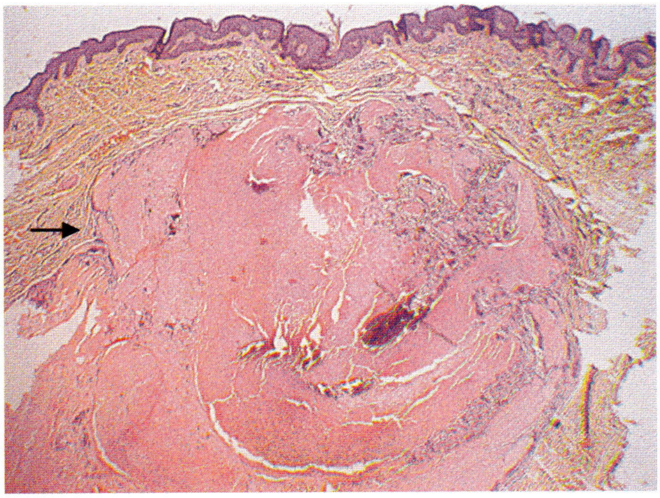

FIGURE 17.1.6.1

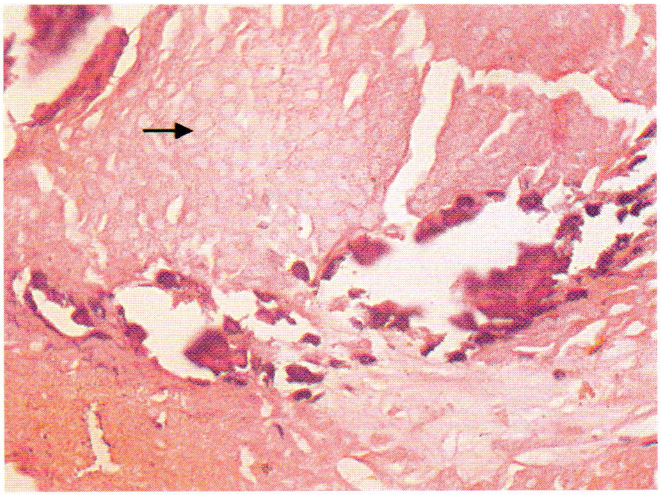

FIGURE 17.1.6.2

17.1.6: Pilomatrixoma/Pilomatricoma

17.1.6.1: Well demarcated tumor in the lower dermis (*Scanner view*)

17.1.6.2: Collection of eosinophilic shadow cells with distinct cytoplasm but no nuclear staining and calcification (*High power view*)

17.1.6.3: Mixed inflammatory cell infiltrate with foreign-body giant cells (*High power view*)

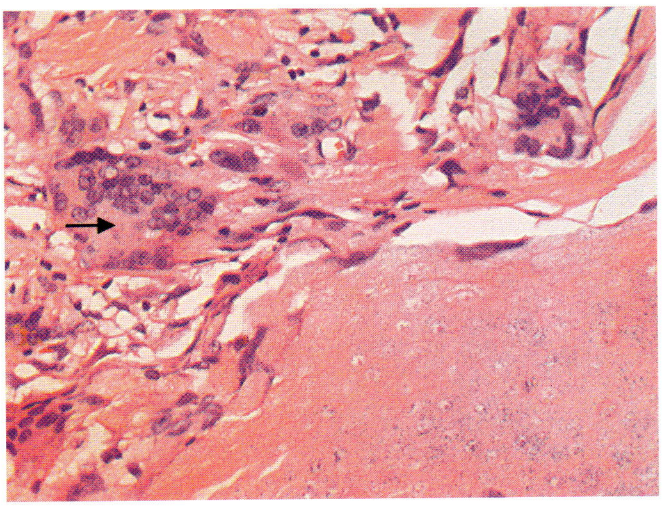

FIGURE 17.1.6.3

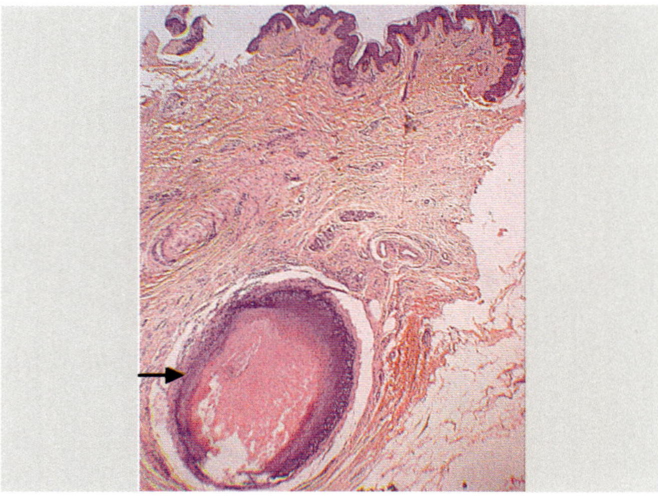

FIGURE 17.1.6.4

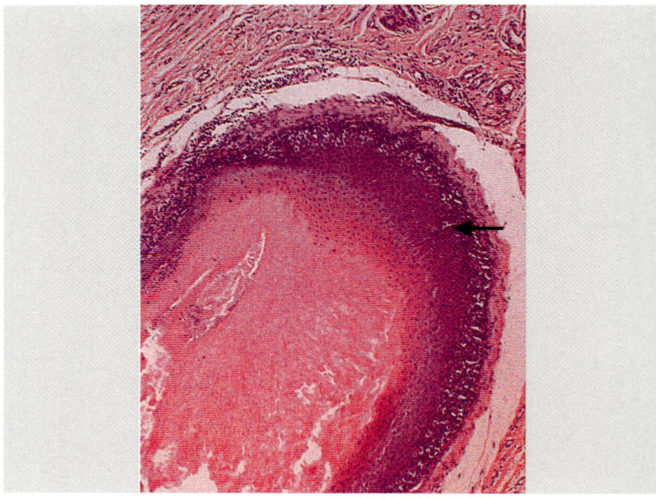

FIGURE 17.1.6.5

17.1.6.4: Another case with tumor island in deep dermis (*Scanner view*)

17.1.6.5: Basophilic cells at the periphery and shadow cells at the center (*Low power view*)

17.1.6.6: Closer view of shadow cells and basophilic cells (*High power view*)

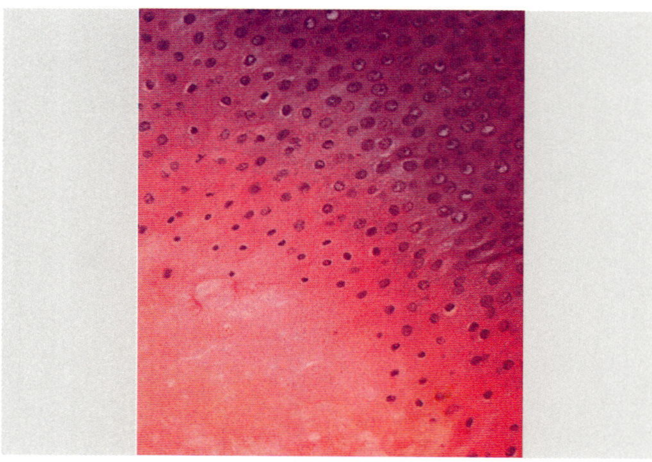

FIGURE 17.1.6.6

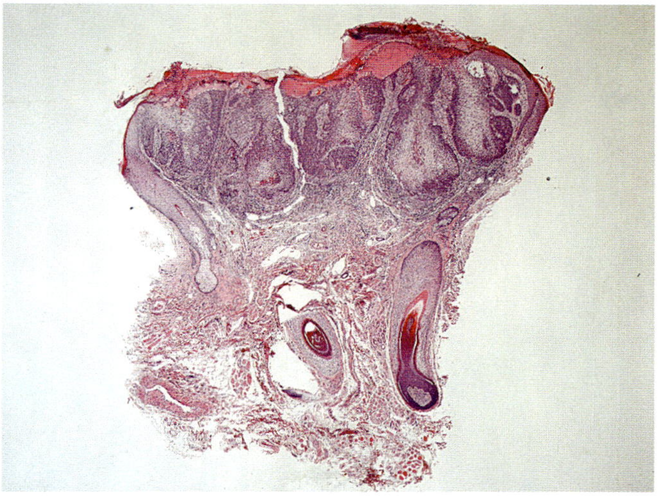

FIGURE 17.2.1.1

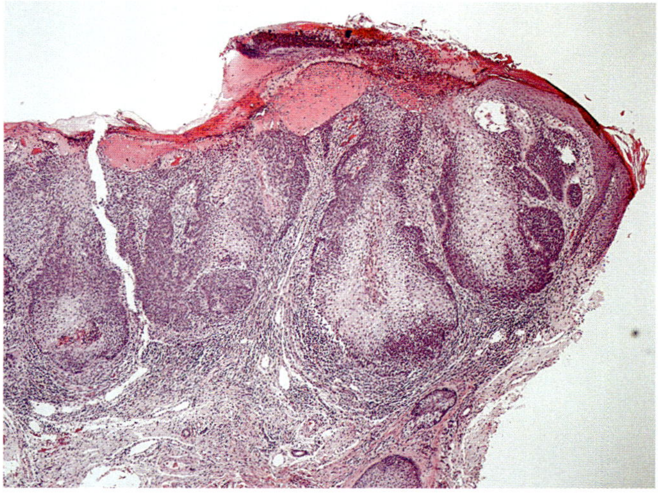

FIGURE 17.2.1.2

17.2: SEBACEOUS DIFFERENTIATION

17.2.1: Sebaceous Adenoma

17.2.1.1: Multilobulated tumor connected to epidermis (*Scanner view*)

17.2.1.2: Multiple sebaceous lobules well delineated with intervening connective tissue septa (*Low power view*)

17.2.1.3: Lobules are composed of peripheral basophilic germinative cells and central mature sebaceous cells with bubbly cytoplasm (*Low power view*)

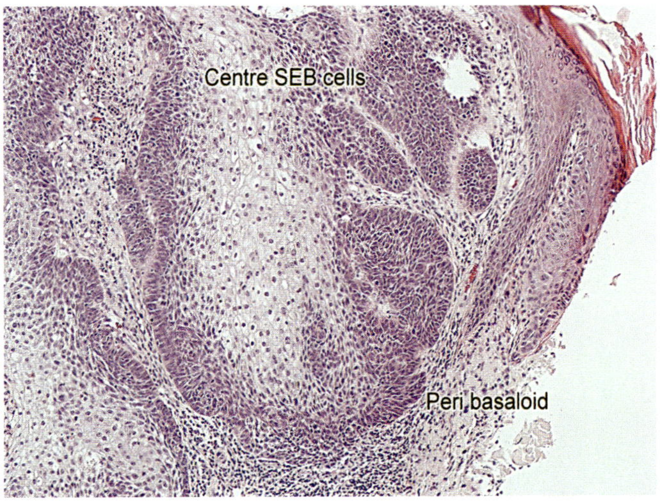

FIGURE 17.2.1.3

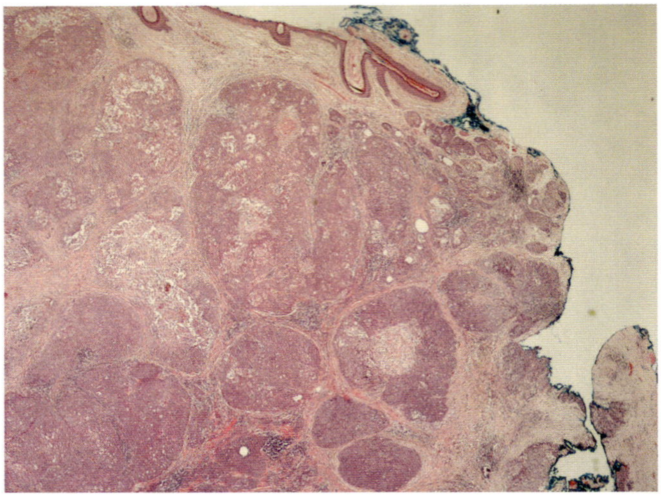

FIGURE 17.2.2.1

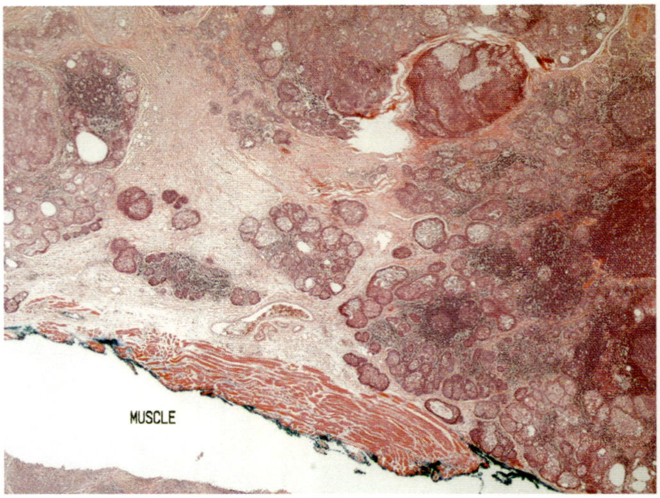

FIGURE 17.2.2.2

17.2.2: Sebaceous Carcinoma

17.2.2.1: Irregular lobules of tumor cells infiltrating the dermis *(Scanner view)*

17.2.2.2: Deep extension into fat and muscle (*Scanner view*)

17.2.2.3: Lobules are composed of basaloid germinative cells and central well differentiated sebaceous cells (*High power view*)

17.2.2.4: Areas showing basaloid cells with pleomorphism and scanty sebaceous cells *(High power view)*

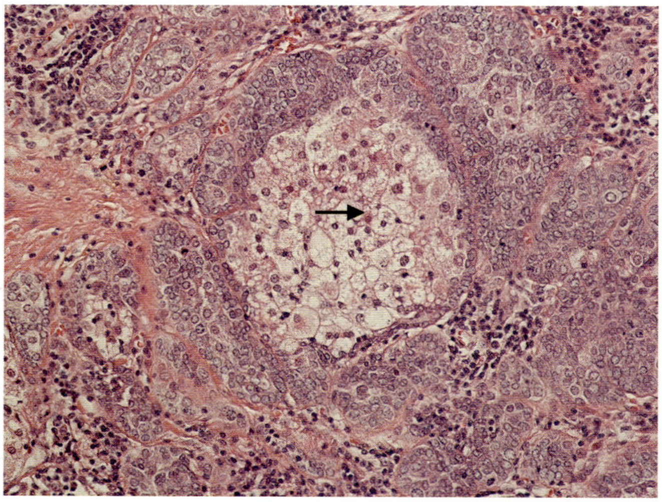

FIGURE 17.2.2.3

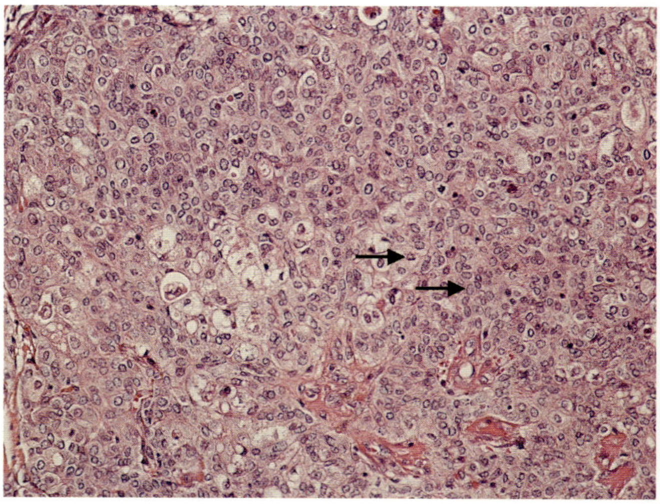

FIGURE 17.2.2.4

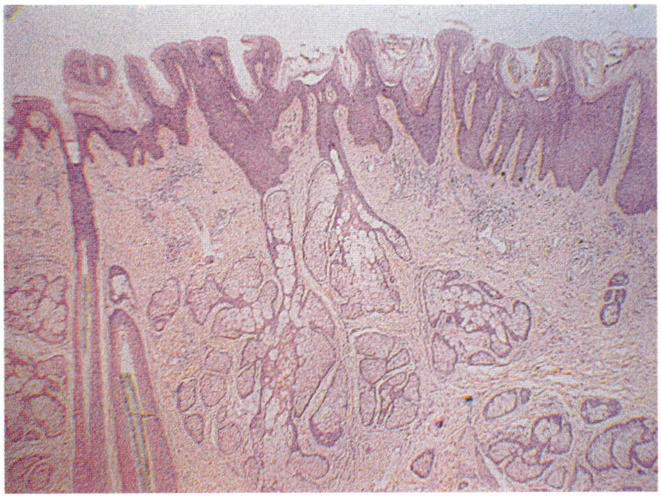

FIGURE 17.2.3.1

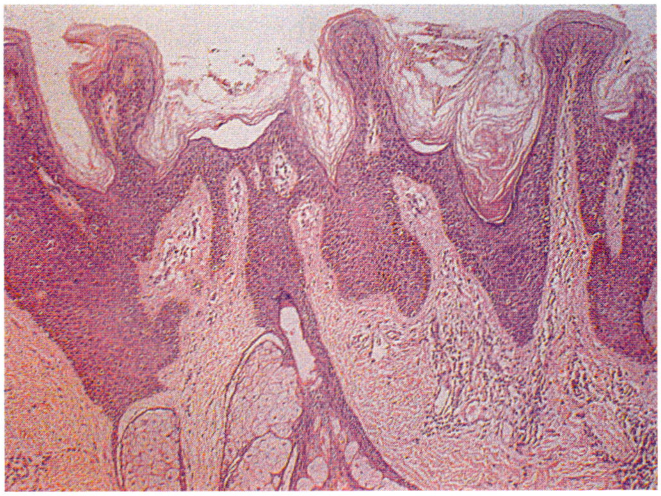

FIGURE 17.2.3.2

17.2.3: Nevus Sebaceous

17.2.3.1: Acanthosis and epithelial papillomatosis with large sebaceous glands (*Scanner view*)

17.2.3.2: Papillomatous hyperplasia closer view (*Low power view*)

17.2.3.3: Apocrine glands, sebaceous glands and hair structures *(Low power view)*

17.2.3.4: Another case with large sebaceous glands and hair follicles (*Scanner view*)

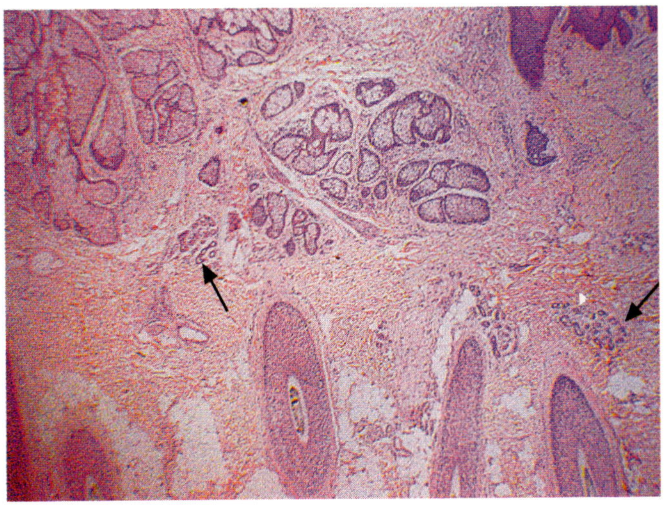

FIGURE 17.2.3.3

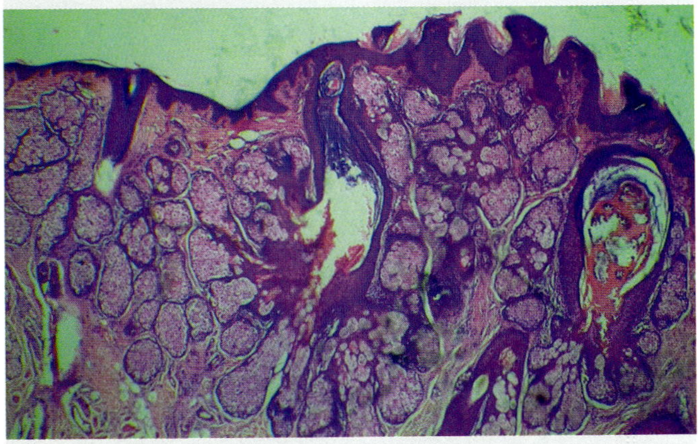

FIGURE 17.2.3.4

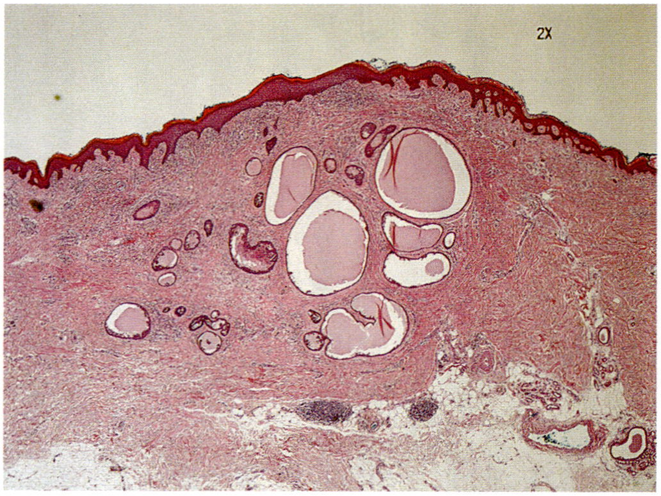

FIGURE 17.3.1.1

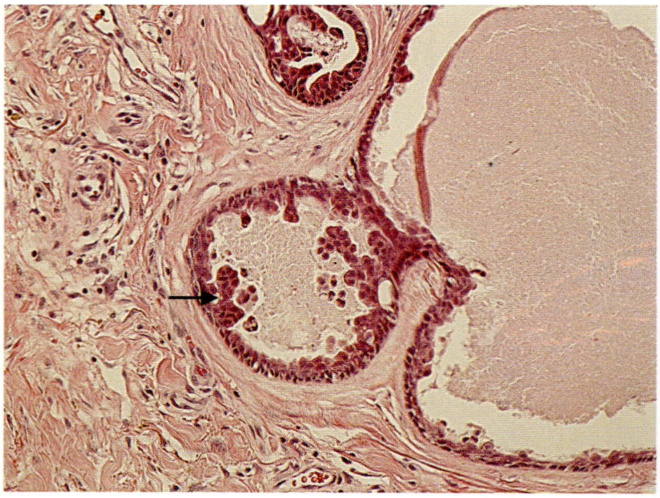

FIGURE 17.3.1.2

17.3: APOCRINE DIFFERENTIATION

17.3.1: Tubular Apocrine Adenoma

17.3.1.1: Circumscribed lobules of dilated variably-sized tubular structures *(Scanner view)*

17.3.1.2: Apocrine cells. Small papillary structures with fibrous stroma *(Low power view)*

17.3.1.3: Apocrine cells. Small papillary structures, tubules lined by two layers of epithelial cells *(High power view)*

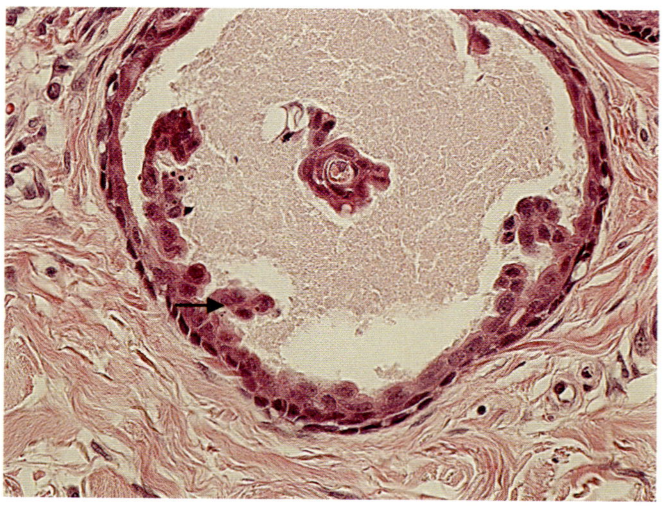

FIGURE 17.3.1.3

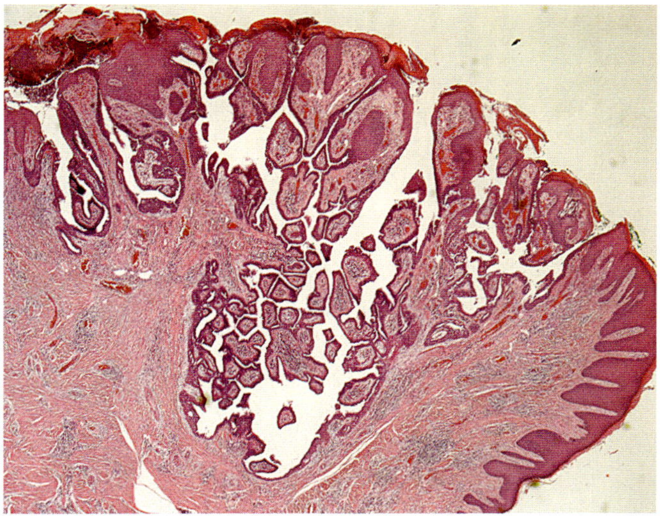

FIGURE 17.3.2.1

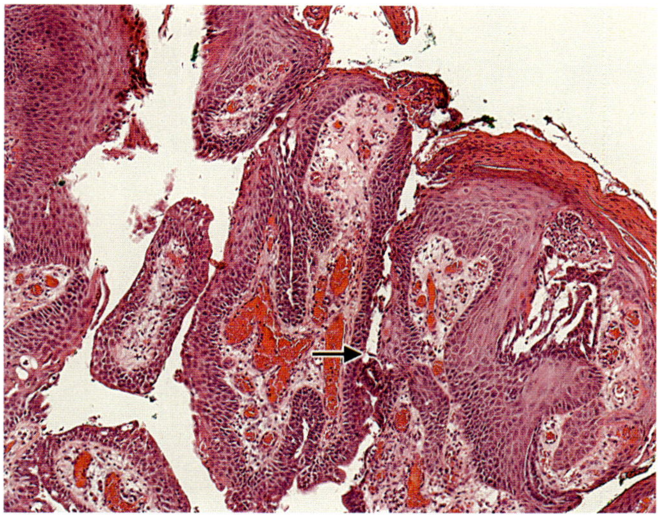

FIGURE 17.3.2.2

17.3.2: Syringocystadenoma Papilliferum

17.3.2.1: Papillary lesion. The surface is covered with squamous epithelium. This tumor developed in a nevus sebaceous *(Scanner view)*

17.3.2.2: Surface squamous epithelium which communicates with ductlike structures *(Low power view)*

17.3.2.3: Papillae are lined by 2 cell layers. The stroma is plasma cell rich *(High power view)*

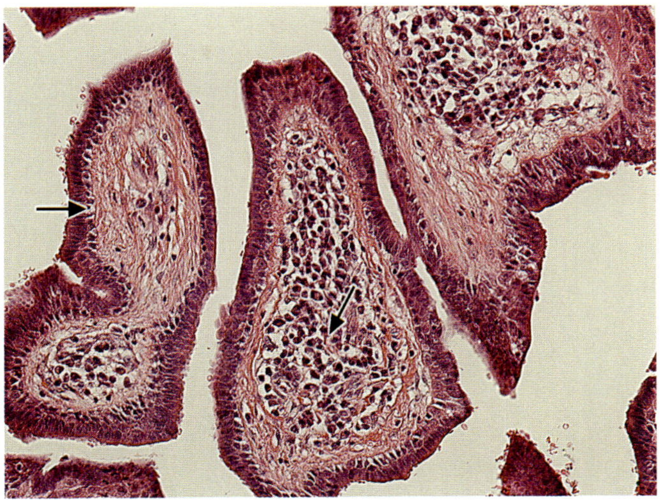

FIGURE 17.3.2.3

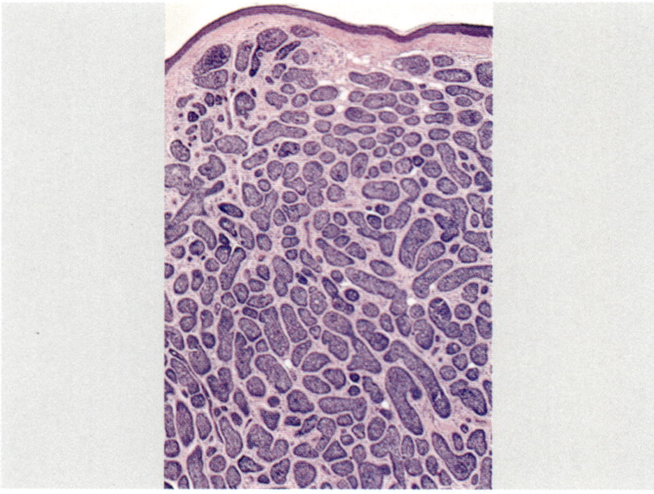

FIGURE 17.3.3.1

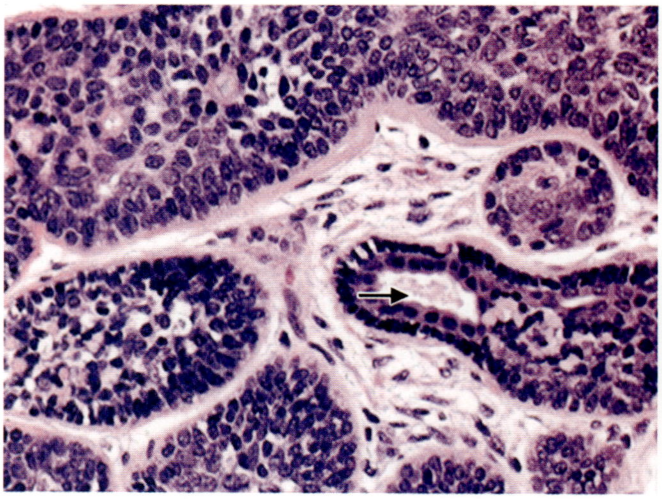

FIGURE 17.3.3.2

17.3.3: Cylindroma

17.3.3.1: Poorly circumscribed dermal tumor which has an appearance of jigsaw puzzle (*Scanner view*)

17.3.3.2: Ductal structures are seen within these tumor masses (*High power view*)

17.3.3.3: Irregularly-shaped islands of basaloid cells surrounded by eosinophilic hyaline bands (*High power view*)

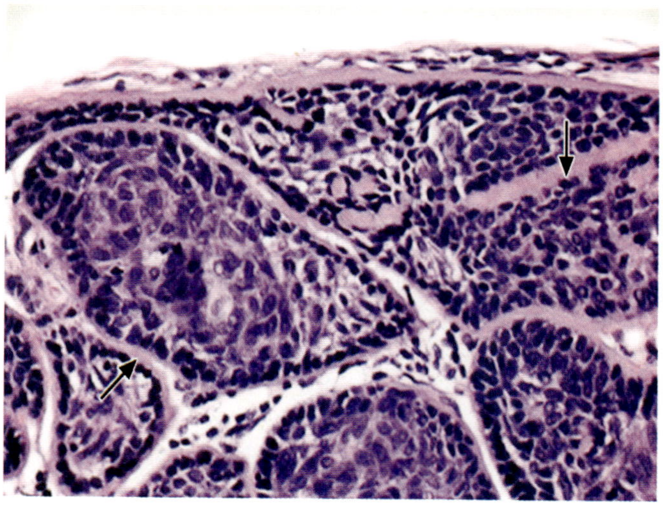

FIGURE 17.3.3.3

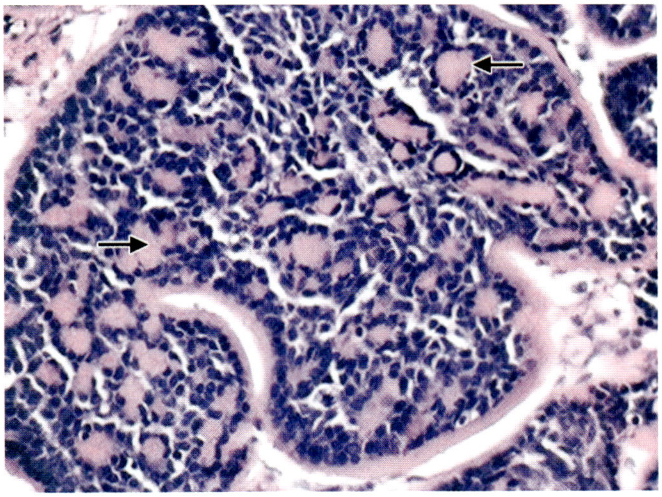

FIGURE 17.3.3.4

17.3.3.4: H & E stain showing pink hyaline material as globules in the tumor (this material stains positive with PAS) *(High power view)*

17.3.3.5: PAS + dense connective tissue sheath called hyaline cylinders *(High power view)*

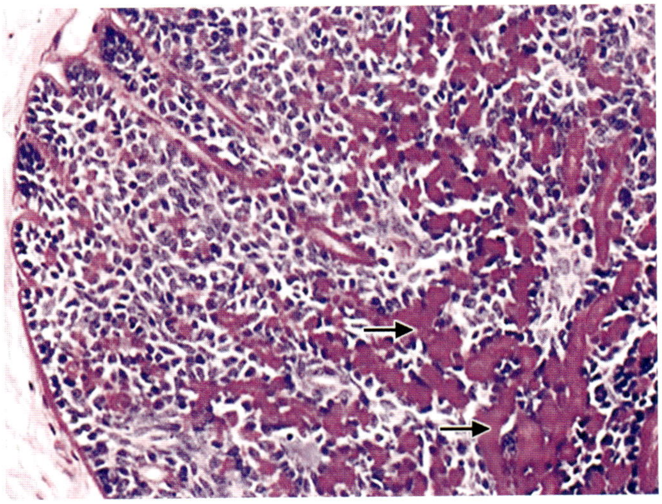

FIGURE 17.3.3.5

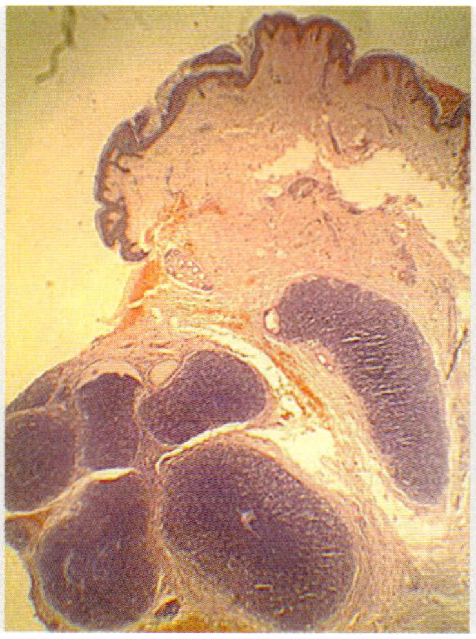

FIGURE 17.3.4.1

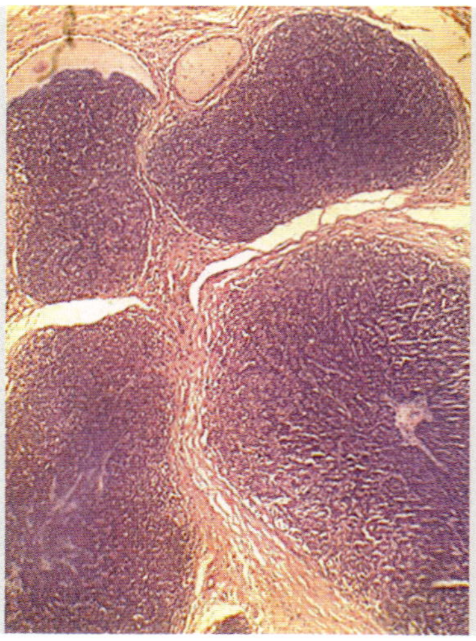

FIGURE 17.3.4.2

17.3.4: Spiradenoma

17.3.4.1: Large, circumscribed basophilic nodules in the dermis separated from epidermis *(Scanner view)*

17.3.4.2: Discrete islands of cells form the nodules *(Low power view)*

17.3.4.3: There are two types of cells—small dark basaloid cells with hyperchromatic nuclei at the periphery and large cells with pale nuclei at the center (*High power view*)

17.3.4.4: Another case with a trabecular arrangement (*High power view*)

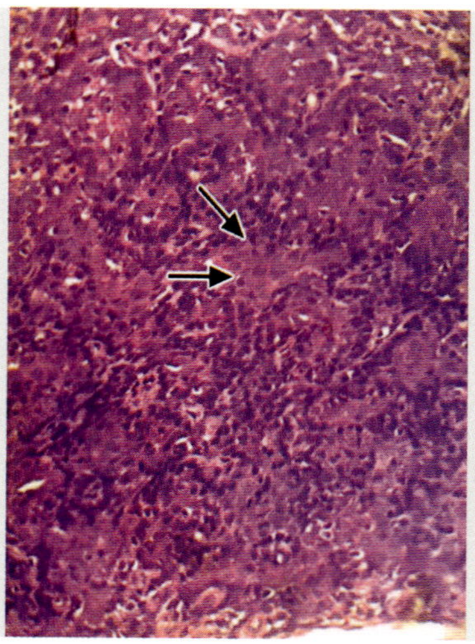

FIGURE 17.3.4.3

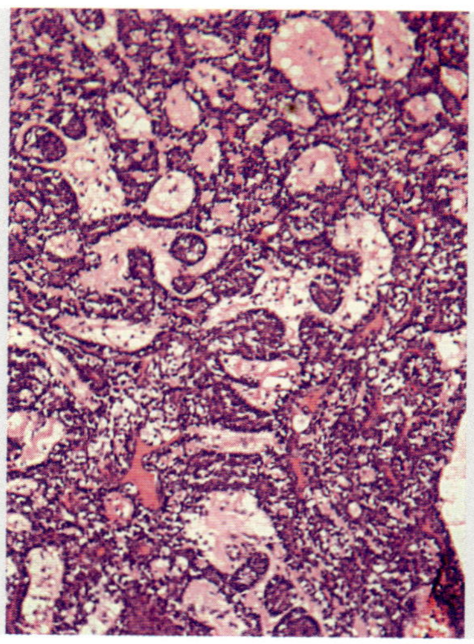

FIGURE 17.3.4.4

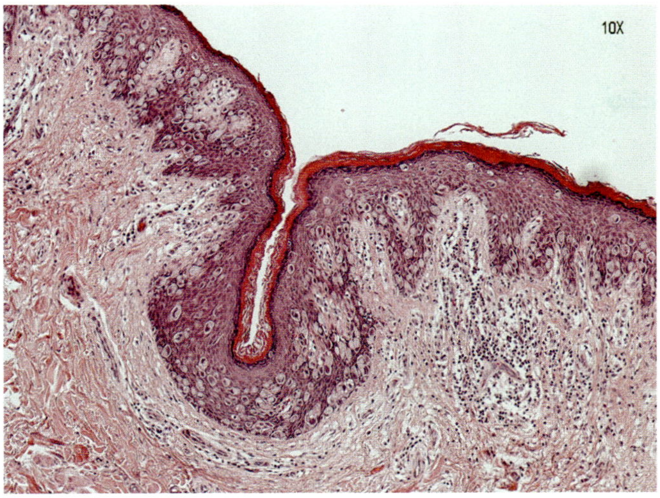

FIGURE 17.3.5.1

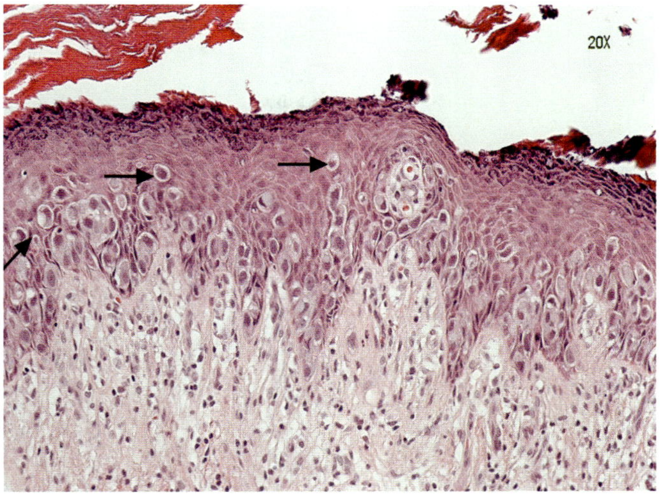

FIGURE 17.3.5.2

17.3.5: Paget's Disease (Extramammary)

17.3.5.1: Large pale cells infiltrating the epidermis, they extend to the epithelium of hair follicles and eccrine ducts *(Scanner view)*

17.3.5.2: Tumor cells with pale cytoplasm at all levels of epidermis *(Low power view)*

17.3.5.3: These Paget's cells show large atypical nuclei, occasional cells have an eccentric nucleus and the appearance of a signet ring *(High power view)*

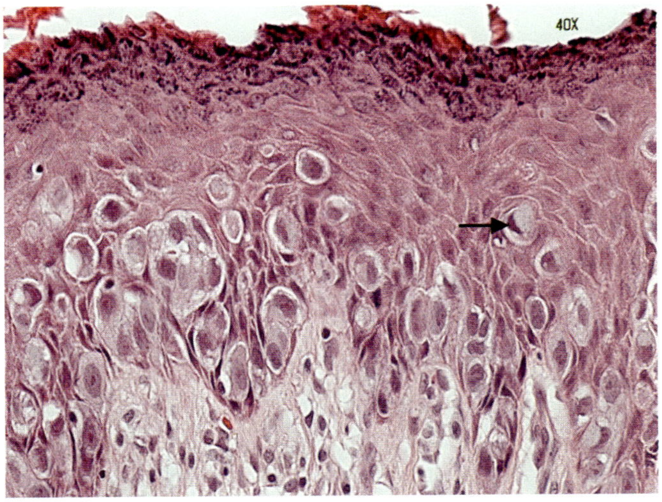

FIGURE 17.3.5.3

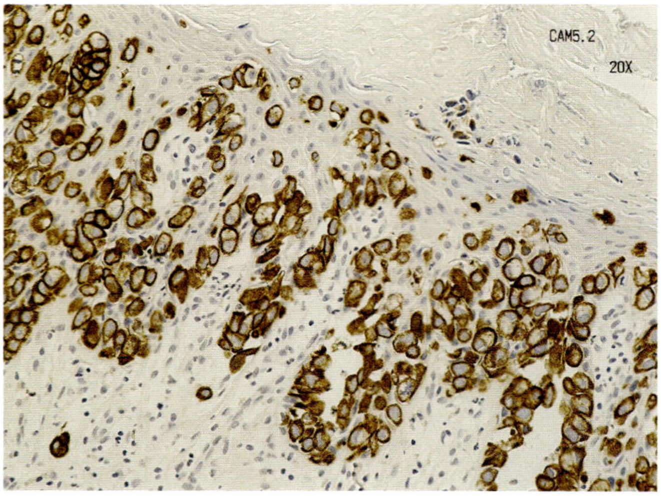

FIGURE 17.3.5.4

17.3.5.4: CAM5.2 positive Paget's cells. The squamous epithelium is negative *(High power view)*

17.3.5.5: Paget's cells CK7+. The squamous epithelium is negative *(High power view)*

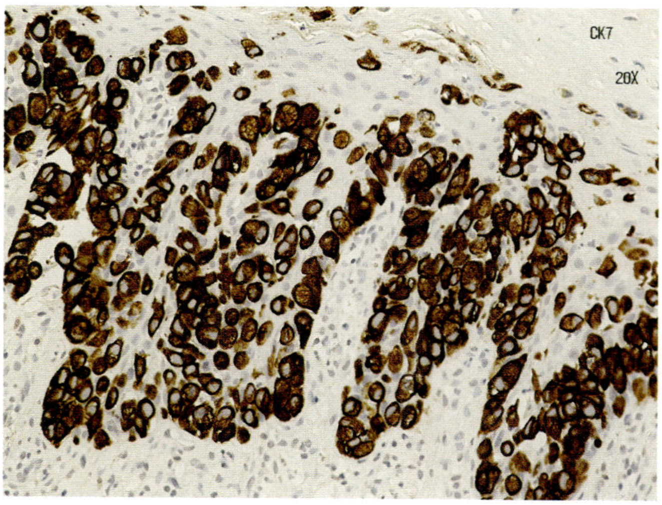

FIGURE 17.3.5.5

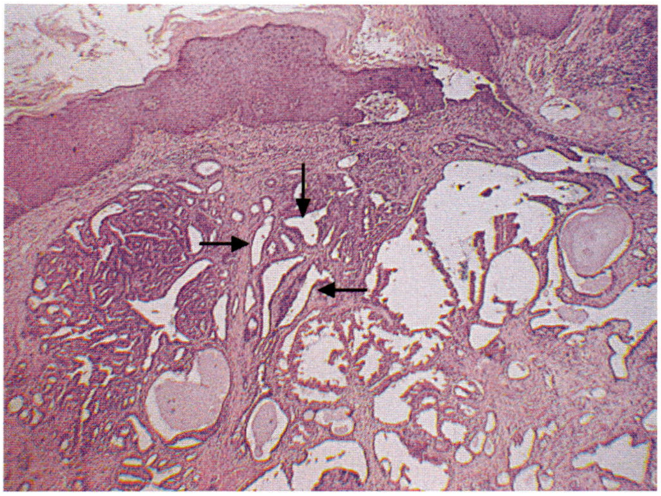

FIGURE 17.3.6.1

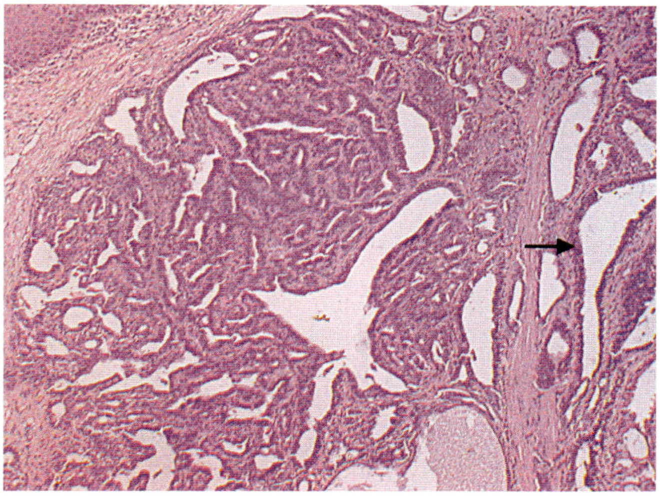

FIGURE 17.3.6.2

17.3.6: Erosive Adenomatosis of the Nipple

17.3.6.1: Ductal proliferation in the superficial dermis (*Scanner view*)

17.3.6.2: Closer view of ductal proliferation (*Low power view*)

17.3.6.3: Showing intraductal papillomatosis and dermal fibrosis (*Low power view*)

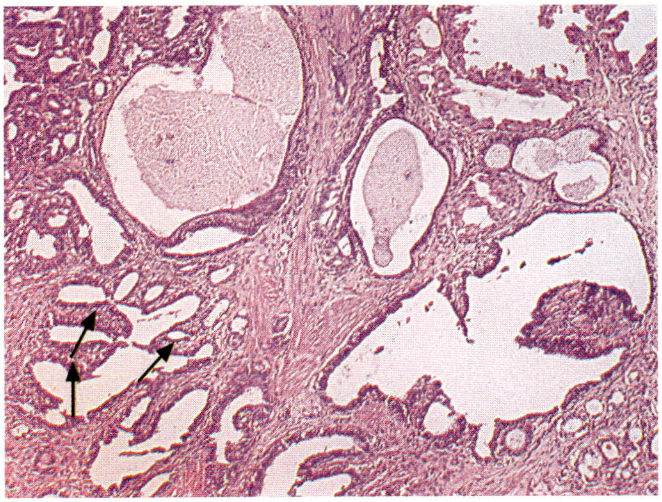

FIGURE 17.3.6.3

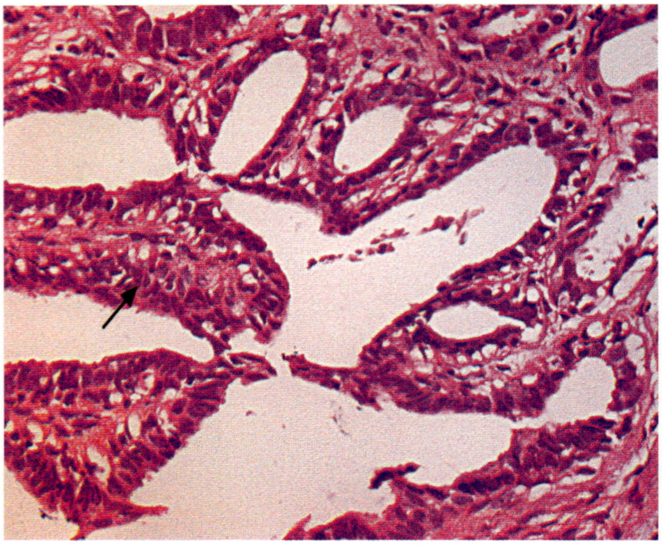

FIGURE 17.3.6.4

17.3.6.4: Closer view of papillary projections (*High power view*)

17.3.6.5: Apocrine decapitation secretion (*High power view*)

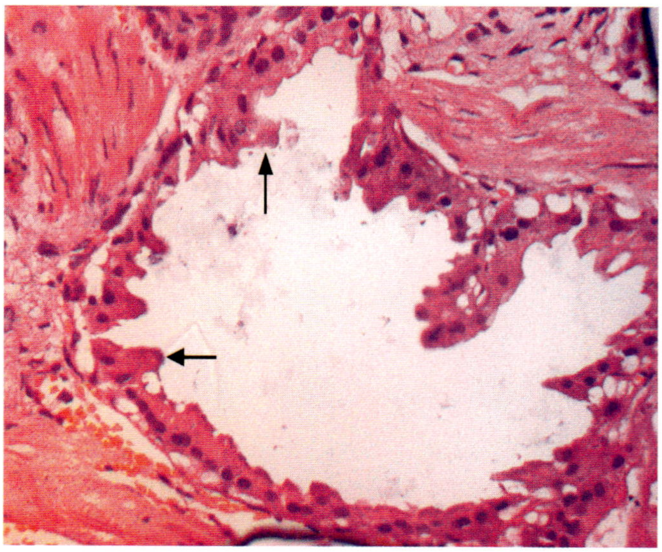

FIGURE 17.3.6.5

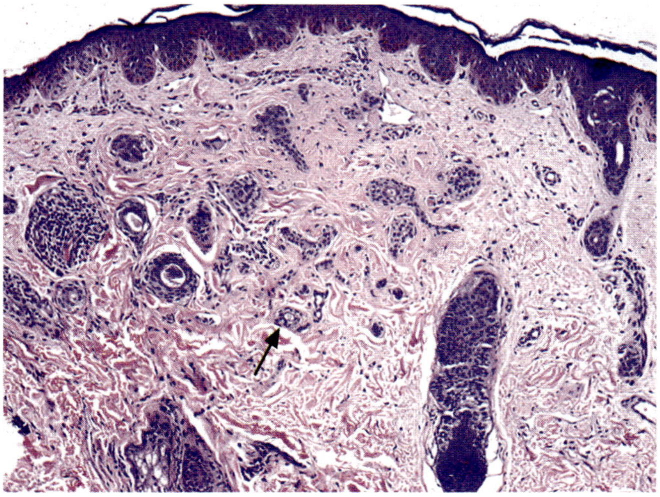

FIGURE 17.4.1.1

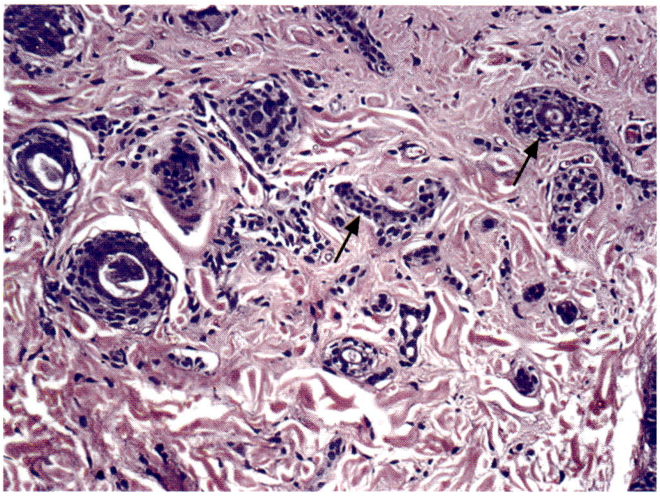

FIGURE 17.4.1.2

17.4: ECCRINE DIFFERENTIATION

17.4.1: Syringoma

17.4.1.1: Tumor in the dermis comprised of multiple small ducts *(Scanner view)*

17.4.1.2: Solid nests and strands of basaloid cells in addition to ducts (*Low power view*)

17.4.1.3: Ducts are lined by two layers of cuboidal epithelium (*High power view*)

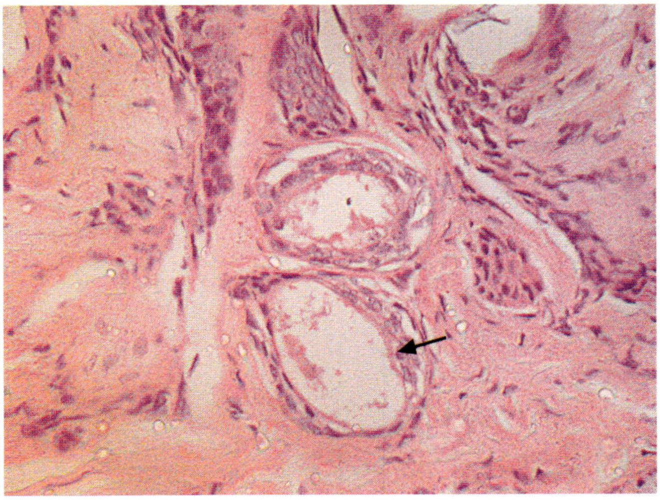

FIGURE 17.4.1.3

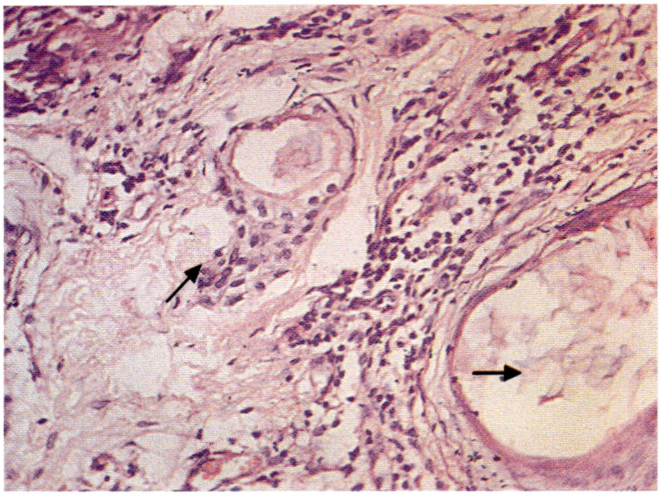

FIGURE 17.4.1.4

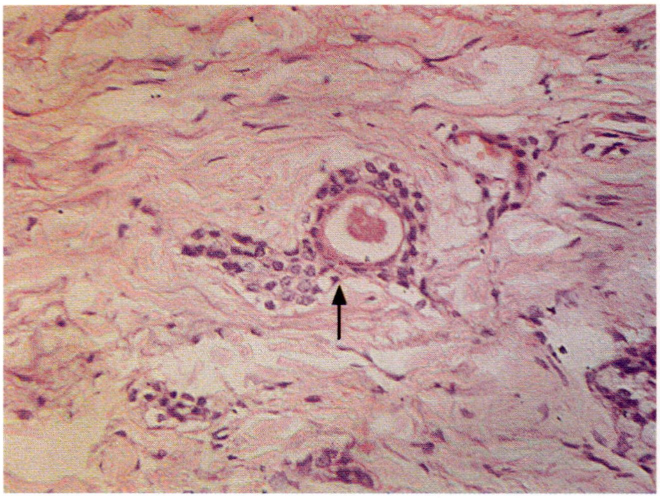

FIGURE 17.4.1.5

17.4.1.4: Ducts have a comma-like tail (tadpole appearance). Ducts are of different sizes and are filled with eosinophilic material (*High power view*)

17.4.1.5: Dense fibrous stroma and tadpole appearance (*High power view*)

17.4.1.6: Chondroid syringoma (*Scanner view*)

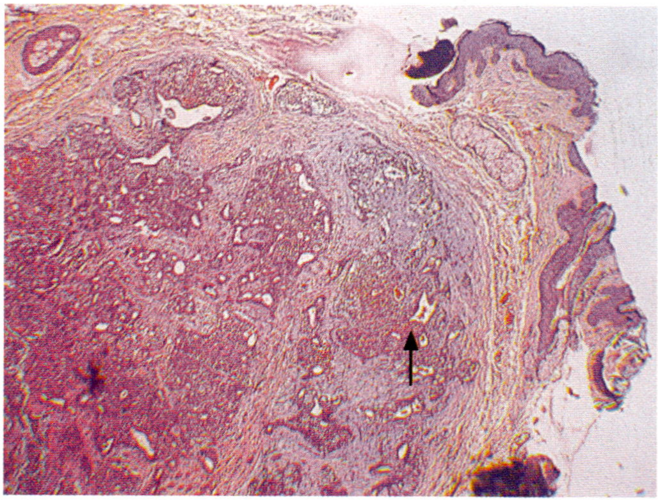

FIGURE 17.4.1.6

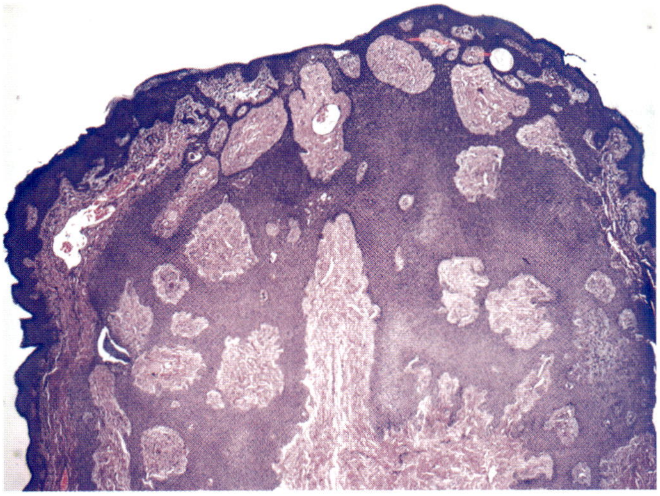

FIGURE 17.4.2.1

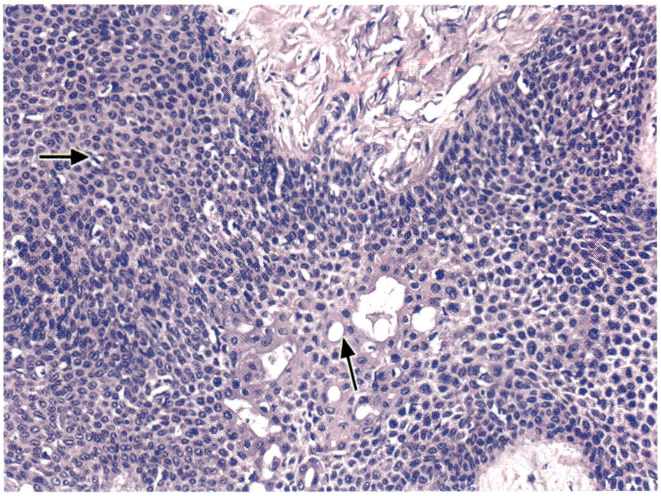

FIGURE 17.4.2.2

17.4.2: Eccrine Poroma

17.4.2.1: Interconnecting epithelium arising from the epidermis, growing downwards to the dermis (*Scanner view*)

17.4.2.2: Poroma cells are small, cuboidal and distinctive from adjacent keratinocytes (*Scanner view*)

17.4.2.3: Poroma cells with intercellular bridges and ductal lumina (*High power view*)

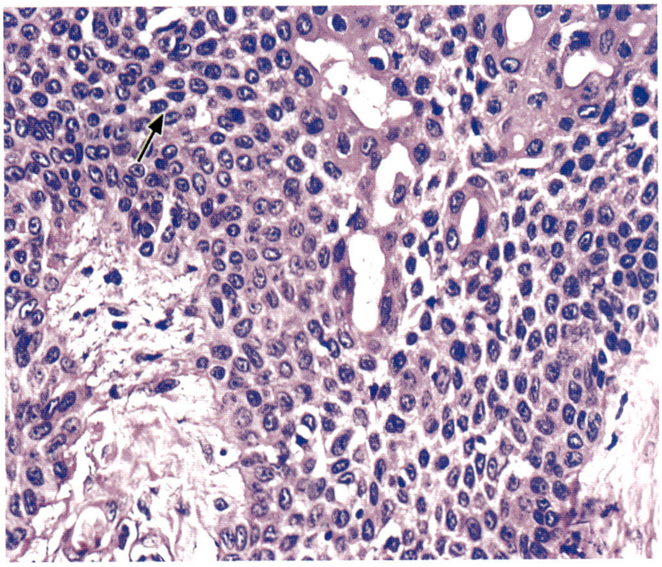

FIGURE 17.4.2.3

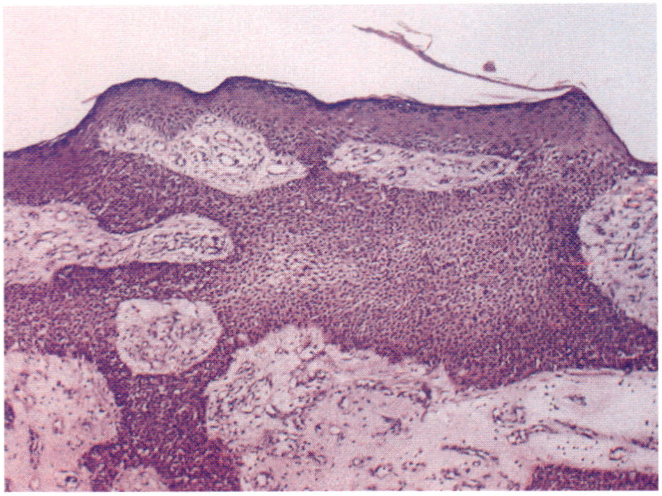

FIGURE 17.4.2.4

17.4.2.4: Another case with down growth of basaloid cells *(Low power view)*

17.4.2.5: The cells are smaller and look different from adjacent keratinocytes (*High power view*)

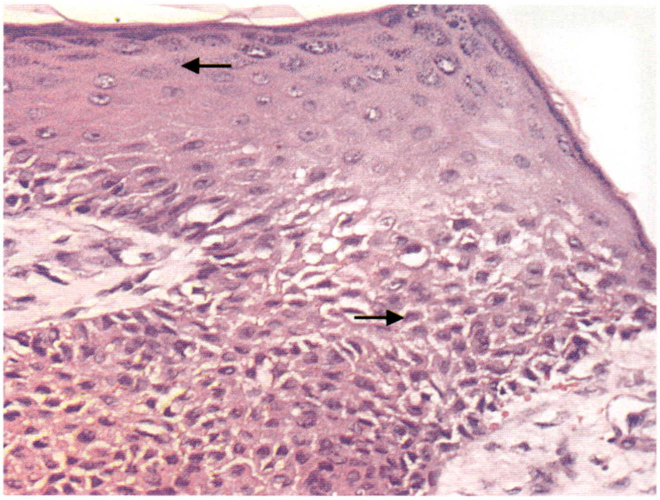

FIGURE 17.4.2.5

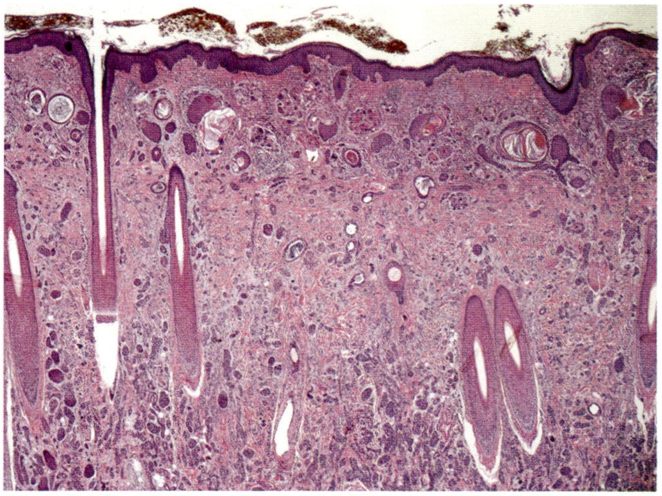

FIGURE 17.4.3.1

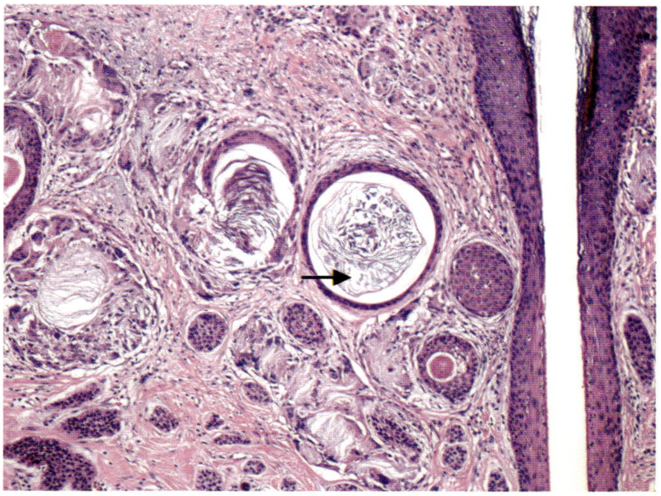

FIGURE 17.4.3.2

17.4.3: Microcystic Adnexal Carcinoma

17.4.3.1: Widely infiltrating tumor into deep dermis (*Scanner view*)

17.4.3.2: Superficial keratinous cysts (*Low power view*)

17.4.3.3: Deep dermis shows infiltrative tumor in cords and strands of basaloid cells with a scirrhous appearance (embedded in a dense, hyalinized stroma) (*Scanner view*)

17.4.3.4: On closer view, the cells show fairly bland morphology (*Low power view*)

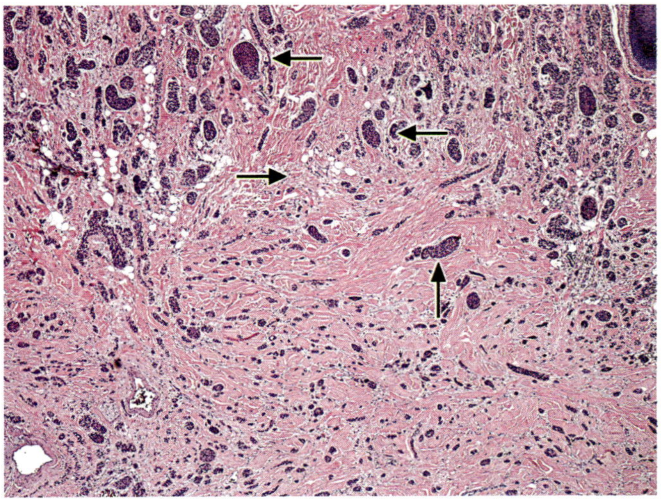

FIGURE 17.4.3.3

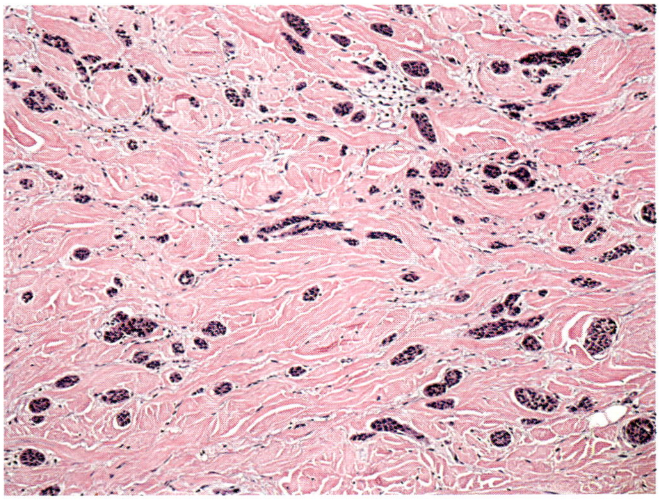

FIGURE 17.4.3.4

DIFFERENTIAL DIAGNOSIS

1. Appendageal tumors with follicular differentiation
   a. Pilar sheath acanthoma
   b. Trichoadenoma
   c. Trichofolliculoma
2. Appendageal tumors with sebaceous differentiation
   a. Sebaceous hyperplasia
   b. BCC with sebaceous differentiation
3. Appendageal tumors with apocrine differentiation
   a. Hidradenoma papilliferum
4. Appendageal tumors with eccrine differentiation
   a. Eccrine porocarcinoma

DIAGNOSTIC PEARLS

1. Transverse sections of biopsies are better for detecting pathological changes in follicular microanatomy.
2. Sebaceous adenoma situated deep in dermis with cystic change may be a marker for Muir Torre syndrome.
3. Multivesicular bubbly cytoplasm differentiates sebaceous carcinoma from other clear cell tumors.
4. Sebaceous and apocrine glands in nevus sebaceous become prominent only after adolescence.
5. Desmoplastic trichilemmomas can be differentiated from SCC and BCC by PAS stain which shows an intact peritumoral basement membrane.
6. The presence of abortive hair follicles and lack of apoptotic foci differentiate trichoepithelioma from BCC.
7. In older lesions of pilomatrixoma, the basaloid cells are completely replaced by ghost cells and dystrophic calcification is seen.
8. Presence of embryonic hair like structures differentiates trichoblastoma from BCC.
9. Mitotic figures are uncommon in microcystic adnexal carcinoma.

Melanocytic Lesions

18

Chapter Outline

18.1: Solar Lentigo
18.2: Melanocytic Nevus
18.3: Blue Nevus
18.4: Spitz Nevus
18.5: Dysplastic Nevus
18.6: Halo Nevus
18.7: Malignant Melanoma

Sara Edward, Ying Guo, Steven Kossard,
Mani Makhija, Alistair Robson

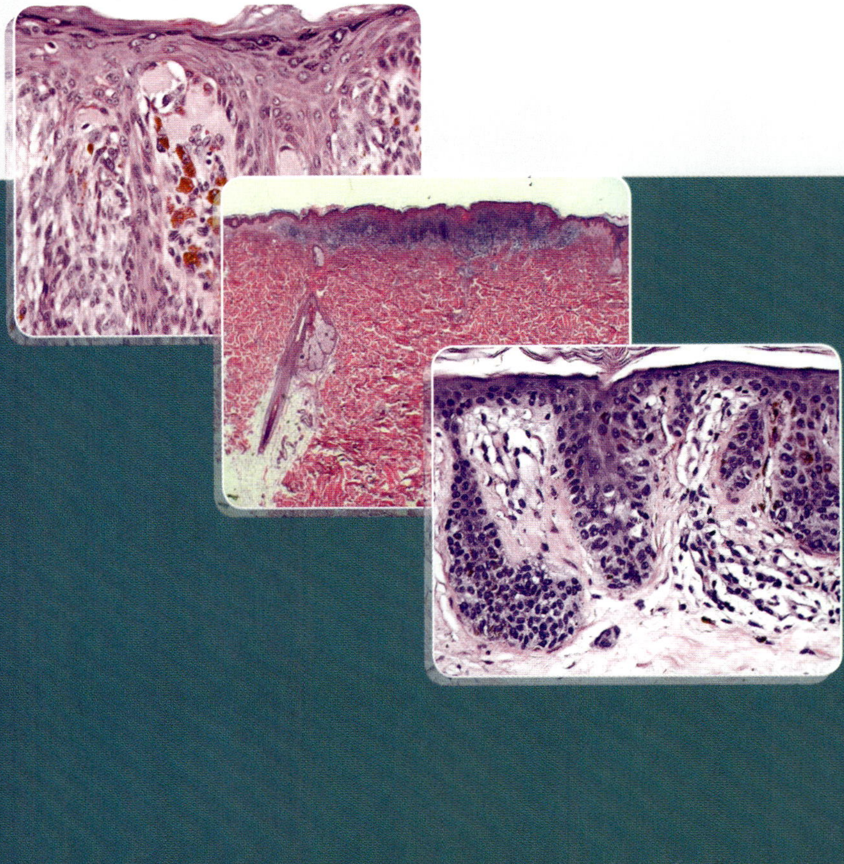

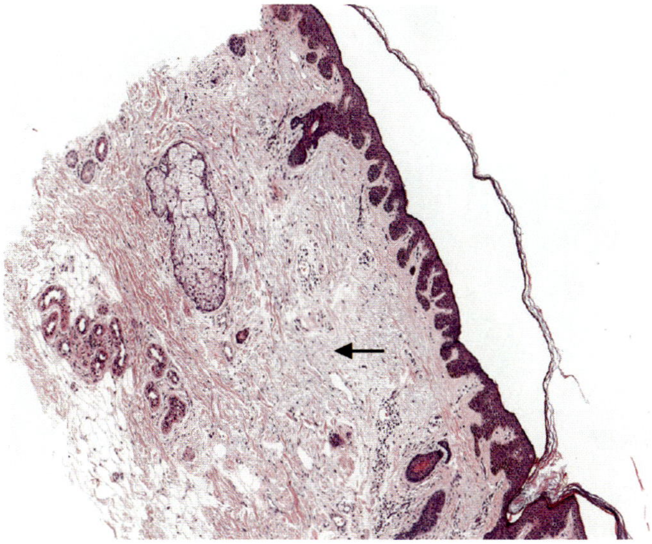

FIGURE 18.1.1

18.1: SOLAR LENTIGO

18.1.1: Hyperplasia of epidermis with club-shaped and elongated rete ridges, solar elastotic changes (*Scanner view*)

18.1.2: Basal hyperpigmentation with an increased number of single melanocytes in the basal layer, the papillary dermis may contain a sparse lymphohistiocytic infiltrate (*Low power view*)

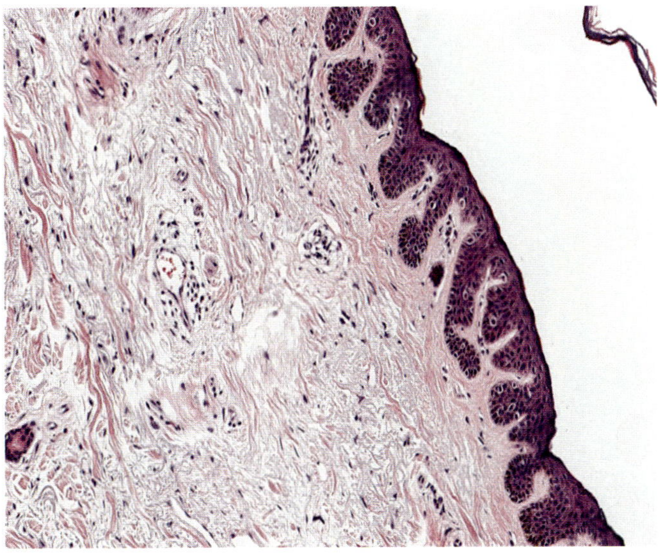

FIGURE 18.1.2

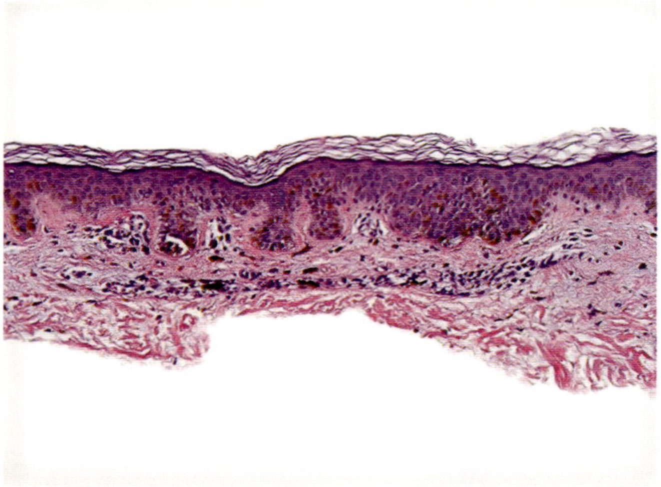

FIGURE 18.2.1

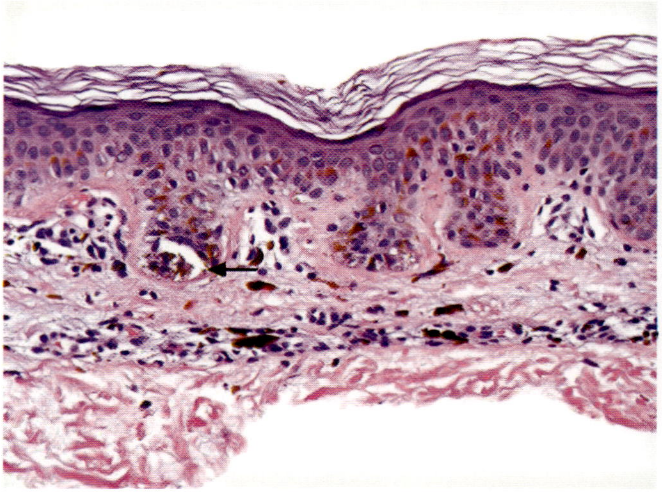

FIGURE 18.2.2

18.2: MELANOCYTIC NEVUS

18.2.1: Junctional melanocytic nevus—discrete nest of melanocytes at the dermoepidermal junction bulging into the dermis (*Scanner view*)

18.2.2: Closer view of melanocytic nest with melanophages and lymphohistiocytic infiltrate in the dermis (*Low power view*)

18.2.3: Intradermal melanocytic nevus—epidermis unremarkable, dermis has nests of melanocytes/nevus cells (*2X*)

18.2.4: The cells have round nuclei and scanty cytoplasm (*4X*)

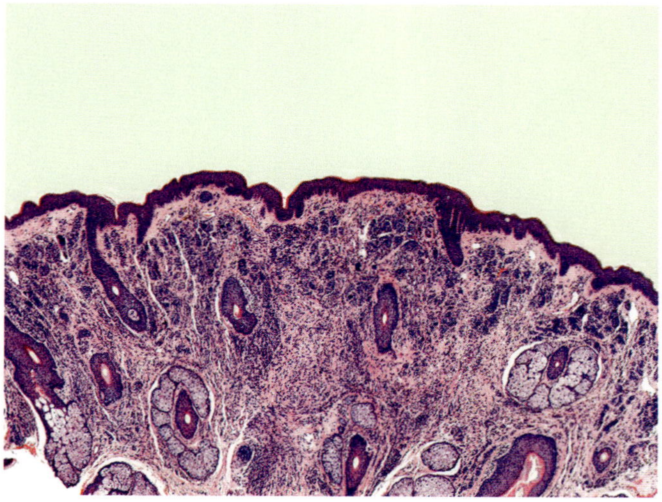

FIGURE 18.2.3

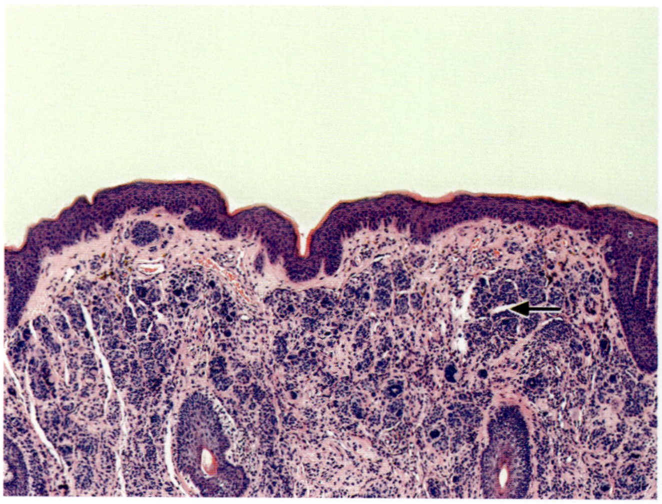

FIGURE 18.2.4

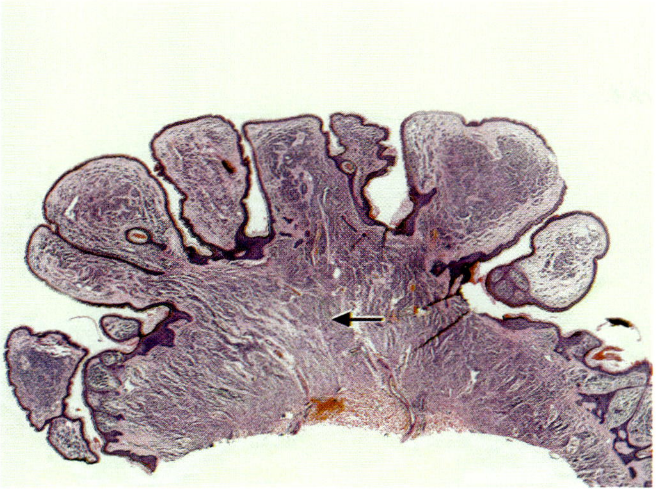

FIGURE 18.2.5

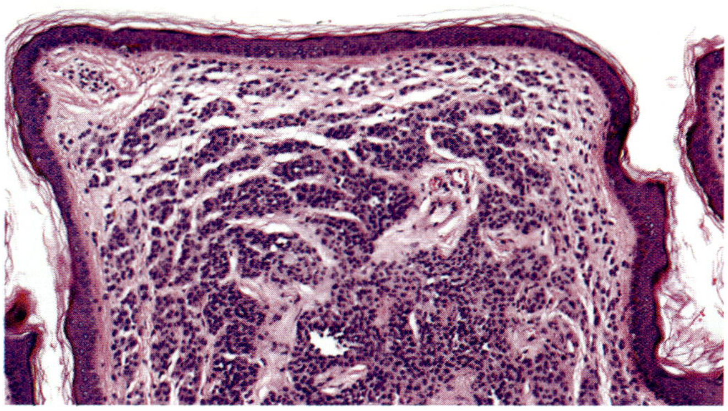

FIGURE 18.2.6

18.2.5: Another case showing nevus cells in the deeper dermis with spindle shape and neuroid appearance *(Scanner view)*

18.2.6: Closer view of elevated epidermis and cuboidal nevus cells (*Low power view*)

18.2.7: Compound melanocytic nevus with both junctional nests and an intradermal component of nevus cells (*Scanner view*)

18.2.8: Orderly nests and cords of nevus cells with melanin pigment. No dysplasia (*Low power view*)

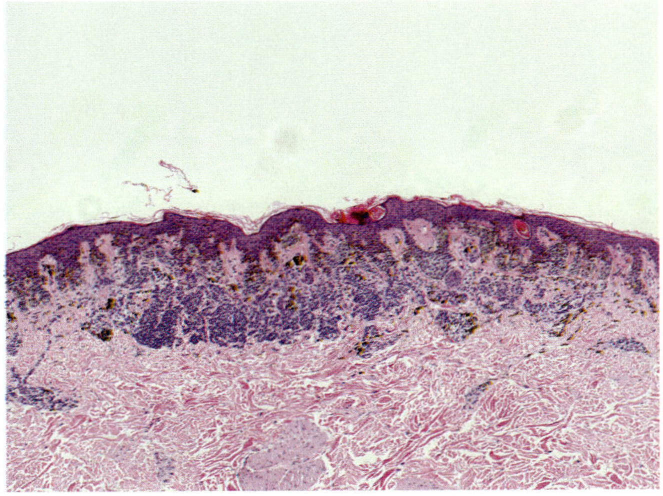

FIGURE 18.2.7

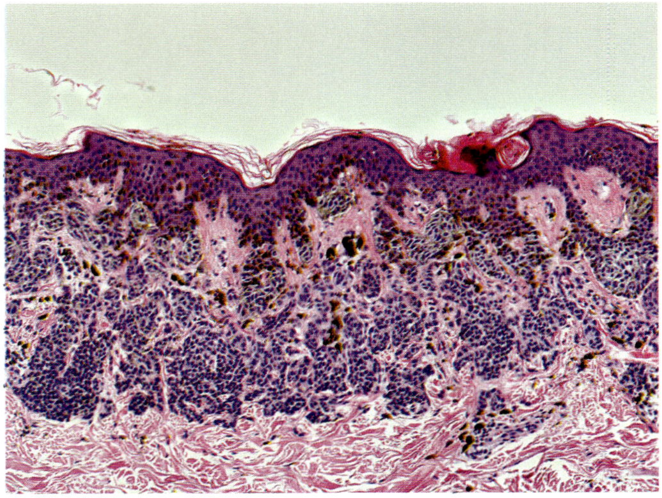

FIGURE 18.2.8

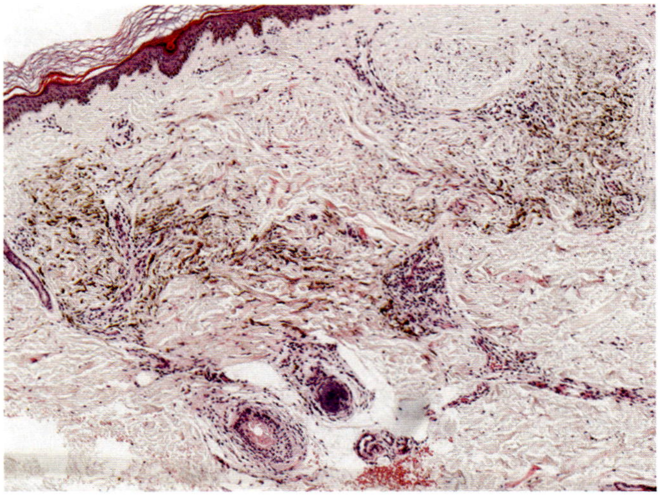

FIGURE 18.3.1

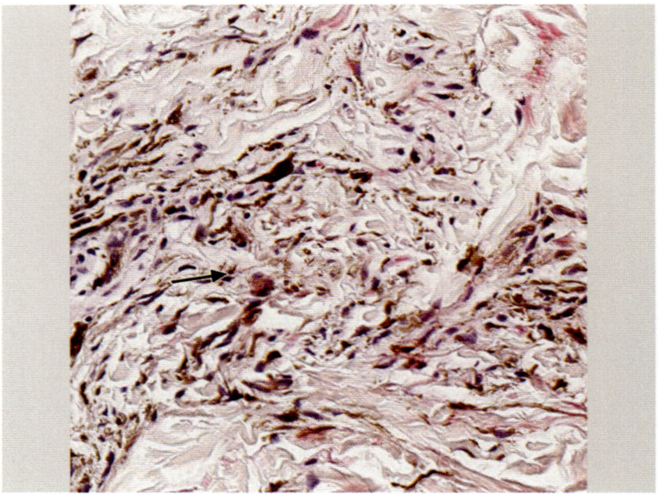

FIGURE 18.3.2

18.3: BLUE NEVUS

18.3.1: Epidermis unremarkable, there are nevus cells with elongated spindle-shaped nuclei in the dermis. The cells usually lie parallel to the epidermis (*Scanner view*)

18.3.2: Cells show elongated nuclei with tapered ends, with abundant melanin pigment. No dysplasia (*High power view*)

18.3.3: Cellular blue nevus—nodular collection of tumor cells occupying entire dermis and extending to the subcutaneous fat (*Scanner view*)

18.3.4: Tumor consists of dendritic melanocytes with epithelioid and spindle cells, abundant cytoplasm and lot of pigment (*High power view*)

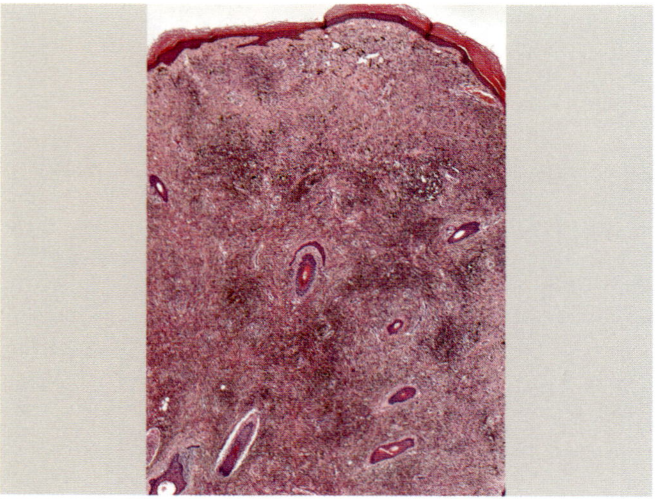

FIGURE 18.3.3

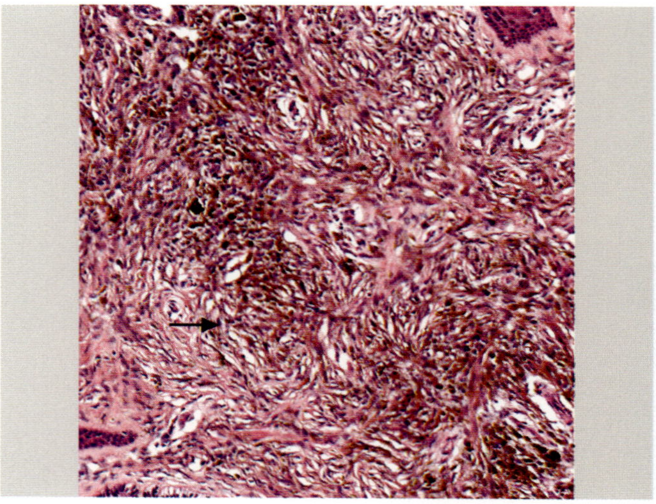

FIGURE 18.3.4

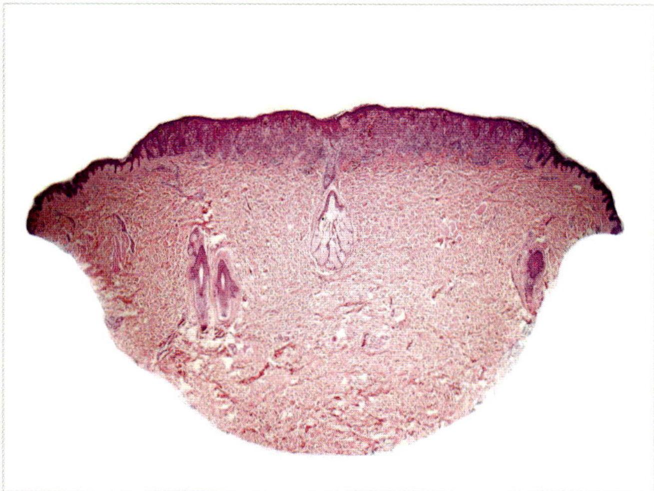

FIGURE 18.4.1

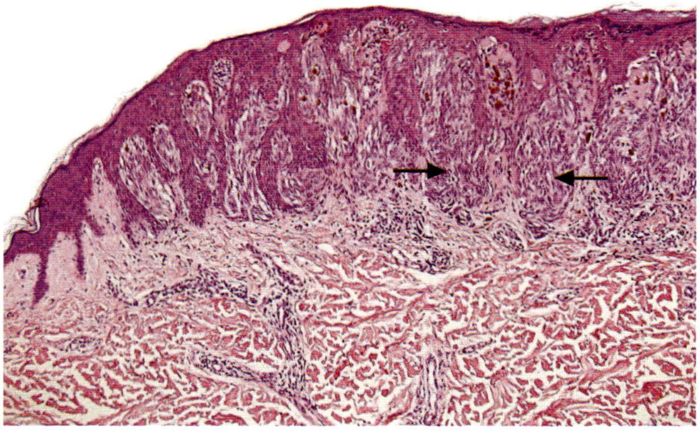

FIGURE 18.4.2

18.4: SPITZ NEVUS

18.4.1: Hyperplasia of epidermis, nests of melanocytes in the epidermis as well as dermis (*Scanner view*)

18.4.2: Confluent nests at the dermoepidermal junction (*Low power view*)

18.4.3: Another case with melanocytes migrating up in the epidermis, nevus cells in the dermis are either epithelioid or spindle shaped (*Low power view*)

18.4.4: Epidermis shows Kamino bodies which are eosinophilic globules composed of basement membrane substance, situated over the tips of dermal papillae, a characteristic feature of Spitz nevus (*High power view*)

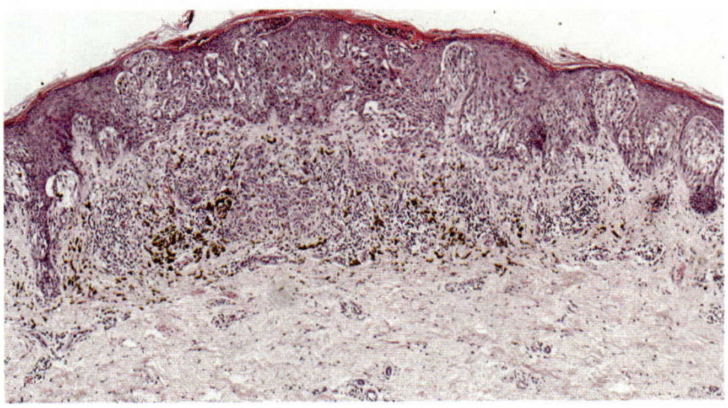

FIGURE 18.4.3

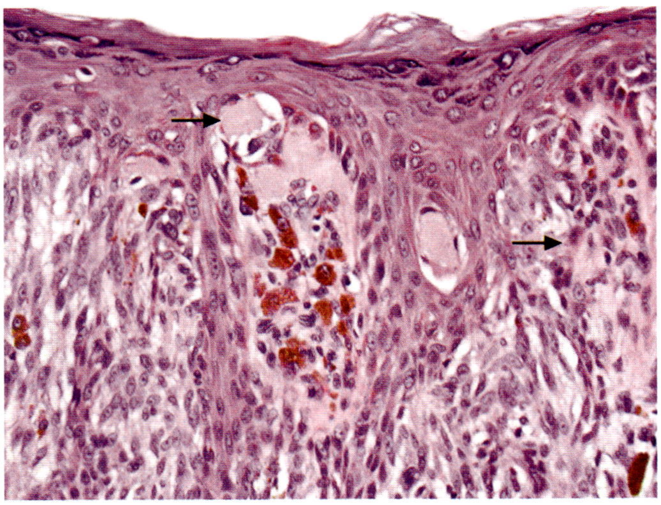

FIGURE 18.4.4

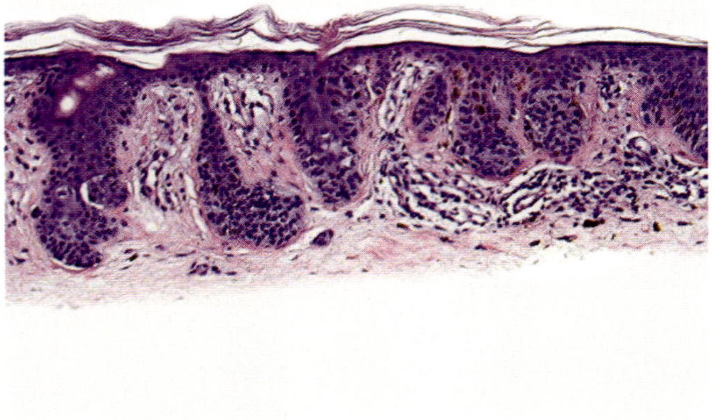

FIGURE 18.5.1

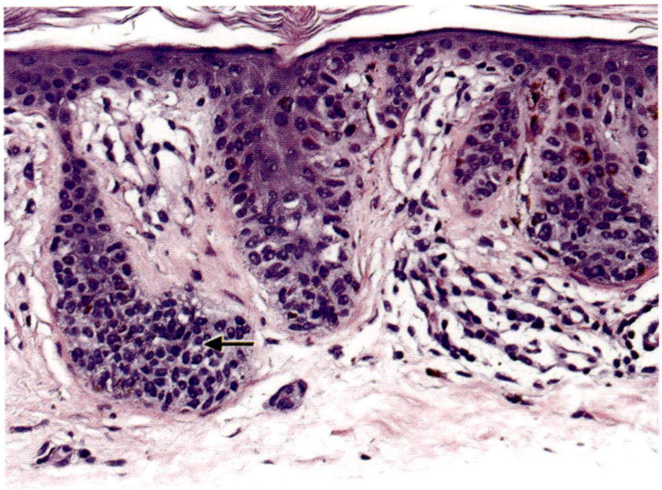

FIGURE 18.5.2

18.5: DYSPLASTIC NEVUS

18.5.1: Nests of melanocytes as well as single cells at the dermoepidermal junction and along elongated rete ridges (*Scanner view*)

18.5.2: Closer view of the nests and perivascular lymphocytes (*Low power view*)

18.5.3: Another case with lentiginous pattern of melanocytes, bridging of rete ridges and dermal fibroplasia (*Scanner view*)

18.5.4: Single cells as well as nests of melanocytes in the dermis (*Low power view*)

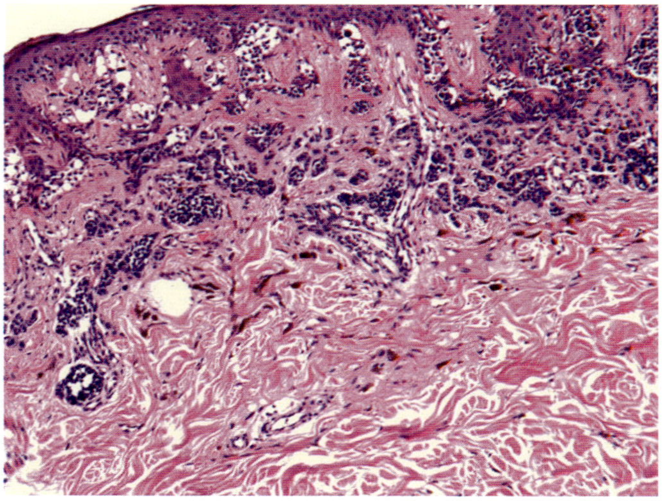

FIGURE 18.5.3

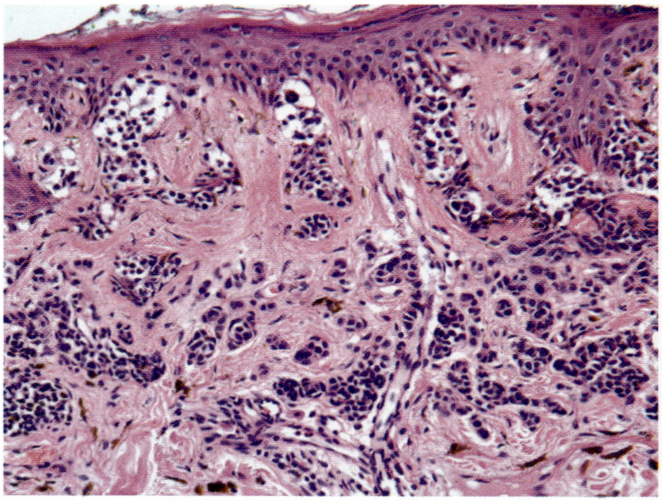

FIGURE 18.5.4

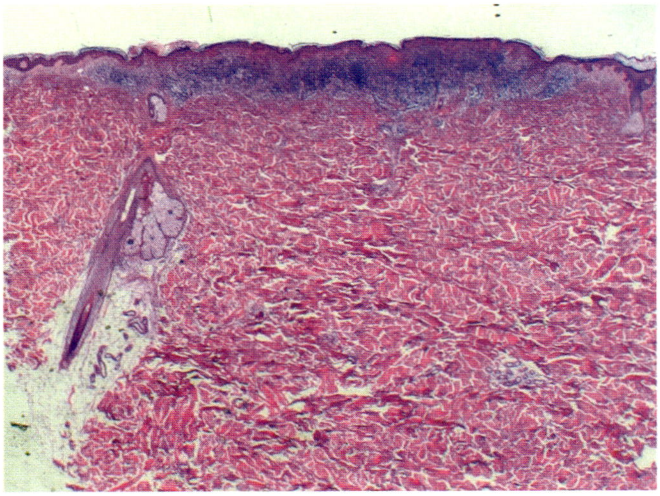

FIGURE 18.6.1

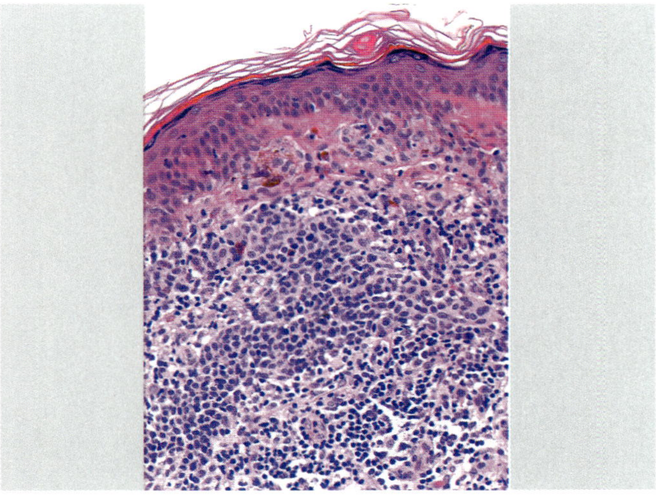

FIGURE 18.6.2

18.6: HALO NEVUS

18.6.1: Well-defined symmetrical lesion with dense lymphocytic infiltrate (*Scanner view*)

18.6.2: Lymphoid infiltrate is admixed with dermal melanocytic nests (*Low power view*)

18.6.3: Dermal nevus cells show mild atypia and an occasional mitotic figure (*High power view*)

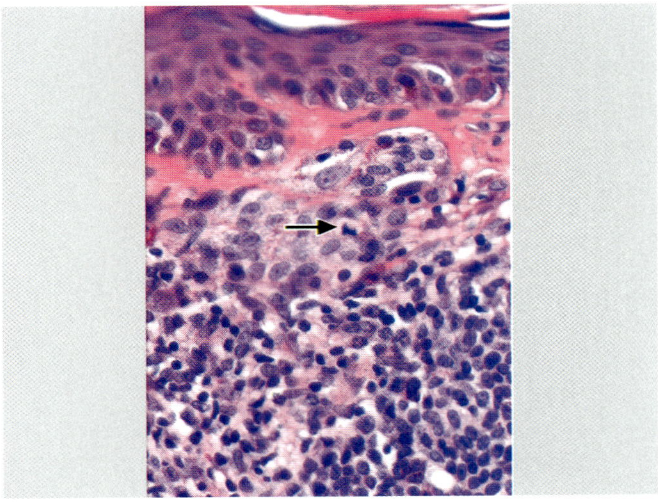

FIGURE 18.6.3

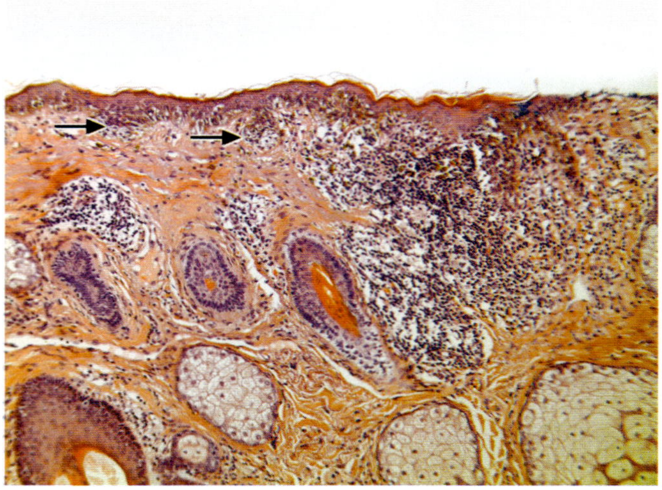

FIGURE 18.7.1

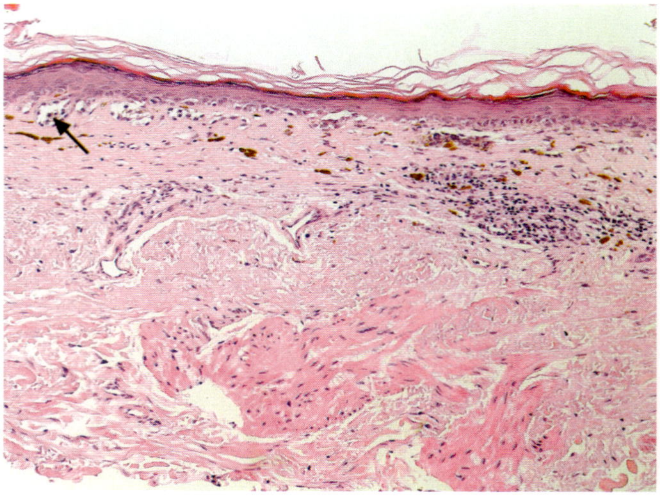

FIGURE 18.7.2

18.7: MALIGNANT MELANOMA

18.7.1: Lentigo maligna—atypical melanocytes lying singly or in nests at the basal layer, may extend upwards in the epidermis (*Scanner view*)

18.7.2: Another case showing epidermal atrophy with confluent single basal vacuolated melanocytes and asymmetric nesting. Host lymphocyte response and fibrosis is a sign of regression (*Scanner view*)

18.7.3: Retraction and prominent regression is seen at the dermoepidermal junction and areas of solar elastosis in the dermis (*Low power view*)

18.7.4: Confluent single melanocytes (immunohistochemistry with microphthalmia transcription factor) (*Low power view*)

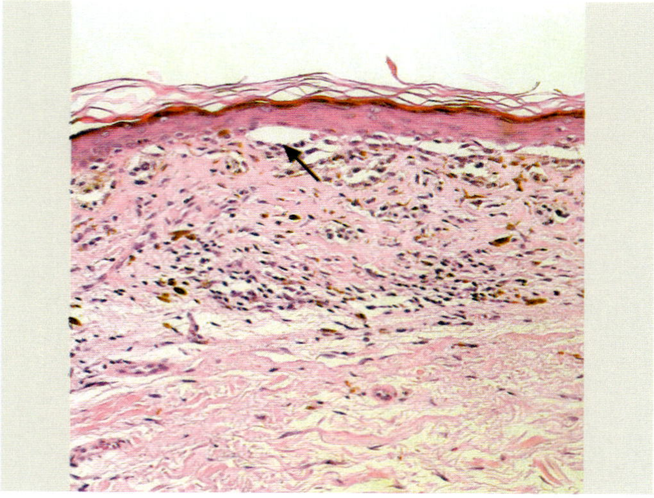

FIGURE 18.7.3

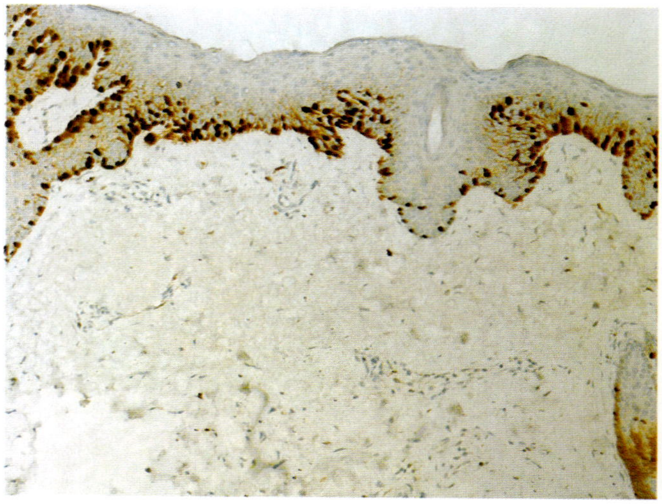

FIGURE 18.7.4

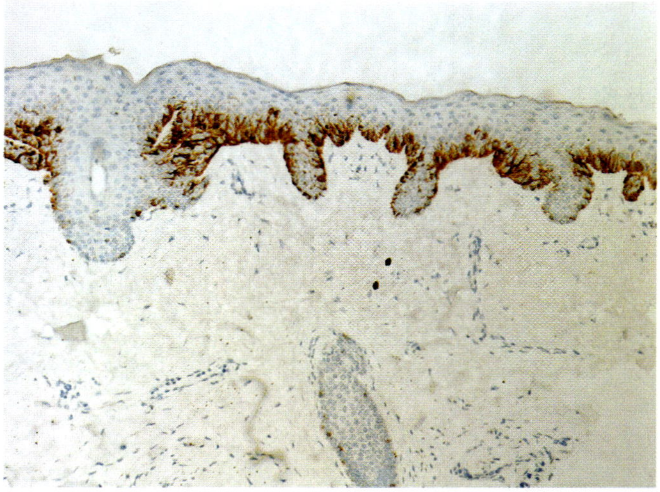

FIGURE 18.7.5

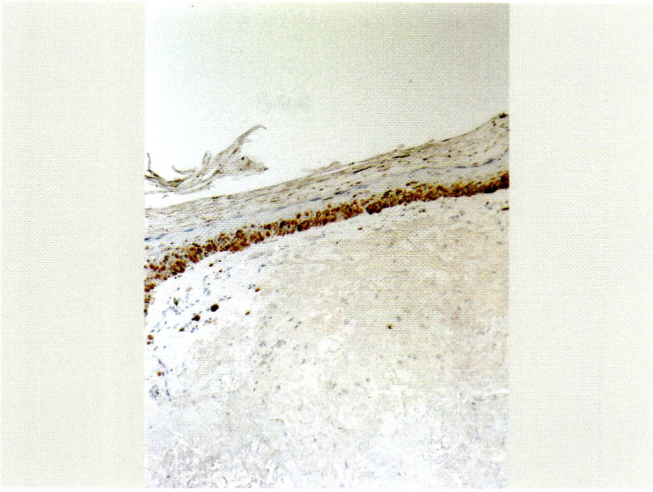

FIGURE 18.7.6

18.7.5: Confluent basal single melanocytes with extension along a hair follicle (Melan-A stain) (*Low power view*)

18.7.6: Confluent single melanocytes (immunohistochemistry with SOX10) (*Low power view*)

18.7.7: Superficial spreading malignant melanoma showing pagetoid "buck-shot" scattered melanocytes, horizontal growth pattern, with invasive component (*Scanner view*)

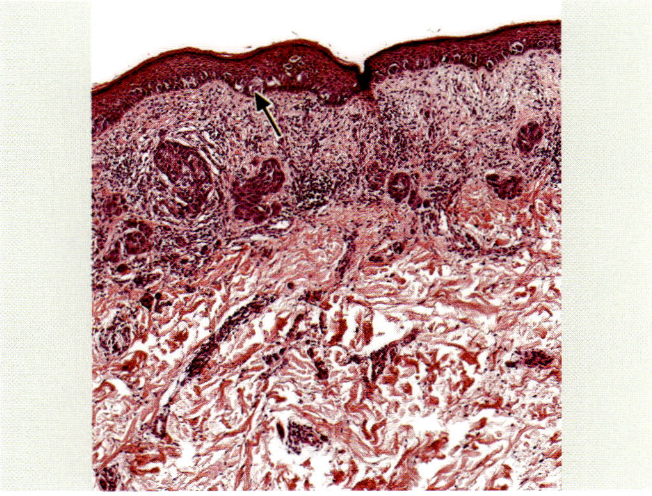

FIGURE 18.7.7

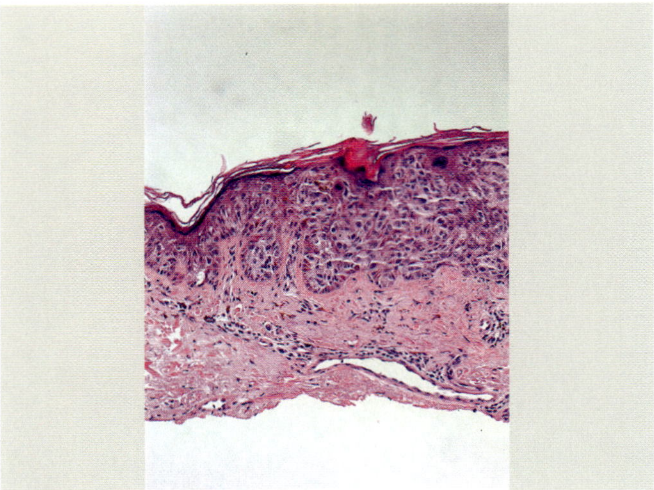

FIGURE 18.7.8

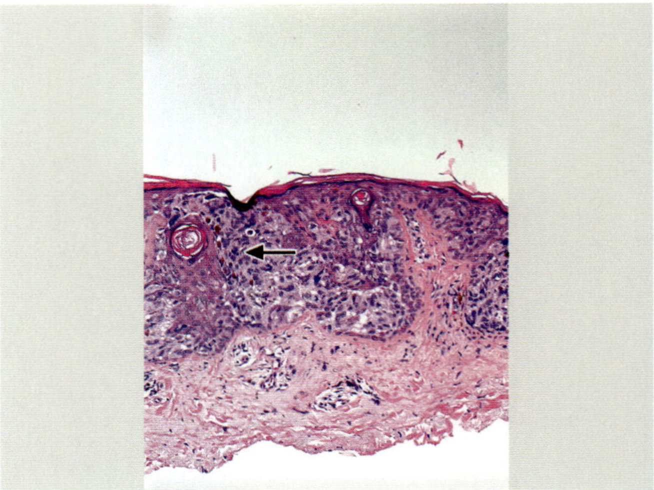

FIGURE 18.7.9

18.7.8: Another case with large irregular nests of atypical melanocytes with pagetoid scatter of single cells in the upper parts of the epidermis. Dermis shows solar elastosis and mild pigment incontinence (*Low power view*)

18.7.9: Irregular nests occupying the epidermis (consumption) with scattering of small groups and single cells at upper levels and also surrounding follicular epithelium. Dermis shows solar elastosis (*Low power view*)

18.7.10: Nodular melanoma—vertical growth pattern, no junctional activity, irregular collections of atypical melanocytes (*Scanner view*)

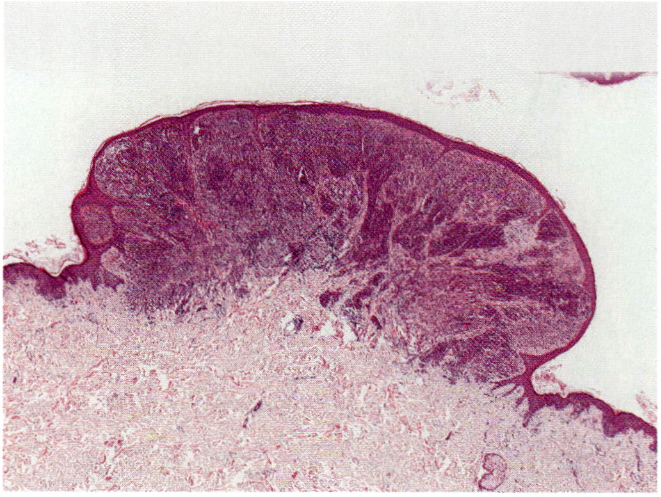

FIGURE 18.7.10

DIFFERENTIAL DIAGNOSIS

1. Melanocyte proliferation at basal cell layer
   a. Lentiginous nevus
   b. Nevus spilus
   c. Recurring nevus
2. Melanocytic proliferation in the dermis
   a. Mongolian spot
   b. Nevus of Ota, nevus of Ito
   c. Phakomatosis pigmentovascularis
3. Histologic differentials of malignant melanoma
   a. Ancient nevus
   b. Atypical Spitz nevi
   c. Site specific atypical nevi

DIAGNOSTIC PEARLS

1. In melanocytic nevi, cells in the deeper dermis are mostly smaller, spindle shaped and contain less melanin.
2. PUVA lentigo shows increase in basal layer melanocytes, which are large and mildly atypical.
3. Spitz nevus—major diagnostic criteria are cell type, symmetrical appearance of the lesion, maturation of nevus cells, lack of pagetoid spread of single melanocytes, presence of Kamino bodies. Minor diagnostic criteria are separation between the epidermis and the nests of nevus cells at the dermoepidermal junctional, pseudoepitheliomatous hyperplasia, an lack of epidermal consumption as in melanoma, superficial dermal edema and telangiectasia, giant nevus cells, and an absence of dysplasia.
4. Nevus of Ota and nevus of Ito show scattered melanocytes in the dermis.
5. Pure nodular melanoma have no apparent radial growth. Angiogenesis in melanoma points towards tumor progression.

19

Vascular and Other Tumors

Chapter Outline

19.1: Capillary Malformation (Nevus Flammeus)
19.2: Cutis Marmorata Telangiectatica Congenita
19.3: Infantile Hemangioma
19.4: Lymphangioma
19.5: Angiokeratoma
19.6: Verrucous Hemangioma
19.7: Angiolymphoid Hyperplasia with Eosinophilia
19.8: Pyogenic Granuloma (Lobular Capillary Hemangiomas)
19.9: Glomus Tumor
19.10: Adenoma Sebaceum (Angiofibroma)
19.11: Kaposi's Sarcoma
19.12: Bacillary Angiomatosis
19.13: Skin Tag
19.14: Dermatofibroma
19.15: Dermatofibrosarcoma Protuberans
19.16: Piloleiomyomas
19.17: Cutaneous Neurofibromas
19.18: Nevus Lipomatosus

Atul Dongre, Uday Khopkar, Pradeep Mahajan, Asha Kubba, Nathan Lee, Jerad Gardner, Jag Bhawan

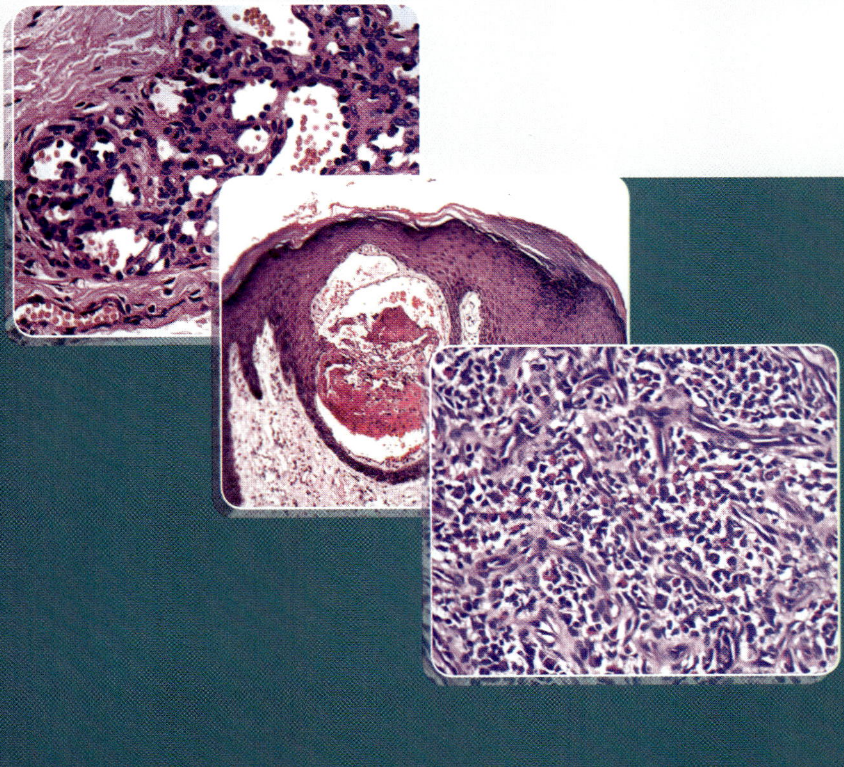

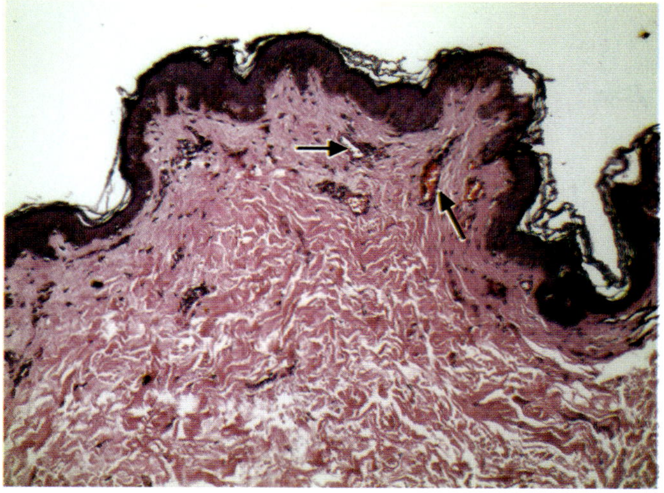

FIGURE 19.1.1

19.1: CAPILLARY MALFORMATION (NEVUS FLAMMEUS)

19.1.1: Dilatation of the thin-walled vessels of the superficial vascular plexus (*Scanner view*)

19.1.2: Closer view of dilated blood vessels in upper dermis containing RBCs (*Low power view*)

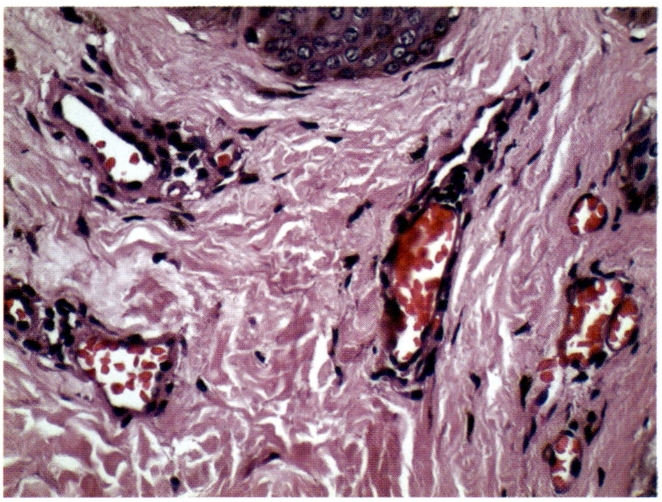

FIGURE 19.1.2

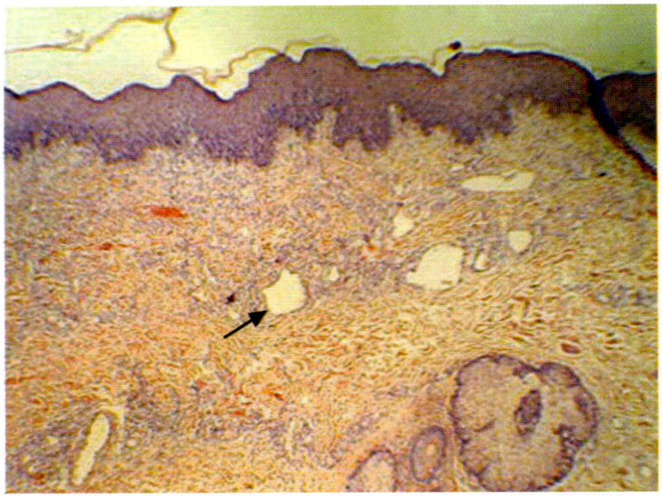

FIGURE 19.2.1

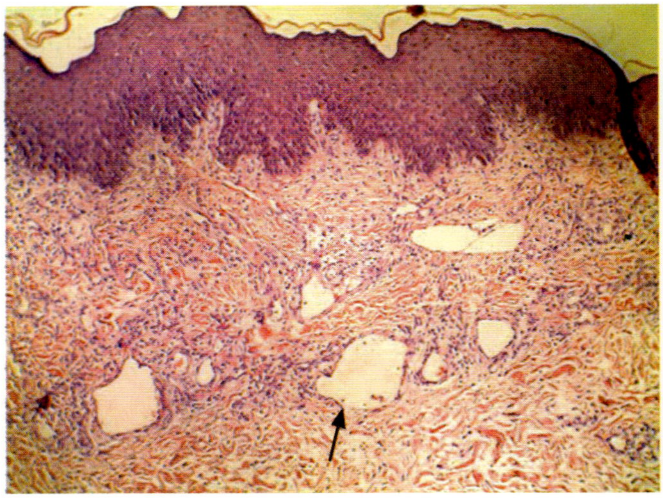

FIGURE 19.2.2

19.2: CUTIS MARMORATA TELANGIECTATICA CONGENITA

19.2.1: Dilated capillaries and veins in the dermis (*Scanner view*)

19.2.2: Closer view of the vessels (*Low power view*)

19.2.3: Dilated capillaries and veins in the subcutis (*Scanner view*)

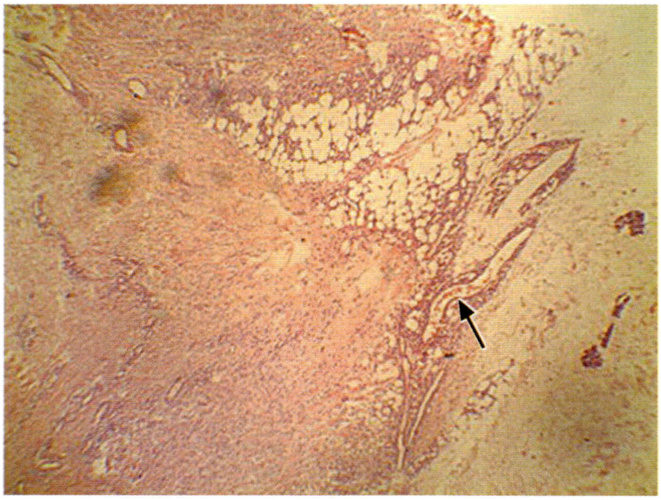

FIGURE 19.2.3

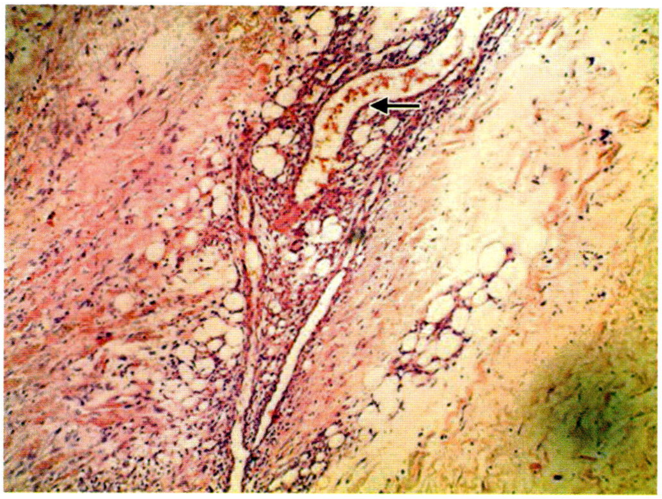

FIGURE 19.2.4

19.2.4: Closer view of vessels (*Low power view*)

19.2.5: Proliferation of vascular channels in the deep (*Low power view*)

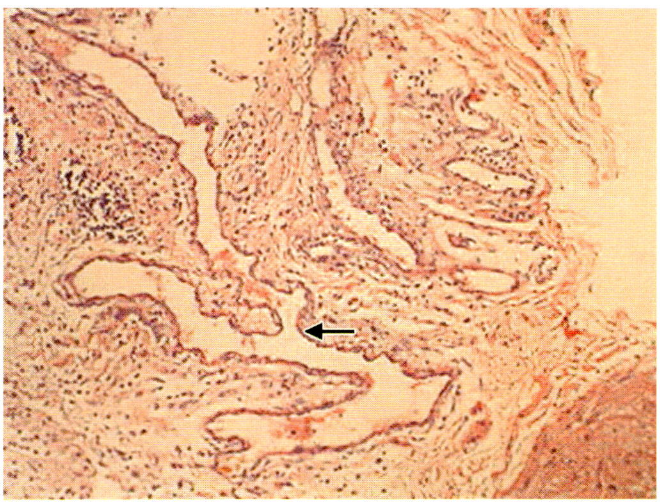

FIGURE 19.2.5

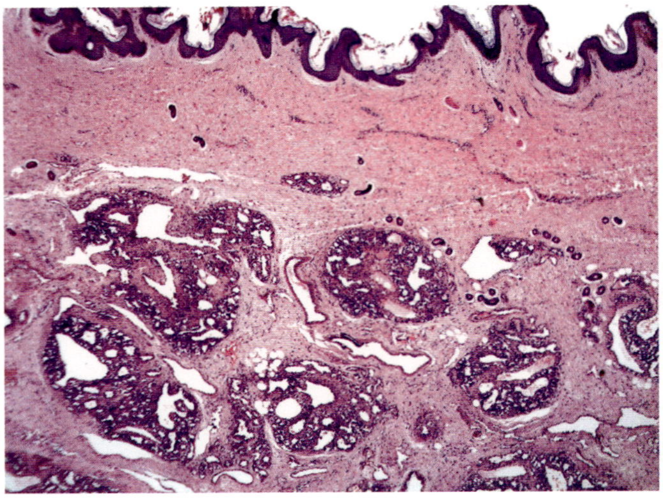

FIGURE 19.3.1

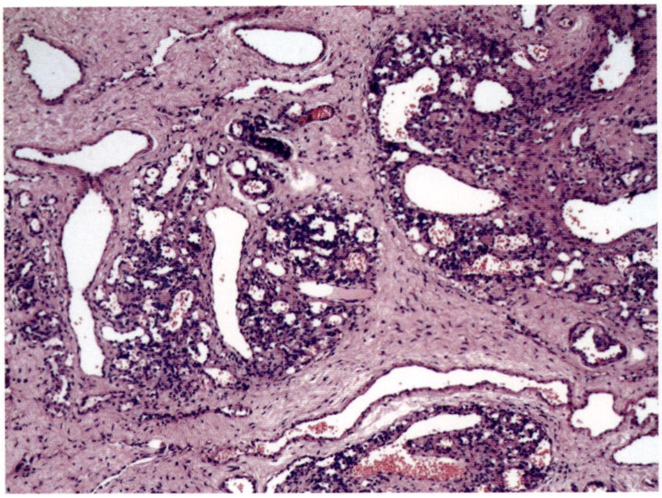

FIGURE 19.3.2

19.3: INFANTILE HEMANGIOMA

19.3.1: The vascular proliferation with lobular configuration (*Scanner view*)

19.3.2: Solid collections of endothelial cells. Vascular lumina lined by plump endothelial cells (*Low power view*)

19.3.3: Closer view of endothelial cells and vascular lumina filled with RBCs (*High power view*)

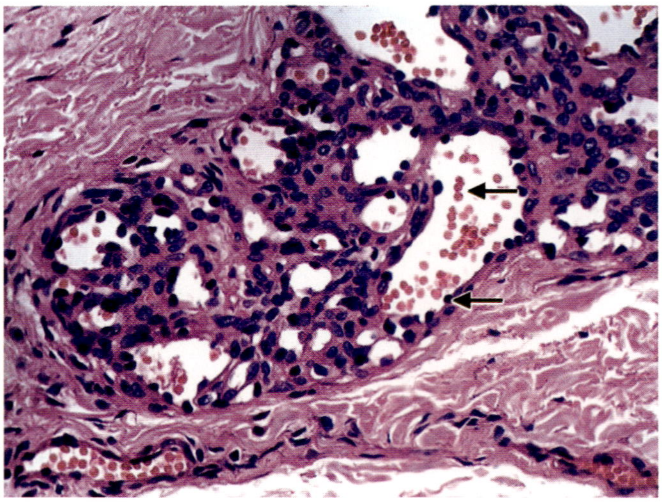

FIGURE 19.3.3

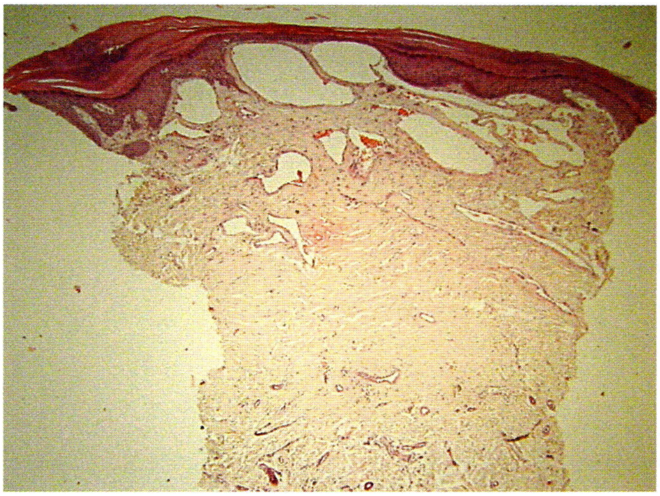

FIGURE 19.4.1

19.4: LYMPHANGIOMA

19.4.1: Multiple dilated thin-walled spaces in the papillary dermis lined by endothelial cells. Epidermis appears atrophic with elongation of rete ridges due to which the lymphatic channels appear to be intraepidermal though they are located in the papillary dermis (*Scanner view*)

19.4.2: The vessels mostly contain lymphatic fluid, but red blood cells may be seen (other features like lymphoid aggregates in the dermis or lymphatic cisterns in the deep dermis or subcutis are seen occasionally) (*Low power view*)

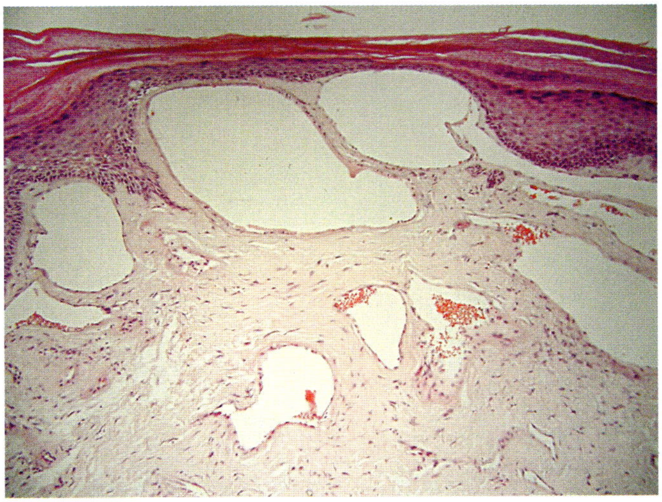

FIGURE 19.4.2

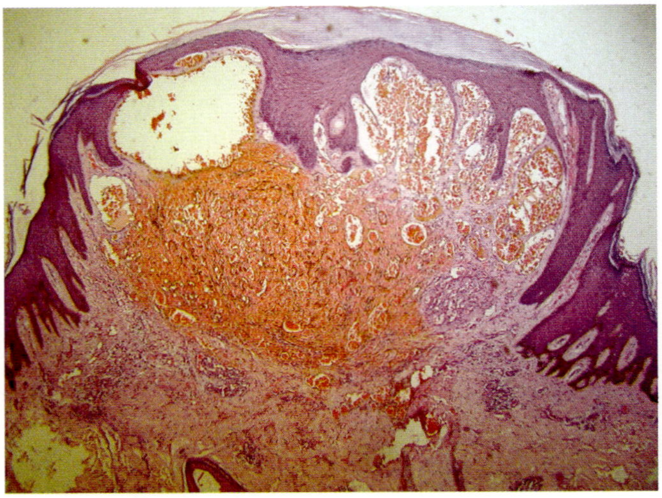

FIGURE 19.5.1

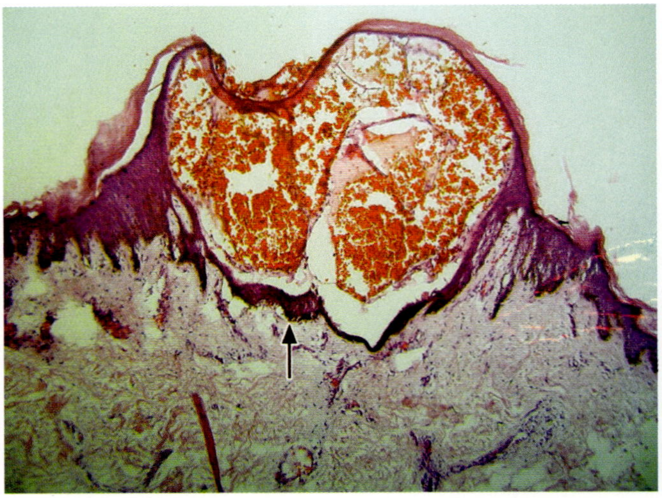

FIGURE 19.5.2

19.5: ANGIOKERATOMA

19.5.1: Multiple large dilated spaces in the papillary dermis containing RBCs (*Scanner view*)

19.5.2: Another case with epidermis enclosing the vascular channels (*Scanner view*)

19.5.3: Epidermis shows hyperkeratosis and irregular acanthosis with rete ridges partially or completely engulfing the vascular channels (*Low power view*)

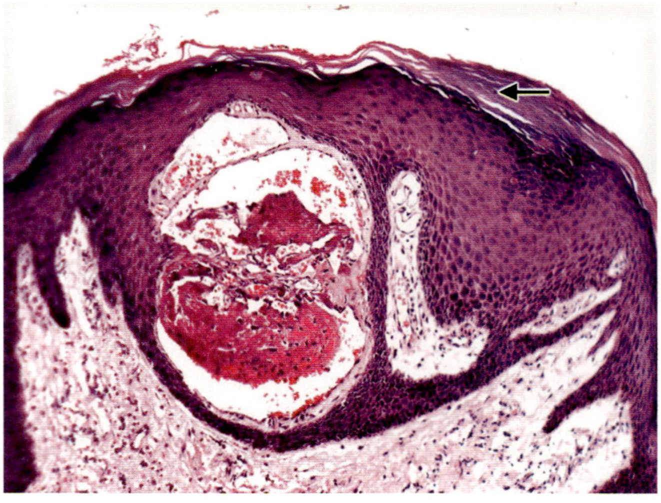

FIGURE 19.5.3

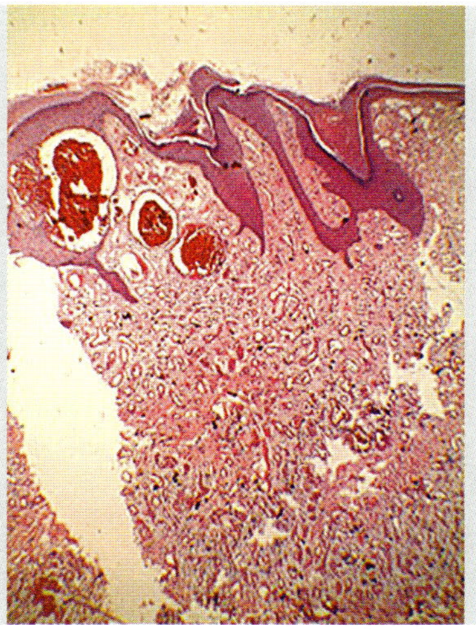

FIGURE 19.6.1

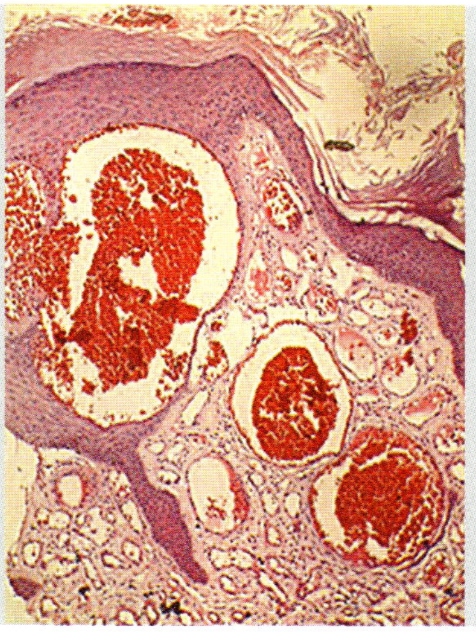

FIGURE 19.6.2

19.6: VERRUCOUS HEMANGIOMA

19.6.1: Many small to large vascular channels are seen in the dermis as well as subcutis (*Scanner view*)

19.6.2: The epidermis overlying the large vascular channels in the superficial dermis shows varying dergree of hyperkeratosis, acanthosis, papillomatosis (*Low power view*)

19.6.3: Vessels in the deep dermis (*Low power view*)

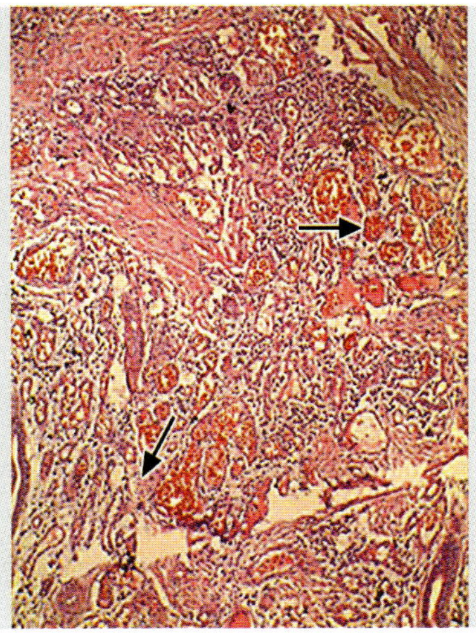

FIGURE 19.6.3

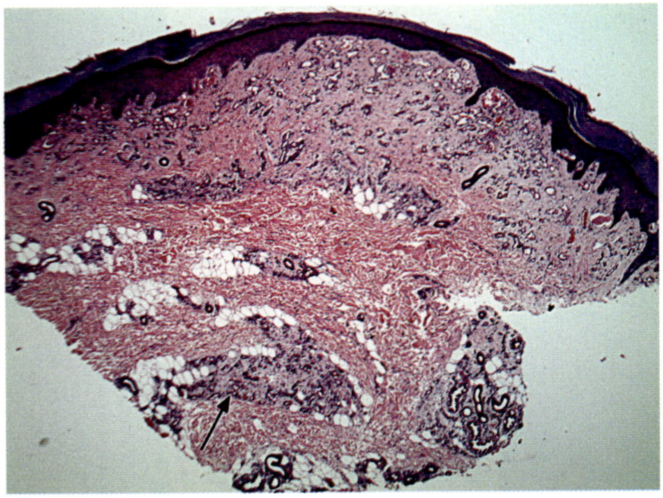

FIGURE 19.6.4

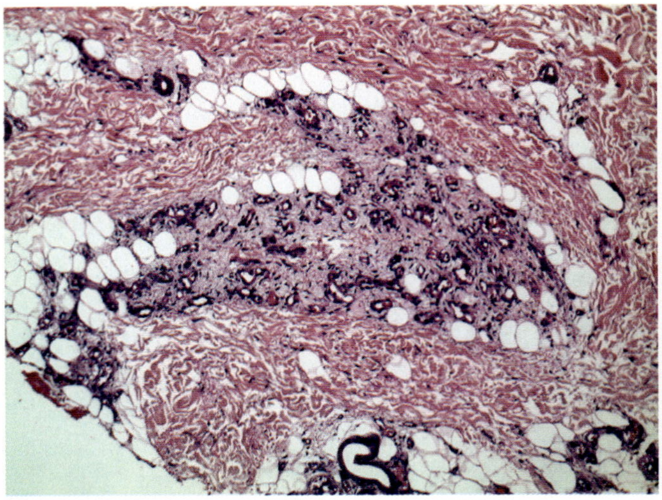

FIGURE 19.6.5

19.6.4: Another case with subcutaneous extension (*Scanner view*)

19.6.5: Closer view of vessels (*Low power view*)

19.6.6: Small blood vessels in the subcutaneous tissue (vs angiokeratomas involve only superficial vessels) (*High power view*)

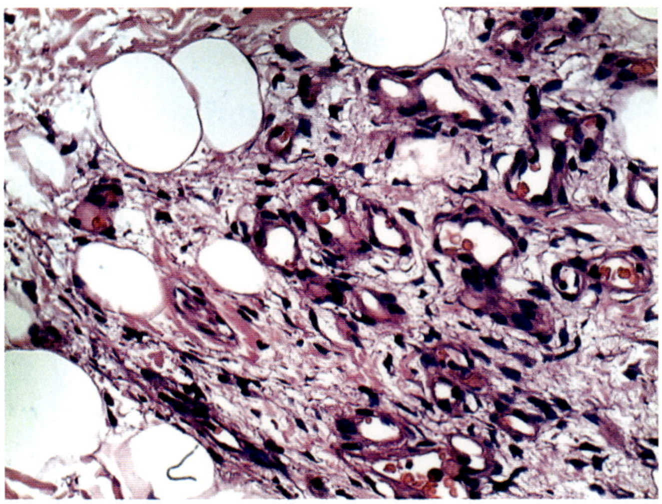

FIGURE 19.6.6

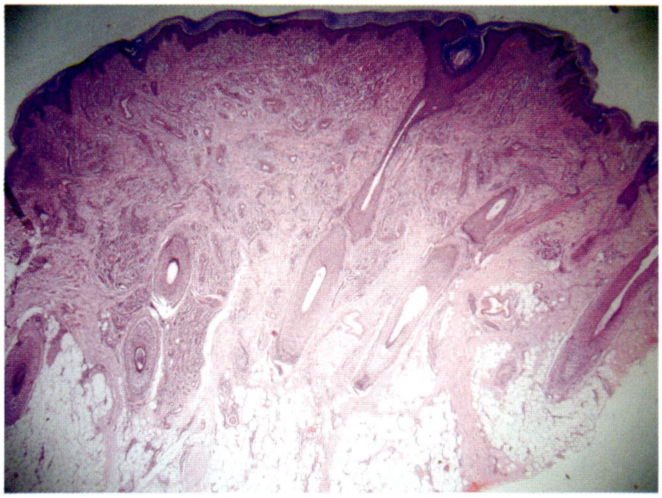

FIGURE 19.7.1

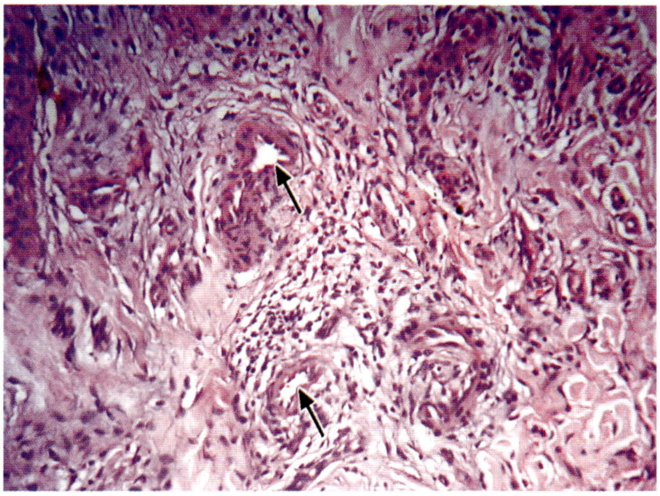

FIGURE 19.7.2

19.7: ANGIOLYMPHOID HYPERPLASIA WITH EOSINOPHILIA

19.7.1: Collections of vessels and inflammatory cells (*Scanner view*)

19.7.2: The section shows increased vascularity with multiple vesssels having varying degrees of thickness lined by plump 'epithelioid' endothelial cells. There are solid collections of endothelial cells also (*Low power view*)

19.7.3: Another case showing circumscribed collections of vessels and inflammatory cells (*Scanner view*)

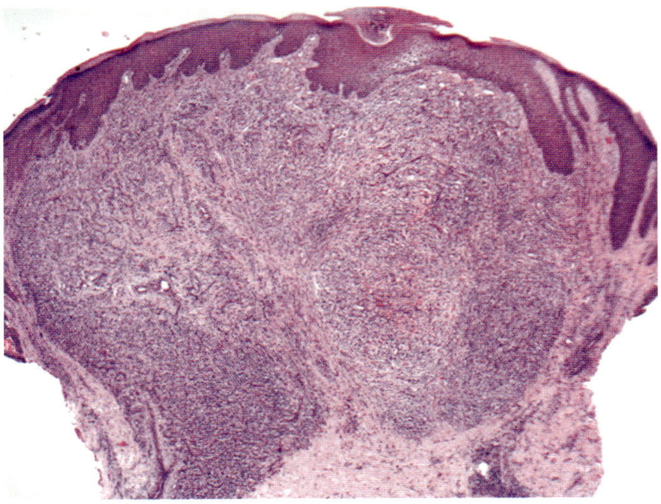

FIGURE 19.7.3

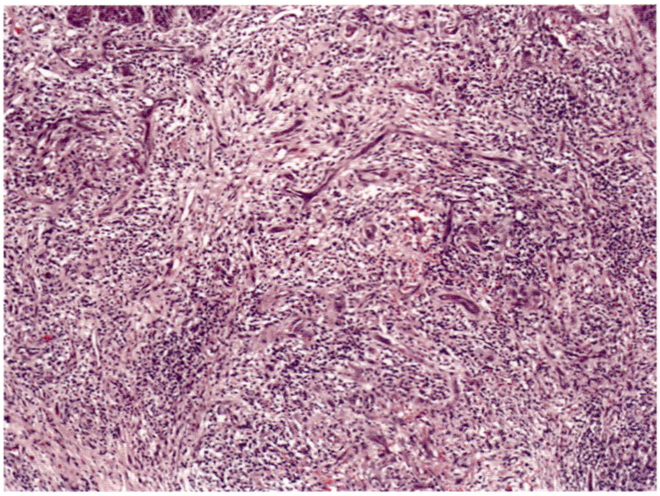

FIGURE 19.7.4

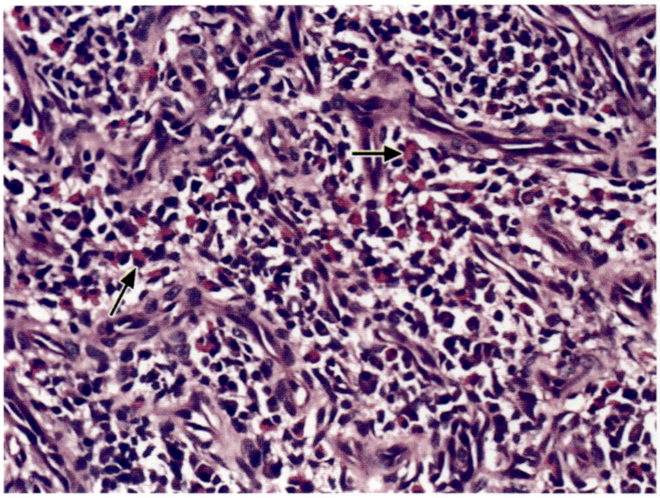

FIGURE 19.7.5

19.7.4: Lymphoid aggregates (*Low power view*)

19.7.5: Plenty of eosinophils (*High power view*)

19.7.6: The endothelial cells lining the vessels show an enlarged nucleus, plenty of eosinophilic cytoplasm with cytoplasmic lumina. Lumina of a few vessels show intravascular proliferations of endothelial cells (*High power view*)

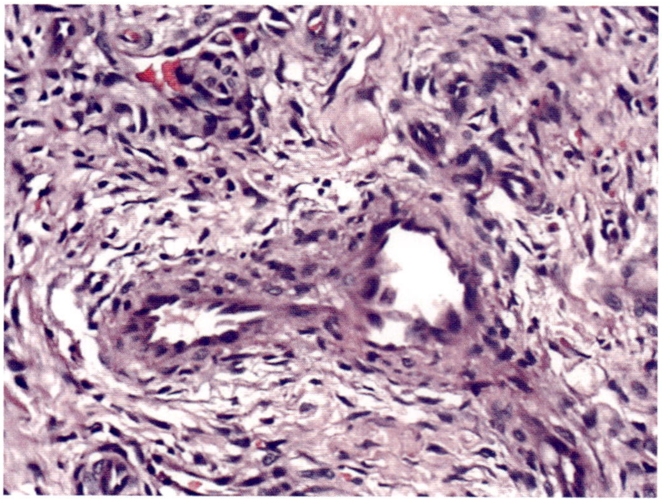

FIGURE 19.7.6

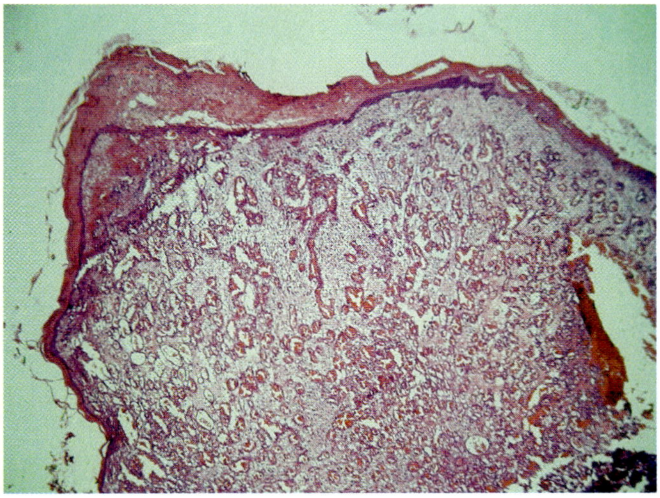

FIGURE 19.8.1

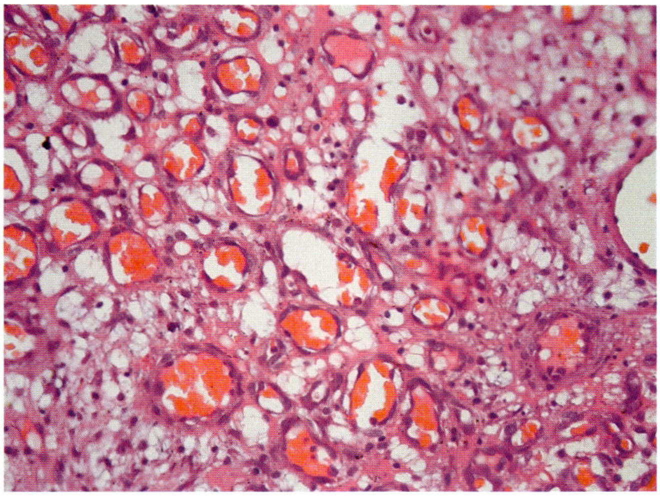

FIGURE 19.8.2

19.8: PYOGENIC GRANULOMA (LOBULAR CAPILLARY HEMANGIOMAS)

19.8.1: Proliferation of vessels, with myxoid or fibrous septa separating the lobules (*Scanner view*)

19.8.2: Closer view of lobulated proliferation of capillary-sized vessels (*Low power view*)

19.8.3: Another case showing loosely packed superficial lobules as opposed to deeper lobules, which are densely packed and cellular (*Scanner view*)

19.8.4: Another case with lobules. Epidermis is thin with elongated rete ridges forming collarette (*Scanner view*)

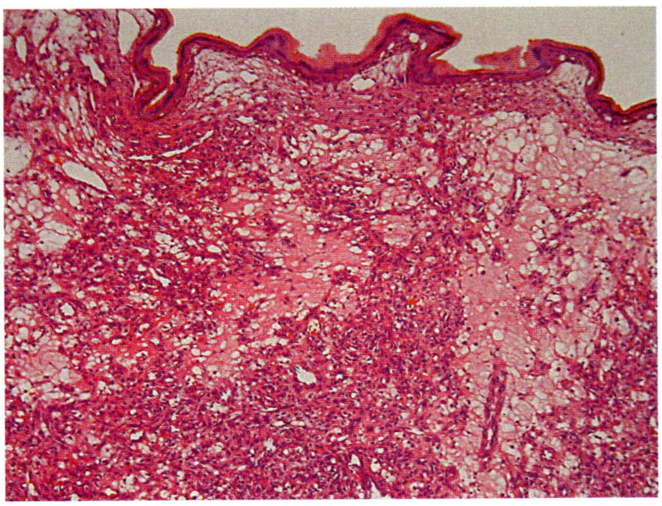

FIGURE 19.8.3

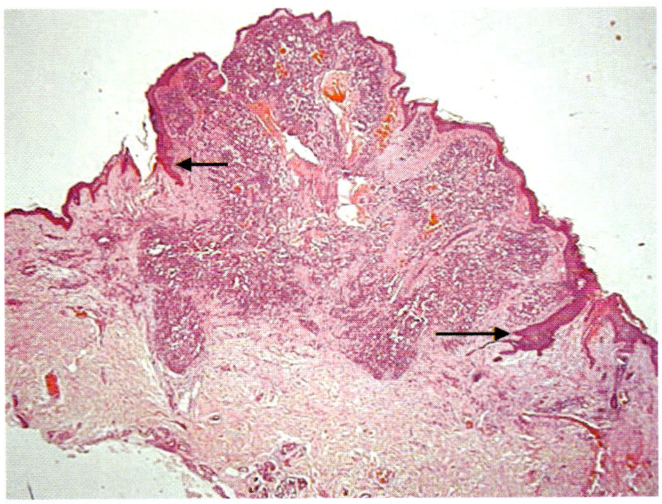

FIGURE 19.8.4

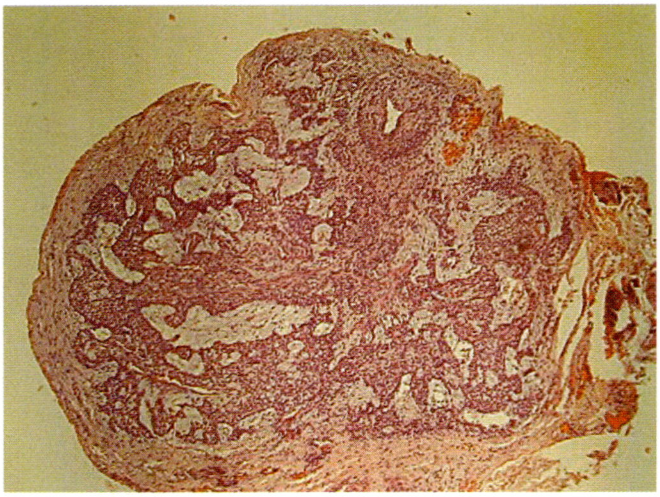

FIGURE 19.9.1

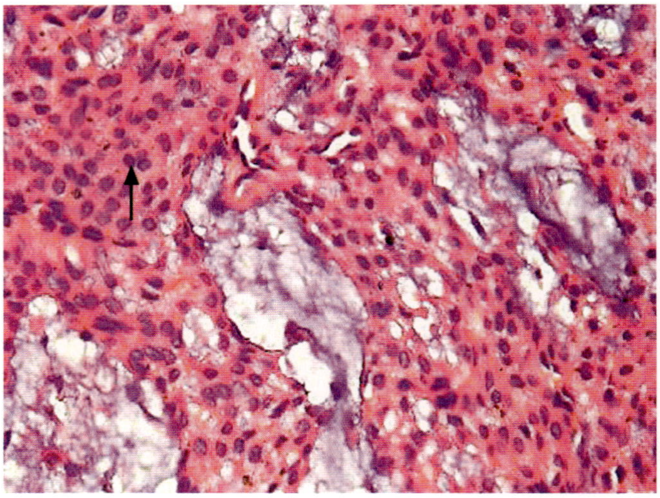

FIGURE 19.9.2

19.9: GLOMUS TUMOR

19.9.1: Well-circumscribed tumor mainly centered in the dermis (*Scanner view*)

19.9.2: Section shows tumor with small capillary-sized vessels encircled by collections of glomus cells in hyalinized stroma. Glomus cells are uniform and round with sharply defined punched out oval nuclei and eosinophilic cytoplasm (*Low power view*)

19.9.3: This tumor contains myxoid stroma and nerve fibers (*Low power view*)

19.9.4: Another case with tumor cells and vessels embedded in a fibrous stroma (*High power view*)

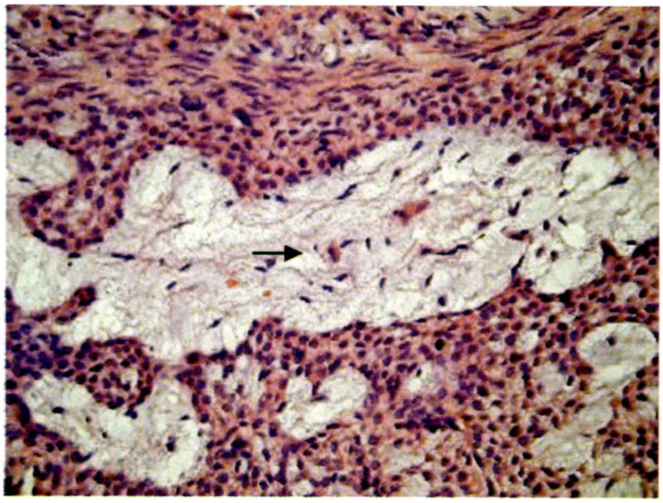

FIGURE 19.9.3

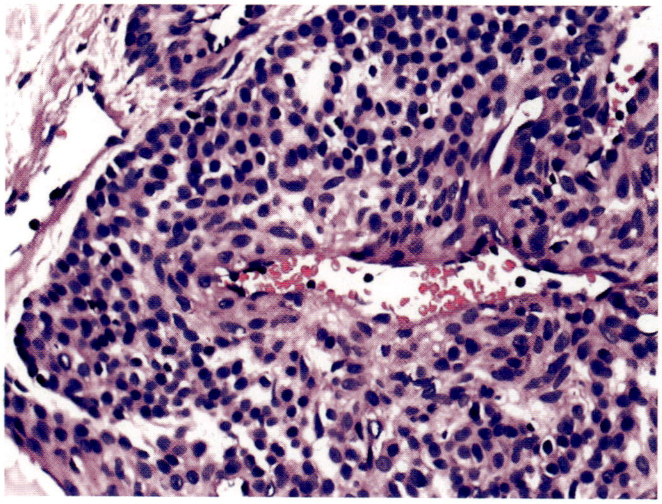

FIGURE 19.9.4

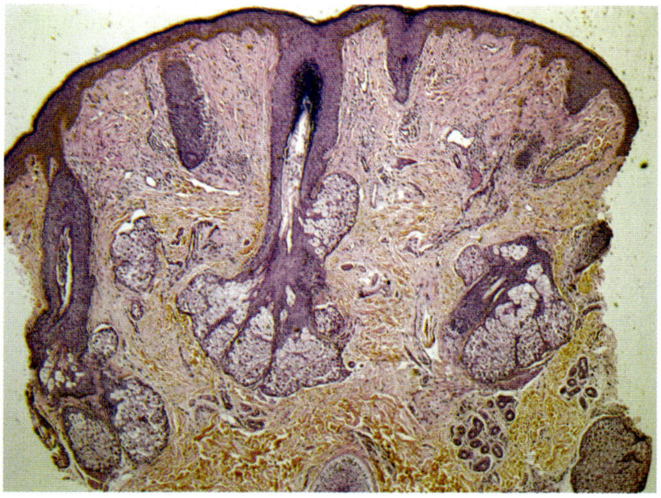

FIGURE 19.10.1

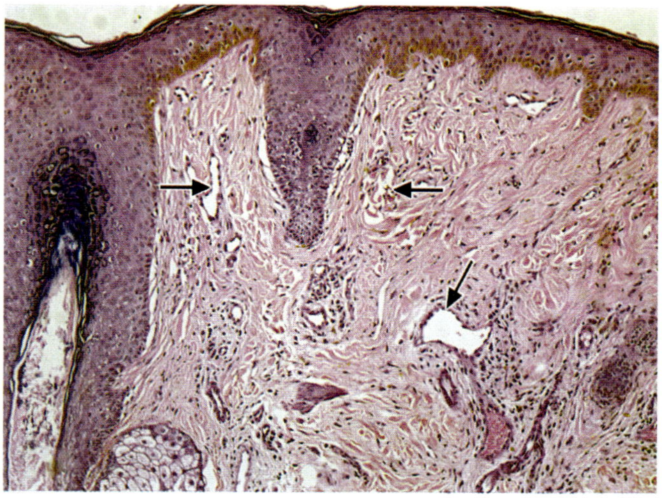

FIGURE 19.10.2

19.10: ADENOMA SEBACEUM (ANGIOFIBROMA)

19.10.1: The section shows flattened rete ridges and increased basal layer pigmentation (*Scanner view*)

19.10.2: Proliferation of blood vessels which look dilated, have irregular shapes and different sizes. There is scant inflammatory infiltrate (*Low power view*)

19.10.3: There is proliferation of fibroblasts and collagen fibers, show concentric arrangement around hair follicles and blood vessels (*High power view*)

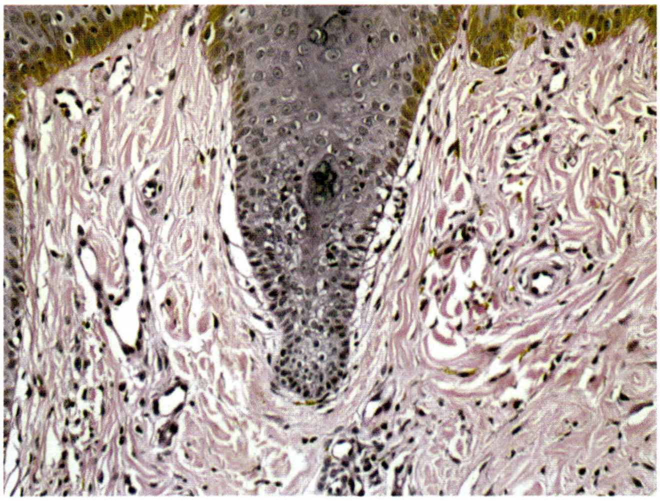

FIGURE 19.10.3

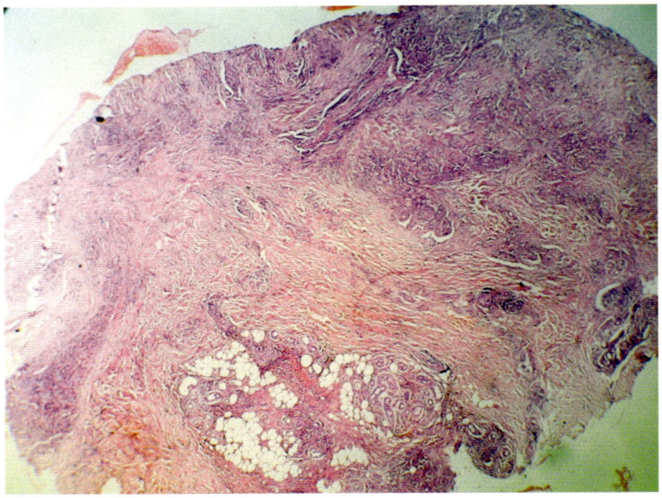

FIGURE 19.11.1

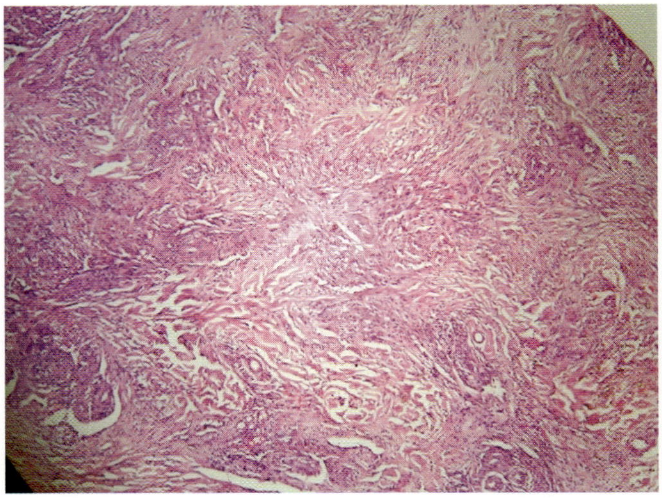

FIGURE 19.11.2

19.11: KAPOSI'S SARCOMA

19.11.1: Dermal tumor extending to the subcutaneous tissue (*Scanner view*)

19.11.2: Predominantly vascular in nature (*Low power view*)

19.11.3: Section shows proliferation of multiple, thin walled, irregular and jagged vascular spaces (*High power view*)

19.11.4: These slit like vascular channels partly surround pre-existing blood vessels or appendage structures in dermis (promontory sign) (*Low power view*)

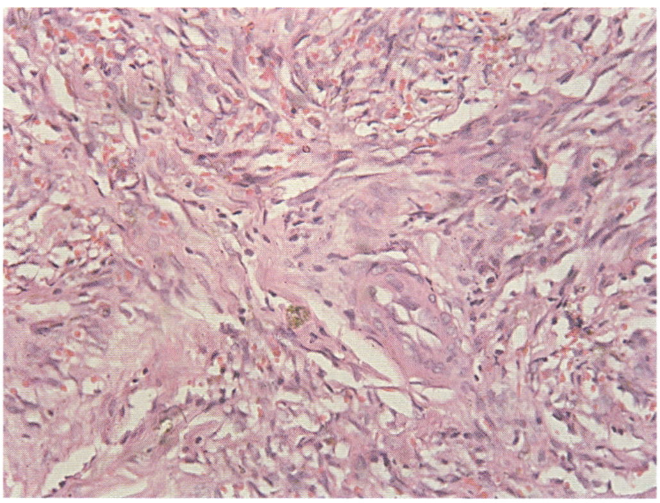

FIGURE 19.11.3

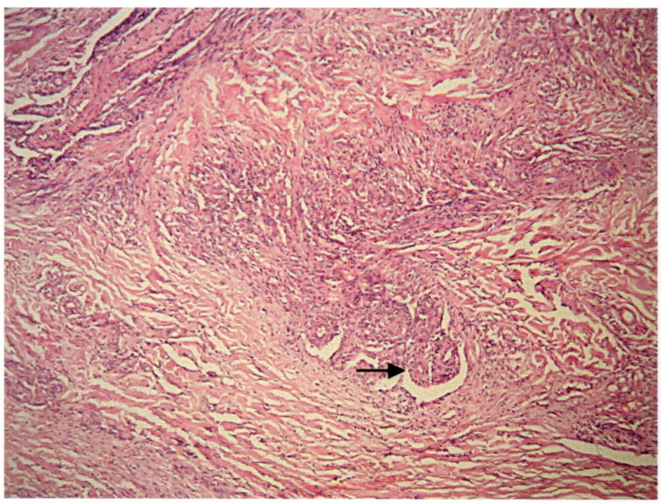

FIGURE 19.11.4

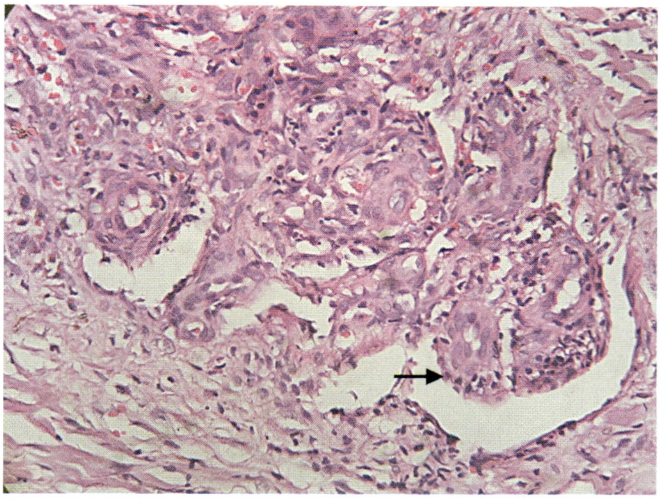

FIGURE 19.11.5

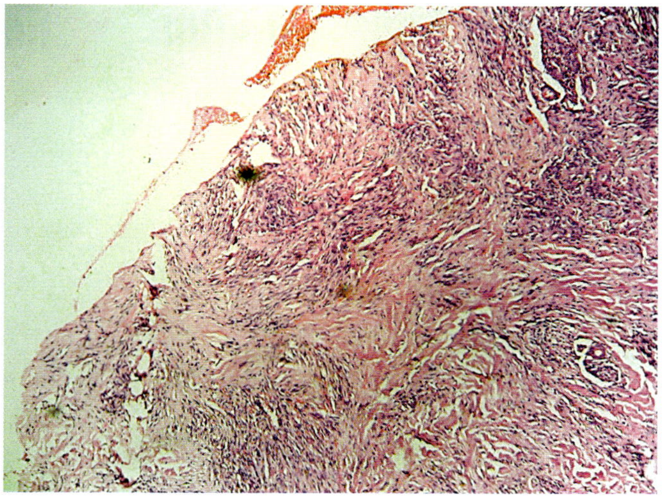

FIGURE 19.11.6

19.11.5: Closer view of promontory sign (*High power view*)

19.11.6: Section shows dermal proliferation of spindle cells (*Low power view*)

19.11.7: Interlacing bundles of spindle cells (which may be pleomorphic) and slit-like vessels (*High power view*)

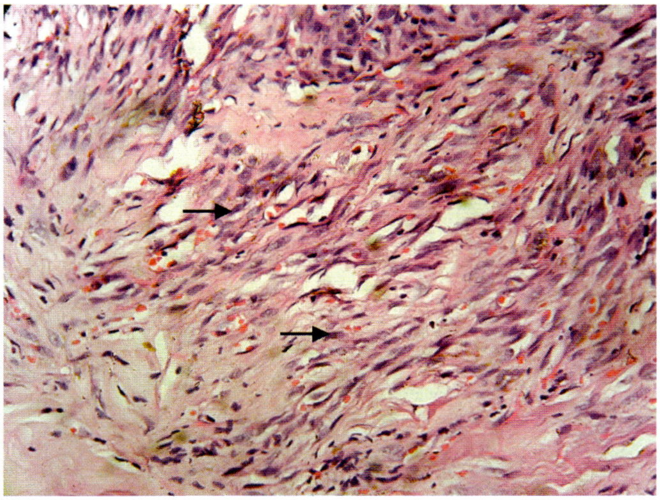

FIGURE 19.11.7

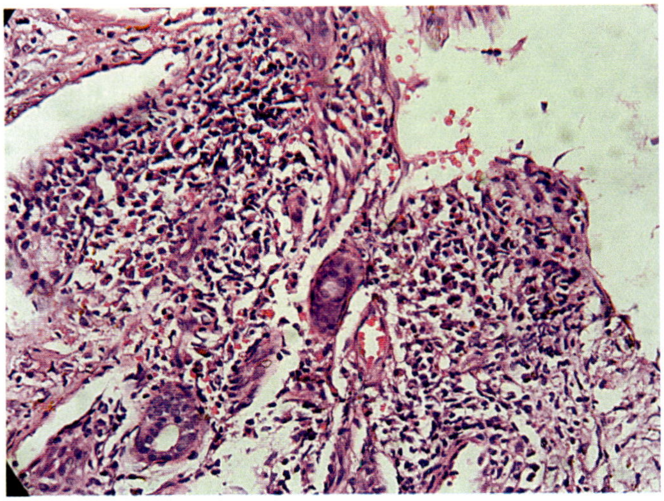

FIGURE 19.11.8

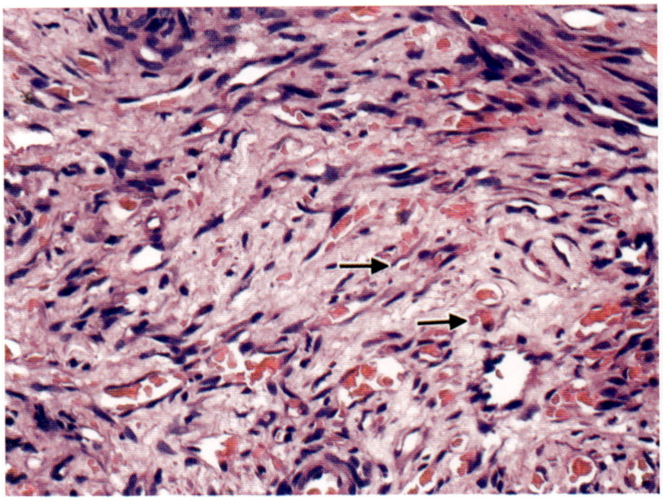

FIGURE 19.11.9

19.11.8: Inflammatory cell infiltrate consisting predominantly of lymphocytes and plasma cells (*High power view*)

19.11.9: Another case showing intracellular and extracellular eosinophilic hyaline globules of varying sizes. They are PAS positive, and represent red blood cell fragments (*High power view*)

19.11.10: Extravasated RBCs and hemosiderin deposits in the dermis (*High power view*)

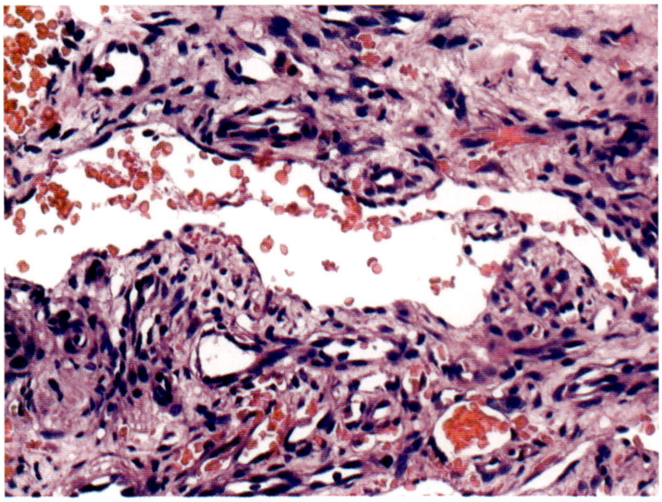

FIGURE 19.11.10

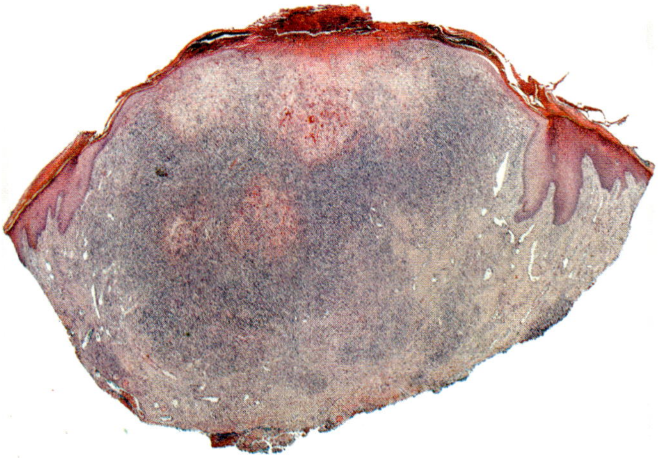

FIGURE 19.12.1

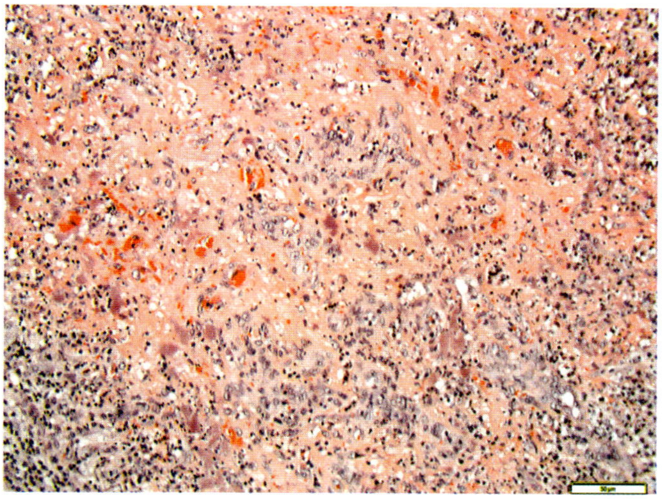

FIGURE 19.12.2

19.12: BACILLARY ANGIOMATOSIS

19.12.1: Section reveals a polypoid vascular proliferation, apocryphally described by Nathan Lee as a "funny looking pyogenic granuloma with extra stuff (*Scanner view*)

19.12.2: Neutrophils are plentiful (*Low power view*)

19.12.3: High power examination demonstrates aggregates of granular basophilic material representing clusters of *Bartonella henselae* bacteria; this finding is pathognomonic for bacillary angiomatosis. Organisms are readily demonstrated by a Giemsa, Warthin–Starry, or Grocott–methenamine silver stain (*High power view*)

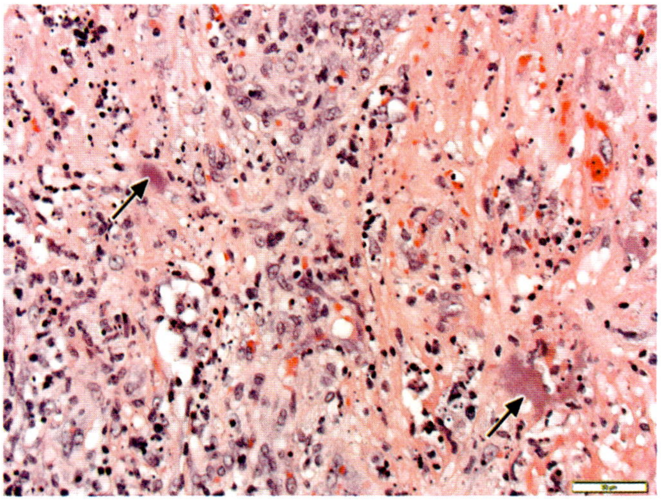

FIGURE 19.12.3

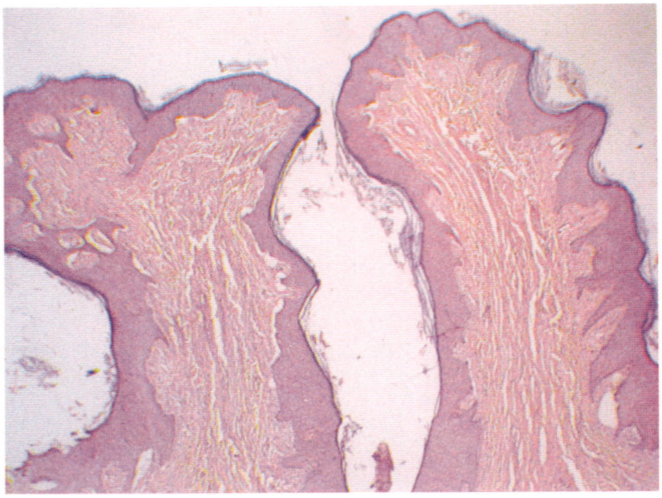

FIGURE 19.13.1

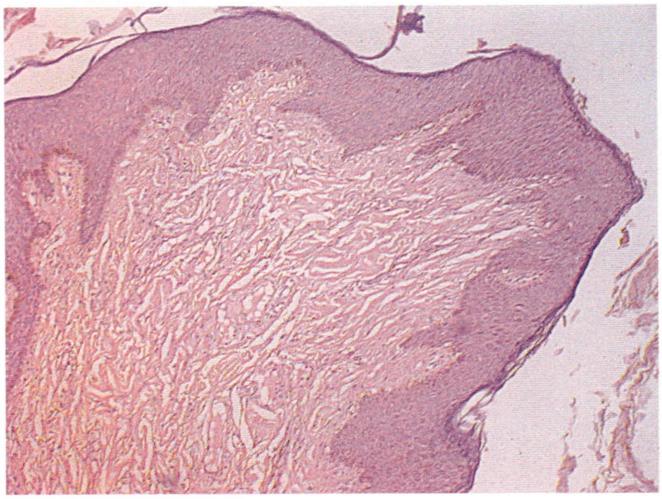

FIGURE 19.13.2

19.13: SKIN TAG

19.13.1: Connective tissue stalks (*Scanner view*)

19.13.2: Mild epidermal hyperplasia (*Low power view*)

19.13.3: The connective tissue stalk is usually composed of loosely arranged collagen and dilated blood vessels (*Low power view*)

19.13.4: Dilated blood vessels (fibroepithelial polyps/fibrolipomas have stroma with central core of adipose tissue) (*Low power view*)

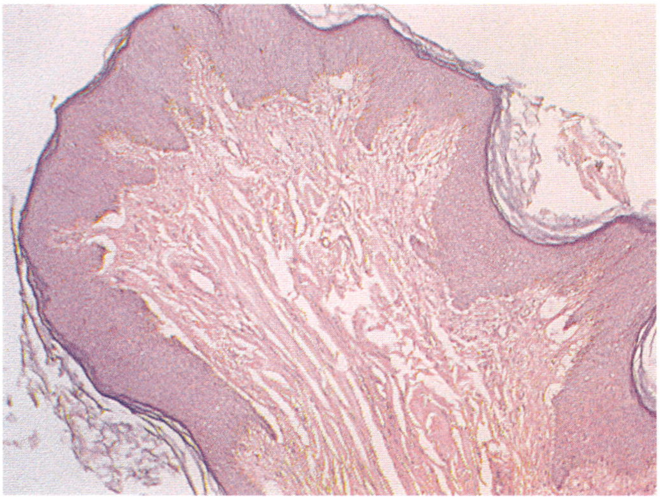

FIGURE 19.13.3

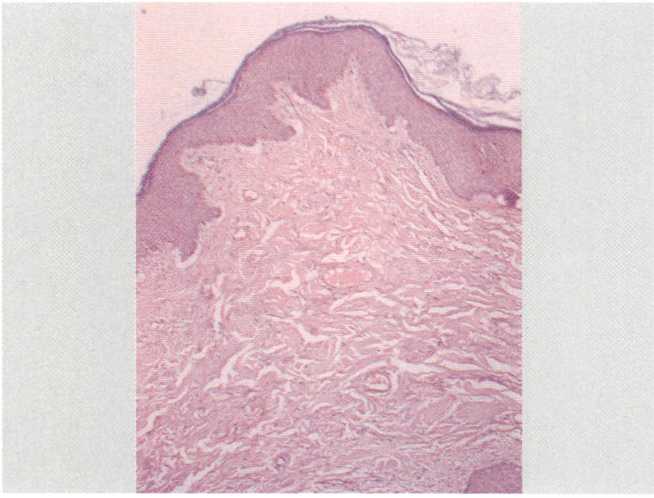

FIGURE 19.13.4

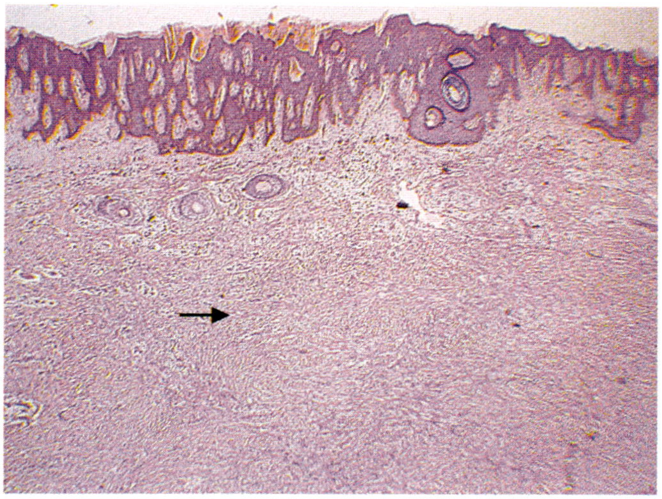

FIGURE 19.14.1

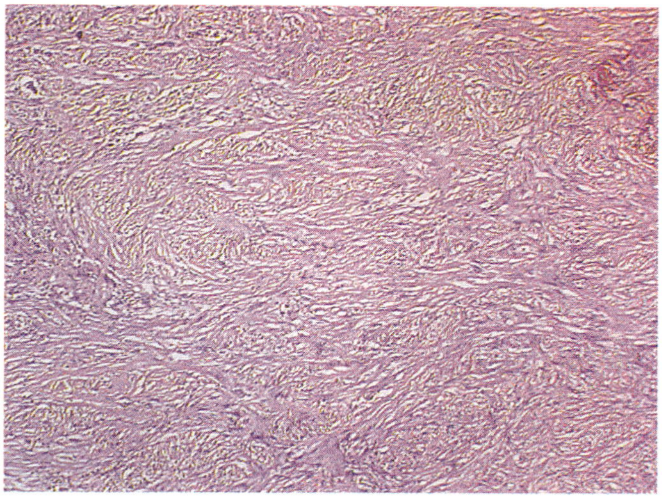

FIGURE 19.14.2

19.14: DERMATOFIBROMA

19.14.1: Non-encapsulated tumors mainly located in the dermis with grenz zone of variable thickness, hyperplasia and increased basal layer pigmentation of the epidermis above (*Scanner view*)

19.14.2: Made up of randomly arranged fibroblast-like cells, histiocytes and blood vessels (referred to as fibrocollagenous, histiocytic, and angiomatous variants according to the major component present. Numerous other variants have also been described) (*Low power view*)

19.14.3: Predominance of collagen and fibroblast-like cells in an irregular, storiform or whorled arrangement. Mitoses are rare (*High power view*)

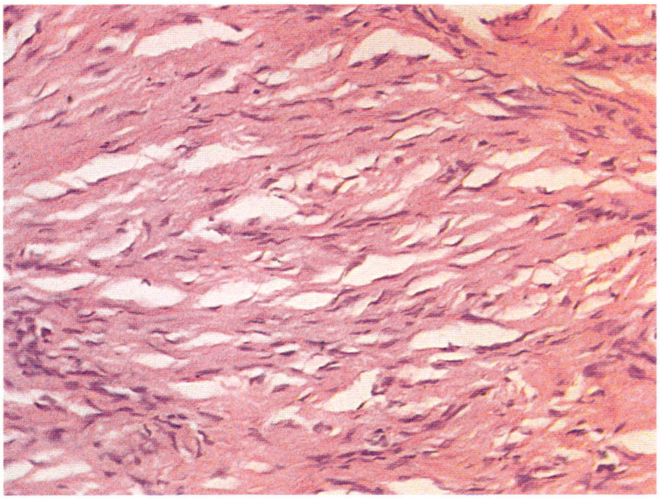

FIGURE 19.14.3

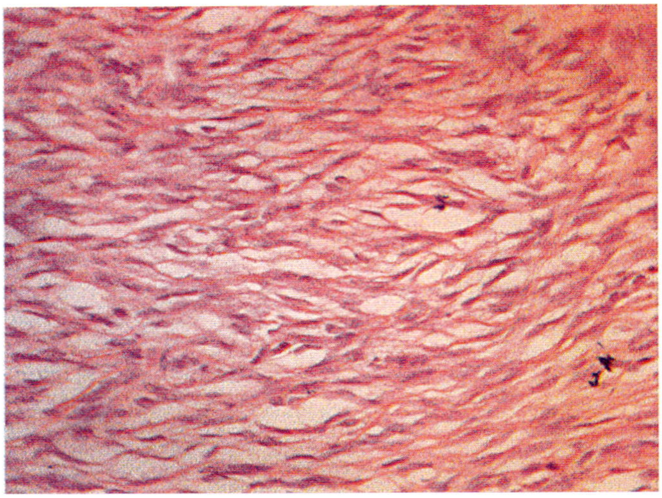

FIGURE 19.14.4

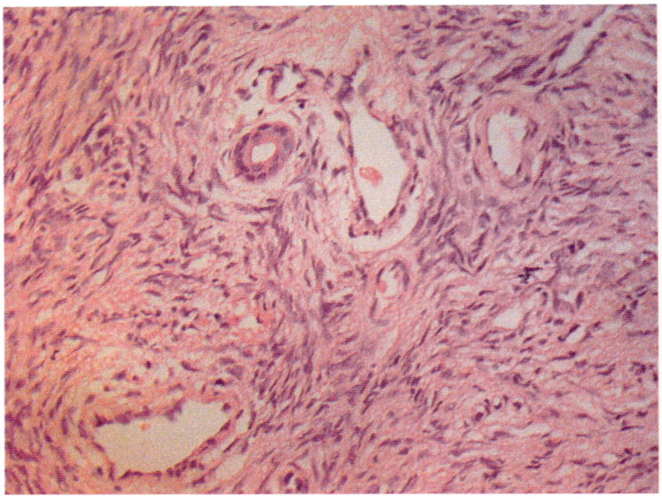

FIGURE 19.14.5

19.14.4: Fibrous histiocytoma shows predominance of histiocytes in a storiform pattern (*High power view*)

19.14.5: Blood vessels (*High power view*)

19.14.6: Blood vessels may have septal extension but usually very less extensive involvement of the subcutis (*Low power view*)

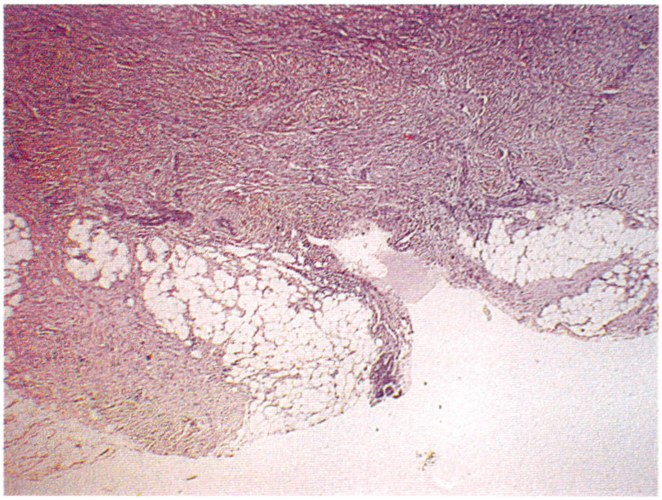

FIGURE 19.14.6

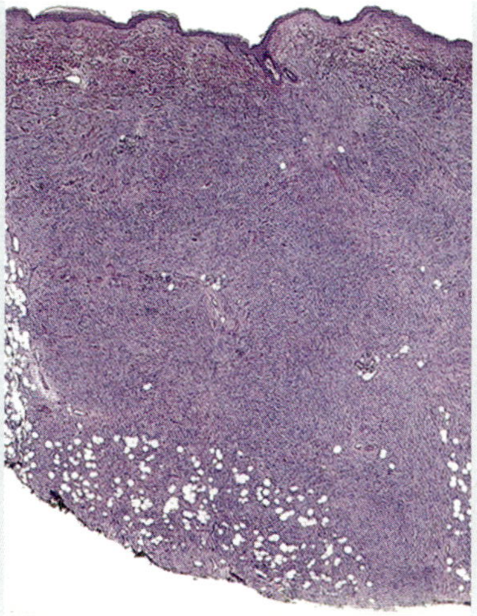

FIGURE 19.15.1

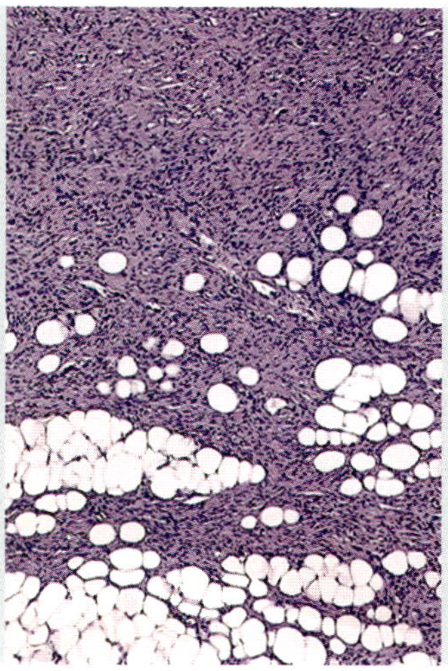

FIGURE 19.15.2

19.15: DERMATOFIBROSARCOMA PROTUBERANS

19.15.1: Dermal tumor with dense and diffuse tumor mass. Grenz zone usual, but involvement of the epidermis is known (*Scanner view*)

19.15.2: Extension of tumor cells into subcutis entrapping the fat cells forming a honeycomb pattern (*Low power view*)

19.15.3: It is a highly cellular tumor composed of fascicles of spindle cells that are arranged in storiform or cartwheel pattern with the cells radiating like spokes of a wheel around a central point usually a vessel (*High power view*)

19.15.4: Section shows monomorphic large spindle cells with plump nuclei. Sparse collagen. Multiple mitotic figures but rarely atypical (*High power view*)

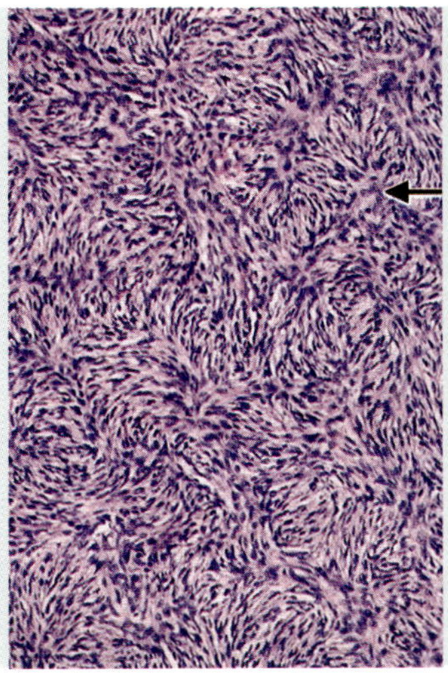

FIGURE 19.15.3

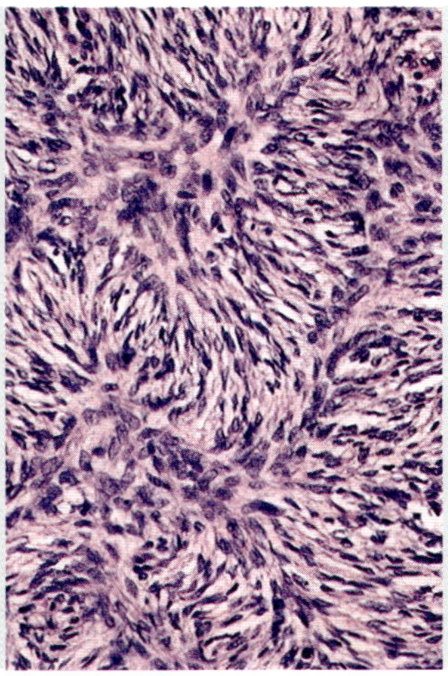

FIGURE 19.15.4

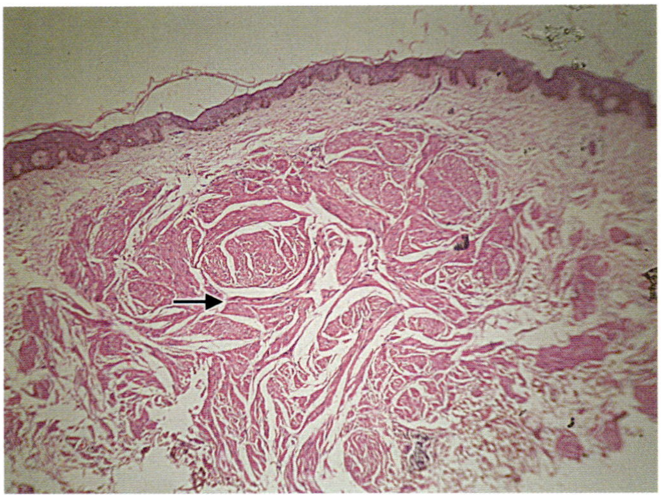

FIGURE 19.16.1

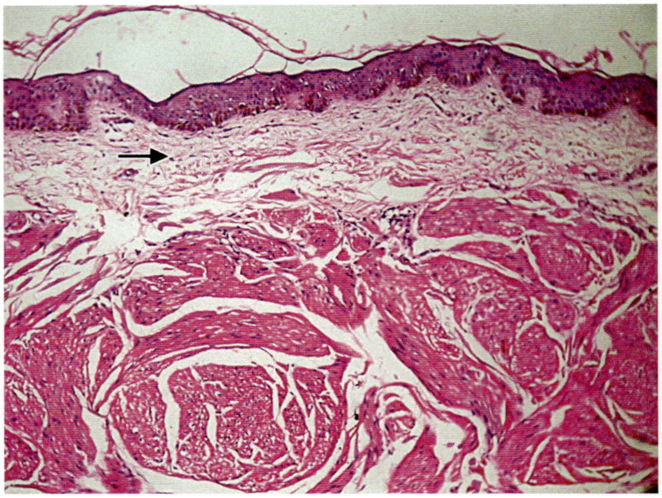

FIGURE 19.16.2

19.16: PILOLEIOMYOMAS

19.16.1: Circumscribed tumor in the dermis arising from the smooth muscle cells of arrector pili muscle (*Scanner view*)

19.16.2: Epidermal changes vary from flattening to hyperplasia. Tumor separated from epidermis normally by a grenz zone (*Low power view*)

19.16.3: The tumor consists of smooth muscle fascicles arranged in haphazard manner lying parallel to the epidermis (*Low power view*)

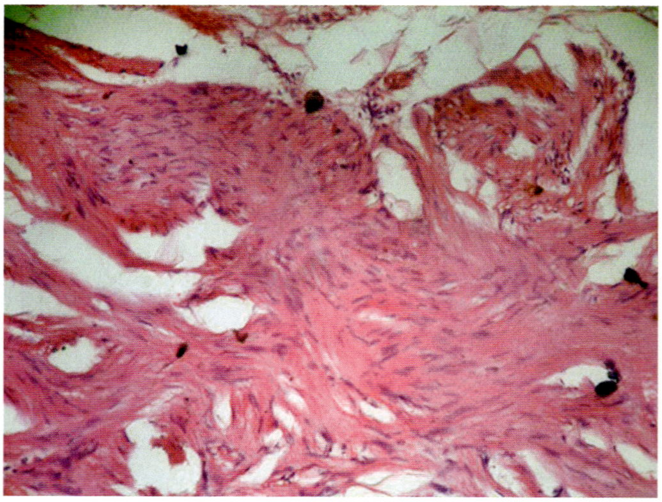

FIGURE 19.16.3

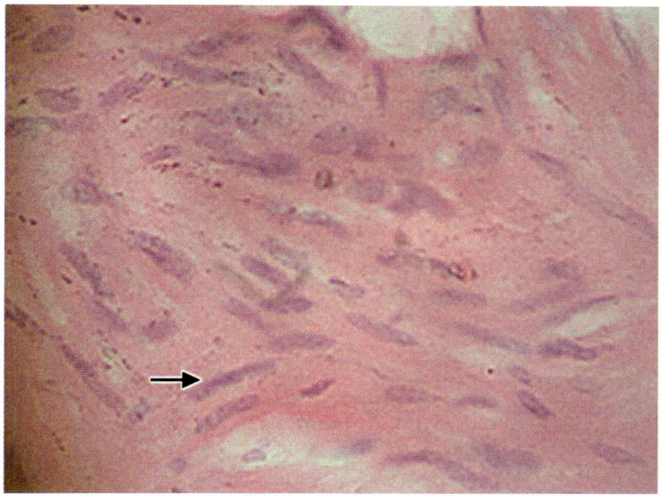

FIGURE 19.16.4

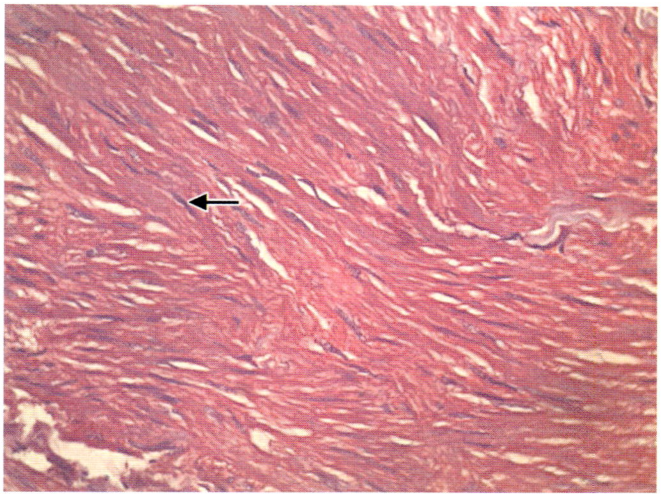

FIGURE 19.16.5

19.16.4: These smooth muscle cells have eosinophilic cytoplasm and cigar-shaped elongated nuclei with blunt ends (*High power view*)

19.16.5: Another case with bundles of smooth muscles and fibrous tissue in the stroma (*Low power view*)

19.16.6: This section shows Masson trichrome stain to confirm the diagnosis of piloleiomyoma (muscle, nuclei—dark red/collagen—blue) (*Low power view*)

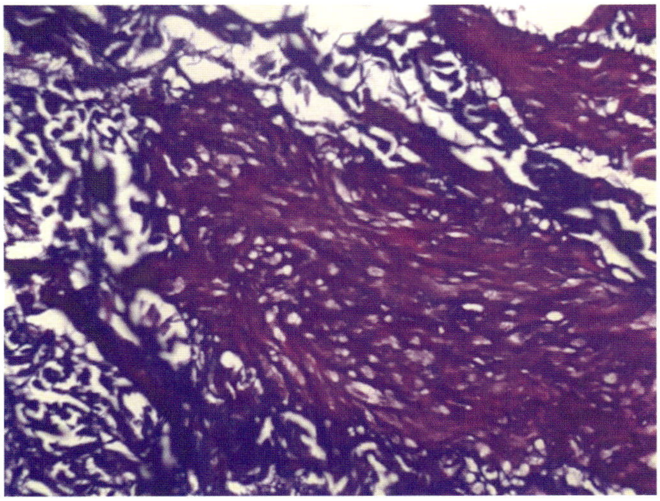

FIGURE 19.16.6

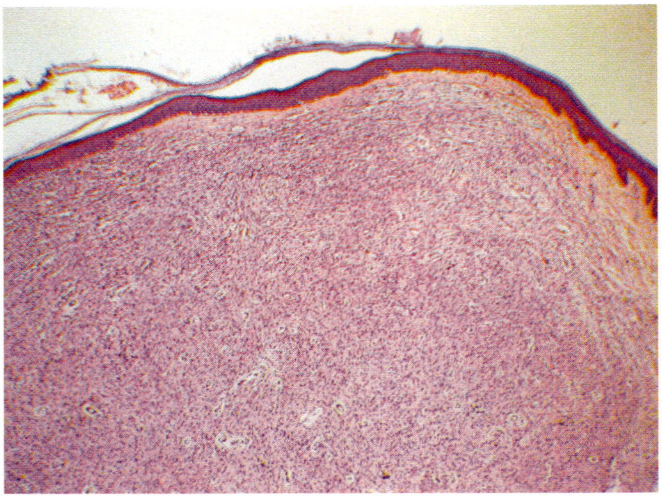

FIGURE 19.17.1

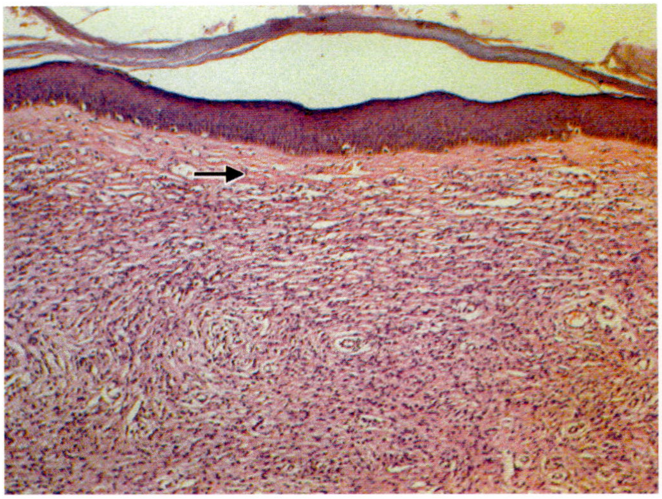

FIGURE 19.17.2

19.17: CUTANEOUS NEUROFIBROMAS

19.17.1: This section shows a circumscribed but non-encapsulated benign tumor made up of spindled cells located in the dermis and subcutaneous tissue, arising from small cutaneous nerves (*Scanner view*)

19.17.2: The lesion is separated from the epidermis by a grenz zone (*Low power view*)

19.17.3: The lesion is composed of delicate fascicles, usually only a single cell thick (*High power view*)

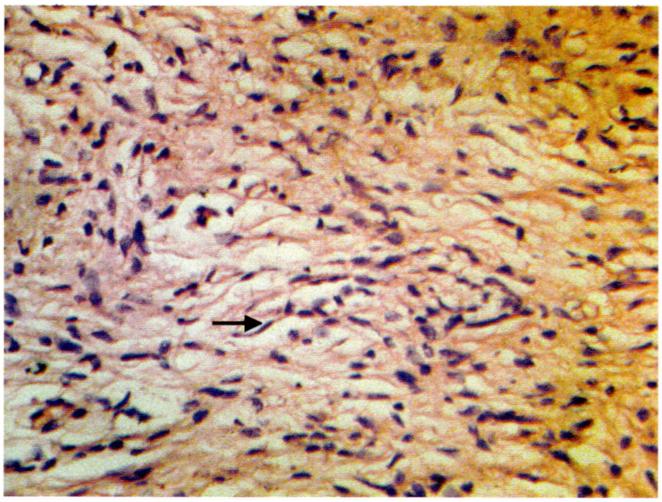

FIGURE 19.17.3

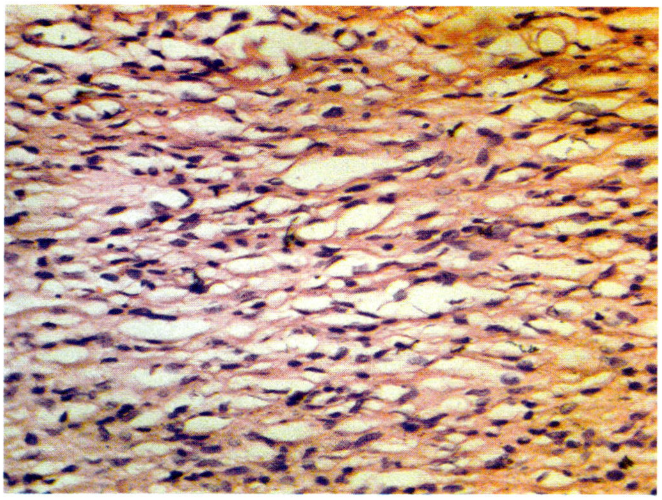

FIGURE 19.17.4

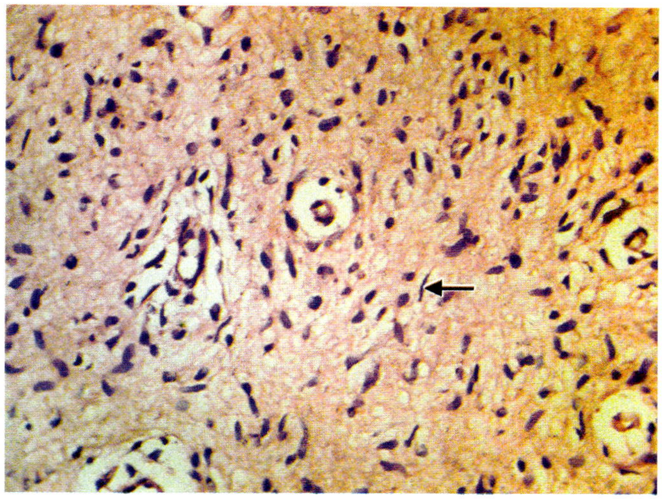

FIGURE 19.17.5

19.17.4: The cells show oval or spindle-shaped nucleus and scant cytoplasm (*High power view*)

19.17.5: Some cells have wavy nuclei. The stroma is pale staining with thin collagen bundles (*High power view*)

19.17.6: Section shows spindle cell fascicles and dilated blood vessels (*High power view*)

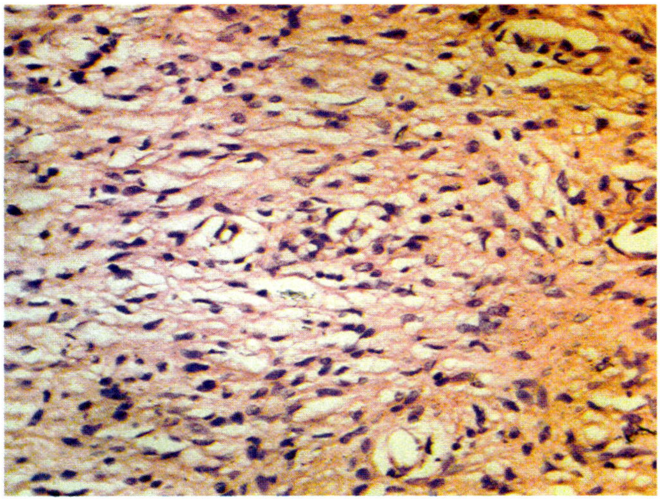

FIGURE 19.17.6

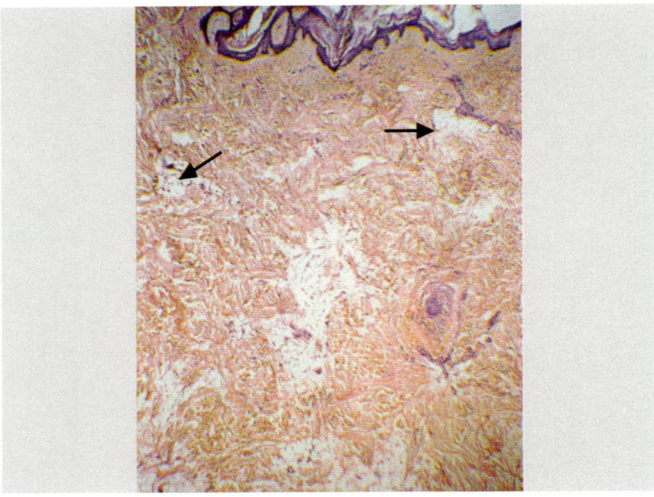

FIGURE 19.18.1

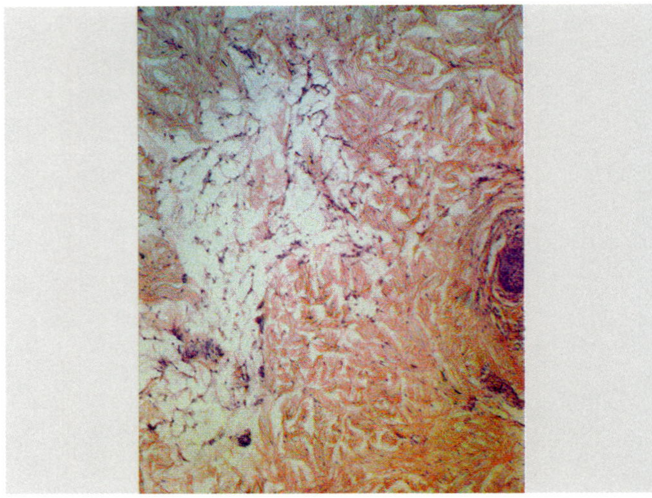

FIGURE 19.18.2

19.18: NEVUS LIPOMATOSUS

19.18.1: There are varying collections of adipose tissue in the dermis. Basal cell layer shows hyperpigmentation and adnexae are atrophic (*Scanner view*)

19.18.2: Closer view shows mature fat cells and thickening of collagen bundles (*Low power view*)

19.18.3: Fat cells also seen around dilated blood vessels (*Low power view*)

19.18.4: Usually, there is no connection of this adipose tissue with the fat of underlying subcutaneous tissue (*Scanner view*)

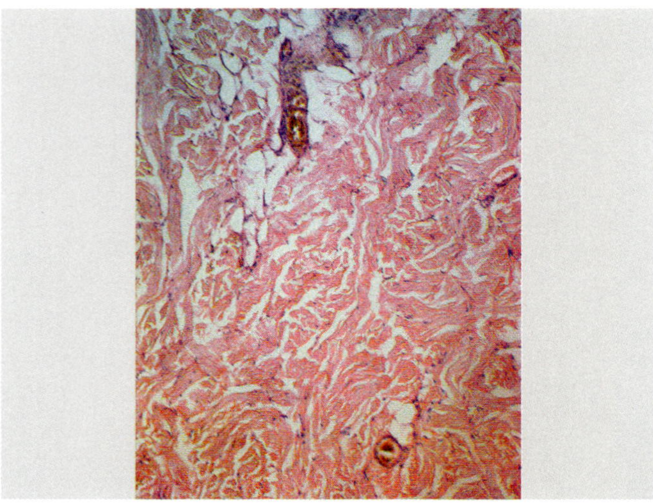

FIGURE 19.18.3

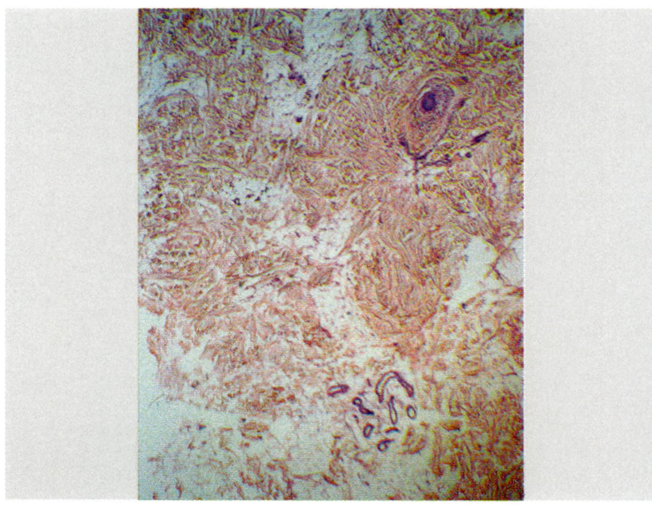

FIGURE 19.18.4

DIFFERENTIAL DIAGNOSIS

1. Cherry angioma
2. Lymphangiectasia
3. Spindle-cell hemangioendothelioma
4. Angiosarcoma
5. Fibrosarcoma
6. Nodular fasciitis
7. Hemangiopericytoma

DIAGNOSTIC PEARLS

1. Lymphangiectasia do not show subcutaneous involvement as against lymphangioma circumscriptum.
2. Angiokeratomas in Fabry disease show vacuolation of smooth muscle in the blood vessels and in the arrectores pilorum.
3. Organisms are not seen in pyogenic granuloma and neutrophils are restricted to the surface of the ulcer as opposed to bacillary angiomatosis.
4. Kaposi's sarcoma shows spindle cells and slit-like vessels where as bacillary angiomatosis demonstrates epithelioid endothelial cells, neutrophils and organisms.
5. Kaposi's sarcoma, glomus tumor and, pyogenic granuloma have different histologic presentations.
6. HHV 8 DNA detection by marker studies is important for diagnosis of Kaposi's sarcoma.

Cutaneous Infiltrates—Nonlymphoid

20

Chapter Outline

20.1: Mastocytosis
20.2: Plasma Cell Infiltrates
20.3: Langerhans Cell Histiocytosis
20.4: Histiocytosis
20.5: Xanthomatous Infiltrates
20.6: Eosinophilic Infiltrates

Pradeep Mahajan, Atul Dongre

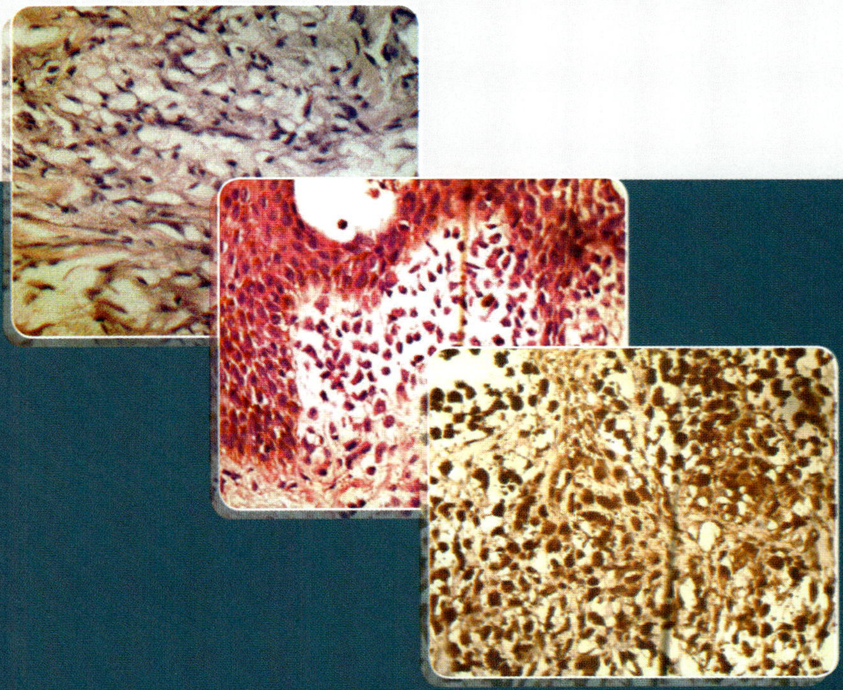

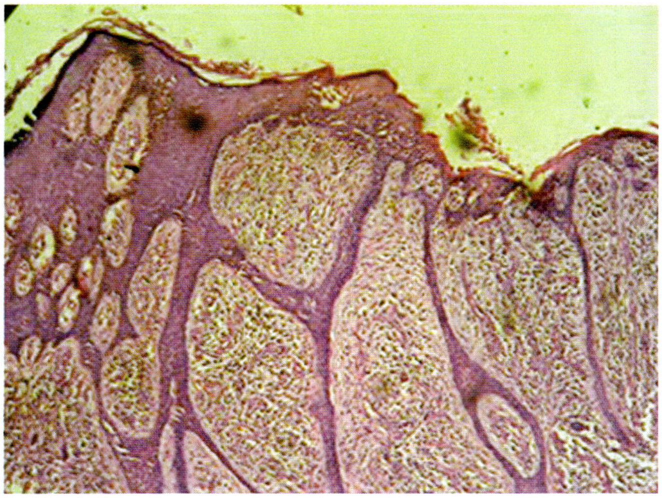

FIGURE 20.1.1

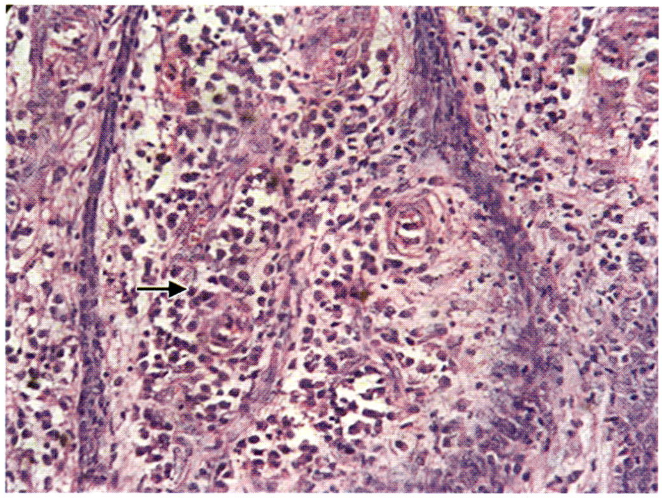

FIGURE 20.1.2

20.1: MASTOCYTOSIS

20.1.1: The mast cell infiltrate is mainly located in the upper dermis and near the dermoepidermal junction (*Scanner view*)

20.1.2: *Urticaria pigmentosa*—variable numbers of mast cells (large cuboidal cells with granular cytoplasm) and scattered eosinophils (*High power view*)

20.1.3: Solitary mastocytoma—dense infiltrate in mid-dermis, extending to subcutaneous (*Low power view*)

20.1.4: Toluidine blue stain highlighting mast cells (*Low power view*)

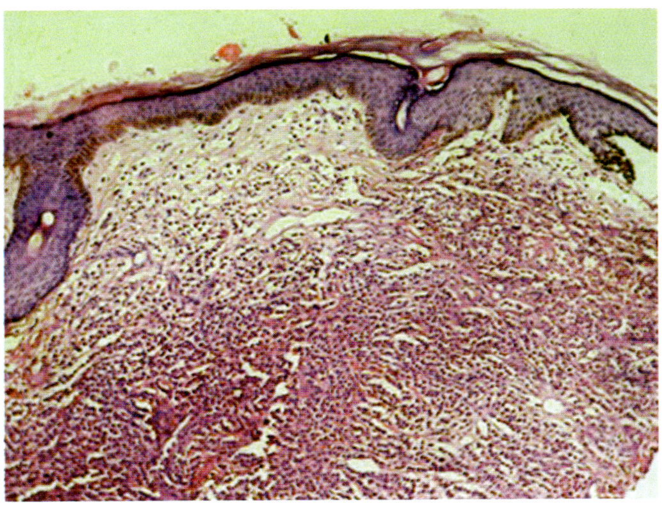

FIGURE 20.1.3

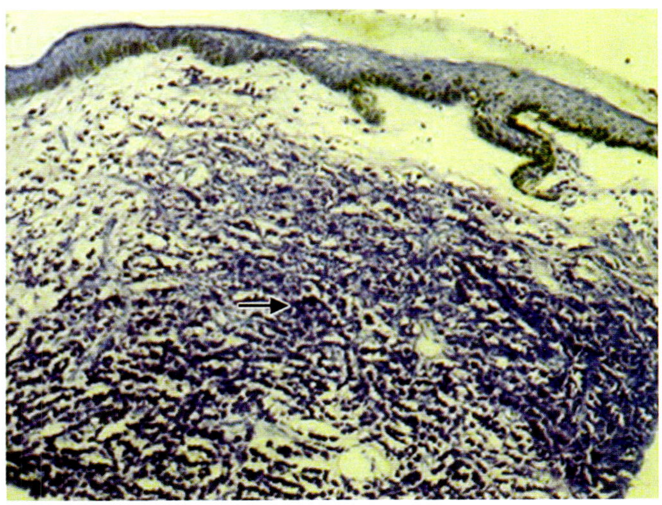

FIGURE 20.1.4

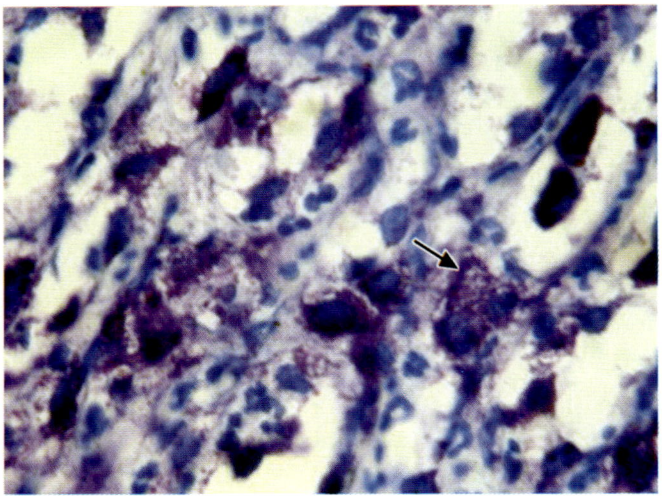

FIGURE 20.1.5

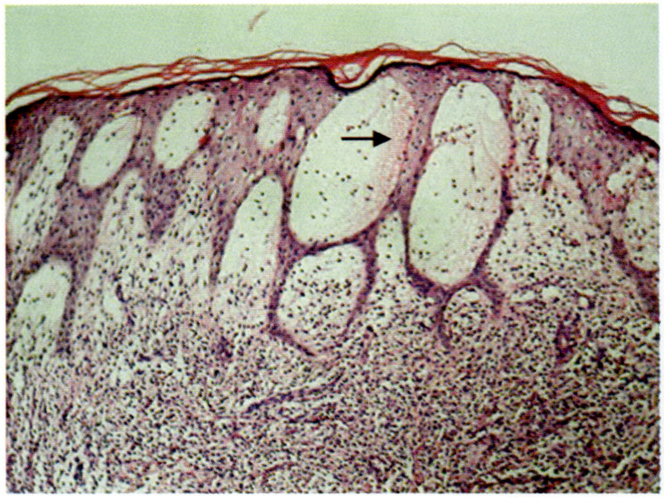

FIGURE 20.1.6

20.1.5: Granules stain metachromatically with toluidine blue (*High power view*)

20.1.6: *Bullous mastocytosis*—intense papillary edema resulting almost in a subepidermal separation with underlying dense collections of monomorphic mast cells (*Low power view*)

20.1.7: Positive toluidine blue stain (*Low power view*)

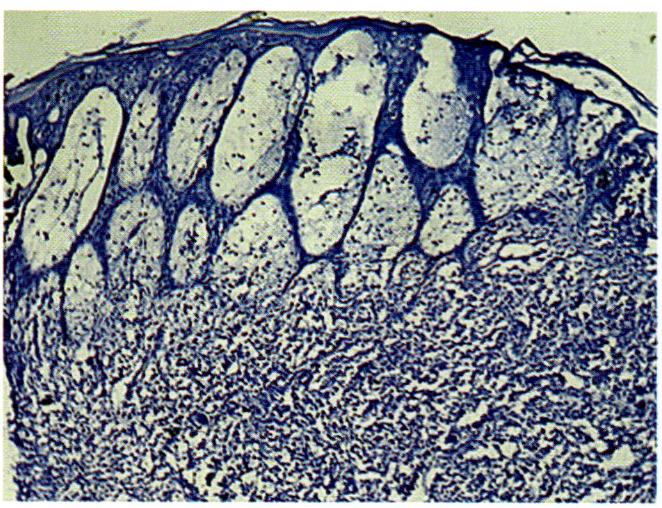

FIGURE 20.1.7

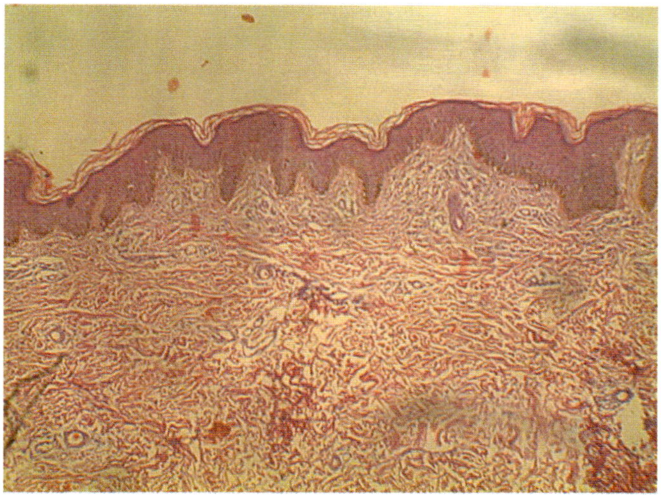

FIGURE 20.1.8

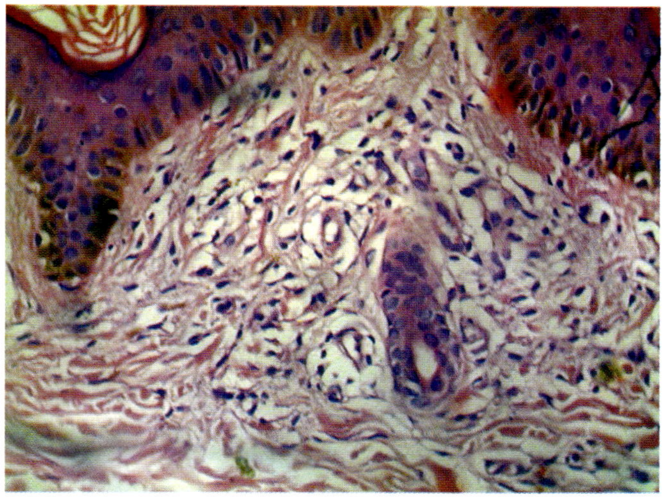

FIGURE 20.1.9

20.1.8: Telangiectasia macularis eruptiva perstans—only slight increase in the number of mast cells admixed with a few eosionophils (*Low power view*)

20.1.9: The epidermis shows increased melanin in the basal layer with ectatic capillaries and little elongated mast cells in perivascular distribution in the dermis (*Low power view*)

20.1.10: Granules stain metachromatically with toluidine blue (*High power view*)

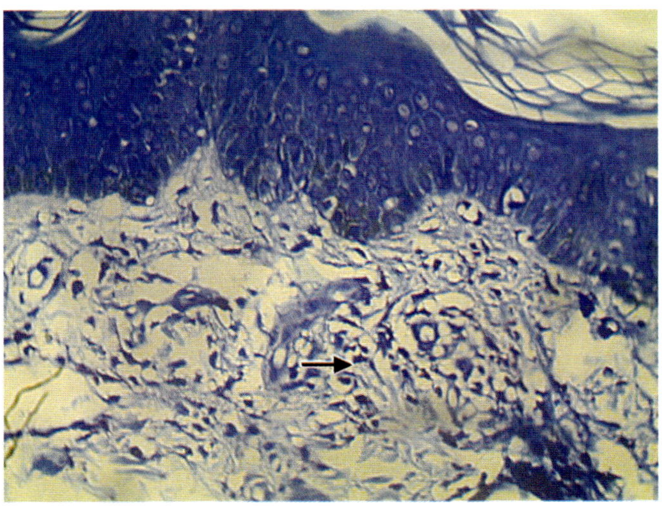

FIGURE 20.1.10

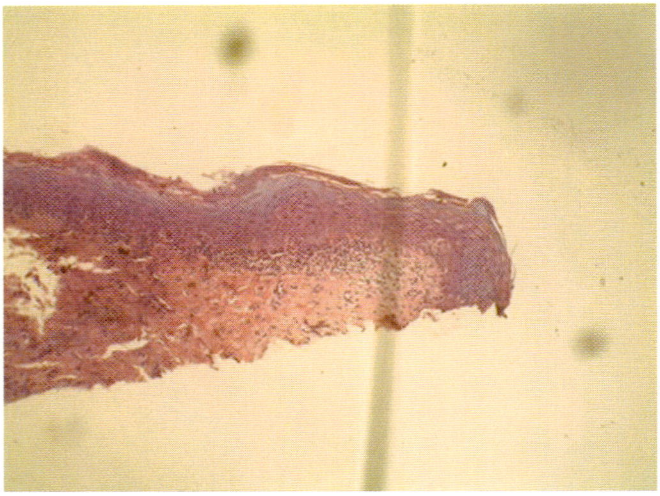

FIGURE 20.2.1.1

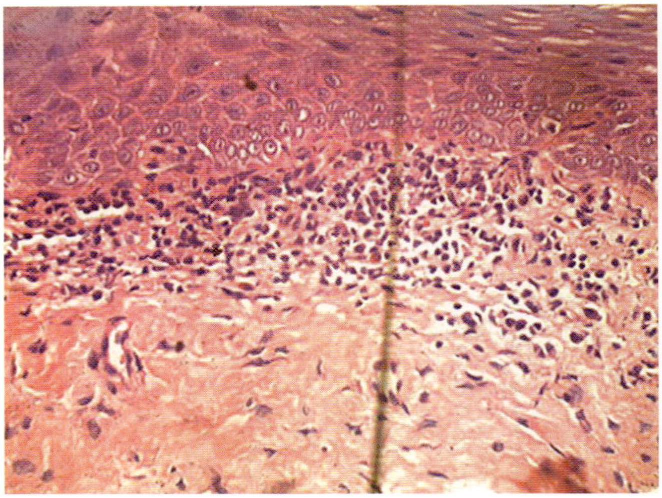

FIGURE 20.2.1.2

20.2: PLASMA CELL INFILTRATES

20.2.1: Plasmacytosis Mucosae (Including Zoon's Balanitis)

20.2.1.1: Stratified squamous epithelium of glans penis with band-like infiltrate in the upper dermis (*Scanner view*)

20.2.1.2: Predominant plasma cell infiltrate with dilated blood vessels (*High power view*)

20.2.1.3: The number of plasma cells vary with the stage of the disease (*High power view*)

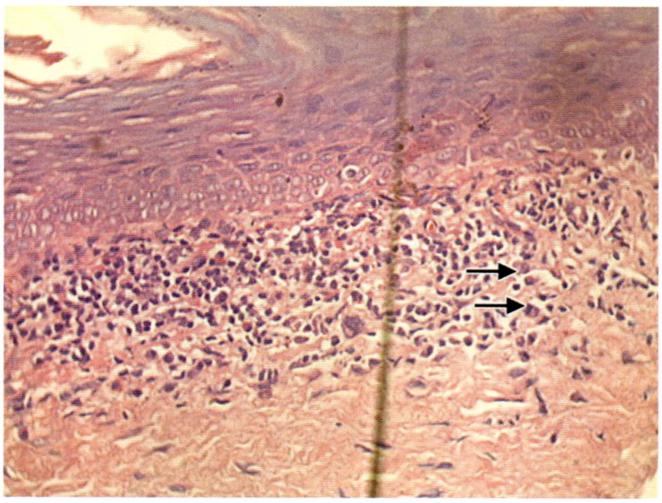

FIGURE 20.2.1.3

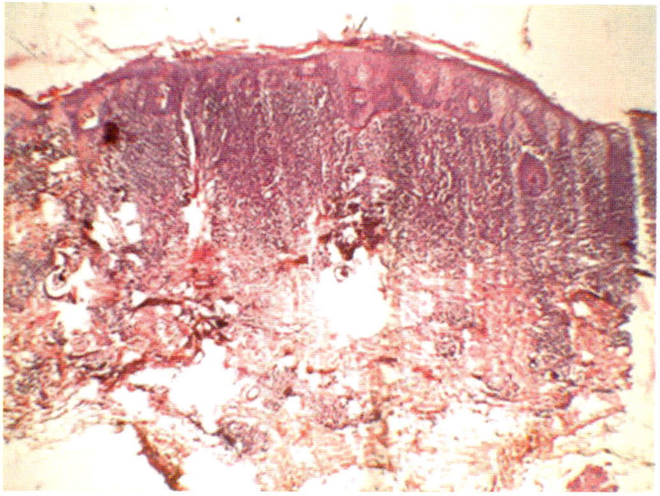

FIGURE 20.2.1.4

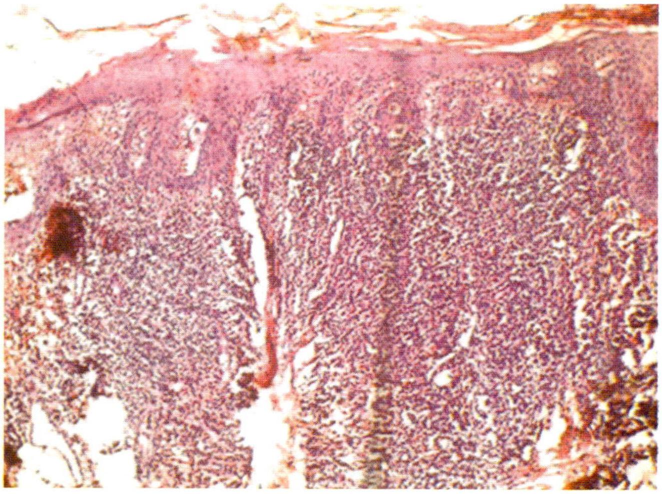

FIGURE 20.2.1.5

20.2.1.4: Another case with biopsy from lip showing dense, band-like infiltrate (*Scanner view*)

20.2.1.5: Infiltrate composed mainly of plasma cells with a few lymphocytes (*Low power view*)

20.2.1.6: Plasma cells and Russell bodies (round eosinophilic inclusions in the cytoplasm) in the dermis (*High power view*)

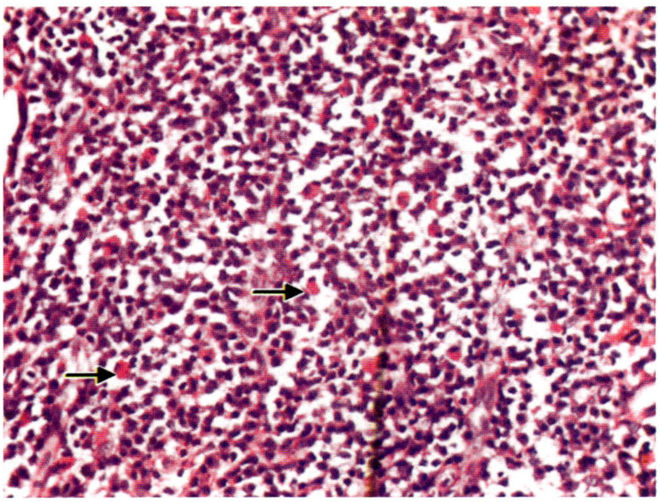

FIGURE 20.2.1.6

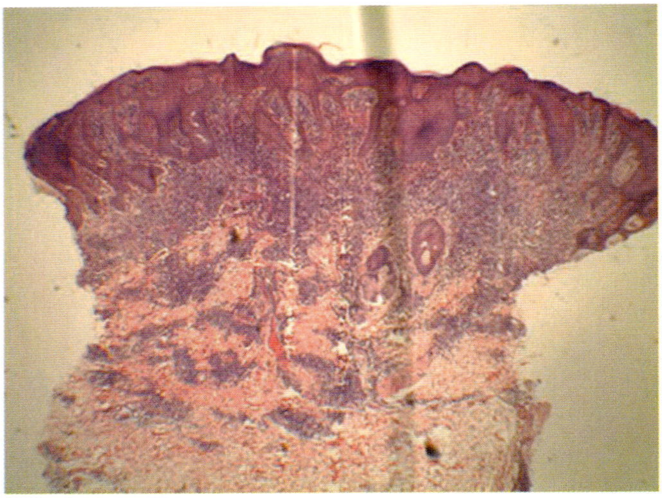

FIGURE 20.2.2.1

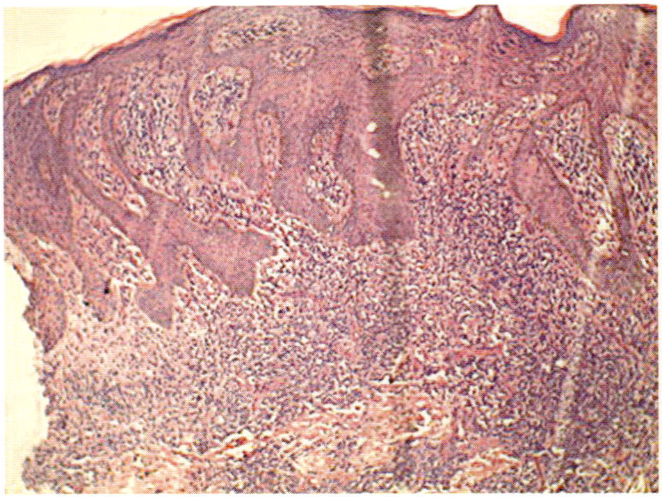

FIGURE 20.2.2.2

20.2.2: Secondary Syphilis

20.2.2.1: Epidermal hyperplasia with moderately dense superficial and deep perivascular infiltrate (*Scanner view*)

20.2.2.2: The infiltrate is composed of lymphocytes, with some histiocytes and variable numbers of plasma cells (*Low power view*)

20.2.2.3: Plasma cell infiltrate with dilated blood vessels and endothelial cell swelling (endarteritis obliterans) (*High power view*)

20.2.2.4: Another view of plasma cell infiltrate with vascular changes (*High power view*)

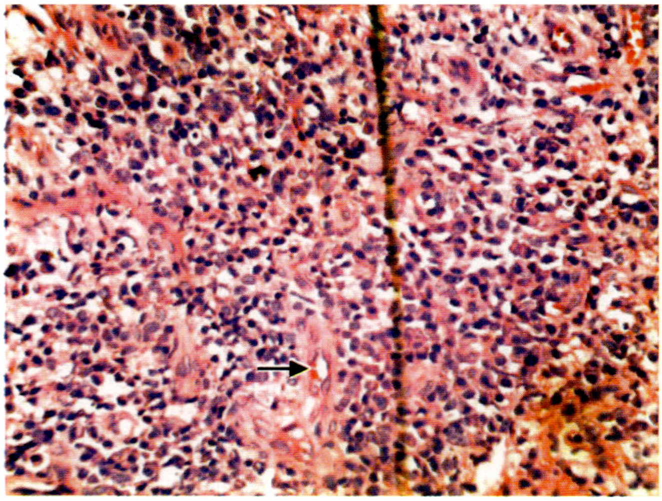

FIGURE 20.2.2.3

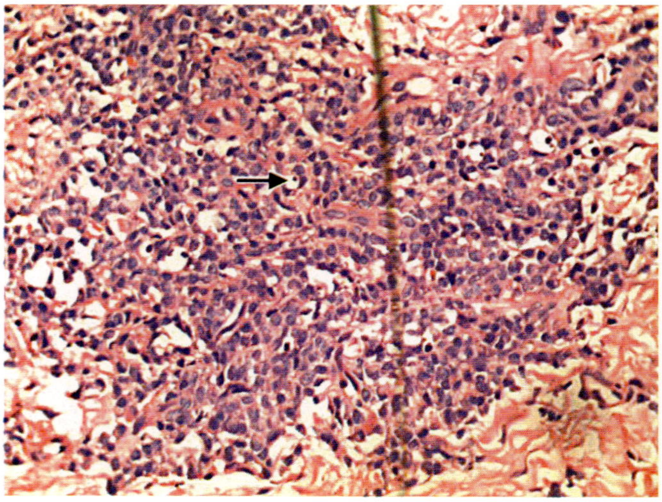

FIGURE 20.2.2.4

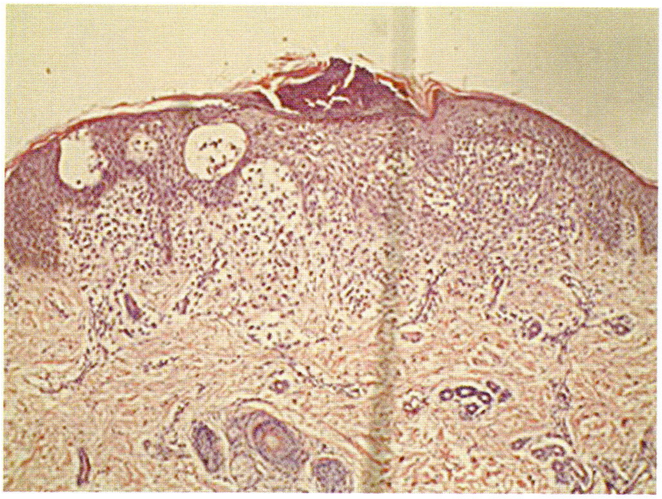

FIGURE 20.3.1

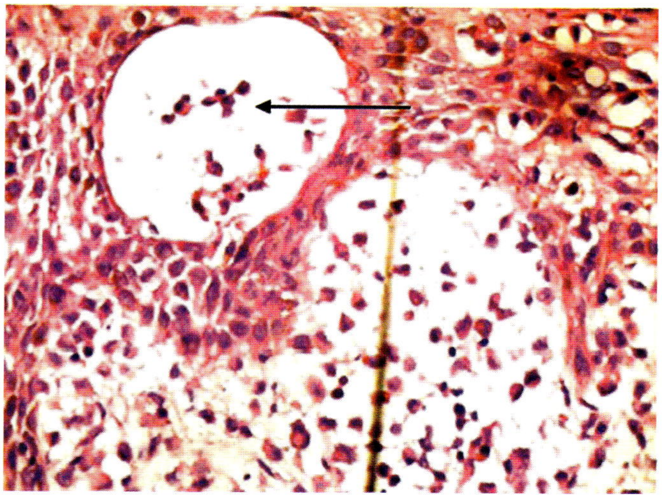

FIGURE 20.3.2

20.3: LANGERHANS CELL HISTIOCYTOSIS

20.3.1: Infiltrate in the upper dermis not extending the reticular dermis (*Low power view*)

20.3.2: The cells invade the epidermis, forming small aggregates in the upper epidermis (*High power view*)

20.3.3: Infiltrate composed of large ovoid cells with eosinophilic cytoplasm and indented nucleus—Langerhans cells (*High power view*)

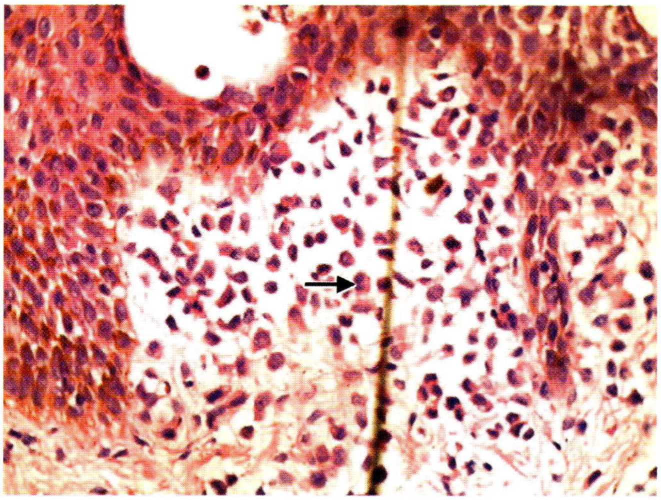

FIGURE 20.3.3

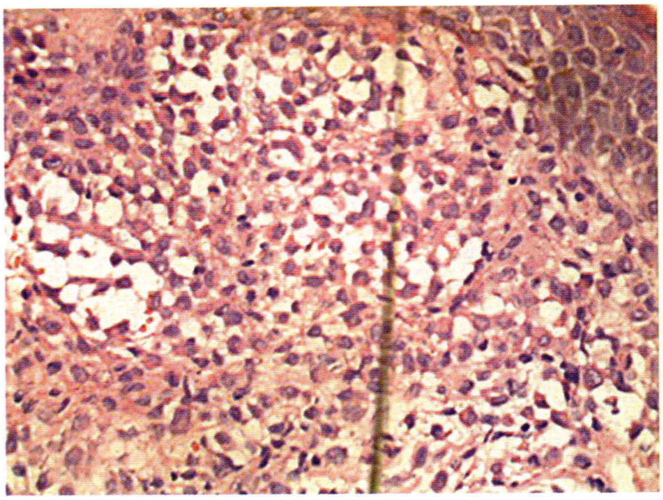

FIGURE 20.3.4

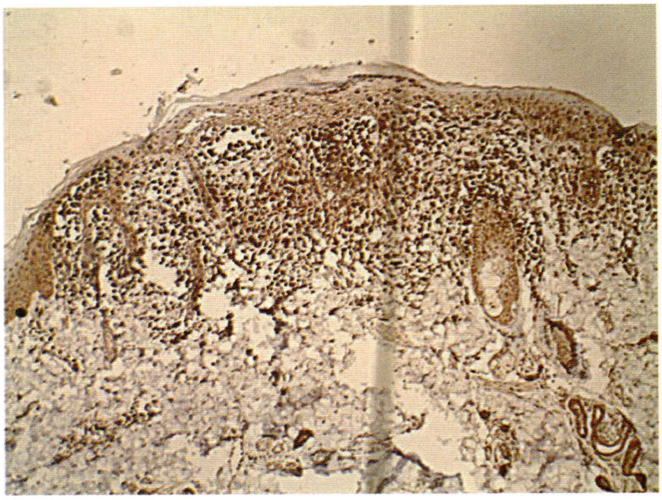

FIGURE 20.3.5

20.3.4: Clusters of Langerhans cells with reniform and eccentric—'coffee-bean' nucleus in the papillary dermis (*High power view*)

20.3.5: Langerhans cell are S-100 positive (other markers are CD1a, HLA-DR, and langerin CD207) (*Low power view*)

20.3.6: Closer view of positive S-100 (*High power view*)

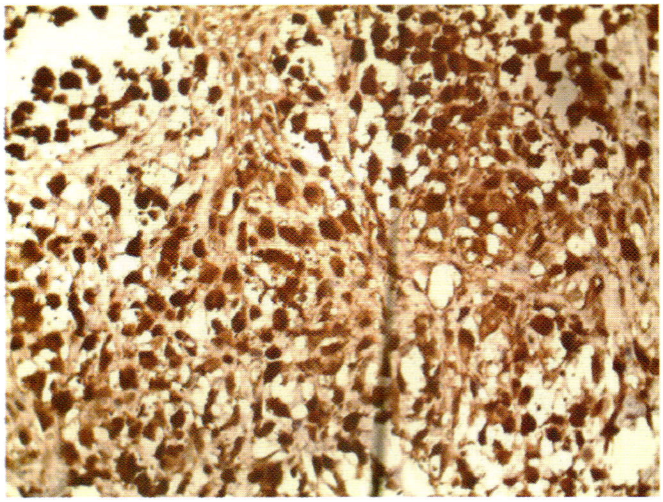

FIGURE 20.3.6

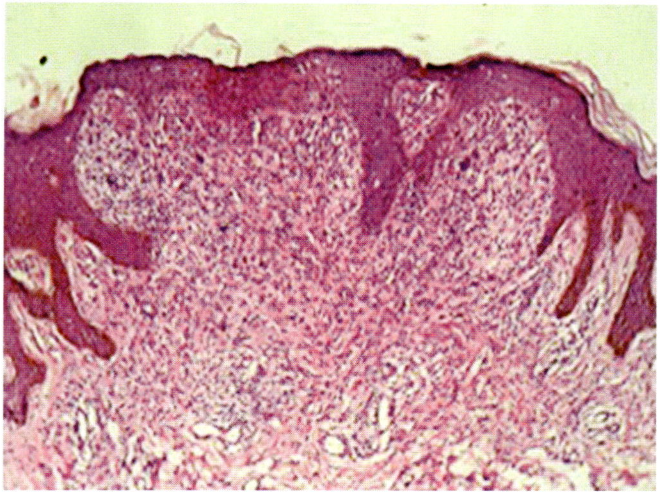

FIGURE 20.4.1.1

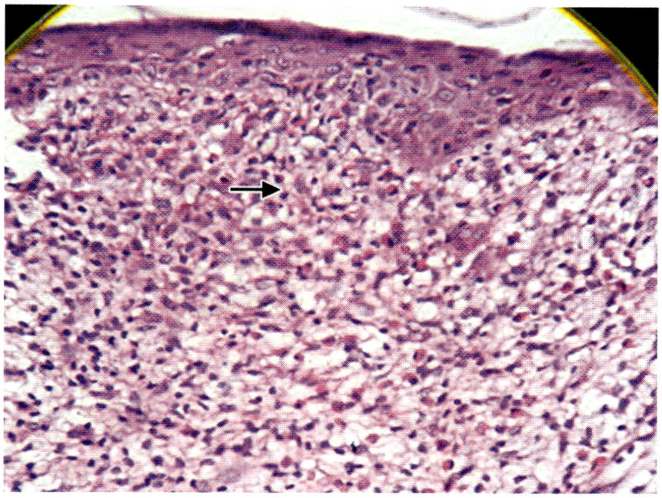

FIGURE 20.4.1.2

20.4: HISTIOCYTOSIS

20.4.1: Juvenile Xanthogranuloma

20.4.1.1: Ill-defined moderately dense infiltrate involving the upper dermis (*Low power view*)

20.4.1.2: Uniform infiltrate composed of histiocytes having vesicular nuclei, eosinophilic cytoplasm and indistinct cytoplasmic borders (*High power view*)

20.4.1.3: Section shows foamy histiocytes indicative of older lesion along with a few eosinophils (*High power view*)

20.4.1.4: Infiltrate also composed of a few lymphocytes and eosinophils (*High power view*)

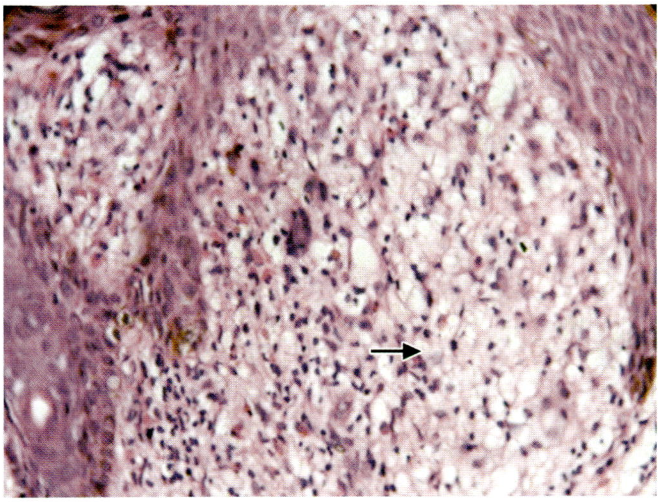

FIGURE 20.4.1.3

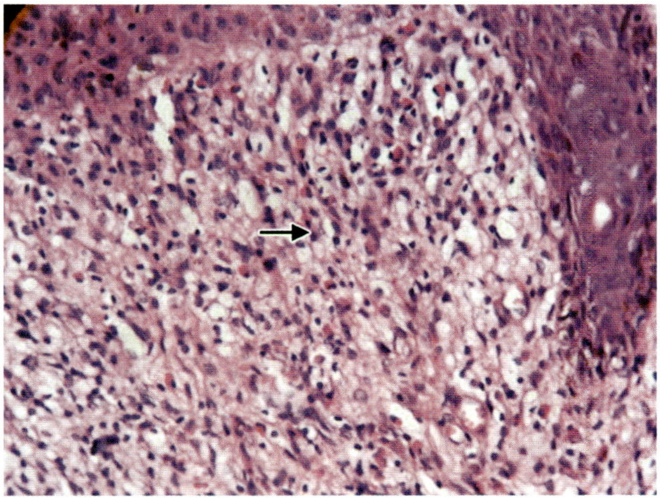

FIGURE 20.4.1.4

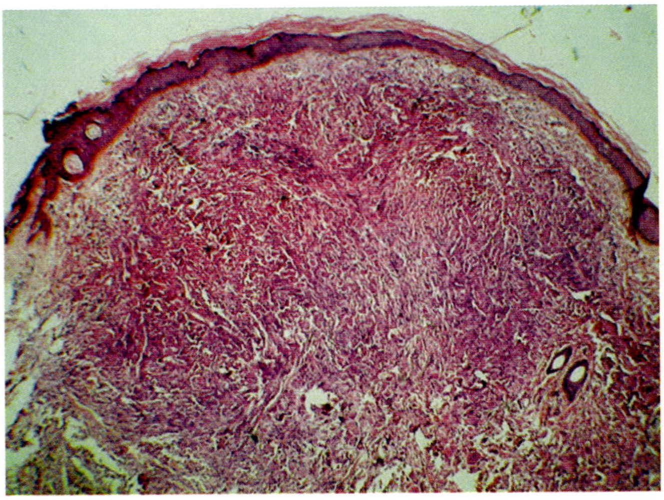

FIGURE 20.4.2.1

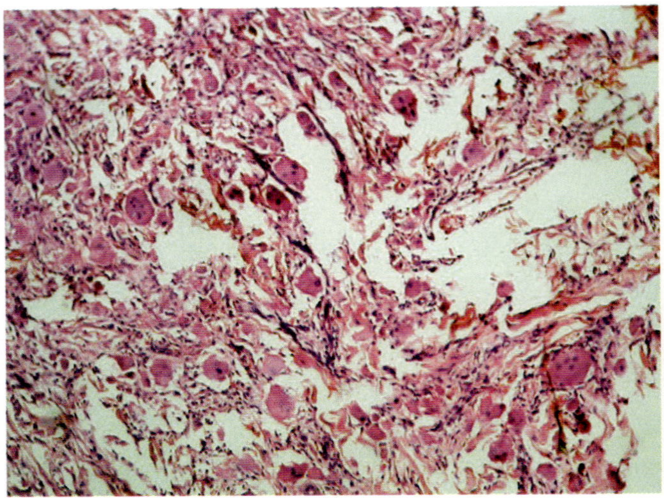

FIGURE 20.4.2.2

20.4.2: Multicentric Reticulohistiocytosis

20.4.2.1: Section shows well demarcated unencapsulated histiocytic infiltrate in the dermis with a narrow grenz zone separating it from overlying atrophic epidermis (*Scanner view*)

20.4.2.2: Infiltrate composed of mononuclear and multinucleate histiocytes and perivascular lymphocytes (*Low power view*)

20.4.2.3: The hallmark of the condition is histiocytes that are large, multinucleated with 4 or more nuclei and eosinophilic, granular cytoplasm referred to as 'ground glass' (*High power view*)

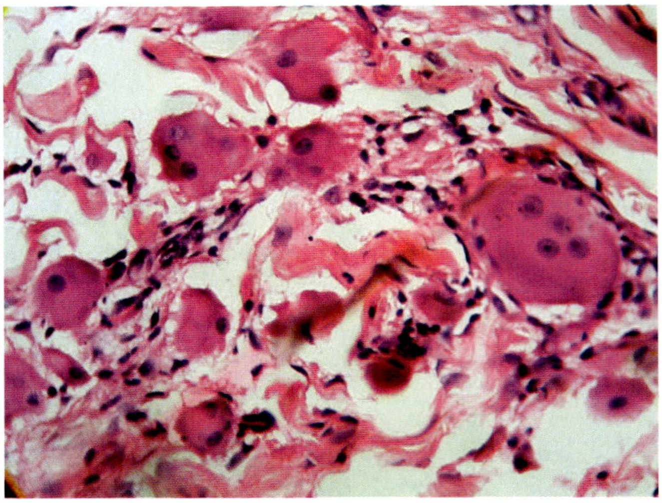

FIGURE 20.4.2.3

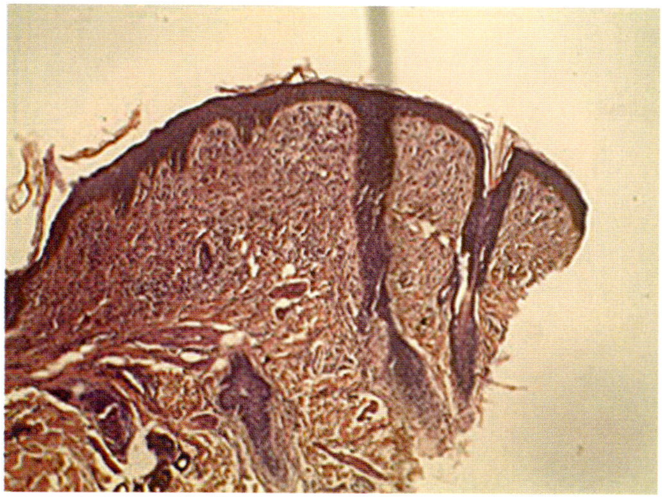

FIGURE 20.4.3.1

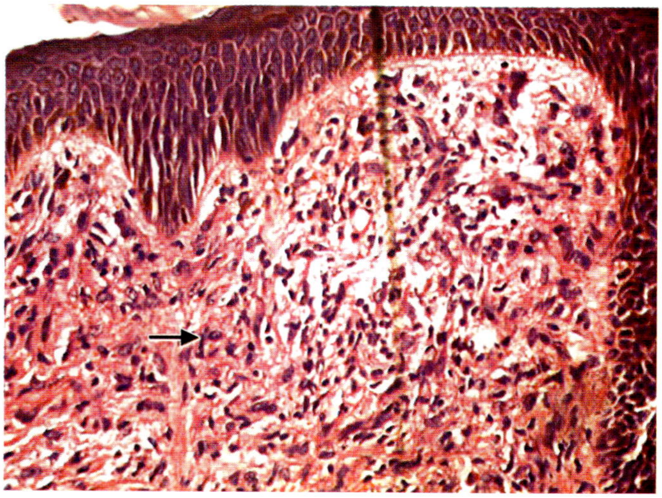

FIGURE 20.4.3.2

20.4.3: Benign Cephalic Histiocytosis

20.4.3.1: Moderately dense and diffuse infiltrate in the upper dermis (*Scanner view*)

20.4.3.2: The infiltrate is composed of histiocytes with an oval vesicular nucleus and ill-defined eosinophilic cytoplasm, but no foamy change (*Low power view*)

20.4.3.3: Closer view of histiocytes. There are scattered lymphocytes within the infiltrate also (*High power view*)

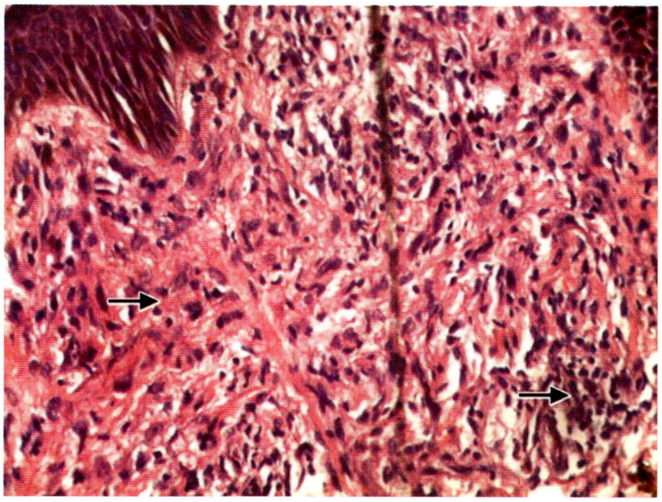

FIGURE 20.4.3.3

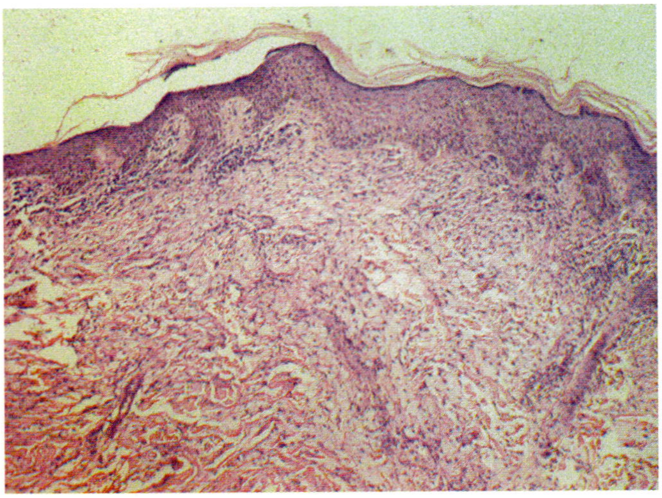

FIGURE 20.5.1

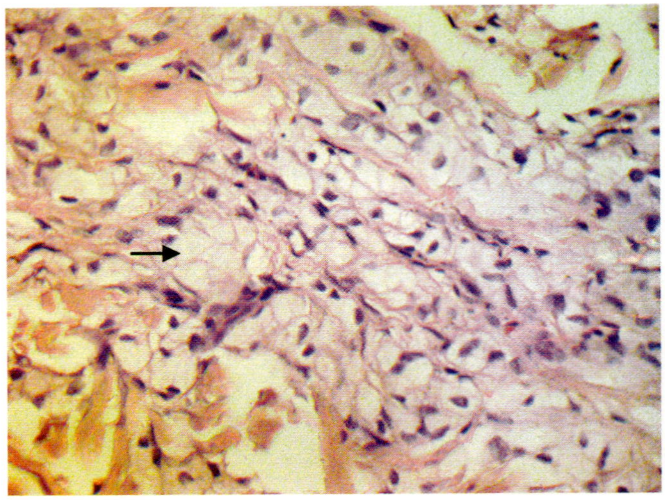

FIGURE 20.5.2

20.5: XANTHOMATOUS INFILTRATES

20.5.1: The cellular infiltrate throughout the dermis (*Low power view*)

20.5.2: In established lesions, there is obvious foamy change of macrophages (due to intracellular lipid deposits) in the infiltrate (*High power view*)

20.5.3: These foam cells are also present between the collagen bundles along with extracellular lipid deposits (*High power view*)

20.5.4: The dermis shows collection of foamy macrophages. The Touton giant cells or eosinophils are absent. Older lesions show fibrosis (*High power view*)

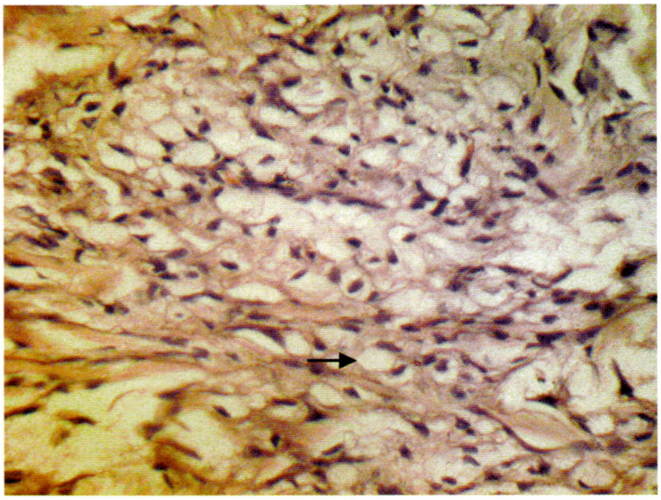

FIGURE 20.5.3

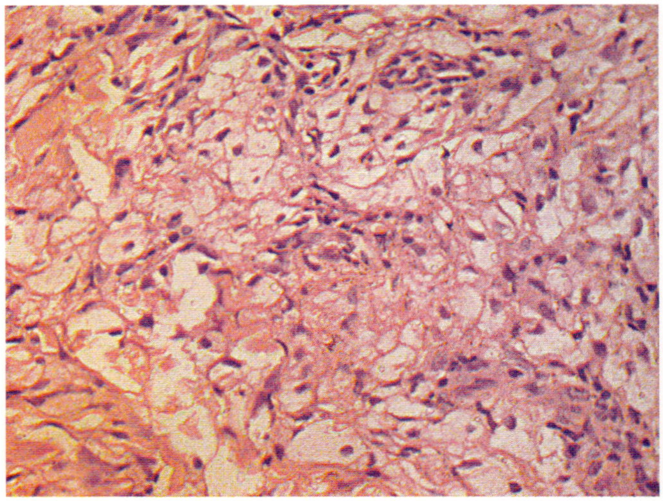

FIGURE 20.5.4

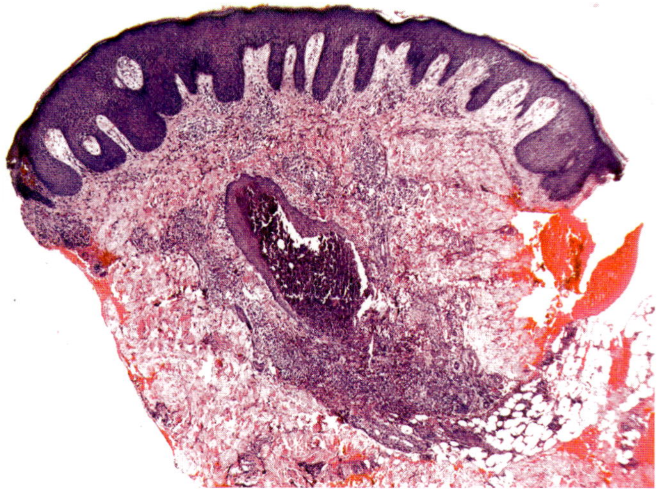

FIGURE 20.6.1.1

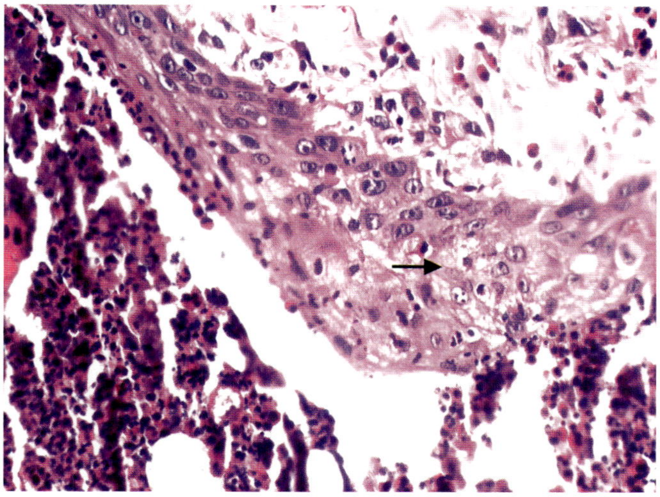

FIGURE 20.6.1.2

20.6: EOSINOPHILIC INFILTRATES

20.6.1: Eosinophilic Folliculitis

20.6.1.1: All the variants show follicular spongiosis and inflammatory infiltrate (*Scanner view*)

20.6.1.2: Some hair follicles may show destruction with necrosis due to inflammatory infiltrate (*High power view*)

20.6.1.3: The inflammatory infiltrate is mainly composed of eosinophils with a few neutrophils and mononuclear cells (*High power view*)

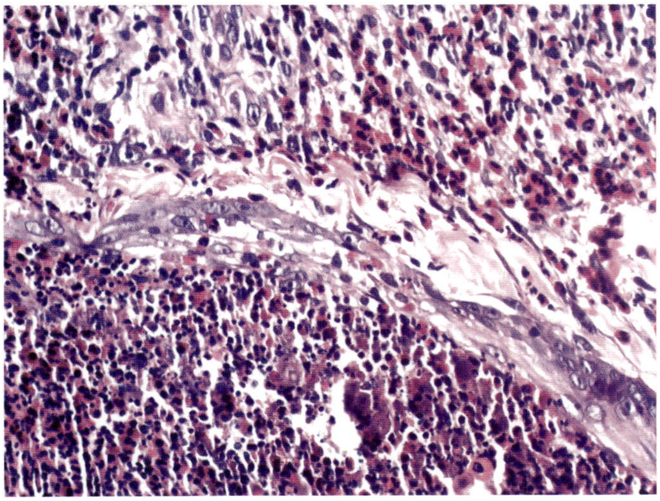

FIGURE 20.6.1.3

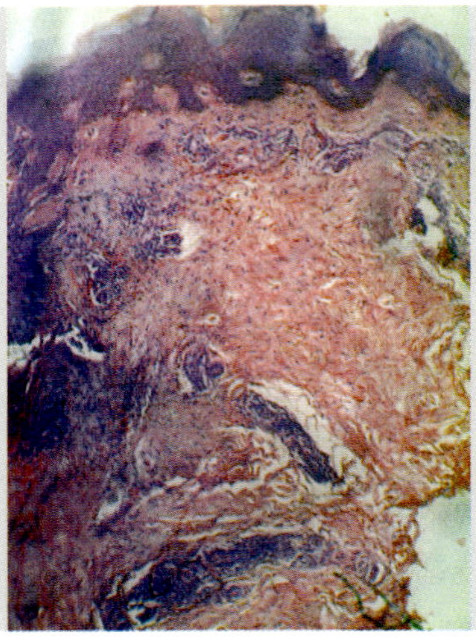

FIGURE 20.6.2.1

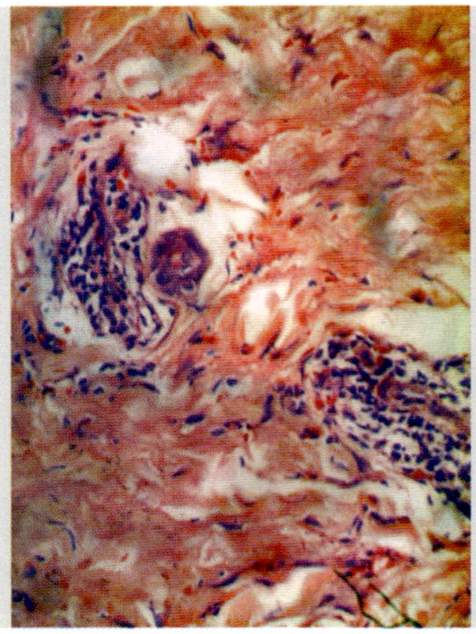

FIGURE 20.6.2.2

20.6.2: Hypereosinophilic Syndrome

20.6.2.1: Hyperplasia of the overlying epidermis with dense perivascular infiltrate throughout the dermis (*Scanner view*)

20.6.2.2: Perivascular eosinophils and lymphocytes (*Low power view*)

20.6.2.3: Another view of the infiltrate composed of eosinophils and lymphocytes but also contains a few plasma cells (*Low power view*)

20.6.2.4: Papillary edema with microthrombi containing eosinophils (*Low power view*)

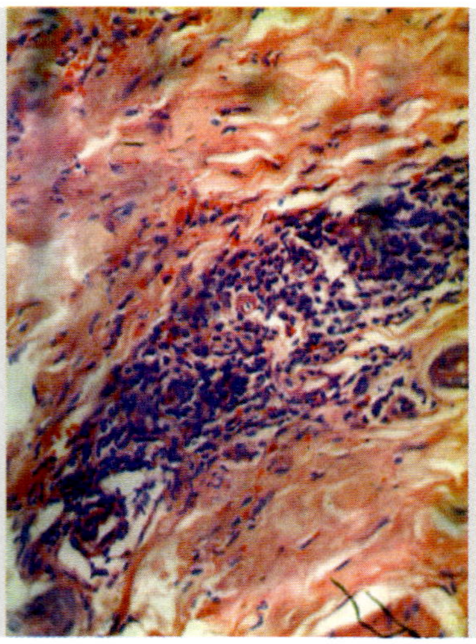

FIGURE 20.6.2.3

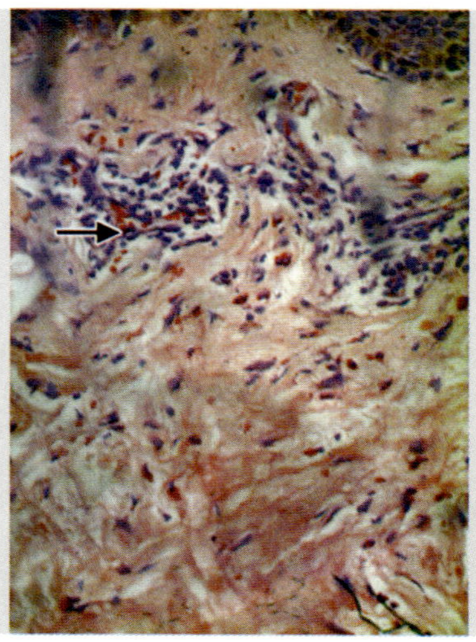

FIGURE 20.6.2.4

DIFFERENTIAL DIAGNOSIS

1. Plasmacytomas and multiple myeloma
2. Xanthoma disseminatum
3. Necrobiotic xanthogranuloma
4. Generalized eruptive histiocytosis
5. Progressive nodular histiocytosis
6. Rosai Dorfman disease
7. Verruciform xanthoma
8. Eosinophilic cellulitis

DIAGNOSTIC PEARLS

1. Specific mast cell marker is CD117 but neoplastic mast cells are positive for CD2 or CD25.
2. Specific marker for Langerhans cells is CD207.
3. Cutaneous xanthomas do not show other inflammatory cells as against xanthogranulomas.
4. Also xanthogranulomas frequently show Touton giant cell but not foreign body giant cells.
5. Flame figures seen in eosinophilic infiltrates are eosinophil granule major basic protein coated on normal collagen.

21 Lympho-proliferative Disorders of Skin

Chapter Outline

21.1: Benign Cutaneous Lymphoid Hyperplasia (Pseudolymphoma)
21.2: Lymphocytic Infiltrate of the Skin (Jessner's)
21.3: Follicular Mucinosis
21.4: Mycosis Fungoides
21.5: Sezary Syndrome
21.6: Folliculotrophic Mycosis Fungoides
21.7: Subcutaneous Panniculitis—Like T-cell Lymphoma (Alpha/Beta T-cell Lymphoma)
21.8: Lymphomatoid Papulosis
21.9: Anaplastic Large Cell Lymphoma
21.10: Primary Cutaneous Diffuse Large B-cell Lymphoma

Nandakumar Gopinath, Uday Khopkar, Chirag Desai, Pradeep Mahajan, Nathan Lee, Jerad Gardner, Asha Kubba

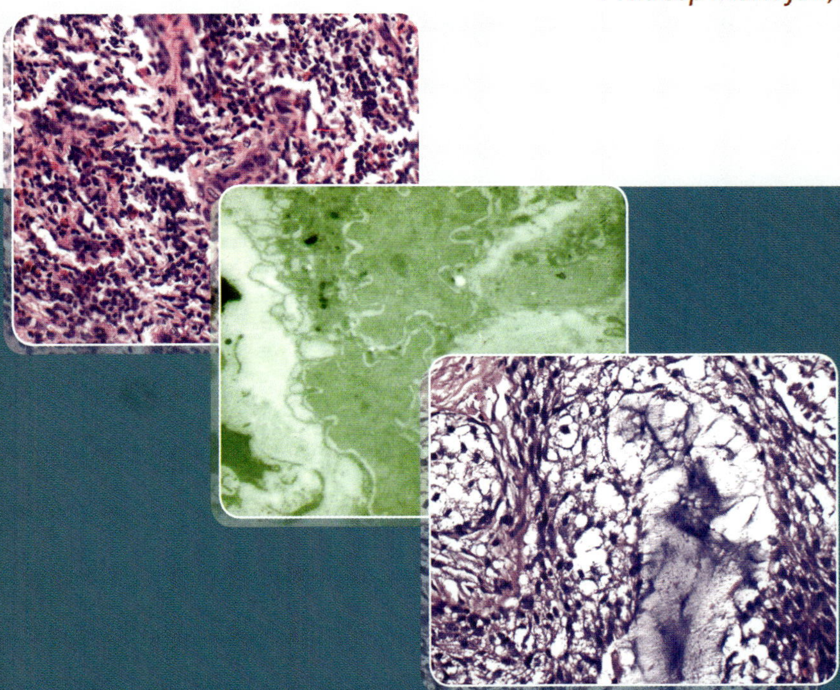

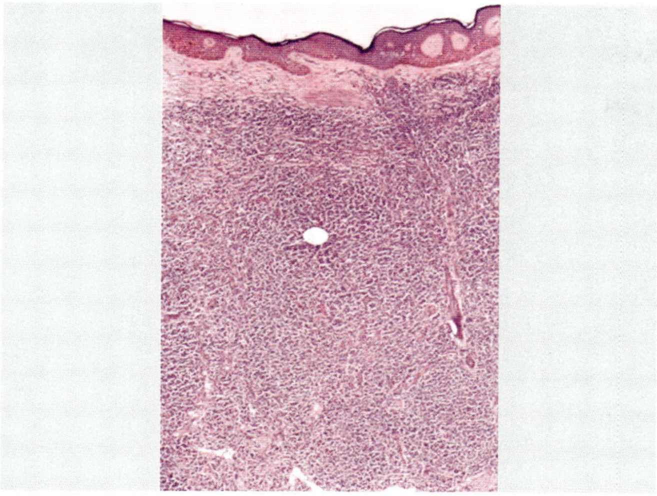

FIGURE 21.1.1

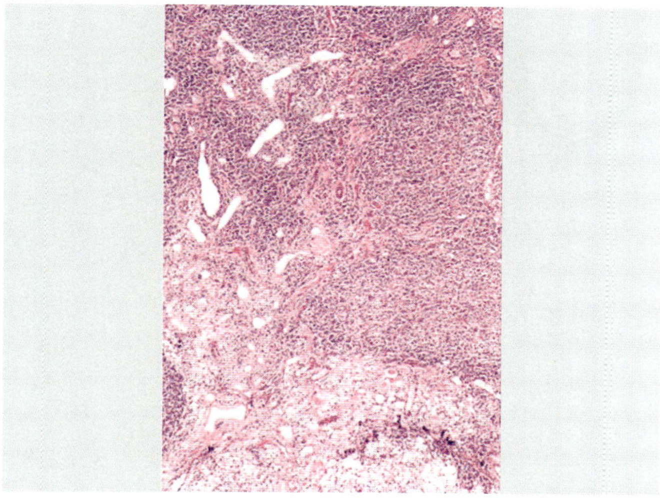

FIGURE 21.1.2

21.1: BENIGN CUTANEOUS LYMPHOID HYPERPLASIA (PSEUDOLYMPHOMA)

21.1.1: A diffuse, top heavy lymphocytic infiltrate in the dermis, a grenz zone is prominently seen (*Scanner view*)

21.1.2: Infiltrate is nodular, perivascular and periadnexal in distribution, extends to the deep reticular dermis and subcutis (*Scanner view*)

21.1.3: Another case showing lymphoid infiltrate similar to reactive lymphoid tissue at lymph nodes or tonsils with uniform looking cells suggesting benign nature (*Low power view*)

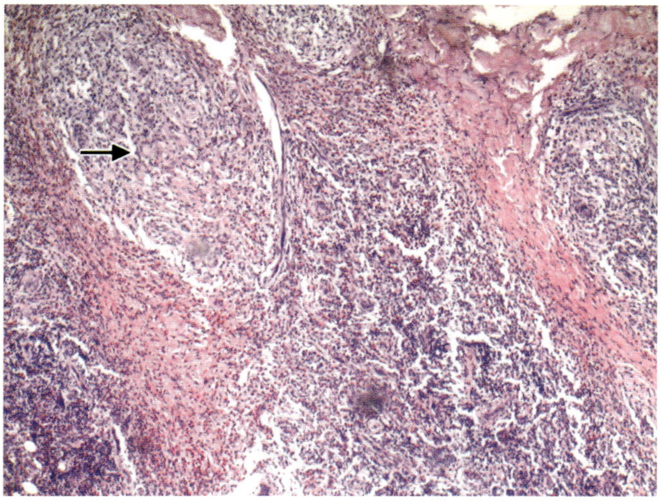

FIGURE 21.1.3

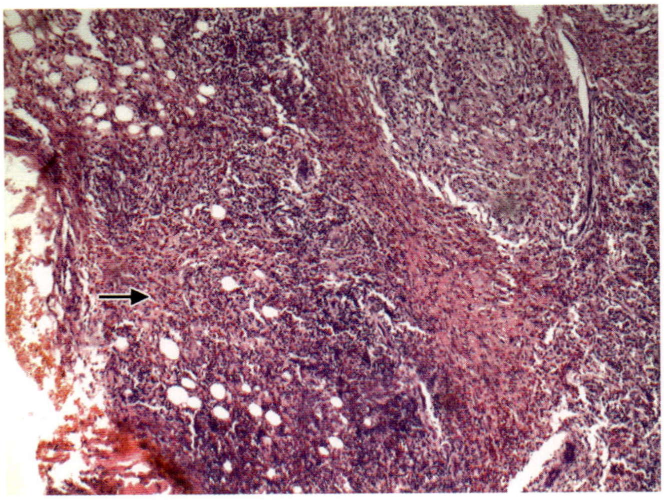

FIGURE 21.1.4

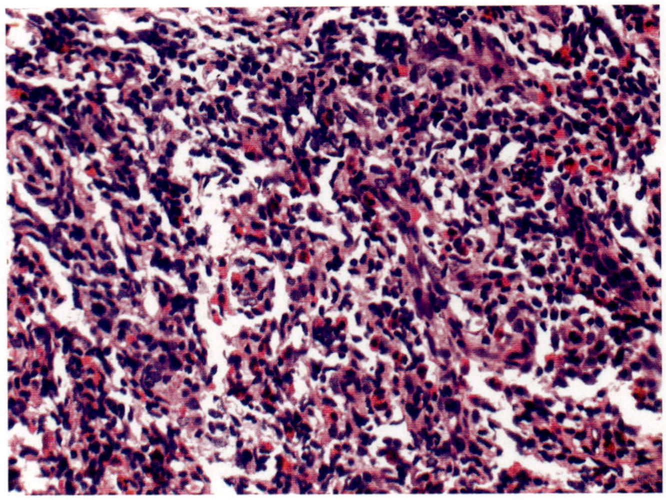

FIGURE 21.1.5

21.1.4: Lymphoid follicles present with darkly staining areas consisting of proliferating centroblasts and lighter areas mainly with centrocytes (*Low power view*)

21.1.5: Germinal centers comprise an admixture of large centroblasts, small and large centrocytes, and tingible body macrophages (*High power view*)

21.1.6: The interfollicular areas are composed of mixed infiltrate with predominant small lymphocytes, scattered blast cells, histiocytes, plasma cells, and sometimes eosinophils *(High power view)*

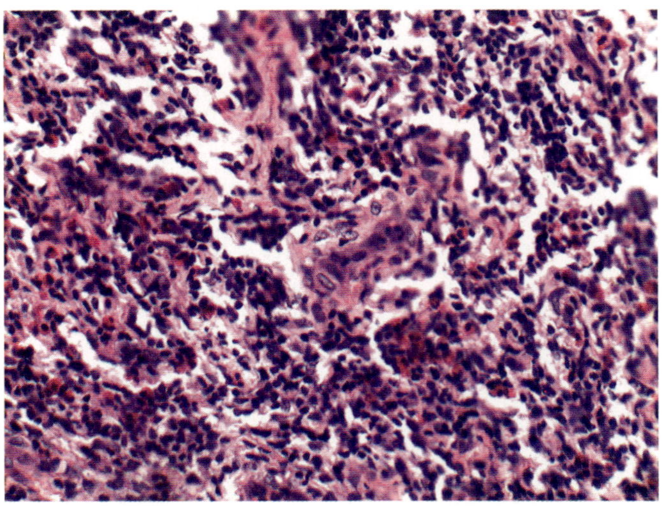

FIGURE 21.1.6

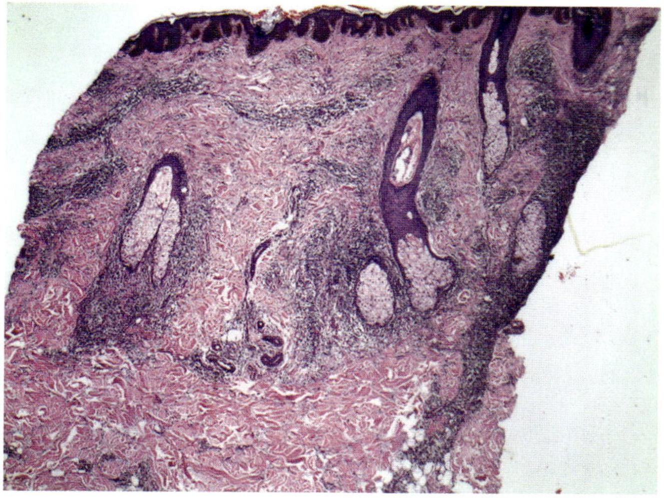

FIGURE 21.2.1

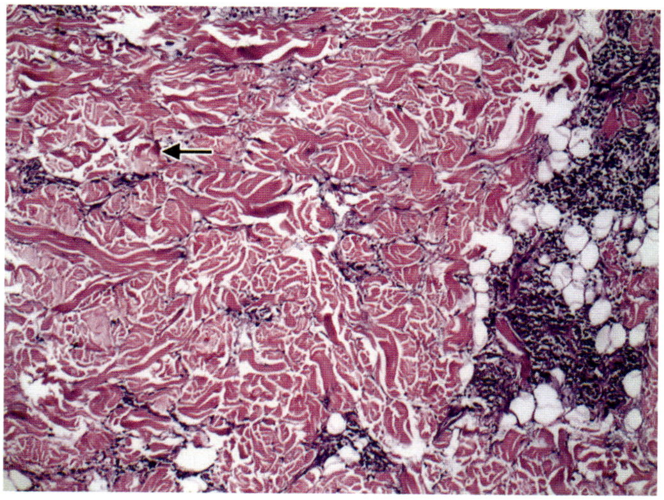

FIGURE 21.2.2

21.2: LYMPHOCYTIC INFILTRATE OF THE SKIN (JESSNER'S)

21.2.1: The epidermis is unremarkable. Dermis shows moderately dense perivascular infiltrate of small mature lymphocytes (*Scanner view*)

21.2.2: There is an increase in dermal ground substance (*Low power view*)

21.2.3: Occasional histiocytes and scattered plasma cells may also be present but lymphoid follicles are not a feature (*High power view*)

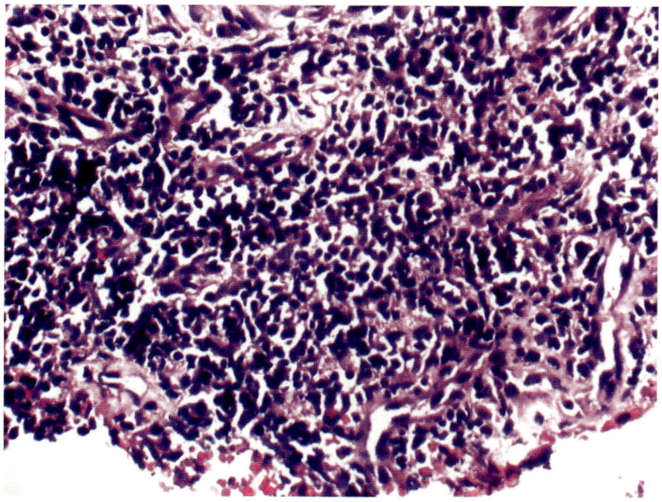

FIGURE 21.2.3

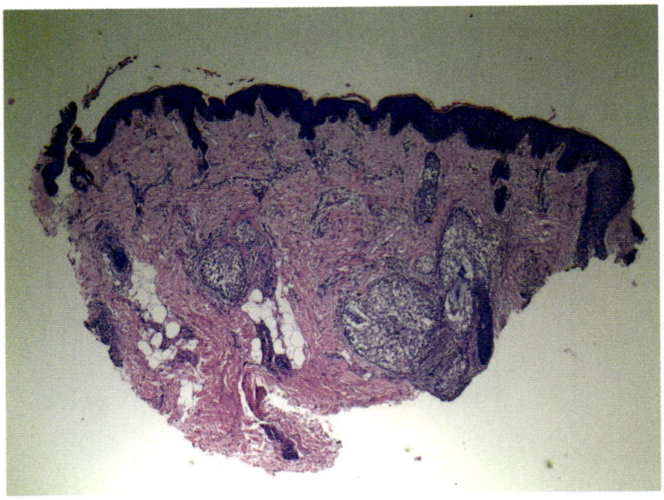

FIGURE 21.3.1

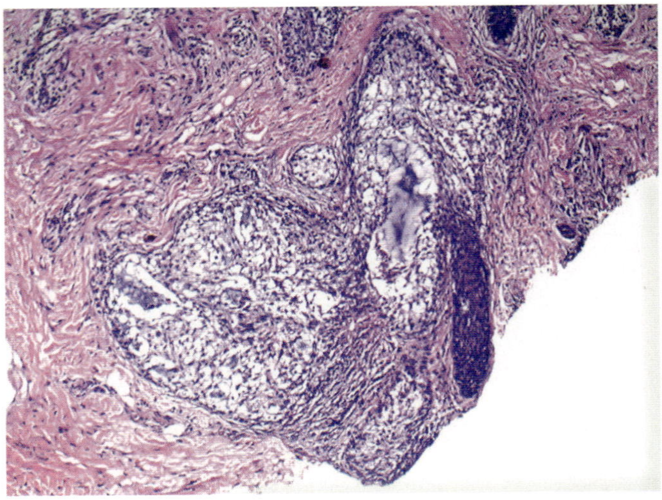

FIGURE 21.3.2

21.3: FOLLICULAR MUCINOSIS

21.3.1: Predominantly periappendageal lymphocytic infiltrate (*Scanner view*)

21.3.2: Distorted follicles with spongiosis and inflammatory infiltrate (*Low power view*)

21.3.3: Follicular degeneration with accumulation of mucin within the follicles (*High power view*)

21.3.4: Another view with infiltrate and mucin (*High power view*)

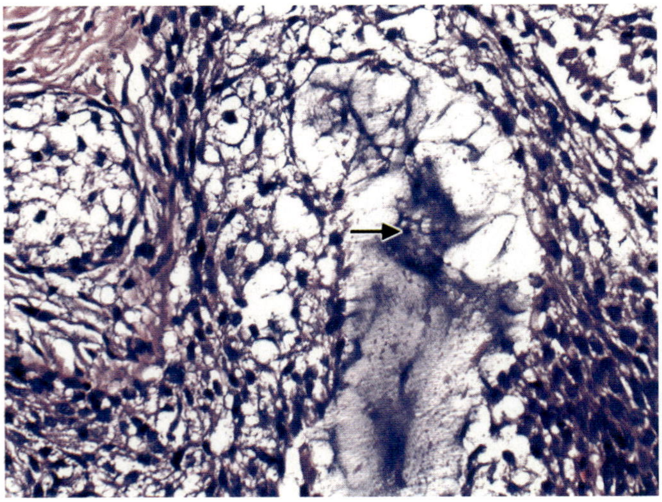

FIGURE 21.3.3

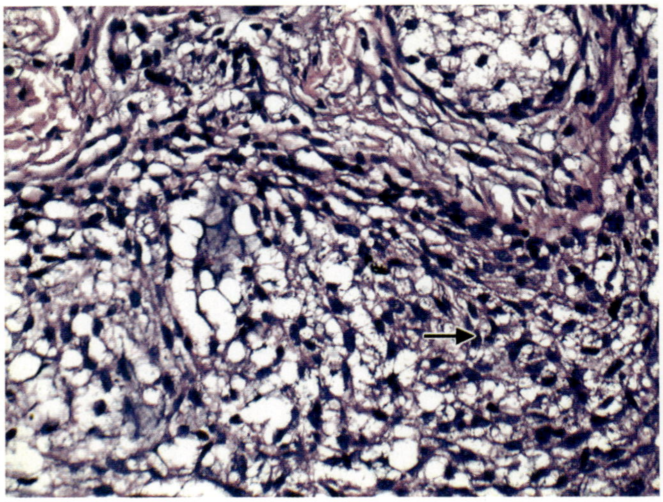

FIGURE 21.3.4

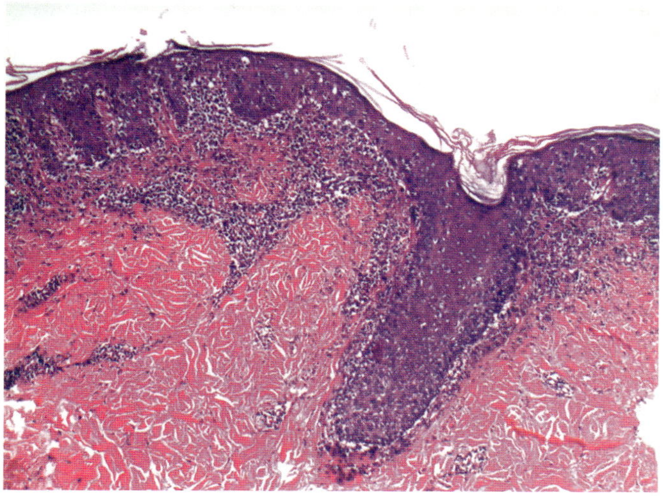

FIGURE 21.4.1

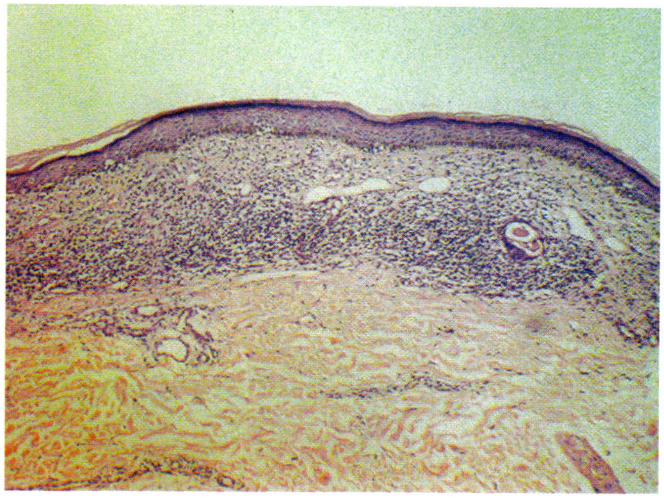

FIGURE 21.4.2

21.4: MYCOSIS FUNGOIDES

21.4.1: Patch stage shows lymphoid infiltrate involving the papillary and superficial reticular dermis difficult to differentiate from inflammatory diseases (*Scanner view*)

21.4.2: In plaque-stage MF, the lymphocytic infiltrate within the dermis is band-like, with lymphocytes at the epidermal–dermal junction (*Scanner view*)

21.4.3: Extension of lymphocytes into the epidermis without much of spongiosis (epidermotropism). Single lymphocytes in the epidermis are surrounded by clear halos (*High power view*)

21.4.4: Lymphocytes lie in a single row within the basal layer of the epidermis (Toy Soldier's appearance) (*High power view*)

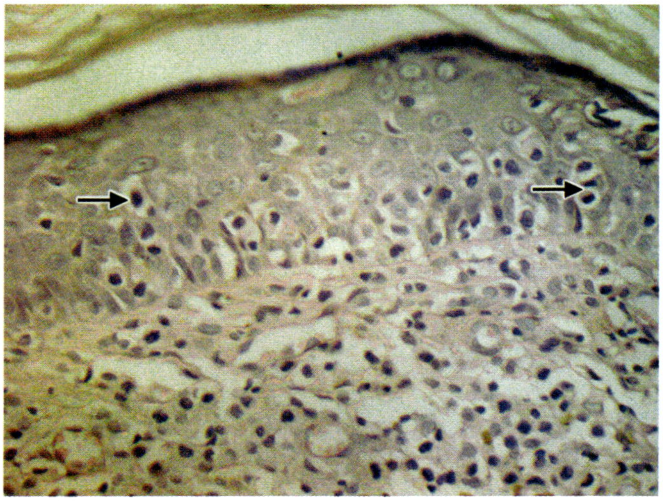

FIGURE 21.4.3

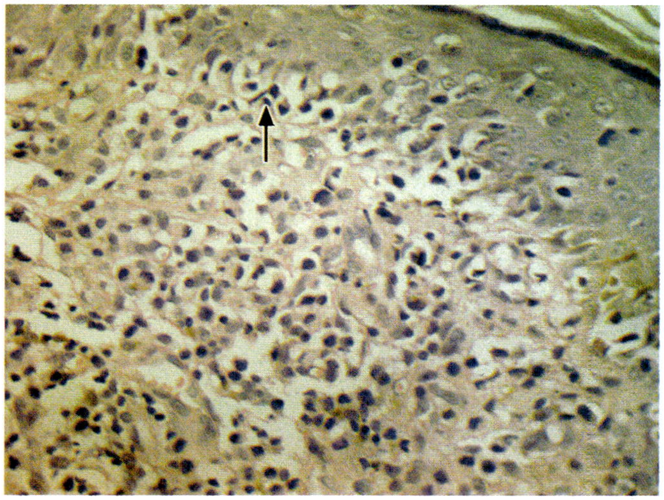

FIGURE 21.4.4

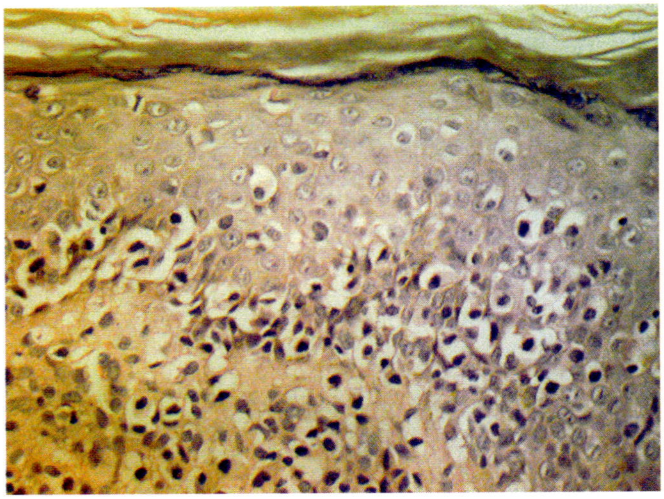

FIGURE 21.4.5

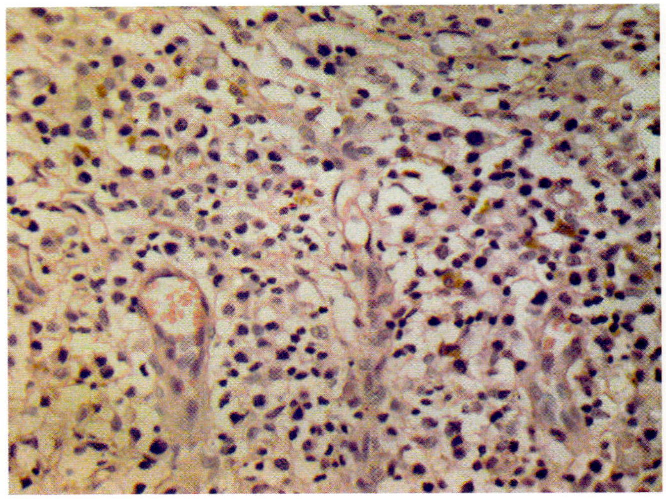

FIGURE 21.4.6

21.4.5: Epidermis shows lymphocytic collections leading to pautrier microabscesses (*High power view*)

21.4.6: Atypical lymphocytes in the dermis and pigment incontinence (*High power view*)

21.4.7: Tumor stage—the lymphocytes diffusely infiltrating the superficial and deep dermis, epidermis uninvolved (*Scanner view*)

21.4.8: Tumor stage—the lymphocytes are of different sizes and have irregular nuclei, mitotic figures are significant (*Low power view*)

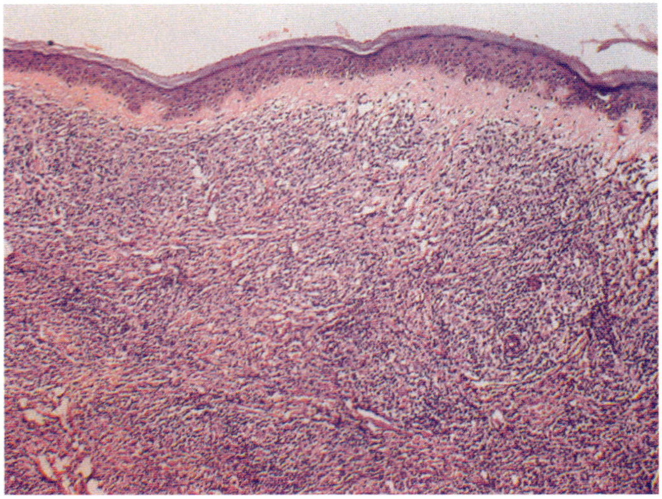

FIGURE 21.4.7

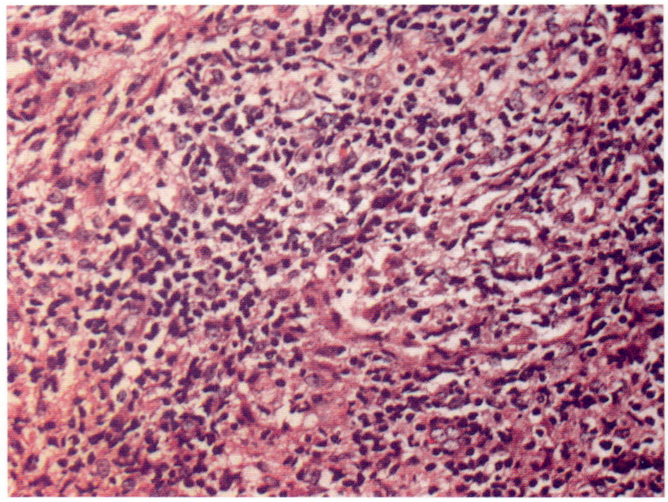

FIGURE 21.4.8

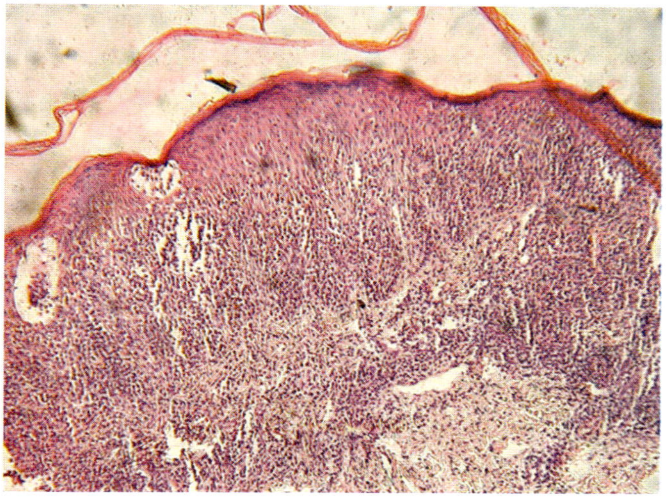

FIGURE 21.5.1

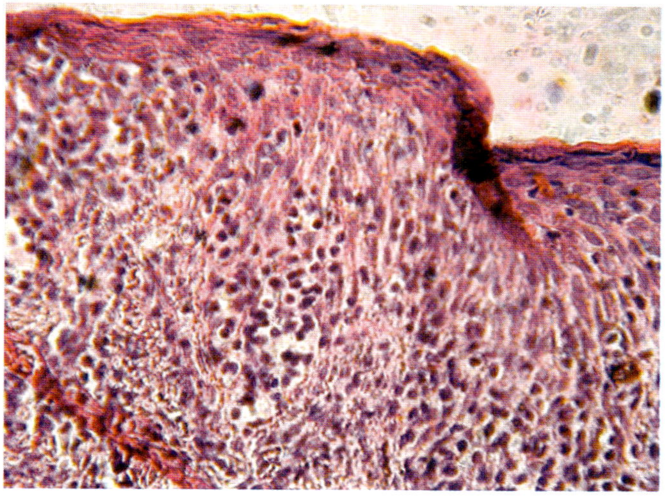

FIGURE 21.5.2

21.5: SEZARY SYNDROME

21.5.1: Extensive lichenoid upper dermal infiltrate (*Scanner view*)

21.5.2: Exocytosis of lymphocytes without much of spongiosis (*Low power view*)

21.5.3: Large/atypical lymphocytes surrounded by a clear halo (Sezary cells) (*High power view*)

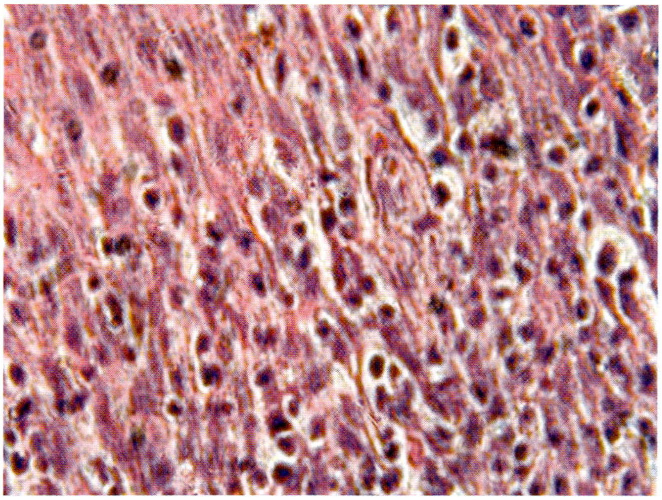

FIGURE 21.5.3

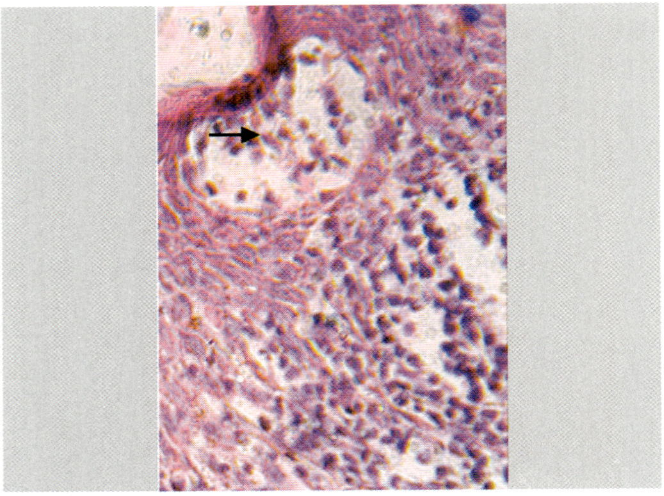

FIGURE 21.5.4

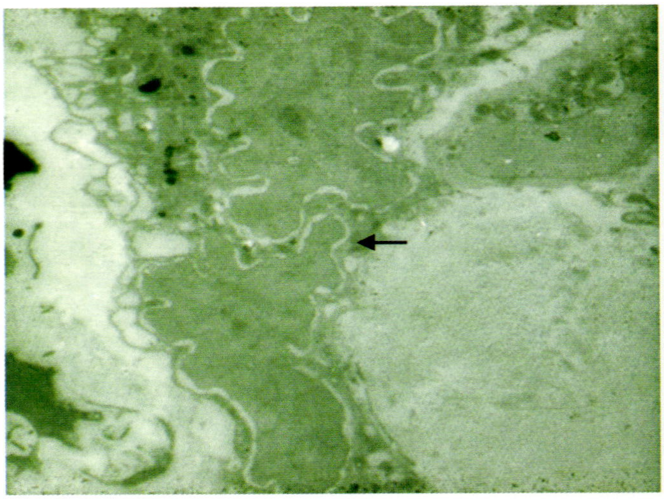

FIGURE 21.5.5

21.5.4: Pautrier's microabscesses (*Low power view*)
21.5.5: Electron microscopy demonstrates cerebriform nuclei of atypical lymphocytes
21.5.6: IHC showing CD4 positivity (*High power view*)

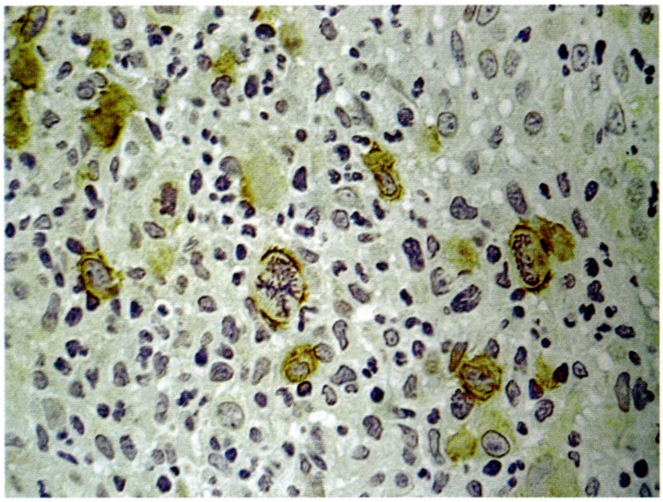

FIGURE 21.5.6

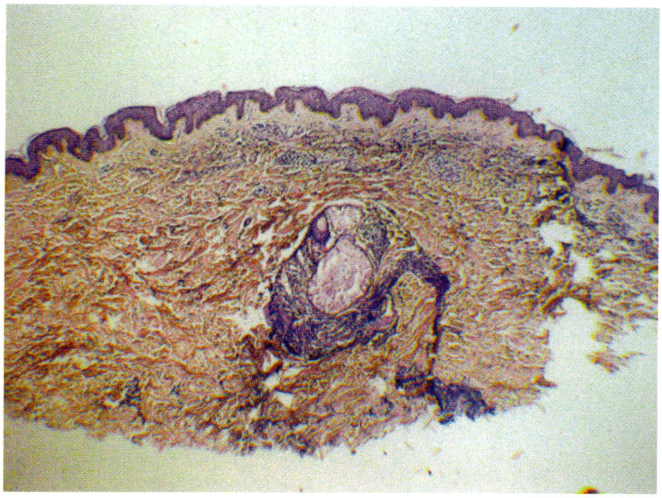

FIGURE 21.6.1

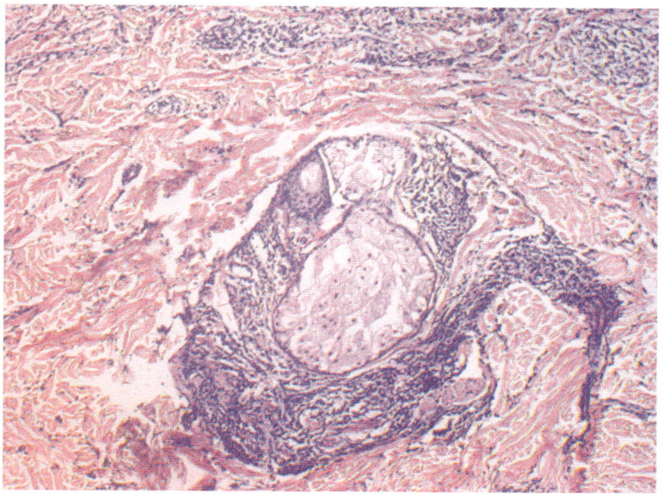

FIGURE 21.6.2

21.6: FOLLICULOTROPHIC MYCOSIS FUNGOIDES

21.6.1: Follicular and perifollicular infiltrate (*Scanner view*)

21.6.2: With or without mucin (*Low power view*)

21.6.3: Infiltrate of small to medium sized lymphocytes (*High power view*)

21.6.4: Nuclei appear atypical/cerebriform (*High power view*)

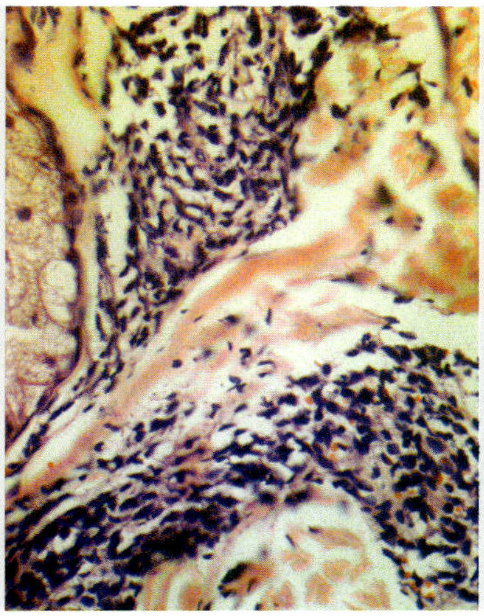

FIGURE 21.6.3

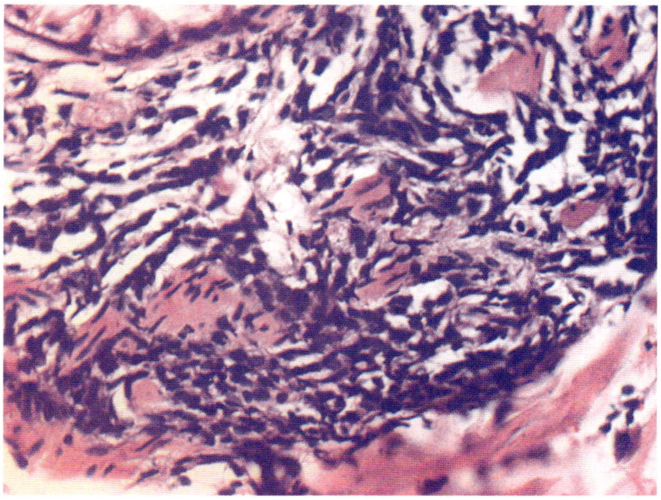

FIGURE 21.6.4

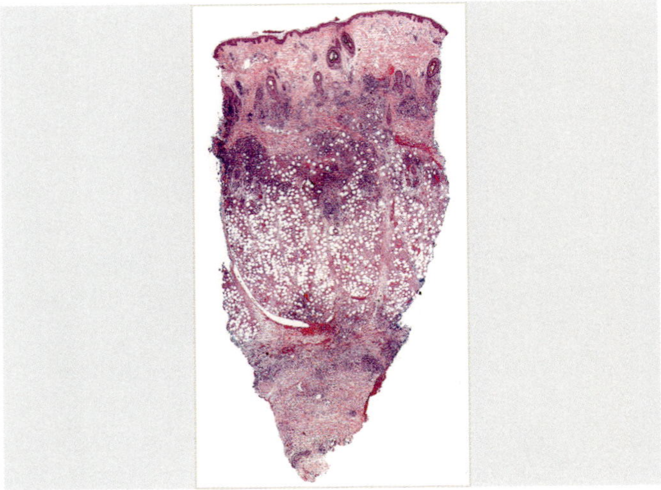

FIGURE 21.7.1

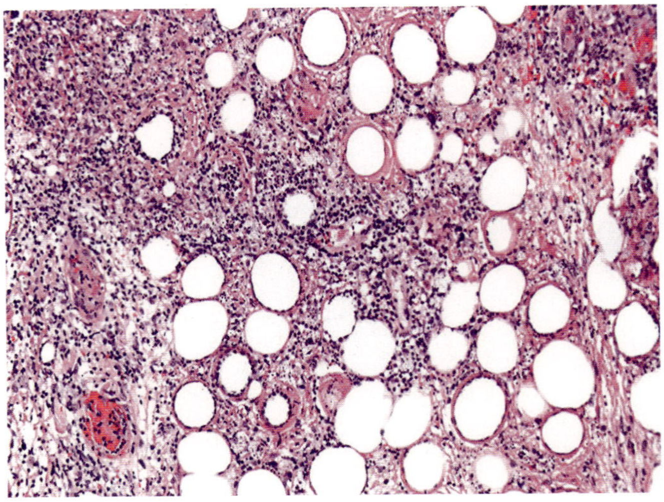

FIGURE 21.7.2

21.7: SUBCUTANEOUS PANNICULITIS—LIKE T-CELL LYMPHOMA (ALPHA/BETA T-CELL LYMPHOMA)

21.7.1: There is dense lobular involvement of the subcutis by T cells with extension into the deep reticular dermis (*Scanner view*)

21.7.2: Fat necrosis and karyorrhectic debris are typically seen (*High power view*)

21.7.3: Membranous circumscription of atypical lymphocytes around individual adipocytes (described at "rimming") is a important clue. The features can be very similar to lupus panniculitis/profundus (*High power view*)

21.7.4: Another view of rimming, alpha/beta lymphoma must be distinguished from the much more aggressive gamma/delta T cell lymphoma, which can also involve the subcutis with a similar pattern to that seen in subcutaneous panniculitis-like T cell lymphoma (*High power view*)

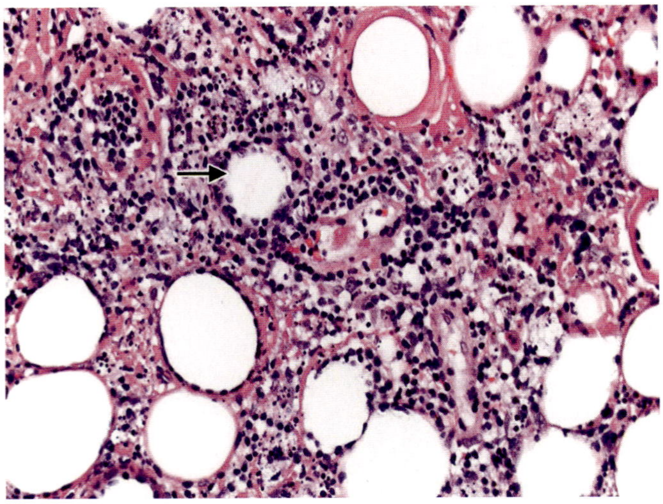

FIGURE 21.7.3

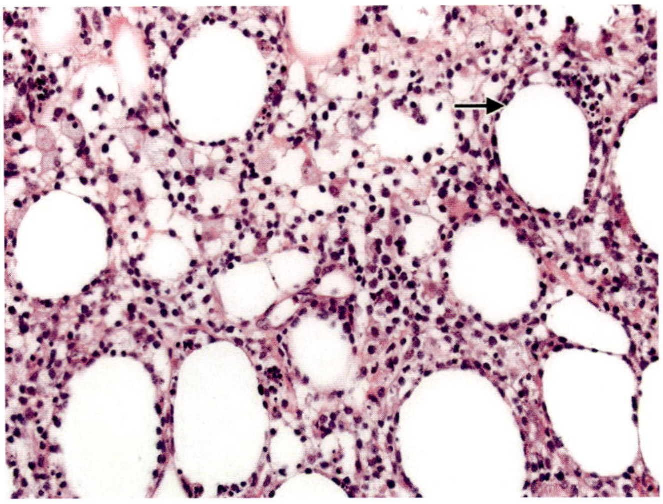

FIGURE 21.7.4

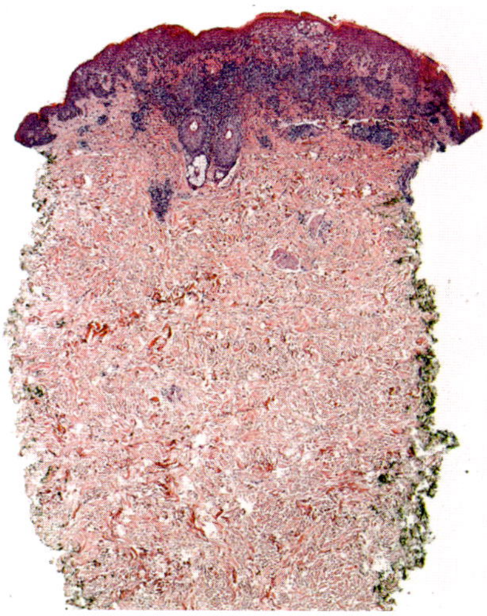

FIGURE 21.8.1

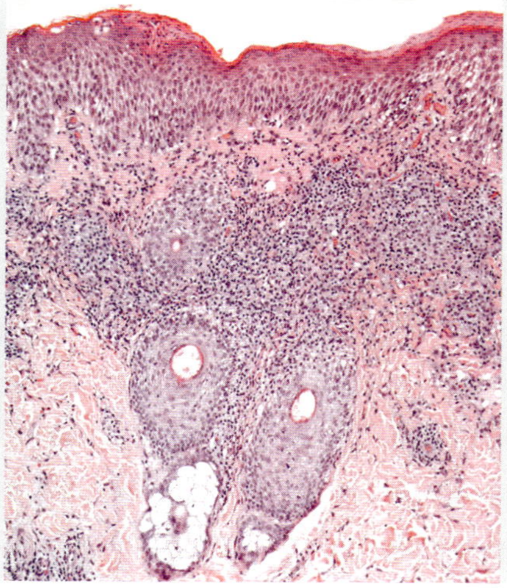

FIGURE 21.8.2

21.8: LYMPHOMATOID PAPULOSIS

21.8.1: A wedge-shaped dermal lymphocytic infiltrate (*Scanner view*)

21.8.2: Closer view of wedge-shaped infiltrate (*Low power view*)

21.8.3: Large atypical lymphocytes, eosinophils are frequent (lymphocytes express CD30 on immunohistochemistry) (*High power view*)

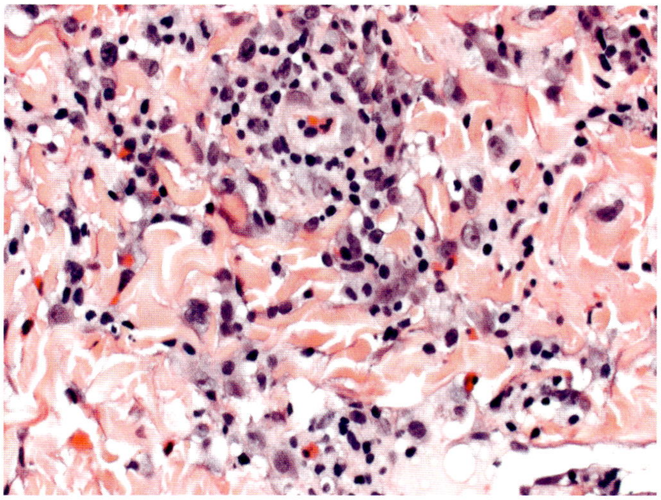

FIGURE 21.8.3

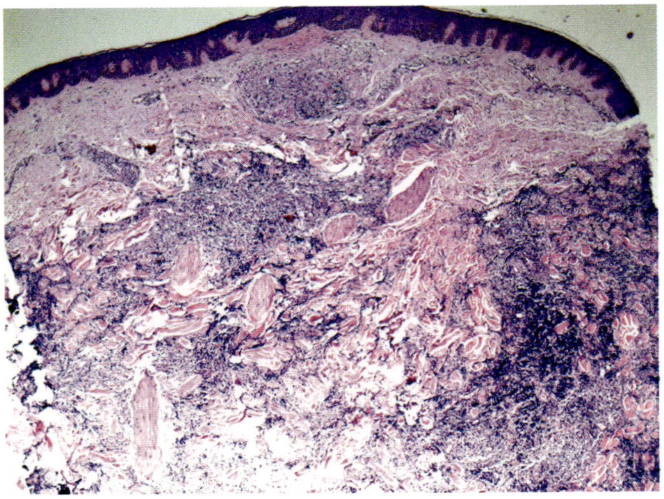

FIGURE 21.9.1

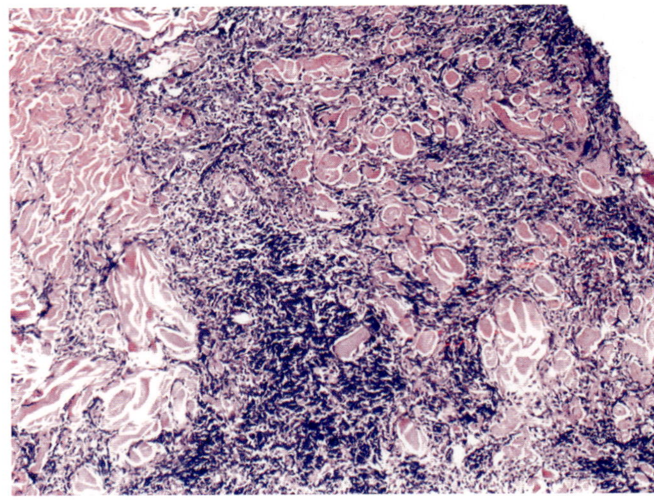

FIGURE 21.9.2

21.9: ANAPLASTIC LARGE CELL LYMPHOMA

21.9.1: The tumor cells grow in large nests. Epidermotropism is often absent but may be seen in up to 40% of cases (*Scanner view*)

21.9.2: There are diffuse sheets of tumor cells commonly showing areas of necrosis (*Low power view*)

21.9.3: The tumor cells display an anaplastic morphology with abundant cytoplasm and pleomorphic vesicular nuclei with clumped heterochromatin and prominent nucleoli. Mitoses including atypical forms are common (*High power view*)

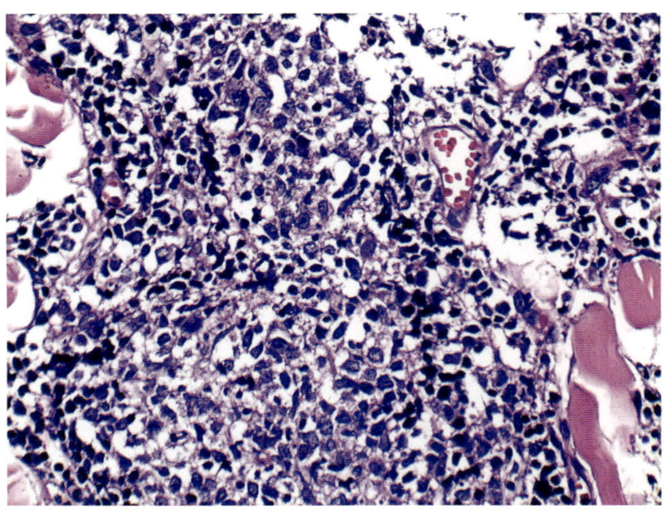

FIGURE 21.9.3

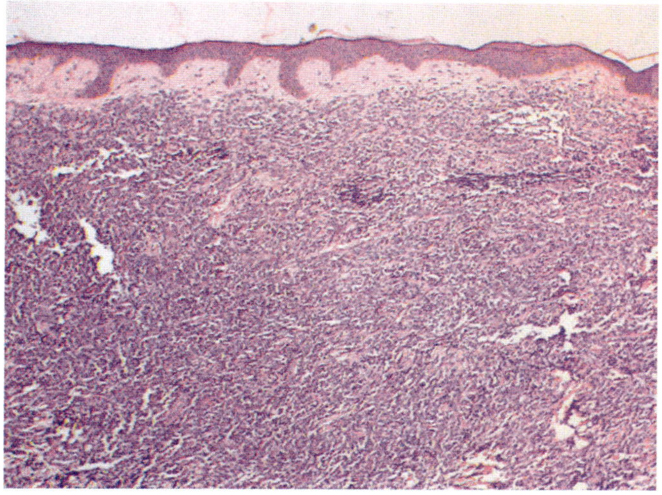

FIGURE 21.10.1

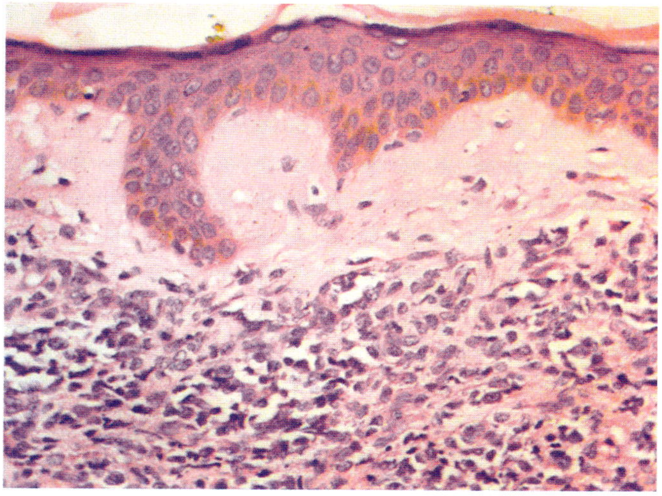

FIGURE 21.10.2

21.10: PRIMARY CUTANEOUS DIFFUSE LARGE B-CELL LYMPHOMA

21.10.1: Biopsy shows a diffuse dermal infiltrate composed of sheets of centroblasts and immunoblasts (*Scanner view*)

21.10.2: A grenz zone is present (*Low power view*)

21.10.3: Centroblasts have little cytoplasm with round to oval vesicular nuclei and multiple small nucleoli (*High power view*)

21.10.4: Immunoblasts have more abundant basophilic cytoplasm and a single large eosinophilic nucleolus, mitotic figures are significant (primary cutaneous marginal zone B-cell lymphoma, the infiltrate contains reactive lymphoid follicles) (*High power view*)

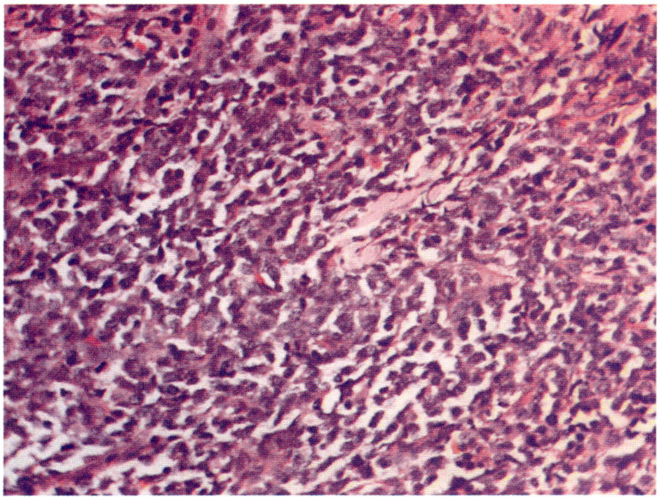

FIGURE 21.10.3

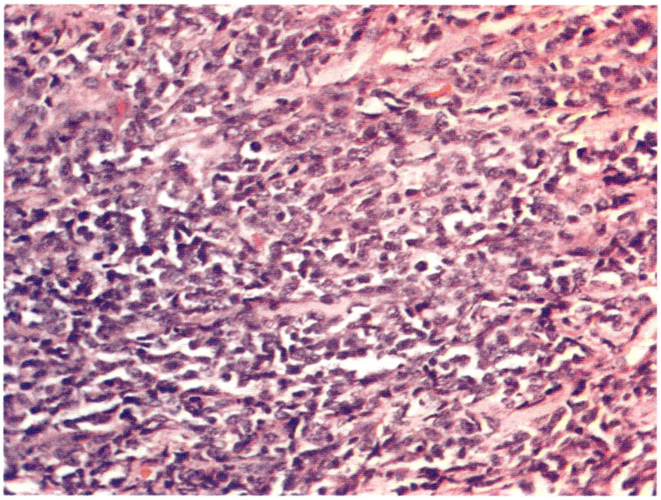

FIGURE 21.10.4

DIFFERENTIAL DIAGNOSIS

1. Pagetoid reticulosis
2. Granulomatous slack skin disease
3. Lymphomatoid granulomatosis
4. Lymphomatoid drug reaction
5. NK/NK T-cell lymphoma
6. Adult T-cell leukemia/lymphoma
7. Primary cutaneous peripheral T cell lymphoma unspecified

DIAGNOSTIC PEARLS

1. The nuclear indentations of Sezary or Lutzner cell are better appreciated in Giemsa stain.
2. Eosinophilic or plasma cell infiltrate is commonly seen in benign lymphoid hyperplasia.
3. Epidermotropism may not be seen in granulomatous mycosis fungoides (MF).
4. Pagetoid reticulosis shows psoriasiform hyperplasia with epidermal infiltration with haloed atypical lymphocytes.
5. The pigmented purpuric dermatoses (PPD) and pigmented purpuric dermatitis-like lesions of MF are many a times difficult to distinguish histologically.
6. Tumor cells usually lack expression of CD7 in MF.
7. Follicle center cell lymphoma and marginal zone B-cell lymphoma represent 90% of all forms of cutaneous B-cell lymphoma.
8. Multiple biopsies over a period of time are often needed for the diagnosis of lymphomas.
9. For diagnosis of lymphoma and to clearly define subgroups; apart from histology techniques like immunohistochemistry, in-situ hybridization, polymerase chain reaction technology, fluorescence in-situ hybridization (FISH), gene rearrangement techniques, flow cytometry for immunophenotyping, etc. are also utilized.

22 Miscellaneous Conditions

Chapter Outline

22.1: Porokeratosis
22.2: Epidermolytic Hyperkeratosis
22.3: Hidradenitis Suppurativa
22.4: Scabies
22.5: Erythema Annulare Centrifugum
22.6: Polymorphous Light Eruption
22.7: Urticaria
22.8: Pruritic Urticarial Papules and Plaques of Pregnancy
22.9: Acrodermatitis Enteropathica
22.10: Cutaneous Metastasis

Nathan Lee, Jerad Gardner, Venkataram Mysore

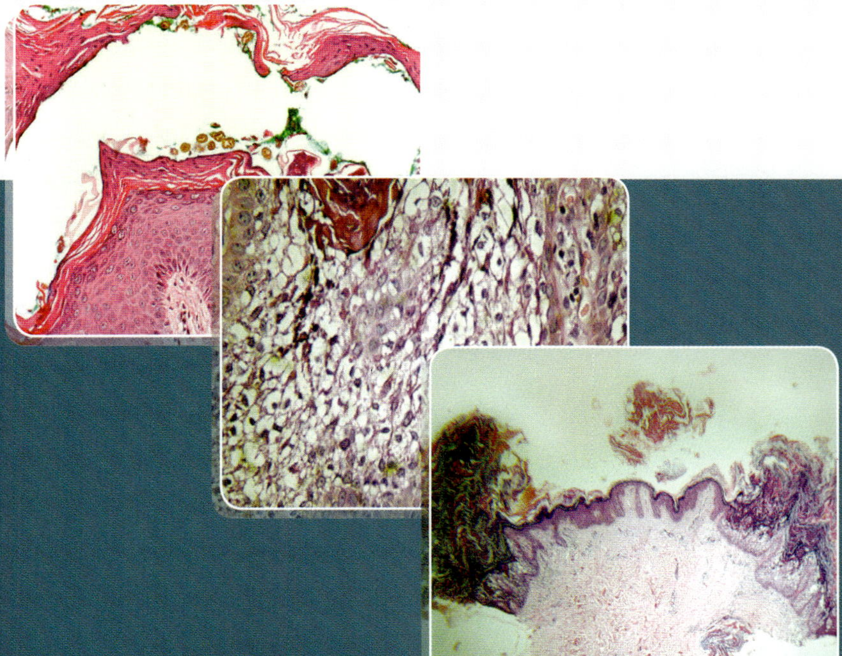

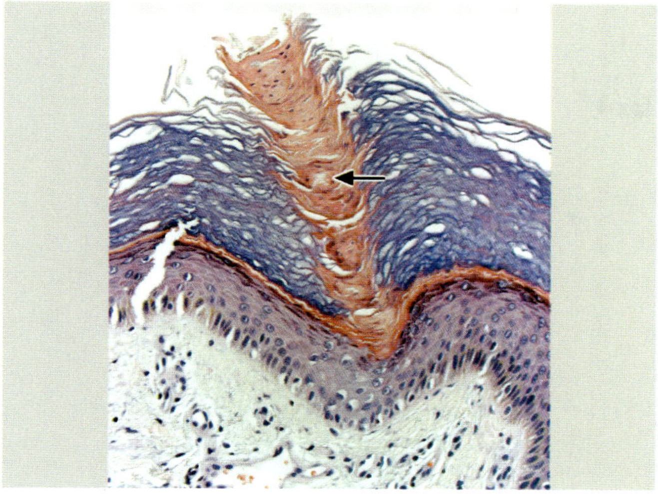

FIGURE 22.1.1

22.1: POROKERATOSIS

22.1.1: Porokeratosis is characterized by tall tiers/columns of parakeratosis referred to as cornoid lamellae (biopsy from the border of the lesion). There is slight epidermal invagination at an angle beneath the cornoid lamellae (*Low power view*)

22.1.2: Granular cell layer is absent below the invagination and there are dyskeratotic cells. The cornoid lamellae bear some resemblance to smoke rising from a chimney or a steam engine train/locomotive (biopsy from the central atrophic part of the lesion usually shows lichenoid tissue reaction) (*Low power view*)

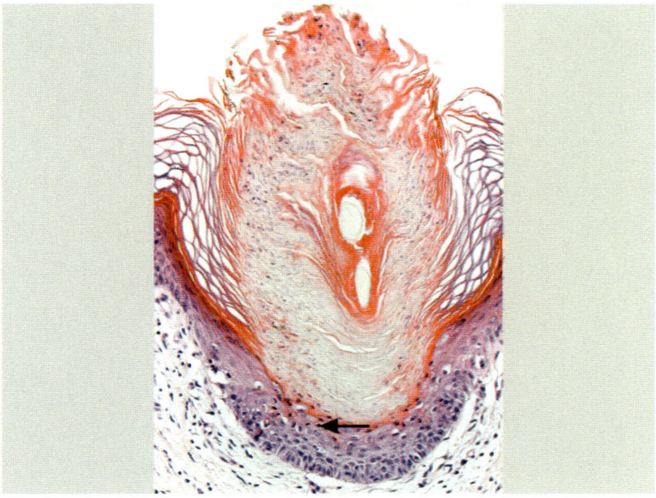

FIGURE 22.1.2

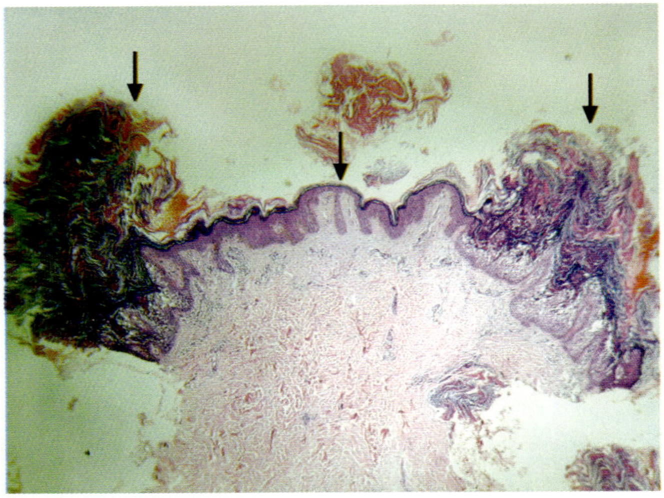

FIGURE 22.2.1

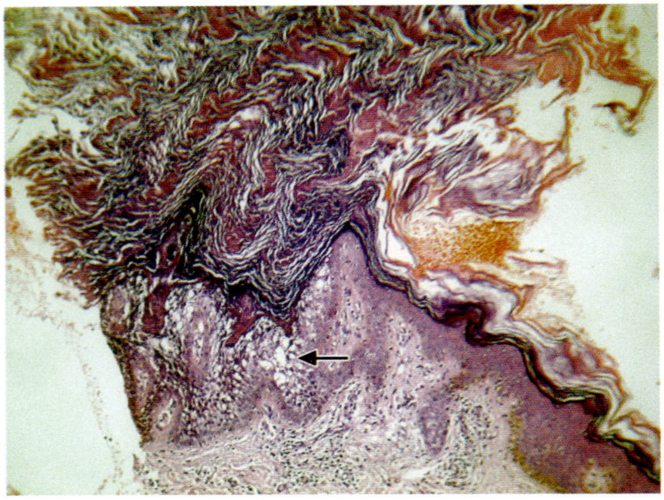

FIGURE 22.2.2

22.2: EPIDERMOLYTIC HYPERKERATOSIS

22.2.1: Localized areas of marked hyperkeratosis and hyperplasia (peaks and valley view) (*Scanner view*)

22.2.2: Vacuolar change in the upper spinous and granular layers, mild dermal infiltrate (*Low power view*)

22.2.3: Keratohyaline granules are coarse and clumped (*Low power view*)

22.2.4: The pale areas represent lysis of the keratinocyte cytoplasm due to mutation leading to misfolding of keratin 1 and keratin 10 proteins. The pink globules represent aggregates of abnormal keratin filaments (*High power view*)

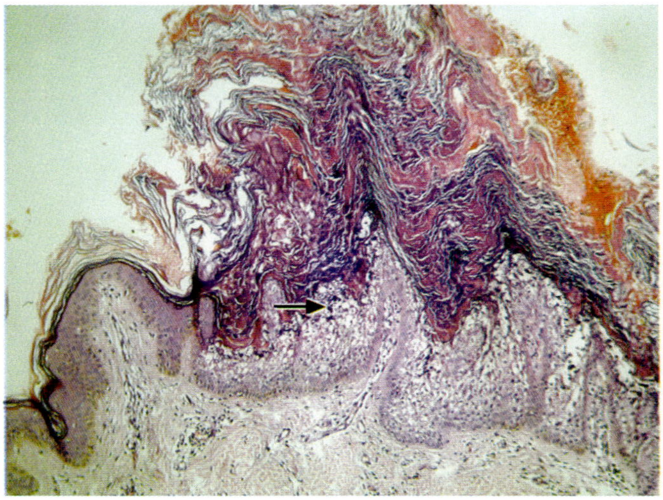

FIGURE 22.2.3

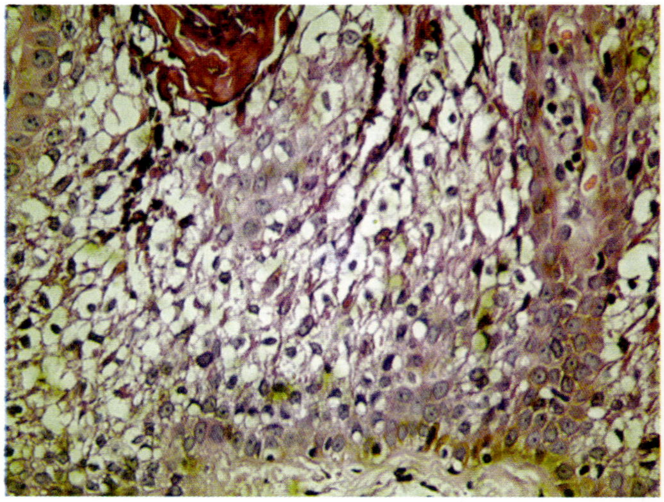

FIGURE 22.2.4

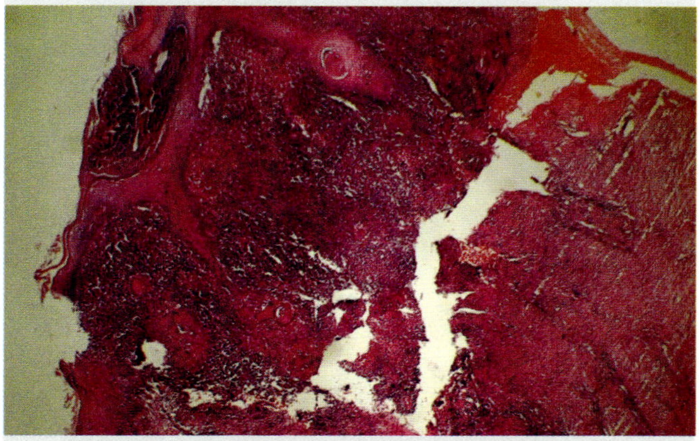

FIGURE 22.3.1

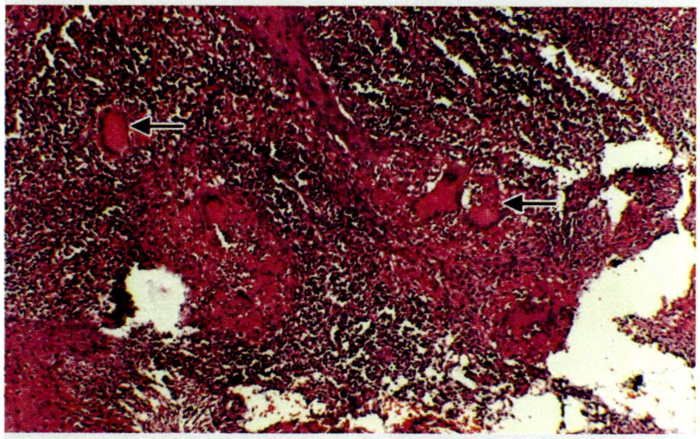

FIGURE 22.3.2

22.3: HIDRADENITIS SUPPURATIVA

22.3.1: Epidermal hyperplasia and dense polymorphous perifollicular infiltrate extending throughout the dermis (*Low power view*)

22.3.2: Giant cells and epithelioid cell granulomas (*High power view*)

22.3.3: Deep dermal and subcutaneous microabscesses (*High power view*)

22.3.4: Dermal edema and accumulation of plasma and collection of neutrophils in the stratum corneum (crusting) (*High power view*)

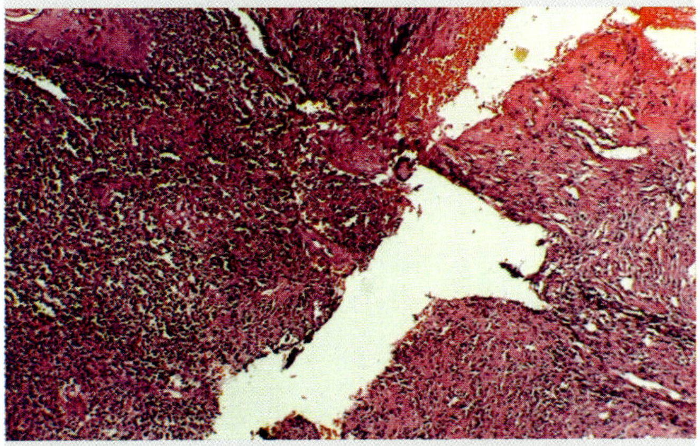

FIGURE 22.3.3

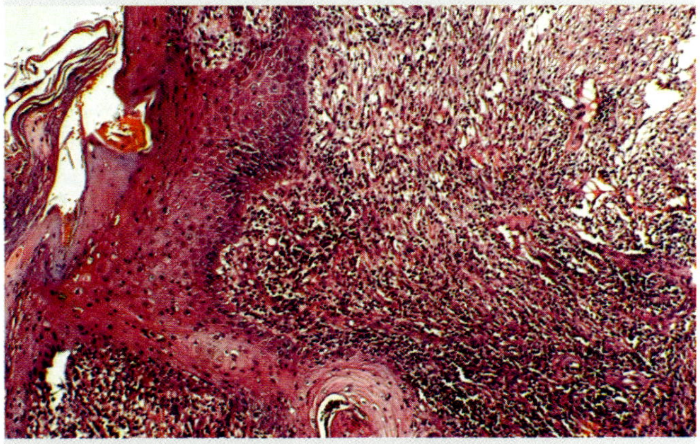

FIGURE 22.3.4

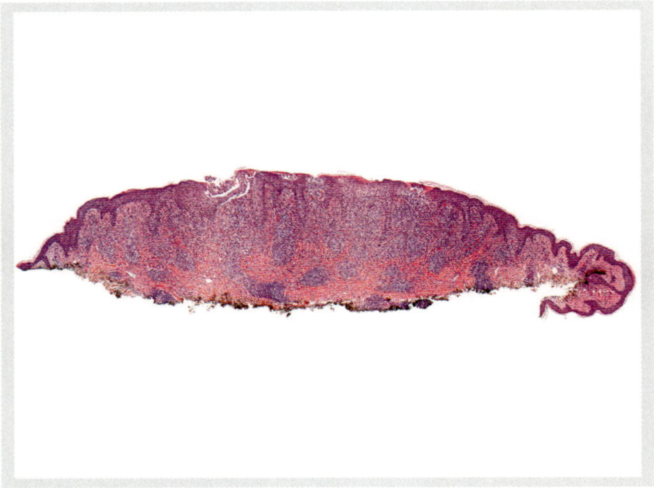

FIGURE 22.4.1

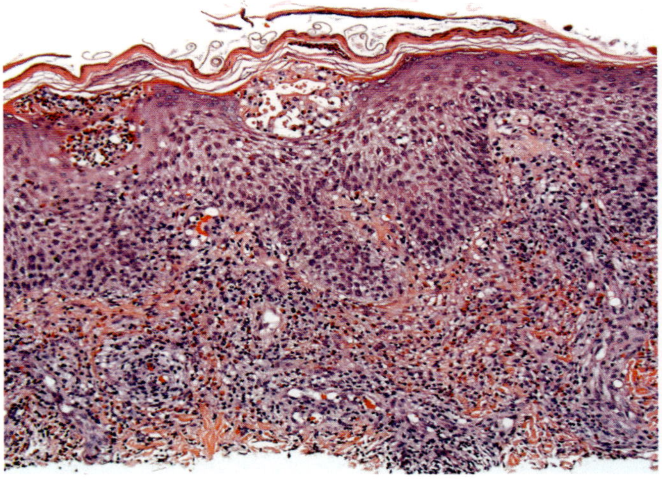

FIGURE 22.4.2

22.4: SCABIES

22.4.1: Spongiotic dermatitis with abundant eosinophils (*Scanner view*) (better appreciated in the next image with higher magnification)

22.4.2: Empty egg casings (resembling "pink pigtails") in the stratum corneum are a good clue for scabetic infestation (*Low power view*)

22.4.3: Crusted ("Norwegian") scabies is a florid proliferation of scabies mites, marked epidermal hyperplasia with hyperkeratosis (*Scanner view*)

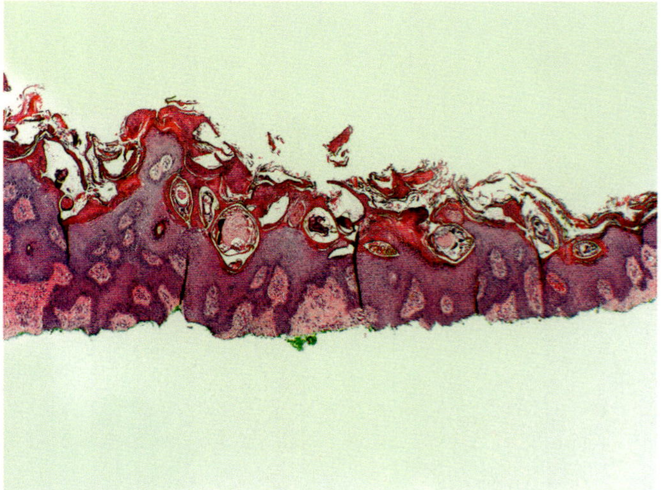

FIGURE 22.4.3

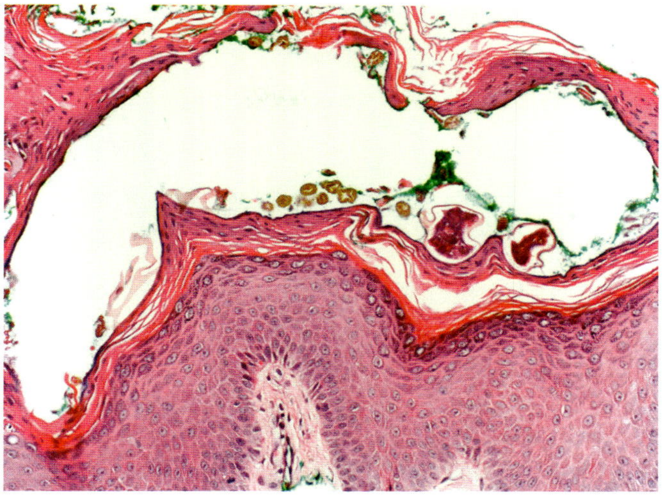

FIGURE 22.4.4

22.4.4: The burrow within the stratum corneum containing small brown globules of scybala (feces) are evidence of scabies infestation even if the mite is not visible (*High power view*)

22.4.5: Adult mites, egg casings, and scybala (feces) are all present in these figures (Examination with polarized light often shows areas of birefringence within the spines, scybala, and some of the internal organs within the scabies mite) (*High power view*)

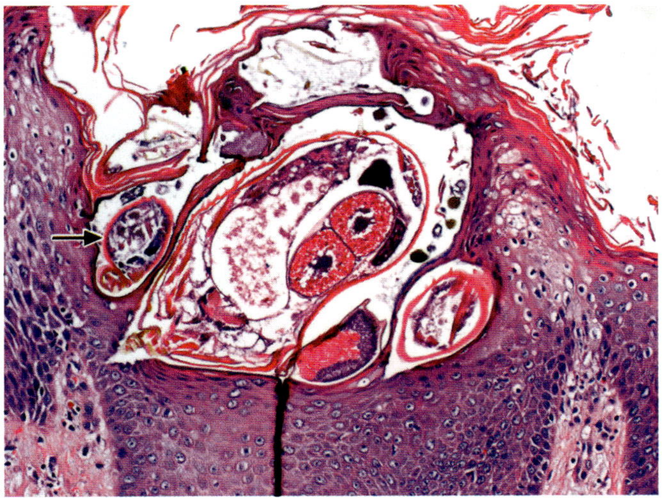

FIGURE 22.4.5

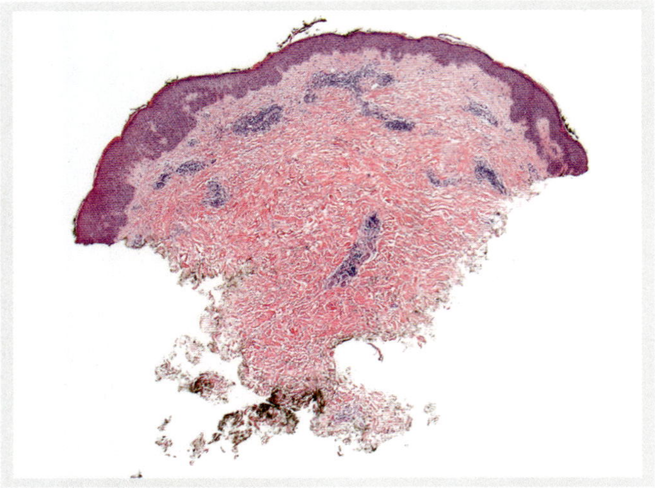

FIGURE 22.5.1

22.5: ERYTHEMA ANNULARE CENTRIFUGUM

22.5.1: Erythema annulare centrifugum demonstrates tight cuffing ("coat sleeves") of lymphocytes around superficial and deep vessels (*Scanner view*)

22.5.2: Closer view of the infiltrate, in deep variant epidermis is normal superficial type epidermis shows spongiosis (difficult to differentiate from pityriasis rosea) (*Low power view*)

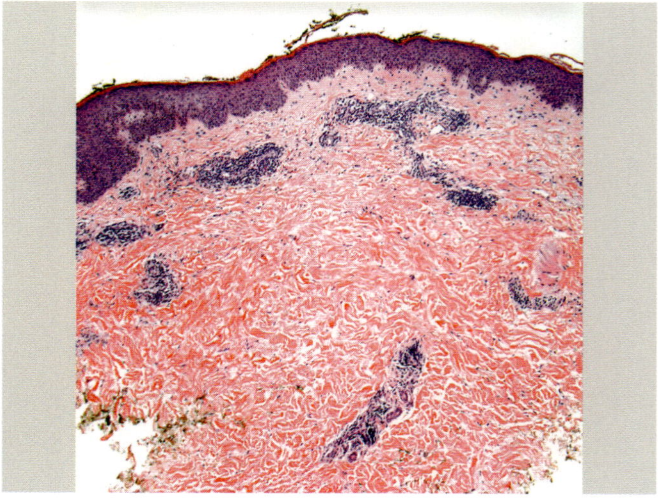

FIGURE 22.5.2

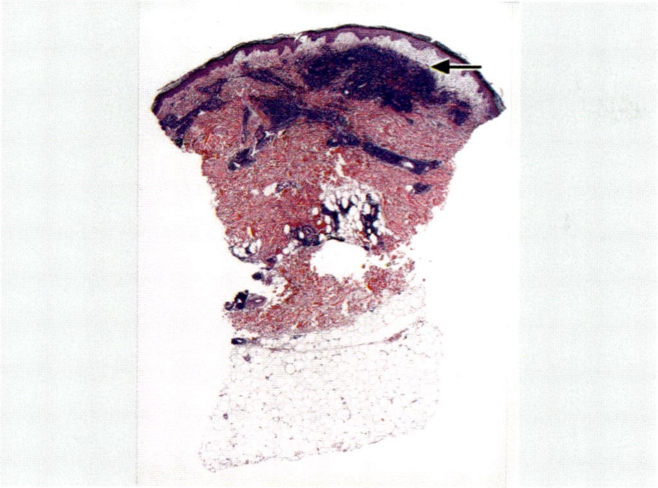

FIGURE 22.6.1

22.6: POLYMORPHOUS LIGHT ERUPTION

22.6.1: Polymorphous light eruption is characterized by extensive edema of the papillary dermis with a prominent underlying superficial and deep perivascular lymphocytic infiltrate (*Scanner view*)

22.6.2: Papillary edema with lymphocytes, intact basal cells, perivascular lymphocytes (*Low power view*)

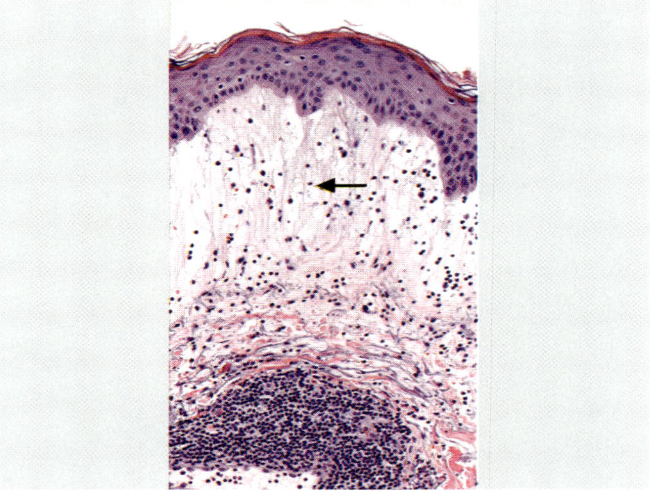

FIGURE 22.6.2

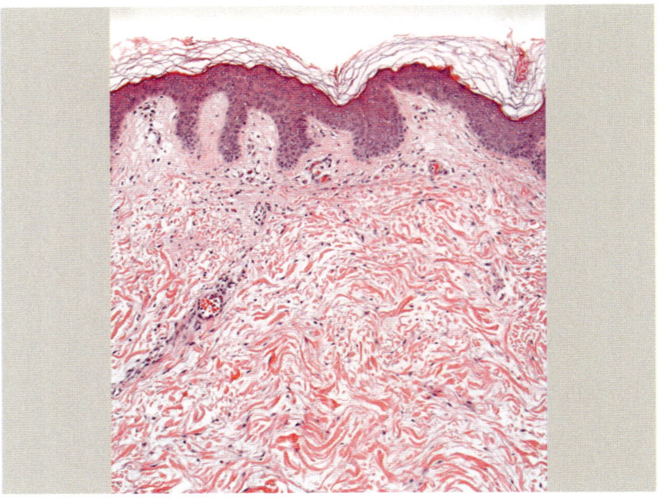

FIGURE 22.7.1

22.7: URTICARIA

22.7.1: The histologic changes of urticaria may be quite subtle. Shows variable amount of dermal edema, which histologically appears as increased white space between reticular dermal collagen bundles (*Low power view*)

22.7.2: Section showing sparse perivascular lymphocytic infiltrate with a few eosinophils and neutrophils scattered in the dermis. Intraluminal neutrophils within small superficial blood vessels, a useful clue to the diagnosis (*High power view*)

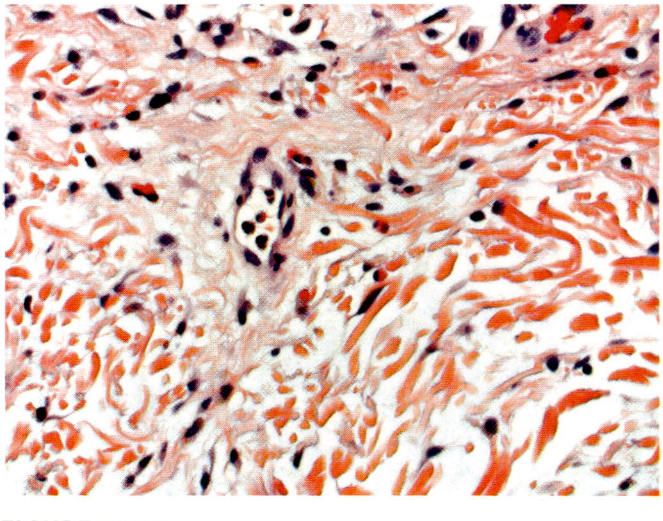

FIGURE 22.7.2

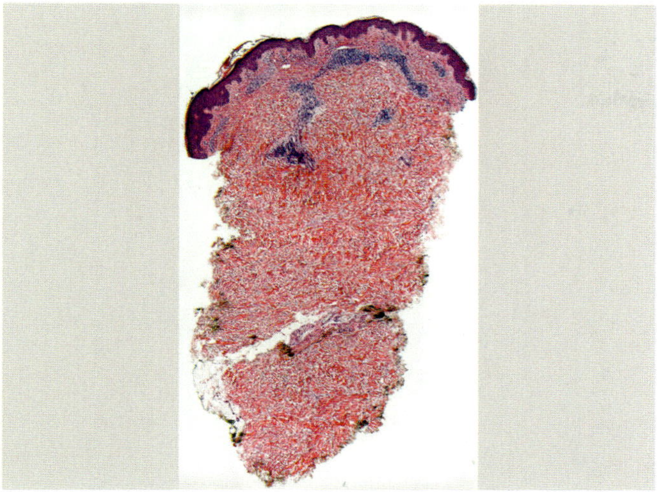

FIGURE 22.8.1

22.8: PRURITIC URTICARIAL PAPULES AND PLAQUES OF PREGNANCY

22.8.1: Demonstrates variable papillary dermal edema, superficial and/or deep perivascular lymphocytic infiltrate (other characteristic is the presence of a few eosinophils in the infiltrate) (*Scanner view*)

22.8.2: Epidermis shows focal parakeratosis (spongiosis is another feature in a few cases) (*Low power view*)

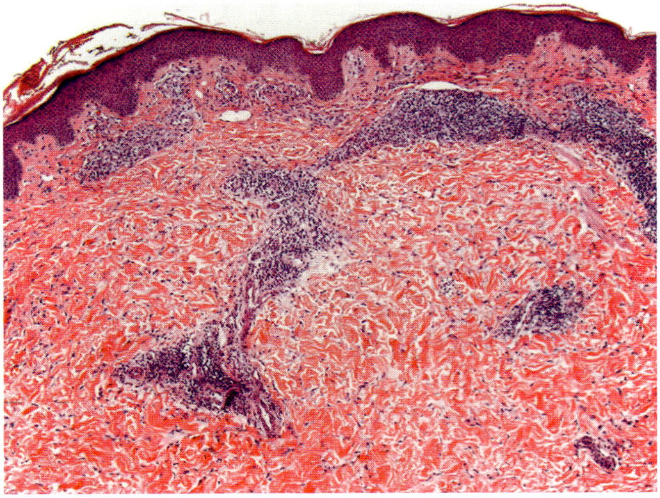

FIGURE 22.8.2

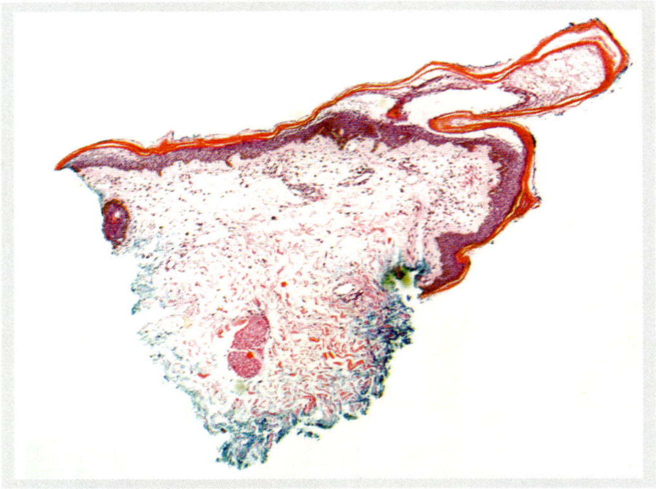

FIGURE 22.9.1

22.9: ACRODERMATITIS ENTEROPATHICA

22.9.1: Section shows parakeratosis, spongiosis and hypogranulosis (*Scanner view*)

22.9.2: The other feature is keratinocyte pallor within the superficial epidermis (in this view extensive edema leading to clefting) dermal edema (older lesions are more psoriasiform). Other forms of nutritional deficiency like pellagra and necrolytic migratory erythema (glucagonoma syndrome) show similar histologic features (*Low power view*)

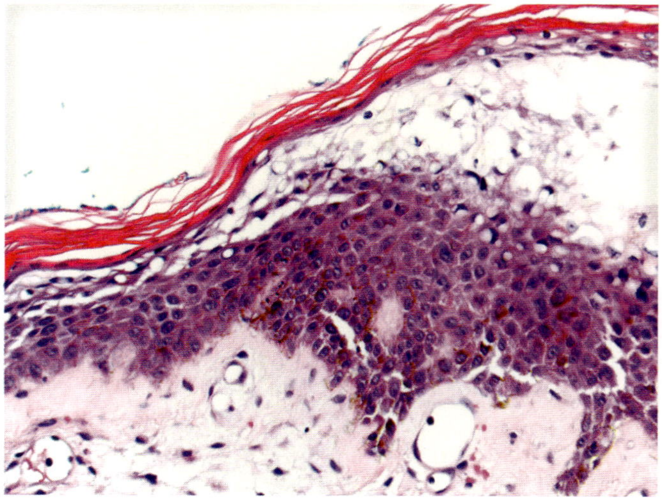

FIGURE 22.9.2

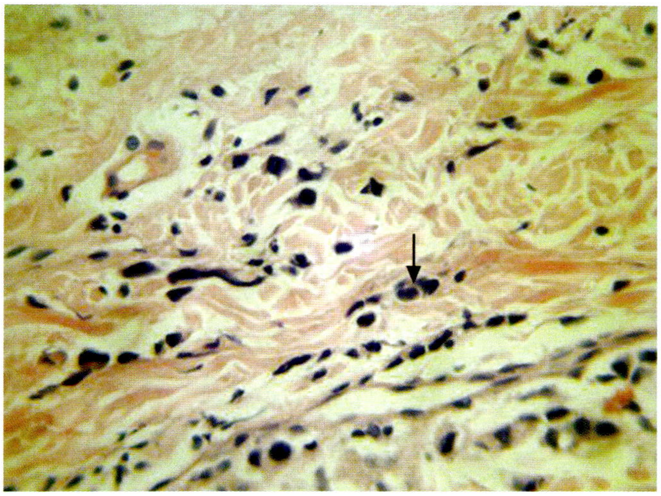

FIGURE 22.10.1

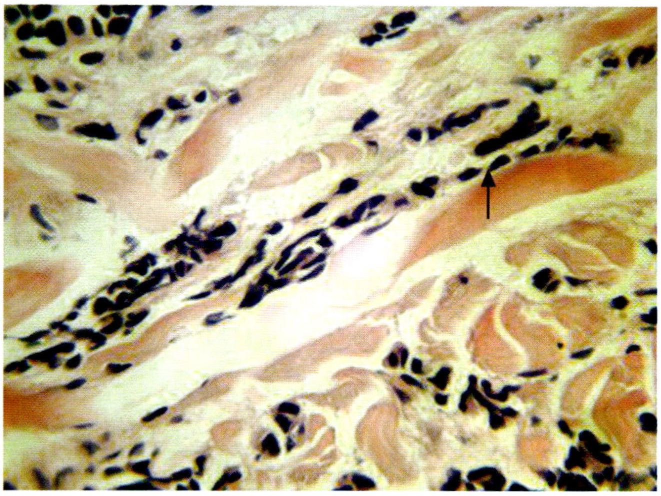

FIGURE 22.10.2

22.10: CUTANEOUS METASTASIS

22.10.1: Atypical cells in dermis, which are large and show mitotic figures (*High power view*)

22.10.2: Atypical cells in single file between collagen fibers (*High power view*)

22.10.3: This is characteristic of carcinoma breast. Note the large cells irregular in shape and size (*Oil emmersion view*)

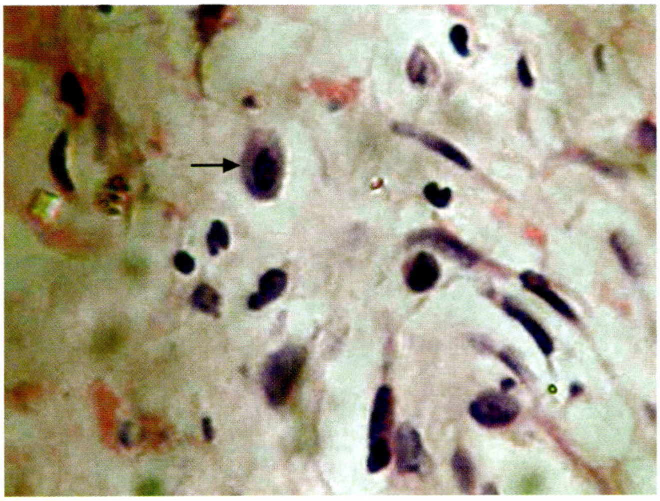

FIGURE 22.10.3

Further Reading

1. Ackerman AB, Boer A, Bennin B, Gottlieb GJ. Histologic Diagnosis of Inflammatory Skin Diseases. 3rd edn. New York: Ardor Scribendi; 2005.
2. Ackerman AB, Briggs PL, Bravo F. Differential Diagnosis in Dermatopathology III. 2nd edn. Philadelphia: Lippincott - Williams & Wilkins; 1993.
3. Ackerman AB, Guo Y, Lazova R, Kaddu S. Differential Diagnosis in Dermatopathology II. 2nd edn. Philadelphia: Lippincott - Williams & Wilkins; 1999.
4. Ackerman AB, Mendonca A. Differential Diagnosis in Dermatopathology I. 2nd edn. Philadelphia: Lippincott - Williams & Wilkins; 1992.
5. Ackerman AB, White WL, Guo Y, Umbert I. Differential Diagnosis in Dermatopathology IV. 2nd edn. Philadelphia: Lippincott - Williams & Wilkins; 1994.
6. Barnhill RL, Crowson AN (Eds). Textbook of Dermatopathology. 3rd edn. New York: McGraw- Hill; 2010.
7. Clarke LE, Clarke JT, Helm KF. Colour Atlas of Differential Diagnosis in Dermatopathology. New Delhi: Jaypee Brothers; 2014.
8. Cockerell, et al. Dermatopathology: Clinicopathological correlations. 1st edn, 2014.
9. Elder DE, Elenistas R, Johnson BL, et al. Lever's Histopathology of the Skin. 11th edn. Philadelphia: Lippincott -Williams &Wilkins; 2014.
10. Elston DM , Ferringer T, et al. Requisites in Dermatopathology. Edinburgh: Saunders-Elsevier; 2009.
11. Grant-Kels JM (Ed). Colour Atlas of Dermatopathology. New York: Informa; 2007.
12. Hood AF, Kwan TH, Mihm MC, et al. Primer of Dermatopathology. 3rd edn. Philadelphia: Lippincott - Williams & Wilkins; 2009.
13. Maize CJ, et al. Cutaneous Pathology. Churchill Livingstone; 1998.
14. McKee PH, Calonje E, Brenn T, Lazar A. McKee's Pathology of the Skin with Clinical Correlations. 4th edn. Elsevier's - Saunders; 2012.
15. Mehregan AH, Hashimoto K, Mehregan DA, Mehregan DR. Pinkus' Guide to Dermatohistopathology. 6th edn. New York: McGraw-Hill; 2001.
16. Patterson JW. Weedon's Skin Pathology. 4th edn. Edinburgh: Churchill Livingstone; 2016.

Index

A

Abscess 294
  dermal 294
Abundant eosinophils 432
Abundant melanin pigment 354
Acantholysis, secondary 278
Acantholytic
  cells 19, 89, 92, 93, 96-99, 306
  dyskeratosis 18
Acanthosis 282, 302, 333, 371
  epidermal 39, 272
  of epidermis 285
Acid-fast bacilli 122
  stain 140
Acne vulgaris 251
Acquired perforating dermatoses 270, 271
Acrodermatitis enteropathica 41, 438
Actinic cheilitis 306
Actinic granuloma 161
Actinic keratosis 18, 305, 306, 319
Actinomycetoma 137
Adenoma sebaceum 377
Adipose tissue 382
Adnexal atrophy 220
Allergic contact dermatitis 73
Alopecia areata 237, 252
Amyloid, deposits of 256
Anagen follicles 237, 240
Anaplastic large cell lymphoma 424
Androgenetic alopecia 239
Anetoderma 226
Angiofibroma 377
Angiokeratoma 370, 391
Angiolymphoid hyperplasia 373
Angiosarcoma 391
Aplasia cutis congenita 234
Apocrine cells 334
Apocrine
  decapitation secretion 342
  glands 4, 5, 333
Apoptotic keratinocyte 55, 59, 66
Appendageal tumors 321
Aquamous eddies 303, 327
Arão-Perkins bodies 252
Arrectores pilorum muscle 189, 239
Arthropod bite reaction 74
Aseptate hyphae 150
Asteroid body 154
Atrophic adnexal structures 219
Atrophic epidermis 55, 64, 65, 131, 132, 219-221, 226, 404
Atrophoderma 234
Atrophy, epidermal 66, 358

B

B cell lymphoma 425, 426
Bacillary angiomatosis 381
  pathognomonic for 381
Bacilli
  multiple 131
  sparse 130
Bacterial infections 292
Banana-shaped fiber 261
Bartonella henselae bacteria 381
Basal cell 93, 435
  carcinoma 311, 319
  damage 45, 46, 48-51
  layer 48, 56, 188, 190, 193, 305, 308
    pigmentation of 108, 111, 191, 192
  pigment in 191
  squamatization of 45
  vacuolation 60, 61, 67
Basal keratinocytes, fragments of 102
Basal layer of epidermis 417
Basaloid cells 301, 303, 304, 332, 336, 343, 346, 347
  islands of 311
  nests of 325
  pigmented 301
  small dark 338
Basaloid germinative cells 332
Basaloid islands 323
Basaloid structures 324
Basaloid tumor 325
  cells 312
Basilar melanocytes 195
Basophilic cells 330
Basophilic cytoplasm 425
Becker's nevus 189
Behcet's disease 177, 213
Biopsy 243, 429
Blaschko dermatitis 85
Blast cells, scattered 414
Blisters, subepidermal 113, 118
Blood vessels 31, 52, 83, 128, 174, 175, 194, 200, 259, 377, 383, 384, 398
  dermal 176
  dilated 365, 382, 390, 400
  in dermal papillae 30
  in superficial plexus 39
  proliferation of 377
  small 83, 372
Body macrophages 414
Borst-Jadassohn phenomenon 303
Bowen's disease 41, 307, 310, 319
Bowenoid papulosis 285
Breast, carcinoma 439
Bubbly cytoplasm 331
Bulla with blister cavity, subepidermal 104
Bullous mastocytosis 396
Bullous pemphigoid 108
  lesion of 110
Bundles of collagen 221

C

Cafe-au-lait macules 195
Calcinosis cutis 255
Calcium 255
  deposits 212, 255
Candidiasis 78, 288
  acute superficial 288
Cell 296
  acanthoma, clear 41
  atypical 439
  cuboidal 395
  in epidermis, groups of large 281
  large pale 339
  large vacuolated 282
  layer
    of basal 96
    of epithelial 334
  palisading of 311
  rich 108
  rupture of 278
  single 356
  subepidermal 57
  types of 338
Cellular blue nevus 354
Cellular tumor 385
Cellulitis 292
Cephalic histiocytosis, benign 405
Cheilitis granulomatosa 162
Cherry angioma 391
Cholesterol clefts 248
Chondrodermatitis nodularis helicis 273
Chondroid syringoma 344
Chondromas 263
Chromoblastomycosis 273
Chromomycosis 141
Church spires 18, 19
Churg-Strauss disease 173
Cicatricial alopecia 243
Civatte bodies 61
Coffee-bean nucleus 402
Collagen
  bundles 157, 221, 229, 390
  disease of 215
  disorders 217
  fibers 217, 377
    irregular 229
  in papillary dermis 194

in stratum corneum 268
tissue nevi 217
Collagenoma 217
Colloid milium 260, 263
Colon biopsy 163
Compound melanocytic nevus 353
Condyloma acuminatum 284
Connective tissue stalks 382
Cornoid lamellation 17, 18
Crohn's disease 163
Cuboidal epithelium, layers of 343
Cutaneous
implants 263
infections 275
infiltrates 393
lupus erythematosus, acute 60
lymphoid hyperplasia, benign 413
nerves 388
neurofibromas 388
tuberculosis 123
xanthomas 409
Cutis marmorata telangiectatica congenita 366
Cylindroma 336
Cyst 235
dermal 249, 250
epidermal 247
formation 251
small 205
wall 248, 249
Cytologic atypia 306
Cytoplasm 278, 281, 296, 329, 387, 399
of cells 277
Cytoplasmic lumina 374

D

Darier's disease 18, 98, 101
Dendritic melanocytes 354
Dense fibrous stroma 312
Dense inflammatory infiltrate in dermis 160, 295
Dense neutrophilic infiltrate 142
Dermatitis
acute 73, 80
atopic 82
chronic 37
superficial 39
herpetiformis 113
Dermatofibroma 383
Dermatofibrosarcoma protuberans 385
Dermatomyositis 64, 69
Dermatopathology 15
Dermatophytoses 78, 286
Dermis
normal 205
superficial 57, 156, 259, 341
reticular 417
upper 33, 38, 401, 403
half of 178
Dermoepidermal junction 46, 51, 56, 109, 117, 355, 356
Diabetic renal failure 271
Discoid lupus erythematosus 62, 244
Dowling-Degos disease 192
Drug
deposits 263
eruption 57
fixed 58
induced vasculitis 168
Dyshidrosiform dermatitis 80
Dyskeratosis 18, 101
Dyskeratotic
cells 19, 98, 285, 307, 310, 429
scattered 75
disease 101
Dysplasia 310
Dysplastic nevus 356

E

Eccrine differentiation 343
Eccrine sweat glands 4, 7
Edema
dermal 64, 134, 162, 431
subepidermal 292
Ehler Danlos syndrome 222
Elastic degeneration, zone of 161
Elastic fibers in dermis 227
Elastic tissue stains 226
Elastin changes 223
Elastin, disease of 215
Elastofibroma 223
Elastomas 234
Endarteritis obliterans 400
Endothelial cell 368, 373, 374
swelling 174, 177, 400
thickening 167
Endothelial swelling 175, 203
Eosinophil 6, 11, 115
Eosinophilic cellulitis 409
Eosinophilic cytoplasm 374, 401
Eosinophilic degenerated elastic fibers 224
Eosinophilic fascitis 234
Eosinophilic folliculitis 407
Eosinophilic globules 355
Eosinophilic infiltrate 407
epidermal 20, 21
dermal 20, 21
Eosinophilic material 209, 260
Eosinophilic microabscesses 97
Eosinophilic nucleolus 425
Eosinophilic spongiosis 20, 21, 75, 76, 85
Eosinophils 74, 93, 94, 97, 101, 108, 109, 125, 169, 170, 173, 175, 201, 374, 403, 408, 414
in dermis 73, 90, 114
perivascular 74, 408
Epidermal junction, dermal 187
Epidermal layer, upper 32
Epidermal malignant conditions 299
Epidermis 331
hyperplastic 137
layers of 99
necrosis of 56, 58
normal 3, 205, 217
portion of 306
Epidermolysis bullosa 102, 103
acquisita 104
Epidermolytic hyperkeratosis 430
Epithelial hyperplasia 269
Epithelial papillomatosis 333
Epithelioid cell 354
granuloma 125, 127, 131, 134, 151, 431
Epithelioid histiocytes 127, 152
Erosive adenomatosis of nipple 341
Erythema
annulare centrifugum 434
elevatum diutinum 175
induratum 202
multiforme 56
nodosum 199, 213
leprosum 135
Erythematous skin 110
Erythroderma 41, 69
Erythroplasia 310
Eumycetoma 139
Exanthematous pustulosis, acute 77
Exocytosis 40
Extracellular eosinophilic hyaline globules 380
Eye liner sign 308, 309

F

Facial idiopathic granulomas 164
Familial benign pemphigus 99
Fat cell 206, 385
degenerated 212
mature 390
necrosis 211
periphery of 207
Fat necrosis 211
Fat, deep extension into 332
Fibers
degenerated 272
of ochronosis 261
Fibrin deposition 176, 182
Fibrinoid
degeneration 167
extravasation 179
necrosis 168
Fibroblast 194, 221, 228
increased 229
like cells 383
Fibroepithelial polyps 382
Fibroplasia, dermal 356
Fibrosarcoma 391
Fibrosing dermatitis 8
Fibrosis, dermal 103, 105, 159, 176, 209, 341
Fibrous
histiocytoma 384
septa, proliferation of 375
tissue 243
tract replacing follicle 242
Filamentous bacteria 137
Filamentous fungi 139
Florid proliferation 432
Fluorescence in-situ hybridization 426
Foam cells 20, 21, 406

Foamy histiocytic, perivascular 132
Focal atrophy of epidermis 60
Focal basal cell
  damage 50
  vacuolation 53, 65, 66, 77
Focal epithelioid granulomas, multiple 129
Focal fat cell necrosis 205
Focal mucinosis 233
Focal parakeratosis 39, 67, 82, 84
Focal spongiosis with exocytosis 84
Follicle containing debris 270
Follicle, rupture of 251
Follicle, upper part of damaged 242
Follicular degeneration 416
Follicular epithelium 48, 94, 270
  disruption of 290
Follicular hyperkeratosis 35, 36, 65
Follicular infiltrate 421
Follicular keratosis 327
Follicular lichen planus 48
Follicular mucinosis 416
Follicular ostia 305
Follicular ostium 81
Follicular spongiosis 407
Follicular wall, disruption of 246
Folliculitis 8, 252, 294
  decalvans 246
Folliculotrophic mycosis fungoides 421
Foreign body
  giant cells 160, 207, 329
  granuloma 160
Fragments, dermal 104
Frontal fibrosing alopecia 252
Fungal
  elements 78, 288
  folliculitis 290
  hyphae 139, 146
  infections 286

G

Gastrointestinal symptoms 163
Giant cell 54, 124, 126, 127, 131, 136, 145-147, 149, 154, 158, 160, 201, 246, 376, 431
  in deep dermis 171
  multinucleated 11, 155, 156, 161, 204, 206, 262
  multiple 159, 160
  reaction 161
Glomus tumor 376
Glucagonoma syndrome 41
Gouty tophi 258
Graft-versus-host disease 59, 69
Gram stain 296
  negative 140
Granular basophilic material 381
Granular cell layer 30, 38, 55, 84, 247, 249, 282, 301, 305, 429
Granular cytoplasm 395
Granular layer 29
Granuloma 124, 136, 152, 161
  annulare 156
    perforating 273
  around nerve 130
  cells 146
  dispersed 134
  extravascular 173
  faciale 174
  in mid dermis 141
  in upper dermis 141, 147
  naked 152
  palisading 156
  suppurative 137
  with giant cells 122, 162, 172
  with multinucleated giant cells 123, 129
  with Schaumann body 155
Granulomatous
  dermatitis 151
  infiltrate in dermis 144
  infiltration
    epidermis 142
    to deep dermis 142
  inflammation 204
  reaction 123, 262
  rosacea 127
  slack skin disease 426
  tissue reaction 119
Grocott's methenamine silver stain 146
Ground substance, dermal 415
Grover's disease 85, 101
Guttate psoriasis 31

H

Hailey-Hailey disease 18, 99, 101
Hair
  cleavage 94
  destruction of 243
  miniaturized 239
  papilla formation 325
  structures 324, 333
Hair follicle 4, 5, 237, 241, 259, 294, 333, 359, 377, 407
  epithelium of 339
  loss of 243
  paucity of 243
  portions of 323
  rupture of 241
  size of 189
Halo nevus 357
Hamartoma 189
Hansen's disease
  borderline
    lepromatous 131
    tuberculoid 130
  indeterminate 128
  lepromatous 132
  midborderline 136
  tuberculoid 129
  type 1 lepra reaction 134
Hemangiopericytoma 391
Hemorrhage 241
Hemosiderin deposits in dermis 380
Hemosiderin in macrophages 183
Henle's layer 4
Henoch-Schonlein type 168
Herpes folliculitis 279
Herpes simplex 278
Herpes zoster 278
Herpesviridae family 278
Hidradenitis suppurativa 431
Histiocytic panniculitis 213
Histiocytosis 403
Histoid leprosy 133
Homogenous eosinophilic bodies 45
Horn cyst 301, 304, 323, 327
  small 192
Human immunodeficiency virus 69
Huxley's layer 4
Hyaline cylinders 337
Hyalinized collagen bundles 219
Hypereosinophilic syndrome 408
Hypergranulosis 37, 47, 283
  wedge-shaped 45
Hyperkeratosis 17, 18, 37, 38, 59, 60, 64-66, 78, 141, 256, 282, 302, 305, 430
Hypermelanosis 195
Hyperpigmentation of basal layer 189
Hyperplasia 37, 76, 79, 189, 256, 430
  epidermal 62, 139, 229, 400, 431
  mild epidermal 382
  moderate epidermal 257
  of epidermis 84, 351, 355
    irregular 75
  with hyperkeratosis, epidermal 432
  with rete ridges 82
Hyperplastic epithelium 326
Hypertrophic scar 221

I

Idiopathic guttate hypomelanosis 195
IGA bullous disease 116
Immunoblasts 425
Immunofluorescence, direct 8, 10, 13, 96, 100, 109
Immunohistochemistry 8, 12, 13
Impetigo foliaceus 118
Incontinentia pigmenti 75
Infantile hemangioma 368
Infiltrate with lobular panniculitis, dermal 202
Inflammation
  chronic 284
  dermal 146, 286
  mild 58
Inflammatory cell 6, 9, 104, 245, 270, 290, 373, 380
  chronic 124
  infiltrate 203, 246, 329
    in dermis 174
    perivascular 220
  mild chronic 290
Inflammatory crust 294
Inflammatory diseases 18, 417
Inflammatory infiltrate 110, 251
  chronic 255
  mild chronic 75
Inflammatory lesions 251
Infundibular cyst 247
Interface dermatitis 43, 56, 57

Interstitial granuloma annulare 157
Interstitial inflammatory dermal infiltrate 74
Interstitial tissue 74
Intimal fibrosis 170
Intracellular
  eosinophilic hyaline globules 380
  lipid deposits 406
  spores of histoplasma 145
Intradermal melanocytic nevus 352
Intraepidermal
  collections of neutrophils 77
  neutrophils 113, 180
  vesicle 80
    formation 101
Isthmus-Catagen cyst 248

J

Junctional melanocytic nevus 352
Juvenile xanthogranuloma 403

K

Kamino bodies 355
Kaposi's sarcoma 378
Karyorrhectic debris 422
Keloid 221
Keratin in cyst cavity 249
Keratinocyte 278, 345
  atypical 55
  disorganized atypical 306
  multinucleated 308
  nuclei melanin 190
Keratinous cysts 347
Keratoacanthoma 317
Keratohyaline granules 282, 283, 285, 430
  formation of 248
Keratosis pilaris atrophicans 252
Kyrle's disease 269, 273

L

Langerhans cell 401, 402
  histiocytosis 401
Lepra bacilli 132, 135
Leprosy 128
  bacillus 128
Leukocytoclasis 167
  with nuclear dust 179
Leukocytoclastic vasculitis 167, 168, 169, 177
Lichen amyloidosis 256
Lichen myxedematosus 229
Lichen nitidus 54
Lichen planopilaris 243
Lichen planus 45
  hypertrophicus 47
  keratosis 55
  pigmentosus 53
Lichen sclerosus 234
  et atrophicus 65
Lichen scrofulosorum 124
Lichen simplex chronicus 37
Lichen striatus 51
Lichenoid contact dermatitis 69
Lichenoid dermatitis 43, 69, 100
Lichenoid drug reaction 50
Lichenoid pattern 8
Lichenoid purpura 69
Lichenoid reaction 58, 123
Lichenoid tissue reaction 45, 50, 51, 54, 55, 66, 55, 256
Lichenoid upper dermal infiltrate 419
Lip
  epidermal 318
  mucosa of 162
Lipodermatosclerosis 209
Lipoid proteinosis 259, 263
Livedoid vasculitis 182
Lobular capillary hemangiomas 375
Lobular panniculitis 63, 135, 203, 205, 209, 213
  causes of 63
Lobules, subcutaneous 202
Lupus erythematosus 60, 64, 69
Lupus profundus 62
Lupus vulgaris 273
Lymph nodes 155, 413
Lymphangioma 369
Lymphocyte 6, 11, 33, 39, 44, 54, 68, 74, 97, 109, 114, 122, 125, 128, 130, 132, 136, 144, 152, 170, 174, 175, 177, 181, 201, 209, 210, 220, 242, 246, 399, 400, 403, 405, 408, 417, 418, 420, 421, 423, 435,
  atypical 418
  cell 380
  extension of 417
  in dermis, perivascular 285
  in papillary dermis 45
  infiltrate of 39
  mature 415
  migration of 67
  number of 134
  peribulbar 238
    infiltrate of 237
  perivascular 61, 73, 82, 104, 134, 159, 356, 404, 435
    infiltrate of 32, 84, 183
  small 414
Lymphocytic infiltrate 65, 194
  mild perivascular 38
  of skin 415
  perivascular 60, 66, 79, 226, 437
Lymphocytic inflammatory infiltrate 47
Lymphocytic vasculitis 183
Lymphohistiocyte 158, 161
  perivascular 163
Lymphohistiocytic infiltrate 128, 131, 351
  nerves 128
  sweat glands 131
Lymphoid follicles 414, 415, 425
Lymphoma 426
Lymphomatoid
  drug reaction 426
  granulomatosis 426
  papulosis 423
Lymphoproliferative disorders of skin 411

M

Macrophages 135, 177
  large 269
Macular amyloidosis 257
Masson's fontana stain 190
Mast cell 6, 395
  granules 10
Meissner's corpuscle 7
Melanin in epidermis 190
Melanocyte 3, 193, 358, 359
  alteration of 187
  cells 352
  collections of atypical 360
  in dermis 356
    nests of 355
  in epidermis, nests of 355
  nests of 356
  normal 191
  proliferation, mild 189
Melanocytic
  lesions 349
  nevus 352
Melanoma, malignant 358
Melanophages in dermis 189
Membranous lipodystrophy 208
Microabscesses 181
  subcutaneous 431
Microcyst formation in fat cells 209
Microcystic adnexal carcinoma 347
Microphthalmia transcription factor 358
Miescher's granulomas 201
Mikulicz cells 296
Mitotic activity 22, 23, 30
Molluscum
  bodies 277
  contagiosum 277
Monomorphic mast cells 396
Mucin
  deposition 228, 229
  disease of 215
  with 421
  without 421
Mucinous capsule 143
Mucosal epithelium 9, 49
Mucous membrane, lesions of 111
Multicentric reticulohistiocytosis 404
Munro's microabscess 32
Muscle
  bundles of smooth 387
  cells 387
    smooth 386
  deep extension into 332
  fascicles, smooth 386
  smooth 249
Mycobacterium chelonae 151
Mycosis fungoides 69, 417, 426
  diagnosis of 22, 23
Myeloma, multiple 409
Myxoid, proliferation of 375

N

Nail bed lichen planus 46
Nail biopsy 287
Necrobiosis 156
  lipoidica 158
Necrobiotic xanthogranuloma 409
Necrosis, epidermal 181
Necrotic debris 272
Necrotic fat cells 212
Necrotic keratinocytes 51, 55-58, 60, 68, 100
Necrotizing vasculitis 171
Neoplastic dyskeratosis 18
Nephrogenic systemic fibrosis 234
Nerve
  dermal 6, 7
  fibers 376
  involvement 136
Neurovascular bundles 131
Neutrophil 6, 9
  abscess, dermal 151
Neutrophilic
  abscess 139, 293, 294
  infiltrate 167, 200, 203
  microabscess in dermis 180
  spongiosis 85
Neutrophils 31-34, 78, 94, 104, 109, 113, 115-117, 146, 148, 170, 173-178, 200, 212, 286, 288, 290, 381
  collections of 113
  in blister cavity 77
  in epidermis 40
  in stratum corneum 431
  number of 114
  perivascular 135
Nevoid hypermelanosis 193
Nevus cells 352-354
  cuboidal 353
  dermal 357
  in dermis 355
Nevus depigmentosus 188
Nevus flammeus 365
Nevus lipomatosus 390
Nevus sebaceous 333, 335
Nevus, blue 354
Nocardia 138
Nodular fasciitis 391
Nodular histiocytosis 409
Nodular melanoma 360
Nodular vasculitis 202, 203, 213
Nonscarring alopecia 237
Non-tuberculous mycobacterial infections 151
Norwegian scabies 41
Nuclear atypia 314
Nuclear dust 168, 169, 175
  formation of 167
Nucleus 401
Nummular dermatitis 79

O

Ochronosis 261
Ochronosis in dermis 261
Ofuji's disease 85
Oral lichen planus 49
Osteomas 263

P

Pacinian corpuscle 7
Paget's cells 339, 340
Paget's disease 339
Pagetoid reticulosis 426
Pallor, epidermal 284
Palmar skin 9, 80
Palmoplantar warts 283
Pancreatic panniculitis 211
Panniculitis, subcutaneous 63, 422
Papilla
  dermal 31, 54, 113, 115, 256, 257, 355
  fibrin in dermal 113
  squirting, dermal 31
Papillary dermal edema 437
Papillary dermis 39, 40, 83, 135, 194, 224, 312, 351
Papillary edema 62, 65, 74, 112, 178, 396, 408, 435
Papillary lesion 335
Papillary mesenchymal body 325
Papillary microabscess 113, 116
Papillary structures, small 334
Papillomatosis 18, 19, 98, 285, 302, 305, 371
  mild 192
Papillomatous hyperplasia 284, 333
Papulonecrotic tuberculid 124
Parakeratosis 17, 18, 32, 35, 38, 40, 50, 51, 55, 77, 79, 81, 284-286
  mounds of 84
Parakeratotic
  cells 270
  columns 36
  hyperkeratosis 38
  keratin 267
Paraneoplastic pemphigus 100
Pas positive organisms 142, 249
Pautrier's microabscesses 420
Pellagra 41
Pemphigus
  foliaceous 89, 118
  vegetans 97
  vulgaris 93, 101
Perifollicular dermis 290
Perifollicular granuloma 127
Perifollicular infiltrate 251, 421
  of lymphocytes 270
Perifollicular inflammation 127, 246
Periodic acid-Schiff stain 61
  dermatophyte 13
  positive 140
    dermatophytes 286
    for fungus 287
Peripheral basophilic germinative cells 331
Pilar sheath acanthoma 348
Piloleiomyomas 386
Pilomatrixoma 329
Pilosebaceous disorders 235
Pilosebaceous follicles 245
Pityriasis lichenoides 67
  acuta 67
  chronica 68
Pityriasis rosea 84, 434
Pityriasis rubra pilaris 35
Pityriasis versicolor 289
Pityrosporum folliculitis 290
Plaque parapsoriasis, small 39
Plasma cell 6, 11, 49, 125, 144, 152, 159, 174, 206, 220, 246, 295, 306, 310, 380, 399, 408, 414, 415
  infiltrate 398, 400
  number of 398, 400
  predominant 398
Plasmacytomas 409
Plasmacytosis mucosae 398
Poikiloderma 66
Polyarteritis nodosa 170
Polymorphonuclear
  cells 317
  infiltrate, dermal 20, 21
Polymorphous infiltrate 295
Porokeratosis 18, 69, 429
Porokeratotic eccrine duct nevus 18
Poroma cells 345
Porphyria cutanea tarda 106
Postinflammatory hyperpigmentation 194
Pregnancy, plaques of 184, 437
Premalignant conditions, epidermal 299
Proliferating trichilemmal cyst 252
Pruritic urticarial papules 184, 437
Pseudo horn cysts 301
Pseudoepitheliomatous hyperplasia 97, 122, 141
Pseudofolliculitis 252
Pseudolymphoma 413
Pseudomembranous fat necrosis 208
Pseudoxanthoma elasticum 224
Psoriasiform hyperplasia 32, 33, 36, 39
Psoriasiform tissue reaction 27
Psoriasis vulgaris 29
Psoriatic plaque 31
Purpuric dermatoses, pigmented 22, 183, 184, 426
Pustular psoriasis 32
Pyknotic nucleus 283
Pyoderma gangrenosum 180
Pyogenic granuloma 375

R

Red blood cells 68, 175, 183, 249, 369
Reiter's disease 33
Reiter's syndrome 41
Renal failure, chronic 271
Reticular dermis 401, 413
Reticulin fibers penetrate granulomas 154
Reticulin stain 153
Rhinoscleroma 295
Rosai-Dorfman disease 409
Russell bodies 295, 399

S

Sabouraud dextrose agar 143
Sandwich sign 286
Sarcoidosis 152
Satellite cell necrosis 59
Scabies 432
  mites 432
Scalp punch biopsy, sections of 240
Scalp skin 9
Scanty cytoplasm 352
Scanty sebaceous cells 332
Scarring alopecias 242
Schaumann bodies 154, 155
Scleredema 220, 231
Sclerodermoid graft 234
Scleromyxoedema 228
Sclerosis, dermal 59
Sebaceous adenoma 331
Sebaceous carcinoma 332
Sebaceous cells 332
  mature 331
Sebaceous cyst 248
Sebaceous differentiation 331
Sebaceous gland 4, 5, 189, 243, 245, 249, 333
  large 333
  structures 239
Sebaceous lobules 331
Seborrheic dermatitis 81
Seborrheic keratosis 301, 319
Septal fibrosis 202, 209
Septal panniculitis 199, 209, 213, 293
Sezary syndrome 419
Shadow cells 330
Shoulders 111
Silver methenamine stain positive 140, 143
Skin
  normal 191
  tag 382
Solar elastosis 225
Solitary mastocytoma 395
Sparse collagen 385
Sparse dermal infiltrate 109
Sparse superficial perivascular infiltrate 64
Sparsity of lymphocytes 132
Spherical yeast 291
  cell 143
Spindle cells 354, 379, 385
  hemangioendothelioma 391
Spiradenoma 338
Spitz nevus 355
Splendore-Hoeppli phenomenon 137
Spongiosis 84
  mild 40, 82
  with eosinophils 73, 75
  with exocytosis 34, 79
  with multiple spongiotic microvesicles 73
  with neutrophils 77
Spongiotic
  dermatoses 71, 101, 432
  disorders 79, 85
  vesicle with fibrin 80
Sporothrix asteroid 148
Sporotrichosis 147
Squamous cell 45, 76
  carcinoma 313, 318, 319
Squamous epithelial cells 316
  nests of 313
Squamous epithelium 247, 248, 250, 335, 340
  of glans penis 398
Stasis dermatitis 83
Steatocystoma multiplex 249
Stellate fibroblasts 190
Stratified squamous epithelium 249
Stratum corneum 288
Stratum spinosum 277
Subcorneal
  blister 89
  neutrophils 91, 92
  pustular dermatoses 91
Suprabasal
  blisters 93
  bulla with mild 93
  lacunae 97
Suprapapillary epithelium 192
Sweat glands 243
Sweet's syndrome 118, 178
Swollen cells 281
  in upper epidermis 280
Syphilis, secondary 41, 400
Syringocystadenoma papilliferum 335
Syringoma 343
Systemic lupus erythematosus 69

T

T cell
  leukemia 426
  lymphoma 63, 422
    alpha 422
    beta 422
Tattoo pigment 262
Telogen effluvium 240
  chronic 252
Telogen hairs 241
Thrombosis of vessels 168
Tissue, subcutaneous 3, 62, 158, 209, 219, 237, 372, 378
Touton giant cells 406
Toxic epidermal necrolysis 57
Toy soldier's appearance 23, 417
Trichilemmal cyst 248
Trichilemmoma 328
Trichoblastoma 325
Trichoepithelioma 323
Trichotillomania 241
Tuberculoid granuloma 121, 124, 126, 127
  formation 201
Tuberculosis 121, 153, 155
  verrucosa cutis 122, 273
Tubular apocrine adenoma 334
Tumid lupus erythematosus 230
Tumor
  cells 313, 332, 339, 354, 376, 385, 424
    islands of 312
  dermal 378
  mass 336
    diffuse 385
  multilobulated 331
  stage 418
Tumoral calcinosis 263

U

Ulcer 177
Unilocular blister, formation of 115
Urticaria 436
  pigmentosa
Urticarial vasculitis 169

V

Varicella 278, 279
Vascular ectasia 292
Vascular plexus, superficial 365
Vasculitis
  endothelial cell 203
  with fibrinoid necrosis 124
Veins in subcutis 366
Vellus hair cyst 250
Verhoeff-van Gieson stain 223, 268, 272
Verruca plana 280
Verruca vulgaris 18, 282
Verruciform xanthoma 409
Verrucous carcinoma 315, 319
Verrucous epidermal nevus 18, 38
Verrucous hemangioma 371
Vesiculobullous disorders 87
Vessels, proliferation of 375
Viral infections 277
Vitiligo 187

W

Warthin-Starry stain 296
Warty dyskeratoma 101
Wegener's granulomatosis 171

X

Xanthoma disseminatum 409
Xanthomatous infiltrates 406

Y

Yeast forms 142

Z

Ziehl-Neelsen stain 132, 133, 135
Zoon's balanitis 398
Zygomycosis, subcutaneous 149